Praise for the first edition of *Healing Lyme*

Anyone touched by Lyme disease – patients, their families, or health care practitioners – will find this insightful and thorough book to be the essential guide for Lyme disease and its treatment. A hopeful, life-altering book.

WENDY LEFFEL, MD

The first 75 pages are as good a review of the scientific literature as I've seen . . . I was impressed by [Buhner's] grasp of the literature. He really did his homework.

RICHARD HOROWITZ, MD

And for Stephen Harrod Buhner's work

In one book after another, Stephen Harrod Buhner has demonstrated new ways of thinking that address the increasing medical dogmatism and uncertainty of our times. We need a wise interpreter and he has proven himself worth of the title.

MATTHEW WOOD, herbalist and author

Brilliant as ever, Buhner once again brings us cutting-edge research about one of the more invasive and misdiagnosed epidemics of our time. *Healing Lyme Disease Coinfections* is not only a resounding wakeup call for all health care professionals but also offers an elegant and potent paradigm of healing disease that is synergistic, broad, and deeply caring. Buhner has created a brilliant, hopeful resource for everyone affected with Lyme and/or its coinfections.

ROSEMARY GLADSTAR, herbalist, teacher, author

An important book that anyone involved with health-care should read. The ideas bridge traditional herbalism, modern phytotherapy, and laboratory and clinical research.

It is a major contribution to the healing of humanity's relationship with bacteria.

DAVID HOFFMAN, FNIMH, medical herbalist

This important, relentless book contains a mine of information and knowledge for the ecologically-minded.

JEREMY NARBY, author of *The Cosmic Serpent*

A sensitive, intelligent, far reaching work . . . This extraordinaty book breaks all boundaries and in doing so reconnects us with our most radical selves. A truly revolutionary message.

SUSUN WEED, herbalist and author

Also by Stephen Harrod Buhner

Ecological Medicine

*Herbal Antibiotics: Natural Alternatives
for Drug-Resistant Bacteria* (second edition)

Herbal Antivirals: Natural Remedies for Emerging and Resistant Viral Infections

*Healing Lyme Disease Coinfections: Complementary and Holistic
Treatments for Bartonella and Mycoplasma*

Natural Treatments for Lyme Coinfections: Anaplasma, Babesia, and Ehrlichia

Pine Pollen: Ancient Medicine for a New Millennium

Herbs for Hepatitis C and the Liver

Vital Man: Natural Health Care for Men at Midlife

The Fasting Path

*Healing Lyme: Natural Healing and Prevention of Lyme
Borreliosis and Its Coinfections* (first edition, 2005)

Natural Remedies for Low Testosterone

The Transformational Power of Fasting

Poetry/Language

The Taste of Wild Water: Poems and Stories Found While Walking in Woods

Ensouling Language: On the Art of Nonfiction and the Writer's Life

Nonfiction

*The Lost Language of Plants: The Ecological
Importance of Plant Medicines for Life on Earth*

*The Secret Teachings of Plants: The Intelligence of
the Heart in the Direct Perception of Nature*

*Plant Intelligence and the Imaginal Realm: Beyond the
Doors of Perception into the Dreaming of Earth*

Sacred Plant Medicine: Explorations in the Practice of Indigenous Herbalism

One Spirit Many Peoples: A Manifesto For Earth Spirituality

Sacred and Herbal Healing Beers: The Secrets of Ancient Fermentation

Healing Lyme

Natural Healing of Lyme Borreliosis and the Coinfections Chlamydia and Spotted Fever Rickettsioses

Second Edition, Revised, Expanded, Updated

STEPHEN HARROD BUHNER

Raven Press

Silver City, NM

Raven Press
8 Pioneer Road
Silver City, NM 88061

Publisher's Cataloging-in-Publication Data
Buhner, Stephen Harrod
Healing lyme: Natural Healing of Lyme Borreliosis and the Coinfections Chlamydia and Rocky Mountain Spotted Fever/ Stephen Harrod Buhner
p.cm.
Includes bibliographical references and index.
Isbn - 978-0-9708696-4-7 - (pbk.)
1. Lyme disease. 2. Emerging infections. 3. materia medica, Vegetable. I. Title.

Printed and bound in the United States of America at Sheridan Books
10 9 8 7 6 5 4 3 2 1
Text design and layout by Sterling Hill Productions

The poem "Ancient Herbals" is copyright Stephen Harrod Buhner, *The Taste of Wild Water: Poems and Stories Found While Walking in Woods*, Raven Press, 2009. By permission of the author.

Pre-printing production costs for this book were quite generously paid for in part by the donations of over 300 people who are or formerly were struggling with Lyme disease and or its coinfections.

For all those people
whose doctors told them
(and keep telling them)
it's all in their head

And for Julie McIntyre
whose dedication to those who are in need
continually inspires me

CONTENTS

FOREWORD

In the beginning (of our understanding and treating Lyme disease) there was the word, and that word was the microbe *Borrelia burgdorferi*. And we thought it was good that we understood that it was a bacteria that was causing these severe symptoms we were seeing in our patients who we labeled "Lyme Disease." So we treated it, like all other bacteria, with antibiotics, sometimes for very long times in massive doses. And some patients got better, so we thought we knew what we were doing.

However, we could not deny that many of our patients did not get better, in fact many got worse with our treatments, so we had to go back to the drawing board. We realized that tick bites (or mosquito or flea bites) were essentially injecting not only *Borrelia*, but also its close friends *Bartonella*, *Babesia*, *Ehrlichia*, and *Mycoplasma* and later realized that by weakening our patients' immune system, it allowed all kinds of dormant microbes like *Chlamydia* and *Rickettsia* to flourish creating an infectious mess.

With the publication of the first edition of *Healing Lyme* in 2005, Stephen Buhner brought a breath of fresh air to a troubled subject. For those of us who were already wrestling with treating these complicated infections Stephen tilted the landscape for us by encouraging us to do something unheard of: *to look at these infections from the microbe's perspective*, not ours. He realized, early on, that these were not the kind of infections we were used to seeing, and that these microbes were profoundly altering our immune system within minutes of beginning the infectious process, and this led to dysregulation of inflammation, which led to severe neurological, arthritic, muscular, endocrine, emotional, and cognitive shifts, which needed to be understood and taken into account so that healing could occur. For those of us in the field, this information was exceptionally useful and allowed us to provide much better medical care for our struggling patients.

In the intervening ten years, I have personally treated over a thousand patients with Lyme disease and its attendant coinfections. We have learned a lot. Mostly we have realized how little we knew, how little we know, and how much we need to learn to do this properly.

In his recently published books, *Healing Lyme Disease Coinfections: Complementary and Holistic Treatments for Bartonella and Mycoplasma* and *Natural Treatments for Lyme Coinfections: Anaplasma, Babesia and Ehrlichia,* Stephen has taken medical and herbal research to a new level of understanding these infections and provides a clear and logical method for treatment.

So it was now necessary for him to update the original *Healing Lyme* manuscript to include the newest information now available to help us to navigate these difficult waters and to include an overview of two underappreciated infections which accompany Lyme: *Chlamydia* and the Rickettsial family of infections.

This book is written for very different readers, whose informational needs are also different: practitioners who treat Lyme and patients who have Lyme. Happily, he has organized this book into sections that will allow these readers to pick and choose which sections will most meet their needs. Despite the technical nature of some of these chapters, I would encourage all readers to plow into them anyway; it is not necessary to grasp the fine points to appreciate what these microbes are doing to us and with us.

Reading these pages, one cannot help but be impressed with the intelligence (yes, intelligence) and consciousness (yes, consciousness) of these organisms. While I have struggled to learn to treat these same organisms, I cannot help but admire my adversary (even awed, at times) and to do so I must understand what it wants and needs from its host. To imagine that merely giving two weeks of an antibiotic will eradicate it for all patients bitten by a tick is tragically missing the boat.

Understanding the physiology of these infections, which Stephen provides us with loving detail, allows us to appreciate his clear approach: learn what structures and cells lines are being infected and protect them, quiet the outpouring of inflammatory cytokines, provide herbs that can modulate the dysfunctional immune system, help the body process the toxins that are being produced by these microorganisms (especially when we kill them with antibiotics), reduce the specific symptoms manifest in that patient, and provide materials that will specifically treat those microorganisms.

Put another way, we must find ways to allow the body's innate healing system to do its job properly (since those systems have been essentially hijacked by the micobes' needs).

Ah, do I hear the echo of an old argument? *But of course, my dear Monsieur Pasteur, eet eez not zee microbe we need to be concerned with, but zee terrain, no?* argues Professor Bernard. Hopefully, we can finally lay that discussion to rest: it is both the microbe and the terrain; in fact, as we can clearly see in these pages, it is the microbe that actively participates in altering, shaping, and creating the terrain.

Moving forward from Lyme disease, Stephen delves into the associated bacterial species of *Chlamydia*, then *Rickettsia*. While some Lyme experts have not yet included *Chlamydia* as one of the usual suspects of coinfection, Stephen clearly shows that it is present in ticks and it will probably not be long before *Chlamydia* is formally included in this group as well. Moreover, previous infections with *Chlamydia* that leave dormant or latent organisms in the body can clearly be reactivated, as can a wide variety of viral infections, when the immune system is dysregulated by *Borrelia*, thus becoming yet another part of the problem.

For me, as a clinician, one of the most important things to understand about *Chlamydia* (other than that it is more common than appreciated: recent research by Dr. Armin Schwarzbach from Germany notes that 86 percent of his Lyme patients test positive for *Chlamydia* as well) is that when we are attacking it, with either antibiotics, herbals, or other supplements, it releases a unique toxin called *porphyrin* into host, which can create what looks like a prolonged Herx (short for Jarish-Herxheimer) reaction in the patient. A typical Herx represents only two to three days of an intense exacerbation of a patient's symptoms caused by excessive release of toxins from the infecting microbe (*Borrelia*, *Bartonella*, etc.) When that reaction, after instituting a new antibiotic or dosage increase, or the use of NAC (N-acetyl cysteine, which specifically can kill the EB form of *Chlamydia*), lasts for a week or more, this is a tip-off to me that we may be dealing with a porphyrin release, which is treated very differently. I would encourage readers to check out the website www.CPNHELP.ORG to learn more.

As Stephen points out, Rickettsial infections are underdiagnosed and undertreated (because: [1] they are underdiagnosed and [2] can become chronic, which often does not get treated). Again, from a clinician's perspective, we are beginning to realize we have not looked hard enough for these infections and are beginning to do so now (and would really appreciate some decent tests so we could make these diagnoses in a more timely fashion).

So, take off your shoes, settle in for the night, and begin to learn the updated version of "Everything You Wanted to Know About Lyme Disease But Were Afraid to Ask." Yes, this information can be overwhelming and scary, but it can also save your life and restore your health.

Neil Nathan, MD

Dr. Nathan is the author of *Healing Is Possible: New Hope for Chronic Fatigue, Fibromyalgia, Persistent Pain and Other Chronic Illnesses.*

HOW TO USE THIS BOOK
AND WHO IT IS FOR

I did as much research as I could and I took ownership of this illness, because if you don't take care of your body, where are you going to live?
Karen Duffy

Illness and death are not optional. Patients have a right to determine how they approach them.
Marcia Angell, MD

My first published exploration of Lyme disease and its coinfections occurred with the appearance of *Healing Lyme* (Raven Press) in 2005. In the years since that early work my increasing exposure to this group of emerging diseases, and the people who suffer from them, has significantly deepened my understanding of both Lyme and coinfections. In consequence, mid-2013 saw the publication of a depth look on two crucial Lyme coinfections: mycoplasma and bartonella (Inner Traditions). Early 2015 saw the publication of a depth look at three other Lyme coinfections: *Babesia, Ehrlichia* and *Anaplasma* (again, Inner Traditions). With the completion of those two books, the five major coinfectious organisms of Lyme now have their own depth analysis and natural treatment protocols. This book, the revised second edition of *Healing Lyme* brings the work, finally, up to date through an expanded, much more comprehensive look at the nature of the Lyme spirochetes and sophisticated protocols for treating them. In addition, the nature and treatment of two lesser known coinfectious organisms are explored, specifically *Chlamydia* and *Rickettsia*, responsible for rickettsioses, the best-known member of which is Rocky Mountain spotted fever.

As with the earlier books on the Lyme group of infections, the second edition of *Healing Lyme* is meant to be used by specific groups of people, i.e., those who are suffering from a difficult-to-treat *Borrelia, Chlamydia,* or Rocky Mountain spotted fever infection, and/or clinicians who themselves treat those who are infected with any of these organisms.

If you are infected with *Borrelia, Chlamydia,* or Rocky Mountain spotted fever. . .

. . . this book is designed to help you understand the infectious organisms as well as understanding some of the approaches that can be used to treat the diseases and the symptoms they cause.

Please understand that some of the book is fairly technical. That is for the clinicians (or for you if you want to delve that deeply into it). An important part of my work in the Lyme disease world has been to: (1) increase understanding of what the disease organisms are and what they do in the body; (2) empower people who are ill to take charge of their own healing journey; and (3) show that contrary to most medical belief, herbal medicines are tremendously sophisticated interventions for chronic conditions such as these. This is *why* portions of the book are so technical. Nevertheless, you can skip the really technical bits if you want. They are not necessary in order for you to treat either of these conditions effectively.

> *If all you want to know is how to treat your Lyme infection*
> *effectively, please . . . just skip ahead to Chapter Eight.*

However, if you are up for it, I think you will find the overview chapters on these infections useful. I have found that once someone understands what the bacteria do in the body, it tends to lessen the fear that these diseases engender. Understanding what the organisms do during infection also makes it easier to understand the treatment regimens I recommend, i.e., just why they help to turn the conditions around. It will also help you generate unique healing approaches of your own, contributions to treating Lyme infections that come out of your own genius. No one person can have all the answers, the Lyme journey needs all of us.

That being said, the deeper technical look at the cytokine cascade and the minutiae of what the organisms do in the body are not really necessary if you just want a cursory overview of the diseases and how to treat them.

This book also contains an extensive look at the natural protocols that are effective for each of the diseases. **Please note:** *These protocols are designed to be used along with antibiotics if you wish to do so.* I don't think you necessarily have to give up either pharmaceuticals *or* natural medicines to find health. However, if you have tried antibiotics and they have failed to help you, the protocols in this book can be used, effectively, all by themselves to treat these three infections.

Also, a note: *The herbs and supplements in this book are* **not** *the only ones in the world that will help.* (Please don't write me and ask why [*fill in the blank*] is not part of the protocol. Just re-read this paragraph.) Use the protocols outlined herein *only* as a starting place, a guideline. Add anything you feel will help you and delete anything that you feel is not useful. Microorganisms, when they enter a human body, find a very unique ecosystem in that particular person. Thus the disease is always slightly different every time it occurs. That means that a pharmaceutical or herb that works for one person may not work or work as well for another. *There is no one-size-fits-all treatment for these particular organisms.*

> **Again . . . there is no one-size-fits-all treatment for Lyme or any of its coinfections.**

Anyone who says there is, is either trying to sell you something or doesn't really understand this group of infectious organisms. *There is no one way to health such that in all times and all places and with all people it will always work.* Life, and disease, and the journey to wellness are much more complex and sophisticated than that. So, trust your own feeling sense and pay attention to what your body is telling you. *You* are the best judge of whether something is working for you or not, whether you need to add something else or not, whether you are getting better . . . or not.

Now, a comment on dosages: I will often suggest a *range* of dosages for the herbs and supplements that can help these conditions. If you have a very healthy immune system, you will probably need smaller doses; if your immune system is severely depleted, you may need to use larger doses. If you are *very* sensitive to outside substances, as some people with Lyme and coinfections are, then you might need to use very tiny doses, that is, from one to five drops of tincture at a time. (This is true for about 1 percent of the people with these infections.) I have seen six-foot five-inch, 280 pound men be unable to take more than five drops of a tincture and a tiny, 95 pound woman need a tablespoon at a time. *Dosages need to be adjusted for each person's individual ecology.*

> **Again . . . dosages need to be adjusted
> for each person's individual ecology.**

And . . . *please be conscious of how you respond to the medicines you are taking. If something disagrees with you, if you feel something is not right in how you are responding to a medicine,* **stop taking it.** Remember: You will always know yourself better than any outside physician. And, just a tiny rant here . . .

Tiny rant

I have been told by a number of clinicians – herbal, naturopathic, and medical – that the majority of people with Lyme and/or its coinfections are too uneducated to understand this series of books, that they are not intelligent enough to determine which herbs to use and which herbs not to use (and, in fact, that many herbs should *only* be discussed or dispensed by properly trained and credentialed herbalists – and yes, that means that most community herbalists and all those who are ill should not), that people with this group of diseases cannot in fact be trusted to be in charge of their own health and journey to wellness, and that I am remiss, even foolish (i.e., stupid, silly, idiotic, witless, brainless, vacuous, mindless, unintelligent, thoughtless, half-baked, harebrained, imprudent, incautious, injudicious, unwise) in supporting members of the Lyme community in their self-empowerment. My feelings about that kind of thinking (and the people who promulgate it – you know who you are and yes, I still know where you live) can be captured in a number of common one-syllable words usually unacceptable in polite company. (Please insert your own favorites here.) For those who strongly disagree with this, you can email me at stephendoesn'tcare@aol.com.

Thus, while it *can* help to have a sophisticated clinician to aid in the journey to welless, it is not always necessary. Further, the truth is, for many people, finding such a person is sometimes impossible, hence taking charge of their own journey to wellness is the *only* option. That is most likely why the Lyme community is as potently informed as they are (much to the dismay of many physicians, paternalistic medical herbalists, and naturopaths).

I do not agree with those clinicians who think you are too stupid to orchestrate your own journey to wellness, that you are too unintelligent or uneducated to understand these books, that you should not be allowed to engage in your own healing without some licensed person overseeing your regimen. In fact, I disagree with that kind of condescending attitude quite strongly.

If you do feel you need a health professional to help you, *then by all means find one.* If you do not feel that you need someone, or that your past efforts with professionals have been unsatisfactory, then again, trust yourself to find what works for you and what does not. In fact, even if you do work with a health professional, I highly recommend that you trust yourself to determine what you are willing to take as medicine and what you are not, to determine for yourself if something is working or if it is not, to engage in self-determination on your journey to wellness. Or as Paul Krugman (2010) once put it . . .

> *When everyone – tout le monde, as Tom Wolfe used to put it, meaning a relative handful of people, but everyone who suppos-edly matters – is saying something it takes a real effort to step outside and say, wait a minute, how do we know that? It's espe-cially hard if you spend your time hanging out with other Very Serious People. . . . This is what you need to know: important people have no special monopoly on wisdom; and in times like these, when the usual rules . . . don't apply, they are often deeply foolish, because the power of conventional wisdom prevents them from talking sense about a deeply unconventional situation.*

If you are a clinician

I have gone into these organisms in depth so that you can begin to under-stand just how complex their actions in the body are. It's my hope that West-ern herbal medicine can begin to emerge as a highly sophisticated form of healing, one *understood* to be highly sophisticated, and one that can deal with the kinds of complexities that are now commonly found in emerging infections. To that end I have introduced the idea of thinking about the synergies that exist between coinfections as well as the concept of examining the kind of cytokine cascades bacteria create during infection.

Cytokines are messenger molecules that act as cellular mediators during the body's immune responses. Each stealth pathogen, during infection, releases certain cytokines to facilitate its infection of the body and, further, to stimulate the breakdown of specific tissues to gain nutrients. Each pathogen decreases certain parts of the human immune system (interfering with an effective immune response) and activates others (stimulating inflammation and cellular breakdown). So while some parts of the immune system become less functional, others become overactive. The overactivity comes from an organism-initiated cascade (think "domino-effect") of inflammatory cytokines.

Each stealth pathogen creates a different kind of cascade, that is, they stimulate certain kinds of inflammation in the body through using the body's immune response for their own ends. This is why infection with these organisms often resembles autoimmune diseases. This is important to understand when designing any kind of elegant, interventive treatment strategy. If you *know* what is happening in the body, you don't have to guess what to do, you know.

And while I don't go into it in any depth in this book, the idea of the complex synergies that exist between herbal medicines is crucial, as well as the understanding of herbal synergists. These are developed in more depth in the revised and expanded edition of *Herbal Antibiotics* (Storey Books, 2012). If you wish to look deeper into plant synergists and herbal synergies, I think you will find that book useful.

As well, time and space limitations made the inclusion of *in-depth* monographs on many of these herbs impossible to include in this volume. I have developed depth monographs on many of these herbs elsewhere – the only ones included in this book are those not included in other books I have written. For those interested, I will note where you can find the depth monographs in the initial pages of the materia medica chapter.

How I arrived at the herbal protocols in this book

The protocols in this book were developed by exploring the dynamics of the diseases themselves, their impacts in people, the experience of clinicians treating them, protocols that those with the diseases have successfully used, thousands of journal papers, a look at the plants' history of usage around the world for treating these and similar conditions, and my own experience with plant medicines over a thirty year period. But please note . . .

The plants herein are just guidelines. The protocols themselves are just guidelines. The dosages are just guidelines. Again: there is *no* one-size-fits-all way to treat these diseases. The intent of this book is to give those who wish one an understanding of the diseases *and* a protocol to begin with so that the diseases can be treated more effectively and with greater sophistication. This is just a beginning, a starting place, so we no longer have to grope along in the dark.

Feel free to alter, add, delete, innovate, think outside the box, argue, insist, and never settle for less than being healthy in the way that you understand it.

And remember: *All* plants are useful as medicinals.

Again, ALL plants are useful as medicinals.

The secret, as always, is in the dose, the timing, and the combination that is used. Just because a plant is not mentioned in this book does not mean it is not useful.

One of the things I have learned from the ill people I have worked with since 1986 (especially those in the Lyme community) is that when a lot of people with a lot of motivation begin looking around themselves, searching for answers, they come up with some truly amazing things. If you lock people in a room with only four ways out, someone will find a fifth way out. *Always.*

Trust yourself, and remember, only *you* know what is health is for you.

WELCOME TO
THE LYME WARS

Similar to other antiscience groups, [Lyme] advocates have created a pseudosceintific and alternative selection of practitioners, research, and publications and have coordinated public protests, accused opponents of both corruption and conspiracy, and spurred legislative efforts to subvert evidence-based medicine. [They] pose a threat to public health.
Paul Auwaerter MD (et al.), Clinical Director, Division of Infectious Diseases, Professor of Medicine, Johns Hopkins

Paul Auwaerter and colleagues compare some Lyme disease activists who use non-evidence-based arguments with anti-HIV or antivaccination extremists. Their Personal View [the column I am responding to] shows that unscientific thinking and malpractice occur in many specialties. Such a focus has unfortunately resulted in suppression of legitimate and necessary scientific debate about the management of syndromes of unclear aetiology, which sometimes occur after a previously proven episode of Lyme disease or tick bites.
Christian Perronne, MD, PhD, Professor of Infectious and Tropical Diseases, Chief, Department of Medicine, Raymond Poincare University Hospital, President of the French Federation of Infectiology, President of the National Council of Universities

In the spring of 2009, I was the 217th person ever to be diagnosed with anti-NMDA-receptor immune encephalitis. Just a year later that figure had doubled. Now the number is in the thousands. Yet Dr. Bailey, considered one of the best neurologists in the country, had never heard of it. When we live in a time when the rate

of misdiagnoses has shown no improvement since the 1930s, the
lesson here is that it's important to always get a second opinion.
. . . While he may be an excellent doctor in many respects, Dr.
Bailey is also, in some ways, a perfect example of what is wrong
with medicine. I was just a number to him (and if he saw thirty-
five patients a day, as he told me, that means I was one of a very
large number). He is a by-product of a defective system that forces
neurologists to spend five minutes with X number of patients a
day to maintain their bottom line. It's a bad system. Dr. Bailey is
not the exception to the rule. He is the rule.
Susannah Cahalan

In 2004, when I began working on the first edition of Healing Lyme, I did not expect to be entering a war zone. But I was. Unfortunately, in 2015, as I now revise that original book, I have discovered that the war, if anything, has intensified. The war is not, however, a conflict between human beings and Lyme disease organisms but a battle between people holding competing theories of Lyme disease and its treatment. During my review of journal papers published since the first edition of Healing Lyme came out, I was particularly saddened to see statements such as this one (Auwaerter et al., 2011) scattered among them.

Advocacy for Lyme disease has become an increasingly important
part of an antiscience movement that denies both the viral cause
of AIDS and the benefits of vaccines and that supports unproven
(sometimes dangerous) alternative medical treatments. Some
activists portray Lyme disease, a geographically limited tick-
borne infection, as a disease that is insidious, ubiquitous, diffi-
cult to diagnose, and almost incurable; they also propose that the
disease causes mainly non-specific symptoms that can be treated
only with long-term antibiotics and other unorthodox and unval-
idated treatments. Similar to other antiscience groups, these
advocates have created a pseudosceintific and alternative selec-
tion of practitioners, research, and publications and have coordi-
nated public protests, accused opponents of both corruption and

conspiracy, and spurred legislative efforts to subvert evidence-based medicine and peer-reviewed science. The relations and actions of some activists, medical practitioners, and commercial bodies involved in Lyme disease advocacy pose a threat to public health.

or this one (Auwaerter et al., 2012) . . .

Tick-borne Borrelia burgdorferi *has been advanced by some as a frequent explanation for medically unexplained symptoms such as continual fatigue, musculoskeletal pains, and subjective neurocognitive dysfunction. Often called "chronic Lyme disease" by adherents of this philosophy, it is loosely defined, and practitioners liberally prescribe nostrums, including prolonged antimicrobial therapies. . . Proponents of this theory have developed their own meetings, literature, activist groups, and substantial internet activities to advance their views. . . . While neither logical nor evidence-based, "Chronic Lyme disease" harnesses corrosive energies that taint modern medicine and society.*

Feelings have regrettably reached religious intensities among many. It has become, in most instances, a rather vicious conflict between different groups of specialists, all with differing paradigms, in all possible combinations: medical/medical, medical/herbal, and herbal/herbal. Caught in the cross fire are those with Lyme disease who are trying to understand what is happening to them and struggling to discover how best to deal with it. This is, in my opinion, reprehensible. The point, as too many healers have apparently forgotten, is finding the most effective way to help people heal. The purpose is not to be right about one's pet treatment regimen or belief paradigm.

A broad review of thousands of peer review journal papers on Lyme disease rather easily reveals that much of the conservative medical world's treatment is not based on any real understanding of the disease. It is, unfortunately, often based *not* on evidence or a clear understanding of the disease organisms in question but merely researcher or physician opinion. As Lee and Vielemeyer (2011) comment in their review of the Lyme treatment guidelines promoted by the Infectious Diseases Society of American (IDSA) between January 1994 and May 2010, "More than half of the current recommendations of the IDSA are based on level III [i.e., personal opinion] evidence only. Until more data from well-designed controlled clinical trials become available, physicians should remain cautious when using current guidelines as the sole source guiding patient care decisions."

Most physicians are in fact basing their understanding and treatment interventions of Lyme disease on incorrect, inadequate, and ineffective information. What is disturbing is that the medical community as a whole appears to have little interest in rectifying the problem.

When I began my initial examination of Lyme disease in 2004, I expected to find a lot of research material on Lyme. And I did. (The intervening years have produced even more.) I expected that nonpharmaceutical approaches to treatment would not be included in mainstream medical practice – and this, too, turned out to be true (and still is a decade later). What I did not expect to find is that significant amounts of reputable research is being ignored by the mainstream medical community. But, I did, and, regrettably, it's still true (though not quite as much as it was), and this troubles me considerably.

Science, though it often is, should never be the plaything of the powerful nor used to control the less powerful simply for the accumulation of power and profit. It is through this perversion of science that science and its practitioners lose the credibility they must have for science to continue to be used effectively in this world.

During the past decade, I and my partner, Julie McIntyre, have had contact with (in the neighborhood of) twenty-five thousand people struggling with Lyme or one of its coinfections. This contact has ranged from minimal email correspondence to in-depth work of a year or more for those with multiple infections and who are experiencing extremely damaging neurocognitive effects. During that time, we have worked as diligently as we can to deepen our understanding of this group of stealth pathogens as well as refining the sophistication of suggested treatment interventions. In the process, we have heard thousands of difficult and often painful stories of the toll the illness has taken on people's lives. Regrettably, many of them included descriptions of disparaging, dismissive, and denigrating treatment by physicians (and sometimes alternative practitioners, most commonly naturopaths). Researchers who take the time to ask Lyme patients about their experience of medical treatment are continually told of such denigration. As Ali et al. (2014) have noted, "Negative experiences were associated with reports of dismissive, patronizing, and condescending attitudes." These revelations are often accompanied by descriptions that include the exhaustion of life savings and terrible descents into nonfunctionality as technological treatment failed to help.

Despite our desires to do so, we have not been able to avoid the Lyme wars, nor will anyone who works to help those with Lyme disease. I wish there was an easy solution. There isn't. The best I can do is to tell you that the conflict exists and that, as you explore the disease more deeply, you will hear a lot of conflicting things about Lyme disease. Some of it will, irritatingly, make little sense – you may begin to feel as if you have been researching the best dieting plan ("*Only* eat elk"). And if you are one of those for whom a short course of antibiotics failed to help, or if you are a practitioner working with Lyme, you *will* spend a lot of time in the midst of the conflict.

You should understand up front that many conservative physicians will not agree with portions of the material in this book; in fact, some will disagree almost violently with it – especially on the subject of herbal medicines, which too many physicians still insist are holdovers from our cave-dwelling, prescientific, superstitious-laden past. (Point to keep in mind: There are no physicians who are trained in the use or understanding of herbal medicines while in medical school in the United States; doctors, as a rule, don't actually know anything about them.)

Some herbal and naturopathic practitioners will have trouble with the material in this book as well, nearly always because they believe they are in possession of "the one true way" to treat Lyme and its coinfections. Nevertheless, the truth is . . . there is no *one* way to healing in the treatment of Lyme disease.

Over the past decade we have found that nearly everything suggested for treating the Lyme-group of disease organisms does help some people and does not help others. Sometimes a short two-week course of antibiotics can completely reverse the disease; sometimes it cannot. Sometimes herbal protocols alone will bring someone back to health, sometimes they won't. Sometimes a combined antibiotic/herbal protocol is the only thing that will work. Sometimes *this* herb will help, sometimes *that* one. For other people, neither of them are any good.

Nevertheless, what I share herein in terms of treatment is based on what I have found by: (1) reading extensively through thousands of peer journals (the references in the bibliography are extensive), especially the work of microbiologists, field researchers, and herbal researchers in countries other than the United States; (2) my own (and my partner Julie's) extensive contact and work with those who have Lyme and/or coinfections; (3) the reports of people's experiences with various treatment interventions; (4) the reports of other practitioners; and (5) the historical use of these kinds of plant medicines (often over millennia) for similar conditions.

A few Lyme war specifics

While things are definitely improving for the better, there is still far too much conflict about this group of disease pathogens. I will talk a bit more about this in different sections of the book but I will just briefly touch on four issues here: 1) rates of infection in the United States; 2) the mode of transmission of the disease; 3) their geographical range; and 4) the effectiveness of antibiotics.

For an extremely long period of time, the Centers for Disease Control and Prevention (CDC) in the United States refused to acknowledge how widespread, and common, Lyme infections were. In 2004 they insisted only 20,000 infections occurred yearly and that such infections were geographically limited. This led many physicians to dismiss their patients' requests for Lyme testing and to insist that the many patients they were seeing with neurocognitive damage could not possibly have Lyme, a coinfection, or a post-Lyme chronic disease condition. So a great many off-the-cuff diagnoses were made, often attributing the symptoms they were seeing to early onset multiple sclerosis or Alzheimer's disease, or psychiatric problems. Many people were inappropriately treated, others, egregiously, were involuntarily hospitalized in psychiatric wards.

Despite the fact that Jonathan Edlow (and other researchers) at Harvard, over a decade ago, noted that, "Epidemiologic data suggest that the actual incidence of Lyme disease could be as much as 10 times higher than CDC data indicate," the CDC refused to alter its official position that only 20,000 new cases of Lyme were being diagnosed per year.

Nevertheless, in 2013, in response to tremendous pressure from activists and accumulating data from research, it altered its position. The CDC now notes that while there are around 30,000 reported cases of Lyme the true incidence is at least ten times that – some 300,000 new infections each year. A CDC release (August 19, 2013) commented that "this new estimate supports studies published in the 1990s indicating that the true number of cases is between 3- and 12-fold higher than the number of reported cases." The most shocking aspect (for me) in that statement, is that the CDC has known this for 20 years but still refused to make it public until researcher and advocate pressure forced them to.

Secondly: Lyme disease is believed to be spread by ticks alone, the main reservoirs for the disease are considered to be mice and deer, and the disease is (still) considered to be geographically limited. Regrettably, this is just as incorrect now as it was in 2004. Although tick transmission appears to be, and probably is, the primary route of human infection, regrettably little research has been conducted on other routes of transmission – and there *are* other routes of transmission. For one thing, *Borrelia* spirochetes are present in a variety of other biting arthropods, such as mosquitos, mites, fleas, and biting flies, and transmission through some of these routes has been documented (e.g., Luger, 1990). Relevant, too, is the presence of coinfectious microorganisms in considerably more than those four biting insects.

Additionally, human-to-human transmission is a great deal more common than physicians realize. For example, *Borrelia* spirochetes, nearly immediately, colonize the urinary bladder of all infected animals – irrespective of species; they are then expressed out of the body in urine; *Chlamydiae* bacteria do this also. (You did wash your hands, didn't you?)

The tendency for the spirochetes to heavily infect just this organ and to pass live out of the body through the urine is not happenstance. Organisms with the length of survival history as Lyme spirochetes do not "accidentally" colonize the urinary bladder and "accidentally" get expressed out of the body in urine. It is a mechanism of both survival and transmission that is common among many bacteria because it works. and it works very well.

To take it a bit further: When they are "starved" or attacked, Lyme spirochetes undergo alterations in their physical form. They change into an encysted form from which they can emerge when conditions improve. (*Chlamydiae* bacteria also utilize this survival strategy.) Ninety-five percent of starved spirochetes can encyst within one minute of expression. These encysted forms have been shown to remain viable for as long as ten months.

Other types of spirochetes have been shown to be viable up to 2.5 years after encysting. Lyme spirochetes in their encysted form have been shown to survive both freezing and thawing and to still be capable of infecting test animals.

These encysted forms of the organism, because of the constant urination of infected animals, liberally cover the soil and plants in areas where Lyme disease is endemic. Animals that then take these encysted forms inside themselves through browsing on ground foliage can be infected by viable spirochetes; Lyme spirochetes do infect in the intestinal tract quite easily and can spread from there throughout the body (*Chlamydiae* organisms do as well). Reconversion to motile forms begins within one hour though it has taken up to six weeks for full reconversion in some studies. There is significant potential for spirochete transmission in urine.

Given this, it is not surprising that, despite contrary assertions by many medical practitioners, the spirochetes are also present in human (and animal) semen and vaginal secretions (e.g., Middelveen et al., 2014). This is why couples are commonly found to be infected with identical *Borrelia* genotypes.

A note here: Despite statistical analysis showing that couples were much more likely to be coinfected with Lyme *Borrelia* than random chance would expect and research that routinely discovered spirochetes (from other genera) in semen and vaginal secretions, *no* PCR analysis or studies occurred with humans until 2013 . . . another casualty of the Lyme wars.

Human breast milk has been found to contain *Borrelia* DNA (Schmidt et al., 1995). Again not surprising as spirochetes (e.g., *Leptospira*) routinely infect animal breast milk (Gordon, 1977; Bolin and Koellner, 1988). And further, spirochete antibodies have been found in tears (Parma et al., 1987), indicating bacterial activity in that medium. Again, no current research has taken this any further, as Middelveen's team did with semen and vaginal secretions in 2013. (My exasperation levels rise again – *all* spirochetes utilize similar infection strategies, why is this so hard to understand?) Some of the Lyme confections are, as well, spread via these routes. (*Chalymdiae*, for example, are now considered to be one of the primary human STD organisms known.) Many of the Lyme-group of diseases, including Lyme itself, have been shown to be transmitted to babies in the womb.

The conventional medical insistence that transmission occurs through ticks alone has stalled research into other modes of transmission *and* the rates of transmission that occurs through them. These other routes play a much greater role than is currently recognized.

Third: A deeper look at this group of pathogens has found, unsurprisingly, that they are not nearly so geographically limited as many people have insisted. They are not just endemic to New England, the Wisconsin/Minnesota area, and Northern California. They are also endemic in the southeastern US, in the Ohio River Valley, in the Pacific Northwest, in Canada, in Texas, and sporadically throughout the desert Southwest. (The organisms are widely present in lizard populations who do in fact serve as reservoirs for the disease.) Most of Europe, especially the northern temperate areas, Eastern Europe, Russia, and parts of Asia, South America, northern Africa, and Australia/New Zealand are also endemic. *Borrelia* are also, counterintuitively, endemic in the Arctic and Antarctic. Despite insistence by numerous physicians and government bodies to the contrary, few places on Earth are exempt from global ecology.

And finally: Antibiotics are thought by most physicians to be highly effective in treating Lyme disease – and for many people they are. I do wish to stress this: *for many people they are.* The turnaround in symptoms for some of the very ill people who take antibiotics is, in fact, (no other word is appropriate here) miraculous. People have gone from being wheel-chair bound and incapacitated as to any normal life to fully functional after a proper diagnosis and a course of antibiotics. Unfortunately, an in-depth review of the literature reveals that antibiotics are not nearly as effective as they are purported to be. Studies show that the effectiveness rates for antibiotics run anywhere from 70–95% depending on the study (and the antibiotic). Rarely included in these statistics, however, is the fact that there is often as much as a 35 percent relapse rate. Additionally, live spirochetes are regularly found in people who have undergone repeated, very potent, more time-limited antibiotic regimens – and even in some who have take antibiotics long term. (Please see the chapter on chronic Lyme disease for more on this.)

The Lyme organism, and the coinfectious pathogens, are highly adaptable and able, in a large minority of instances, to evade antibiotic regimens – even those of long duration. Continual antibiotic dosing can sometimes keep the organisms at low levels in the body (or counteract borrelial inflammation), but studies regularly find that it often does not eradicate them. The longer a Lyme (or co-) infection is untreated, the greater the chance that it will not respond to antibiotic therapy. Given the difficulty of early diagnosis (the characteristic bull's-eye rash only appears in about one-third of those bitten by ticks, only *some* bacterial genotypes generate it), the numbers of those who are treated within one month of infection are low. After this time period (one week to one month), the disease becomes progressively harder to eradicate.

I admit to a bias. In general I am not a fan of antibiotics, and I have written about their overuse and antibiotic-resistance problems in a number of my books, in most detail in *Herbal Antibiotics,* second edition, and *The Lost Language of Plants*. Antibiotics, like many pharmaceuticals, are terribly overused in the United States, and despite what advertisers say, our health as a nation is not the better for it. We are far down on the list of the industrialized nations in both life expectancy and our quality of life. Antibiotic resistance among some very dangerous organisms is a growing problem because of antibiotic overuse. And despite regular alerts from such organizations as the CDC, nothing seems able to slow that use in either hospitals or among physicians.

My standard criteria for antibiotic use, very different than the majority of physicians, is that they should not be used except in instances where there is a strong possibility of death or disability. Otherwise, as most bacterial researchers have stated, we will soon not have them as a treatment option at all. That has ramifications that few of us really wish to contemplate.

Nevertheless, the level of disability that can occur during Lyme infection makes the use of antibiotics warranted in this disease (even by my criteria). Again, antibiotics are spectacularly effective for many people. This does not mean they work for everyone or even a large majority of people who use them. It is, in part, that failure of effectiveness that drives the need for alternatives that are well considered and that can help in the treatment of the disease.

There is a reason so many Lyme sufferers seek out alternative treatments. It is not because they are insane, uneducated, overly hysterical, stupid, or gullible. It is because they are ill, they know they are ill, and conventional medical treatment has not worked for them. (Just because someone is ill does not mean that, as far too many physicians think, they have suddenly become stupid.) Too often, when they turn to their physicians for help after antibiotics fail, they are told it is all in their heads or that they will just have to live with their reduced functionality or that they actually are better – they just can't tell. Too often they find themselves in the middle of the Lyme wars where the paradigm of treatment becomes more important than the health and happiness of the patients themselves.

Healing is possible in Lyme disease, we have seen it over and over again – even in the most intractable cases.

There is hope, don't give up.

CHAPTER ONE

LYME DISEASE AND OTHER BORRELIAL INFECTIONS

Since its original description, Lyme disease (Lyme borreliosis) has risen from relative obscurity to become a prototypical emerging infectious disease. The path to notoriety began with a little noticed epidemic of oligoarthritis in the mid 1970s, mainly in children, in several rural communities clustered about the town of Lyme in southeastern Connecticut, USA. Physicians misdiagnosed many of these children as having juvenile rheumatoid arthritis, leading two astute mothers to seek the assistance of investigators at nearby Yale Univeristy (New Haven, Connecticut). . . . Shortly thereafter, a novel spirochete was isolated from the skin, blood and cerebrospinal fluid specimens obatins from patients with erythema migrans.
Radolf et al., 2012

Some pathogenic strains belonging to the B. burgdorferi sensu lato complex have a worldwide distribution, yet they are rarely considered or tested for.
Christian Perronne, 2014

Nothing about Lyme disease is simple.
Sharon Levy, 2013

Lyme disease is caused by a particular kind of bacterium, a spirochete. The word "spirochete" literally means "coiled hair," and this does describe their appearance to some extent. However, they actually appear to the eye, more than anything else, like a tiny, very active worm. Spirochetes are some of the most ancient bacteria on Earth; they have been around billions of years longer than human beings, and they are very smart.

The spirochetes within the phylum *Spirochaetes* are, similarly to most living organisms on Earth, suffering at the hands of *Homo taxonomisii* (also known as taxonomists), one of the least enjoyable life-forms within the *Homo* genus. In other words, taxonomists are rearranging the Earth's family trees to suit themselves. In the first edition of *Healing Lyme*, just ten years ago, I listed eight different genera (or primary groups) of spirochetes, among which were the *Borrelia*. There are now fifteen groups. These are divided among the four families (larger clans, essentially) in the phylum: *Spirochaetaceae, Brachyspiraceae, Leptospiraceae, Brevinemataceae*. In other words, there are some spirochetes *here*, others over *there*, and still others *here*, all of whom belong in the phylum *Spirochaetes*. (Some members of *Homo taxonomisii* want to put the *Borrelia* into their own family, the *Borreliaceae*. It will probably happen sooner or later.)

The fifteen spirochetal genera, spread among the four families, contain perhaps three hundred different species; there are likely thousands more. New ones are being found all the time. As human experience with Lyme disease the past few decades has shown, people really don't know all that much about these kinds of bacteria. One thing that is known, however, is that spirochetes are extremely common in nature. They live in a wide diversity of habitats. As Gupta, et al. (2013) observe . . .

> They live in marine sediments, deep within soil, commensally in the gut of arthropods, including termites, as well as in vertebrates as obligate parasites. They can also be free-living or host-associated, pathogenic or non-pathogenic, and aerobic or anaerobic. There is also enormous variability in the genome sizes.

Most of them, as Lynn Margulis once put it, have much more important things to do than make us ill; they are integral to the functioning of the planet. Many of the spirochetes are essential coevolutionary partners of other life-forms. They live quite happily, for instance, in a wide variety of intestinal tracts – including our own. Up to twenty different kinds, for example, live in the termite gut where they help process the wood fibers that termites eat. (Without them, the termites would die of starvation and a lot of old wood would not biodegrade.) All these different spirochetes, the helpful and the disease causing, descended from a common spirochetal ancestor billions of years ago.

Still, we tend to be most concerned with the ones that make us sick and there are plenty enough of them to go around. Among the fifteen genera (as of 2015), there are four that have, so far, been found to cause human disease: *Treponema* (syphilis bacteria are its most famous members), *Borrelia* (Lyme spirochetes are its most famous members), *Leptospira,* and *Brachyspira*.

Whether any of the other, new-to-science spirochetes can infect human beings is still unknown. But trends indicate it is very likely – new spirochetal sources of human disease are being found yearly. Researchers are suspecting spirochetes may be the cause of a number of common human ailments for which no known agent has yet been identified, such as some cancers, Alzheimer's disease, and so on. (I will talk more about this in a bit.)

The kind of spirochetes that cause Lyme disease belong to the genus *Borrelia*. (More than one genus is, counterintuitively, not genuses but rather genera.) The way Latin terminology works is that the first name – of a bacteria or a plant, for instance – is the genus name. It's similar to the way your last name indicates the family into which you were born. The second is the species name, similarly to the way that your first name indicates which member of the family you are – it's just that taxonomists do everything backward.

The borrelial organism most associated with Lyme disease is called *Borrelia burgdorferi*. *Borrelia* is the genus, *burgdorferi* the species name, that is, the particular kind of *Borrelia* we are talking about. Sometimes for ease this Latin terminology is abbreviated *B. burgdorferi* or even, when talking about Lyme disease, *Bb.* It often gets more complicated than this, as things of this sort inevitably do, mostly because of the presence of *Homo taxonomisii* in our midst.

Unlike nearly every other human-infectious group of related microorganisms on the planet, the Lyme disease organisms are referred to in a very strange manner. (Leading, inevitably, to more confusion.) Very different species of *Borrelia*, each causing human infections, instead of being referred to by their own unique species names, are regularly and irritatingly lumped in with *B. burgdorferi*. So, if you begin reading about Lyme infections, you will, inevitably, run into the terms *Borrelia burgdorferi* sensu stricto and *Borrelia burgdorferi* sensu lato (sometimes abbreviated s.s. and s.l.). The first term means "in the strict sense" and refers solely to the *B. burgdorferi* species itself. The second term essentially means "in the broad sense" and refers to *all* the *Borrelia* that cause Lyme-like human disease. Not only is this a strange departure from the norm, it's unfortunate. It confuses people who are struggling to understand the disease, and more dangerously, it acts to linguistically hide the very different effects that each of the various Lyme species have when they infect a human being. (And yes, they do cause very different kinds of infections depending on the particular species, subspecies, or strain involved.)

Most Lyme disease bacteria are believed to be transmitted to people via hard ticks, but that picture is, as well, a great deal more complex. As with most things Lyme, it is simultaneously true and not true. (And yes, I will talk about that in a bit, too.)

An important note: infections with *Borrelia* bacteria really should not be referred to as "Lyme disease" (and most certainly not "Lyme's disease"). They should more properly be called borreliosis, which simply means a disease caused by *Borrelia* bacteria. (And one of these days they probably will be.) The name "Lyme" is really a holdover from the early days of the disease, before much was understood about it. It's called Lyme disease because it was first noticed as a unique disease complex in the late 1970s in Lyme, Connecticut, where it emerged as an arthritis cluster in children in that town. So, it is actually named after a *town*, hence *Lyme* disease. (And Canada geese are not *Canadian* geese, they were named after a person whose last name was Canada. The fact that they go back and forth between Canada and the rest of the Americas is just one of life's ironies. My mind is a junkyard of useless but sometimes, when drinking tequila, interesting facts.)

To make all this more complicated, there is actually another *type* of borrelial organism that infects people. It, too, is part of an emerging disease complex in the United States and throughout the world. The members of this group are called the relapsing-fever *Borrelia*. They do very much the same thing during human infection as the Lyme-group do but with one major difference: they cause a relapsing fever syndrome much as malarial and babesial parasites do. They have long been presumed to *only* be transmitted by soft ticks – which, btw, only need a few minutes to transmit the bacteria as opposed to the (most of the time) hours the hard ticks need. But, as with the Lyme-group of spirochetes, the situation is considerably more complicated than that. (The infection caused by these *Borrelia* should then be called relapsing fever borreliosis to distinguish it from nonrelapsing fever infections.)

Borrelia burgdorferi got its unique species name because it was initially identified by a researcher named Willy Burgdorfer, and as often occurs in the taxonomic world, someone named it after its finder.

And, to take this further, the coinfections of Lyme really should not be referred to as Lyme coinfections. They all belong to what should more properly be called the arthropod-transmitted infectious group. (ATIG for those who love acronyms.) There are important reasons for this, which I also will get to in a bit. (Probably in a rant of one form or another.) Other members of the Lyme-Borrelia group, rather than being named for a person, are named for the place they were discovered as *Borrelia carolinensis* is.

(These names can actually reveal a lot about how researchers think. But, when you get into it you will find that it's not that sophisticated really. By no means rocket surgery – hepatitis, for example, just means inflamed liver: it is very much *not* a disease description; it is a *symptom* description. Researchers, it is important to remember, are just people like you and me . . . well, usually. The ones with pen protectors in their pockets actually *are* different.)

Some *Borrelia*, e.g., *Borrelia hermsii* – one of the relapsing fever *Borrelia*, are named, not for its finder (much to his dismay), or for a geographical area (to its dismay), but rather for the species of vector or tick the bacteria live within and which spread them. The way this works is that the species of *Borrelia* that infects people and the species of tick that transmits it have the same species name – *hermsii*. The vector of *Borrelia hermsii* is the tick *Ornithodoros hermsii* hence B. *hermsii*.

Borrelial infections – they aren't new

It is often said that Lyme borreliosis is an emerging disease (true) and that it is a fairly recent one (false). Although Lyme disease seemed to suddenly appear out of nowhere, borrelial organisms have been infecting people as long as people have been. The reason Lyme seemed to so suddenly appear is that it was the first time that specific bacteria were found to be the cause of, in this instance, arthritis. Once the bacteria began to be noticed, it was soon discovered that they were causing a lot of different "diseases." But, regrettably for reductionists, it turned out they were all the *same* disease.

Because of what they do in the body, borrelial organisms can cause an extremely wide range of symptoms. They are very similar to syphilis bacteria in this respect, which is why syphilis infection (and, to some extent now, Lyme disease) was often referred to as the great imitator. Prior to their identification, the diseases caused by borrelial bacteria were simply thought to be different *conditions* that some people got from time to time: arthritis, heart disease, neurological dysfunctions of various sorts – including Alzheimer's, or even cancer. It is just that nobody knew what caused them; no one knew the root cause was a spirochete.

Another reason for the sudden emergence of Lyme disease is that there really has been a huge increase in the numbers of people getting infected. This is primarily due to ecological factors, mostly from two causes: (1) significant increases in human population and resultant land use alterations; and (2) climate change, especially increased warming. (See the section on ecology for more on this.) In a sense, Lyme disease is teaching human beings two things: (1) we don't really know all that much about disease and healing in the West; and (2) it's not nice to fool Mother Nature.

While the earliest accounts of the disease in the medical literature date from the late 1880s (examination of tick specimens from then does show that Lyme borreliosis was present in ticks at that time), it's unlikely that was the first time the pathogen infected human beings. Genomic analysis shows that Lyme spirochetes long ago split off as unique organisms, at minimum some 100 million years ago. Lyme *Borrelia* have been well established in ticks and other vectors for a very long time – they cannot live without a host; they do not exist in the wild. So for some 100 million years, Lyme disease spirochetes have lived in vectors like ticks, and they have infected mammals, and lizards, and birds – pretty much anything a tick can get away with biting.

Research suggests that Lyme borreliosis infection was common in the Louisiana Tchefuncte Indians between 500 BCE and 300 CE. As well, the heavy presence and complexity in the genomic variety of Lyme borreliosis species in Vladivostok in Northeast Asia suggests transfer across Siberia into Alaska between 30,000 and 10,000 BCE. The prevalence and unique genome alterations of the primary American borrelial organism (*Borrelia burgdorferi*) found in Europe also suggests spread *from* the Americas after the heavy European contact that began in 1492. And the oldest known

person infected with Lyme disease is the man found frozen and mummi-
fied in the Tyrolean Alps (Otzi the iceman). He lived approximately 5,300
years ago. Researchers found that when he died, he was infected with Lyme
spirochetes.

So, the *Borrelia burgdorferi sensu lato* group has been around a long time,
and its members have infected people for a long time. It was just not possible
until very recently to isolate the organism, to see it under a microscope, or
to grow it in a laboratory. The litany of symptoms that the organism causes,
for example, arthritis and neurological complications, have been with the
human species for millennia. Many of these conditions have, until now,
been considered idiopathic, that is, from no known cause. Lyme disease is
not a new disease to human beings.

Nevertheless, what *is* true is that borreliosis is in fact an emerging disease.
Specifically, it is moving into the human species in heretofore unknown levels.

The recent history of Lyme *Borrelia* organisms, as researchers have
commented, "appears to have been genetically turbulent," revealing that
the bacteria and their "plasmids are currently in a state of rapid evolutionary
change." Like many pathogenic bacteria, the spirochetes that cause borreliosis are feeling tremendous environmental pressure from the massive
environmental alterations and antibiotic usage that currently accompany
human civilization. They are altering themselves very quickly in response
to those pressures, and the human species is feeling the impacts.

Members of the Lyme-group

When I wrote the first edition of *Healing Lyme*, three species of borrelial
spirochetes in the Lyme-group were believed to be the primary causes of all
human Lyme disease: *Borrelia burgdorferi*, *B. afzelii*, and *B. garinii*. As with
most things Lyme, this has proved to be both true and untrue.

Traditionally, *Borrelia burgdorferi* has been considered to be the primary
agent of Lyme borreliosis in the United States while *B. afzelii* and *B. garinii*
are considered to be the primary agents of European and Asian Lyme
disease. Very simplistically, *B. burgdorferi* has been thought to be the primary
cause of Lyme arthritis, *B. afzelii* of dermatoborreliosis (severe Lyme skin
disease), and *B. garnii* of neuroborreliosis (central nervous system Lyme
disease). This, too, like many definitive statements about Lyme disease, is
overly simplistic and often incorrect.

B. burgdorferi is more common in the United States, the others more common in Europe, but all (and many others besides) exist on both continents, and infections with more than one type of spirochete commonly occur. All of them can cause markedly different symptom pictures at different times in different people in different places. They are not limited to continents or one symptom picture.

All the various borrelial organisms are moving around the world with a great deal of freedom – airplanes are used by more life-forms than just people. Birds (nature's airplanes) are primary carriers of borrelial organisms as well. We live in a world awash with borrelial bacteria; they exist on *every* continent. The pictures we have been given about them so far are not very accurate.

It is important to keep in mind that most researchers and physicians (not all, but most of them) are trying to fit the Lyme-group of microorganisms into a specific kind of rather tiny box. In other words, they are trying to make them fit into the worldview they were trained in when they went to school and became doctors and scientists. Unfortunately, these organisms don't fit very well into that box. This is a large part of the reason for the Lyme wars. Those who are holding onto a restrictive paradigm of what the world is and how it works are doing their best to keep that paradigm in place, no matter what the reality of the world actually is. This is also why, as research deepens and more people with less investment in a restrictive worldview get involved, the information you find about Lyme seems to, sometimes, change so substantially. Very little of the picture built up in the early Lyme days about the spirochetes and the disease complexes they cause (most of which is still insisted to be true) is in fact accurate to reality except in a very simplistic way. (It's old-Lyme thinking.) And that includes the number of borrelial species that can cause Lyme infections.

As Rudenko et al. (2011) comment, the Lyme-group now includes "18 named spirochete species and a still not named group proposed as genomospecies 2. Descriptions of new species and variants continue to be recognized, so the current number of described species is probably not final." And, no, it is not final, not even close. *Borrelia chilensis*, for example, was formally identified in 2014 in Chile.

In 2005, in the initial edition of *Healing Lyme*, there were twelve species believed to exist within the Lyme-group. Most were thought to *rarely or never* cause human infection. By 2011 that number had increased to eighteen, most of whom are now known to cause human infection. And, in 2015, as I write this updated version, the species number is hovering around twenty . . . it is important to note, however, that there are a large number of as-yet unnamed species that are *not* included in that count.

The current members of the Lyme-group are: *B. afzelii, B. americana, B. andersonii, B. bavariensis, B. bissettii, B. burgdorferi, B. californiensis, B. carolinensis, B. chilensis, B. garinii, B. genomospecies2, B. japonica, B. kurtenbachii, B. lonestari, B. lusitaniae, B. sinica, B. spielmanii, B. tanukii, B. texasensis, B. turdi, B. valaisiana, B. yangtze.* (*Note: B. genomospecies2* will probably get its own name eventually as *Borrelia genomospecies1* is now known as *B. americana.*) Each of these species of borrelial bacteria cause a slightly to very different spectrum of symptoms, depending on the species. *B. lonestari*, for instance, causes what is called, not Lyme disease, but southern tick-associated rash illness (STARI), which causes, obviously, a rash-like illness. Still, a rose by any other name . . .

In addition to the known species, there are scores of unique *subspecies* of each of these bacteria. A subspecies, btw, is a borrelial organism that has a different genetic structure from the species it is a subspecies of. It is just that the genetic difference is not considered substantial enough to consider it an entirely different species. And then to make things even more complicated, each species and subspecies has numerous *strains*. A strain, similarly to a subspecies, has a different genetic structure than the parent species, but it is even more similar to the parent than a subspecies is.

Each of these subspecies and strains possess slight variations on the core genome; all cause slightly or very different symptom pictures. I will talk about this more later – but what is true is that each borrelial species, during infection, produces bacterial offspring that have slightly to very different genetic structures. In other words, when you get Lyme disease, you don't have just one bacterial species in your body making you sick but rather an infectious *swarm* of similar but not identical genetic variants. This is one of the reasons why antibiotics are less than perfectly successful at treating Lyme infections.

Some of the subspecies and strains stabilize and become persistent entities in their own right. *B. burgdorgeri*, for instance, is known to have a number of *major* strains, for example the ospC strains B, G, H, and L. Each of those dominant strains, during infection, create still more not-quite-exact copies of themselves, creating even more strains. Each of the major strains differs in its infectivity, virulence, symptom picture, and treatment outcome.

And, to reiterate, there are other borrelial species who don't yet have their own unique name – they usually are just assigned numbers of one sort or another. These include *Borrelia* sp isolate SV1 which will possibly become *B. finlandensis* one of these days. Then there are: *Borrelia* sp tAG158M; various unnamed lizard-borne *Borrelia* that, yes, do cause human infections; a group of unnamed tick-borne *Borrelia* isolated from imported turtles; five, China-found, *Borrelia valasiana*-related strains with such unique genomes they will probably get their own species names; and a number of unnamed species recently found in rodents in California.

And there is still another spirochete, whose genetic structure places it someplace intermediate between the relapsing fever group and the Lyme-group. It has been named *B. myamotoi,* and it also causes human disease – a lot of it actually. It is usually placed in the relapsing fever group (but not always, though that is where I will put it today). So, please keep in mind that *the number of borrelial species that are known increases each year and this is not likely to end anytime soon.* Again, *all* these difference species, subspecies, and strains cause some form of Lyme disease.

The relapsing fever group

There are fifteen species of *Borrelia* bacteria that cause relapsing fever in human beings that have been named (again, more are being found all the time) and a number that have not yet received a species name. Traditionally, these organisms were considered to *only* be transmitted by soft as opposed to hard ticks. (The disease that these cause is often abbreviated TBRF for tick-borne relapsing fever.) However, *B. miyamotoi,* a rather serious emerging infection in the United States, is transmitted by hard ticks and, as research has deepened, more relapsing fever *Borrelia* are being found in hard ticks. As researcher A. G. Barbour (2014) comments, "The discovery of *Borrelia* species that were related to the agents of relapsing fever but were transmitted by hard ticks rather than soft ticks challenged previous taxonomies based largely on microbe-host specificities and geographic considerations." (This is part of the reason that *B. miyamotoi* occupies an odd position somewhere between the traditional relapsing fever *Borrelia* and the Lyme-group.) This group is considered to cause *endemic* relapsing fever.

Borrelia recurrentis is (relatively) unique in that it is primarily transmitted by body lice rather than ticks. It is the source of what is called, variously, louse-borne relapsing fever or urban relapsing fever or, even, *epidemic* relapsing fever.

The named members of the relapsing group are, at present: *Borrelia caucasica, B. crocidurae, B. duttonii, B. graingeri, B. hermsii, B. hispanica, B. johnsonii, B. latyschevii B. mazzotti, B. miyamotoi. B. parkeri, B. persica, B. recurrentis B. turicatae, B. venezuelensis.* (There are, of course, numerous subspecies and strains of every one of the members of this group.) There are others that are believed to *never* cause human disease (where have I heard this before) such as *B. anserina* and *B. coriaceae.* Then there are a number of relapsing fever organisms that, similarly to those in the Lyme-group, have not yet been named. (I have found five so far.) Exact numbers, irritatingly, are difficult to find. Oddly enough, there is no definitive list (that I can find) of all the members of this group.

The sort-of-relapsing fever/Lyme-group *Borrelia*

A movement is on by a number of taxonomists to create yet another group of *Borrelia* distinct from the relapsing fever and Lyme groups; they will probably do so one of these days. This is a group of borrelial organisms transmitted by hard ticks but whose genome differences puts them someplace in between the two groups. The candidates for inclusion in this group, so far, are *Borrelia miyamotoi, Borrelia lonestari,* and *Borrelia texasensis.* (Other taxonomists insist they are *in* the relapsing fever group and that all these organisms shall now be called the *Borrelia miyamotoi sensu lato* group – fisticuffs at 11:00 out behind the high school.) As analysis of the borrelial organisms in hard ticks deepens, it seems inevitable that some sort of new group will emerge and contain the bacteria transmitted from hard ticks that cause unique symptom pictures. It will lie somewhere between Lyme and relapsing fever group. For now, I have put them into either the Lyme or the relapsing fever (RF) group, depending on which (authoritative) journal papers I read first.

The mosquito/biting fly borrelial group

Bacterial members of the Lyme-group have also been found, in relatively small numbers so far, in both mosquitoes and biting flies (as well as mites and fleas). Transmission to humans has been documented from biting flies (Connecticut and Germany), from mites (Russia), and to hamsters by mosquitoes.

Lyme-group spirochetes are durable in mosquitos. Research has shown that they can be transmitted from adult mosquitos to new generations via infected eggs. The spirochetes have also been found to survive mosquito overwintering.

However, to make the situation more difficult, other borrelial spirochetes with unique genetic structures – but very similar to both the Lyme and relapsing fever group – have now been found to be rather common in mosquitoes and biting flies. (And yes, they can transmit the bacteria to people, but no, no one has yet studied this in any depth.) These particular *Borrelia* possess major genetic differences, making them distinct from those in the Lyme/relapsing fever groups.

These unique borrelial organisms have not yet been given their own species names only designations, for instance: BR91, BR149, BR151, BR173, BR177, BR193, BR208, BR 231. From the little research conducted so far, it appears that this group represents a distinct branching of the *Borrelia* genetic tree. It is almost certain that infections from this group occur in people; however, the nature and scope of those diseases, at this point, are completely unknown. This group of mosquito-borne spirochetes have been found to cause a typical Lyme-group antibody response in lab animals.

Other *Borrelia*

There are many other borrelial bacteria that involve themselves in our lives. Virtually no one tests for these other spirochetal organisms, or even knows much about them. An example is *Borrelia vincentii*, which is commonly found in our mouths. It is most famous for causing "trench mouth," which afflicted soldiers in World War I. This bacterial organism can also go systemic, infecting the brain, heart, tonsils (acute tonsillitis), and other organs similarly to other members of the Lyme-group and causing similar symptoms.

And yes, this one can be transmitted by kissing. All borrelial organisms utilize strategies to facilitate their survival and spread. This includes sending multiple bacterial forms into the bladder (and hence the urine) as well as infecting the salivary glands. No one has studied whether or how commonly other types of borrelial bacteria infect human salivary glands, but they should. It's a common behavior in the borrelial world, ignoring it is, well . . . what is the word I am looking for here . . . ?

As time progresses, what researchers discover about the emerging borrelial groups is unlikely to be in our favor. As researchers Rebaudet and Parola comment (2006) . . .

> *Future data may change current concepts. New* Borrelia *species related to the RF spirochetes group have recently been isolated from hard ticks, such as the emerging human pathogen* Borrelia lonestari *that has been identified in* Amblyomma americanum *[ticks] in the USA. Other relapsing fever-like spirochetes have been isolated from hard ticks of the genus* Ixodes *in Japan (*Borrelia miyamotoi*), northern America, Germany, and France. More recently, a further* Borrelia *species has been isolated from hard ticks infesting Turkish tortoises. A phylogenetic tree . . . demonstrated that this spirochete isolate from* Hyalomma aegyptium *[ticks] was related to Lyme-disease-related and RF-associated* Borrelia *but formed a different cluster.*

In short, despite the research that has occurred over the past four decades, humans know very little about infectious spirochetes. What is true is that there are a great many more of them than has been suspected; there are large groupings, whole families of them (to misuse the taxonomic term) that are unique, about whom little is known, and still others whose existence we do not suspect at all. A great many more than currently suspected are going to be found to be the agents of human disease. The future is going to be challenging.

Arthropod transmission

Arthropod comes from "arthro," i.e. joints (hence arthritis) and "pod," i.e., feet (hence podiatrist). In essence the term means jointed feet or in other, more useful terminology "bugs." Specifically, it refers to insects, spiders (which can indeed transmit some coinfections and perhaps borrelial bacteria as well), crustaceans, and so on. Bug-like organisms. Within the Lyme world, it means generally biting, blood-sucking insects of one sort or another. (And no, no matter how much you want to include them, lawyers and politicians are not included in this group.) The reason I use "arthropod" rather than "tick" is that borrelial organisms are transmitted by many organisms other than ticks.

Still . . . everybody "knows" that hard ticks, primarily those in the *Ixodes* genus, transmit Lyme disease, that there are three stages of development of those ticks (larvae, nymphs, adults) – the first, the larval stage being so small as to be almost unseeable, that each stage can transmit the disease, and that the ticks need to be attached for twenty-four to forty-eight hours for transmission to occur.

As with most things Lyme, these statements are both true and untrue; in other words, they are tremendously oversimplified and, in many respects, wrong. The picture is much more complex. I am not going to talk much about the ticks here, at least not in the way most people do ("We're all gonna die"). Instead, I will go into some of the things that really are true about borrelial transmission, most of which you will have rarely, if ever, heard. (I will talk more about the ticks themselves in the traditional way when I talk about the ecology of Lyme disease.)

There are some important complexities that are involved during tick transmission, most importantly the impacts of tick saliva on human immune function, that I will go into during the depth chapter on Lyme disease. (In its simplest, tick saliva shuts down important parts of our immune response; the Lyme bacteria take advantage of this and then initiate further immune suppression in order to keep themselves hidden from immune cells.) You don't really *need* to understand this in any depth (unless you wear pen protectors in your shirt pocket). However, if you do want to go deeper into it, I think the process fascinating and it does help understand some of the autoimmune-like processes that occur during Lyme disease.

In this section I'll just go into two of the transmission aspects that you are, most likely, not going to hear about.

1. *There are a great many more biting insects that transmit borrelial organisms than* Ixodes *hard ticks.*

Hard ticks have been said (and thought) to be the primary transmitters of what we call Lyme disease. Unfortunately, that picture is not as simple as the CDC and many physicians think, or perhaps wish, it to be. More accurately: the Lyme-group are *most often* transmitted by hard ticks.

Originally, the Lyme bacteria were thought to *only* be transmitted by one kind of hard tick, those in the *Ixodes* genus, and a rather limited number of them at that. In the northeastern and middle United States that usually means *Ixodes scapularis* (once upon a time called *Ixodes dammini* – name changed due to discomfort with Lyme advocates cursing in public). In the western and southern US, the primary species is *Ixodes pacificus*. In Europe it is *Ixodes ricinus*, and in Asia it is *Ixodes persulcatus*.

Unfortunately, Lyme bacteria have been found in at least twenty-five other *Ixodes* species and in, at least, fifteen other kinds of ticks, including genera as diverse as *Amblyomma, Boophilus, Dermacentor, Haemaphysalis, Hyalomma, Rhipicephalus, Argas,* and *Ornithodoros*, these last two genera being soft ticks. All these ticks do in fact transmit borrelial organisms to people. For example, the dog ticks (*Rhipicephalus* and *Dermacentor* genera) rather commonly transmit Lyme disease to both dogs and their owners.

The bacteria that cause Lyme infections are, as noted, also found in soft ticks. Borrelial transmission from soft ticks can and does occur (though it usually tends to be relapsing fever rather than Lyme *Borrelia*). This is important because soft ticks transmit Lyme organisms much more quickly than hard ticks. (Though transmission times in hard ticks are a great deal faster than we have been told.)

Further, Lyme bacteria are found in mites, fleas, mosquitoes, and biting flies and, importantly, tick and other arthropod *feces*. Egregiously, very little exploration has been done on these other routes of infection. To just touch on this, tick feces contains unique borrelial biofilms and encysted forms of the bacteria that, when you remove the tick, allows fecal transmission to occur via the break in the skin at the tick bite location. (The ticks, irritatingly, poop continuously when they are feeding.) This is true of all three developmental stages of the tick.

    2. *The transmission times for active infection that nearly all sources*
      list are wrong.

The transmission times that are commonly accepted (and quoted endlessly) are based on some of the very early papers on Lyme disease (e.g., Falco et al. and Piesman et al., quoted in Cook, 2015). Those papers made statements such as "removal of attached *Ixodes scapularis* ticks within 48 hours will effectively prevent Lyme disease" or that ticks "removed during the first 2 days of attachment do not transmit infection to tick bite victims" (Cook, 2015, see also Hynote et al., 2012). Thirty years later a researcher, Michael Cook in the UK, decided to actually examine the accuracy of those figures. Unsurprisingly, they did not hold up. In fact, even in those early studies *some* of the lab animals were infected with tick attachment of less than twenty-four hours.

Here is what is actually true: transmission of borrelial organisms occurs with a tick attachment of somewhere between ten *minutes* and seventy-two hours (transmission in less than sixteen hours is *very* common). The factors involved are complex and include:

1. *Type* of hard tick. *I. persulcatus* ticks, for example, transmit organisms much faster than *I. scapularis*, about twice as fast on average.

2. *Location of spirochetes in the tick*. It's been commonly believed that a transformation of the borrelial bacteria needs to take place before transmission can occur. In essence, once the tick attaches and begins to take a blood meal, the blood has to make its way to the tick midgut before the *Borrelia* can begin altering their form so they can survive in the new animal host. (The ticks analyze the blood, figure out what kind of animal it is, then alter their genetic structure to allow them to infect the new host.) This is only partially true. Nearly all ticks have some spiro-chetes already present in their salivary glands, *some ticks and tick species more than others*. Although these generally exist in lower numbers than in the midgut, these bacteria begin to move into the new host immediately upon tick attachment.

3. *Partially fed ticks* transmit borrelial organisms much more quickly. These are ticks that have fed awhile, dropped off, and then found a new host to feed upon. Partially fed ticks transmit bacteria into new hosts within as little as *ten minutes* of new attachment. Importantly, most ticks engage in partial feeding. That is the norm, not the exception.

4. *Ticks coinfected with other transmissible bacteria* – again, the
   norm not the exception – have much faster transmission
   times than ticks that are not coinfected.

5. *Species, subspecies, and strain* of the borrelial organism
   involved strongly affects time of transmission. The more
   aggressive the borrelial type, the faster the transmission
   time.

6. Soft ticks, biting flies, mosquitoes, and so on have very fast
   transmission times (as anyone who has been bitten by a
   mosquito or biting fly knows). Doctors routinely discount
   transmission from these routes; few people are aware they
   exist.

7. *The health or weakness* of the individual's immune system
   plays a major role. The stronger the immune system, the
   slower the transmission time. The weaker, the faster.
   Note: The most important single thing you can do to
   minimize borrelial infection is to keep your immune
   system as strong as possible. (Yes, this is covered in the
   book.)

Coinfections

I talk in some depth about this in the Appendix, so just a short note here.
We are really dealing here with a complex *group* of arthropod-transmitted
stealth infections, not merely Lyme and its coinfections. Coinfection in all
biting arthropods is common; *it is not an exception.* Coinfection does make
symptoms, diagnosis, and treatment much more complicated.

The most common coinfectious pathogens include anaplasmal, babesial,
bartonellal, chlamydial, ehrlichial, mycoplasmal, and rickettsial organisms. There are a few others that are emerging as concerns as well. These
include *Yersinia, Wolbachia,* and *Leptospira* – this last genus is beginning to
be found in hard tick species around the world, and yes, transmission has
been documented.

Unfortunately for people, depth examination of *Ixodes* ticks has found they
can carry up to 237 *genera* of microorganisms that are infectious to vertebrates. The numbers of coinfectious genera and species are going to continue

to grow. At this point, however, the most common coinfections, in terms of numbers, are *Bartonella, Chlamydia, Mycoplasma,* and *Babesia* bacteria.

Infection statistics

In 2004, as I was writing the first edition of this book, the CDC was insisting that only 20,000 new Lyme infections were occurring yearly . . . this despite the fact that Germany, a significantly smaller country, was reporting 30,000 new infections each year. Still, even then, Harvard researchers were insisting that infections were, at minimum, ten times the CDC number, in other words, at least 200,000 infections per year. In response to tremendous pressure from both researchers and Lyme support groups, in 2013 the CDC altered that figure, finally agreeing that, at least, 300,000 infections were occurring every year in the United States.

Unfortunately, this is almost certainly still too low. Given the wide range of borrelial species that are now known to infect ticks and other biting insects *combined* with the extremely poor ability of technological medicine to identify borrelial infections, yearly statistics are bound to be significantly higher. As the French researcher Christian Perronne (2014) puts it, "The lack of a gold standard for diagnosis makes producing accurate statistics difficult." A nicely put understatement.

Proper extrapolation, in my opinion, puts infection rates in 2015 somewhere between five hundred thousand and one million per year in the United States. This does not include coinfections whose infection numbers (see the *Bartonella/Mycoplasma* book for example) run into the millions.

Infections caused by this group of organisms are not likely to go away anytime soon, especially since ecological disruption and population increases are foundational drivers of the process.

Geographical distribution of Lyme infections

Although the majority of physicians in the United States tend to use the concept of geographical limitation to diagnose Lyme disease in the people who come to them, the truth is that *every state* is endemic for borrelial infections.

Again, every state is endemic for Lyme disease

Unfortunately, lack of awareness of this fact (which is carefully hidden in easily accessible online peer review journals) results in many physicians telling Lyme-infected patients that they cannot possibly have Lyme disease since they don't live in, nor have traveled to, a Lyme-endemic area.

Most sources still list the major Lyme endemic areas in the US as the Northeast, the central areas of Wisconsin/Minnesota, and Northern California. This is old-Lyme thinking, and it isn't very accurate. There is a major endemic region, for instance, in the Southeast; increasing numbers of infections (insisted by physicians, for years, to *not* be Lyme) are being reported from that region. This is one of the major areas of infection by *Borrelia lonestari* (the source of southern tick-associated rash illness, i.e., STARI). Researchers have found that *B. burgdorferi, B. americana,* and *B. andersonii* are extremely common in the Southeast as well. As Clark et al. (2014) note, "The study findings suggest that human cases of Lyme disease in the southern USA may be more common than previously recognized and may also be caused by more than one species of *B. burgdorferi* sensu lato."

More accurately, Lyme is endemic in the very large region from the Atlantic seaboard to the Rocky Mountains (east/west) and from the Gulf coastal states (north/south) into Canada. The hot spots in the Wisconsin/Minnesota region, in the Northeast/New England states, and in the Southeast is only where infections in that region are most dense.

Northern California is the hot spot for infections in the Pacific West, but that infectious range runs from mid-California upward into Canada and eastward to the Rocky Mountain range.

The endemic area with the fewest numbers of infections is in the Southwest and upward through the desert regions into Nevada and Utah. Still, lizards act as reservoirs of borrelial bacteria in those regions, and transmission does occur. Further, those areas are endemic for a large number of the major coinfectious bacteria (e.g., *Rickettsia*).

There is no region in the US that is exempt from the Lyme-group of infections. **This is also true of the rest of the planet.** It does not matter the species of *Borrelia* or which coinfections you are speaking of – they really are everywhere. (Again, see the ecology section for more on this.)

Symptoms of Lyme borreliosis

Most sources still tend to separate symptom pictures by what are considered the main infectious species in North America and Europe/Asia. I am not going to do that here. Borrelial bacteria *tend* to be geographically focused, but in reality all these organisms can be found every place on the planet. And each species can cause a similar range of symptoms. What symptoms they cause does depend to some extent on the species, but the factors involved are considerably more complex.

In our work, the past decade, we have generally seen people who are infected with *B. burgdorferi*, which is (tiresomely) insisted by experts to be the primary cause of arthritic symptoms. However, nearly all the people we have had contact with in this group have neurological problems. Very few have had arthritis as their primary presenting symptom. The symptom separation that is generally used, based on species of organism, is deeply inaccurate and very misleading for practitioners.

In general, all members of the Lyme-group tend to show the same spectrum of symptoms during infection. The early symptoms are essentially flu-like. Then as the bacteria spread further into the body, the symptoms they cause are usually lumped into three main areas: the skin, the joints, and the neurological system. However . . .

Lyme borreliosis can mimic nearly every disease complex known, including diseases that occur in many different organs, including the heart and kidneys. *This mimicry, and the poor diagnostic tests that are available, are what makes Lyme diagnosis difficult, if not impossible, for many doctors.*

Many physicians tend to use what is called *differential* diagnosis when trying to figure out what disease someone has. That is, they focus on the symptom *differences* that various diseases have from one another. (To see how poorly this often works in practice, see the rather grim story in the diagnostic section of the rickettsiosis chapter.) Lyme and the many coinfections will often have no significant differences from other diseases that cause similar symptoms. This is why so many with Lyme disease have been (mis)diagnosed with multiple sclerosis, or Alzheimer's disease, or schizophrenia and treated inappropriately, resulting in years or decades of poor health.

For many people who become infected with borrelial organisms, the wide range of symptoms, and the inept responses of physicians, generates tremendous fear – simply from not knowing how one disease can cause so many effects throughout the body. The answer is very simple.

> *The most important thing to understand about Lyme disease is that the bacteria have an affinity for collagenous tissues. This is at the root of every symptom they cause.*

Borrelial bacteria are parasites. They cannot make very many of the substances they need to live, so they harvest them from their hosts. As Margulis et al. (2009) comment, "Human tissue provides food and other conditions of growth for . . . *Borrelia burgdorferi* spirochetes." The majority of the food they need is to be found in collagen-like tissues throughout the body. Wherever they feed on those tissues is where the symptoms occur. If they find them in the joints, it's arthritis. If they find them in the skin, various skin manifestations emerge. If in the heart, heart disease. If in the nervous system or the brain, neurological symptoms.

For example, the nerves in our brains are covered by myelin sheaths, much like electrical wires are covered by thin plastic insulation sheaths. As with electrical wire, this keeps the nerves protected, insulated. Once borrelial bacteria attach to those sheaths, they use a variety of substances to break them down into a kind of soup of nutrients from which they feed. Once demyelinated, the nerves begin to produce aberrations in nervous system function. This is at the root of most of the neurological symptoms the bacteria cause.

Every symptom someone gets comes from a similar process. Once you understand this, the disease is not then so mysterious or frightening. It is understandable. And more importantly, it's easier to treat. (If you protect the collagen structures of the body, the symptom picture begins to disappear.)

What follows is as complete a symptom list as I could find going through several decades of journal papers on Lyme infections. One note here, however. The journal papers are filled with phrases such as "an example of a rare symptom of Lyme," or "unusual skin manifestation of Lyme." After several hundred of those, it began to be clear that most researchers were engaging in an habitual overuse of the words "rare" and "unusual." ("I don't think that word means what you think it means.")

General symptoms

Arthropod-spread infections, if they are going to cause symptoms (they don't always), generally present as "the flu." This is because our immune systems respond to infections by creating a generalized response we have come to call the flu. Usually, this means a sudden onset of feeling "under the weather," with accompanying fever, chills, headache, general muscle pains, fatigue, and weakness.

Nearly all Lyme books and web sources emphasize the "bull's-eye rash" that sometimes accompanies Lyme-group infections. Unfortunately, this rash is only present in about 30 percent of infections (again, only some genotypes generate the rash during infection). Many physicians base their diagnosis of Lyme on two things: the bull's-eye rash and whether you live in what they consider to be an endemic region. *Neither is a reliable diagnostic indicator for ruling out a Lyme infection.*

Some people have *no* early symptoms, others have a bout of "the flu," which then goes away, others rather quickly get very ill indeed – often with neurological problems, and still others have what are considered an unusual presenting symptom – sudden hearing loss, "tight" skin, trouble walking (loss of balance, i.e., ataxia), and so on. Table 1.1 lists the symptoms that have been found to occur during Lyme-group infections. Any of these can occur as the *only* presenting symptom of a Lyme infection.

Pregnancy and Lyme

Borrelial spirochetes can be transmitted to the unborn child during pregnancy, and adverse outcomes do sometimes occur. Adverse pregnancy outcomes are much more common among those who do not respond to single course antibiotic treatment. Loss of the pregnancy and cavernous hemangioma are the most common outcomes. The children *may* (not *will*) be born with a Lyme infection, which can, sometimes, linger for years.

Relapsing fever symptoms

RF symptoms generally begin between four and fourteen days after an arthropod bite. The initial symptoms are usually a three-day episode of high fever and fatigue accompanied by high levels of RF bacteria in the blood. This is normally followed by a seven day, fever-free interval, then a three-day recurrence, and so on, *ad irritatum.*

Both RF and LD infections share a range of clinical symptoms: arthritis, carditis, and neurological damage are the most common. There are, however, a number of symptoms that occur more often with relapsing fever than Lyme. Abdominal pain and vomiting are more common, diarrhea occurs in ~ (i.e. approximately) 25 percent of those infected. Anemia and disruption of sleep patterns are also somewhat common.

The infected, as Dworkin et al. (2008) comment, "are more likely to have jaundice; petechiae on the trunk extremities and mucus membranes; central nervous system involvement; epistaxis; and blood-tinged sputum." Less common are "iritis, acute respiratory distress syndrome, uveitis, irodocyclitis, cranial nerve palsy and other focal neurologic defects, myrocarditis, and rupture of the spleen." (*Note:* Rupture of the spleen is usually uncommon during Lyme infections. Because of this potential in RF borrelia, protection of the spleen with either *Ceanothus* or *Salvia miltiorrhiza* is crucial.)

Children and women tend to have a more severe infection; spontaneous RF-initiated abortion can occur in up to 50 percent of pregnant women. As with Lyme infections, a large range of symptoms can occur. As Dworkin comments, "One patient may present as having meningitis, another may appear flulike, whereas others may have a febrile gastrointestinal illness or no physical findings." Unfortunately, septic shock can also occur during RF infections, something that is much rarer in Lyme disease. Fatality, in the untreated, runs 2 to 5 percent.

A listing of the most common symptoms includes: headache (94% of people), myalgia (92%), chills (88%), nausea (76%), arthralgia (73%), vomiting (71%), abdominal pain (44%), confusion (38%), dry cough (27%), eye pain (26%), diarrhea (25%), dizziness (25%), photophobia (25%), neck pain (24%), rash (18%), dysuria (13%), jaundice (10%), hepatomegaly (10%), splenomegaly (6%), conjunctival injection (5%), eschar (2%), meningitis (2%), and nuchal rigidity (2%).

Symptoms of *Borrelia miyamotoi* (the most common RF bacteria in the US) are usually a bit slower at coming on: generally 10-15 days after a tick bite. The main clinical signs are high fever, fatigue, headache, chills, and sweating. Functional impairment of the liver (50% of the infected, indicating the necessity for supportive herbs), kidney, and heart are relatively common.

A note on the cytokine dynamics of RF *Borrelia*: I will talk in depth about the cytokine dynamics of Lyme borreliosis (and not so much RF); however,

TABLE 1.1 SYMPTOMS FOUND TO OCCUR DURING LYME-GROUP INFECTIONS

Skin Symptoms

erythema migrans (bull's-eye rash) with single or multiple lesions
pityriasis rosea
painful skin
erythematous livid discoloration (feet and legs)
reticular varices
corona flebectatia paraplantaris medialis
pitting edema
lymphocytoma
primary cutaneous marginal-zone B-cell lymphoma
acrodermatitis chronica atrophicans (usually in very late stage infections)
erythema gyratum repens
erythema nodosum

erythema annulare centrifugum
lymphocytic infiltration of the skin
morphea
anetoderma
atrophoderma of Pasini and Pierini
lichen sclerosus et atrophicans
scleroderma en coup de sabre
panniculitis
eosinophilic fasciitis
necrobiotic xanthogranuloma
alopecia
interstitial granulomatous dermatitis
cutaneous sarcoidosis
necrobiosis lipoidica
sarcoidosis

Joint/Tendon Symptoms

oligoarthritis
rheumatoid arthritis
lumbosacral spondylosis
supraspinatus tendinopathy
synovitis
ruptured synovial cysts

cartilage damage
Baker's cysts
oedema of metatarsal heads II–IV, forefoot pain
interstitial granuloma annulare
chronic dermatitis
colagenosis

Neurological Symptoms

peripheral nerve palsy
hyperalgesic radiculitis
aseptic meningitis
cranial nerve involvement
meningovasculitis
meningoencephalitis
brainstem encephalitis
encephalomyelitis
cranial nerve palsies
severe dysphagia
muscle weakness (bi- or unilateral)
cognitive dysfunction
diplopia, blephaloptosis
horizontal nystagmus
palatoplegia
dysarthria
ataxia (bilateral, acute, cerebellar)
Alzheimer's disease
progressive dementia

brain atrophy
hoarseness/soft voice
laryngeal nerve paralysis
bilateral vocal cord paralysis
respiratory paralysis (requiring tracheostomy)
lymphocytic meningitis
trigeminal palsy
silent thalamic lesion
peripheral facial palsy (Bell's palsy)
dizziness, vertigo
bilateral hearing loss (over time)
sudden sensorineural hearing loss
alexithymia
depression (including suicide attempts)
homicidal rage (often from bartonella coinfection but also present in Lyme)
extreme mood swings
memory dysfunction
painful sensory radiculo-neuritis

multifocal motor radiculo-neuritis

multiple mononeuropathy

chronic unremitting headache

abducens palsy

Alice in Wonderland syndrome (metamorphosia, auditory hallucinations)

multiple sclerosis associated with primary effusion lymphoma

tremor

seizures

epilepsy with multifocal brain lesions

psychosis

(Possible autism-related disorders)

various nervous system lesions

poliomyelitis-like syndromes

radiculalgia

pseudotumor cerebri

brief, recurrent, spontaneous episodes of loss of consciousness

recurrent laryngeal nerve palsy

cerebral vasculitis

regional leptomeningeal parasthesia

transverse myelitis

sleep disorders (no sleep, always sleep)

acute disseminated encephalomyelitis, hypotonia, dysarthria,

(Possible Tourette's syndrome, associated with)

myasthenia gravis

avellis syndrome

acute brachial neuritis (neuralgic amyotrophy)

subacute anterior horn disease

central nervous system lymphoma

lupus-like syndrome

distal axonal polyneuropathy

pontine tumour

intracranial lymphoma

hypersomnia

paralytic strabismus

Organ Symptoms

Prostate carcinoma with painless paraparesis vasculitis

multiple ischemic strokes, acute ischemic pontine stroke

cerebral sinuvenous thrombosis

various nephritic syndromes (glomerulonephritis, mesangioproligerative IgA-nephritis, minimal change disease, acute kidney failure, bilateral obstructive ureteral calculi, neurogenic bladder)

loss of sense of taste and various other taste disorders

non-Hodgkin's (mantle cell) lymphoma

carditis and various cardiomyopathies

atrioventricular block (sometimes complete, sudden onset)

atrial fibrillation

escape rhythm with bundle-branch block morphologies

pericarditis, myocarditis, degenerative valvular disease, endocarditis, aaortic valve stenosis, dilated cardiomyopathy, diastolic heart murmur,

sudden cardiac death

dyspnoea

supraventricular cardiac arrhythmia

multiple organ failure

bruxism (and other malfunctions in the masticatory organ)

temporomandibular joint inflammation and pain

hepatitis

elevated liver enzymes

necrotizing granulomatous hepatitis

various ophthalmic disorders (ocular inflammation, uveitis, panuveitis, retinal vein occlusion, episcleritis, vertical binocular diplopia, serous retinal detachment, choroidal inflammation, chorioretinal folds, ospoclonus, orbital myositis, nystagmus, retrobulbar optic neuritis, conjunctivitis, ptosis, photophobia, ocular flutter, paralytic strabismus, sudden painless vision loss, keratopathy, papillitis, corneal thinning, eyelid erythema)

abdominal wall weakness/distension

lumboabdominal pain

abdominal aortic aneurysm

lumbar rigidity

nocturnal back pain

lymphoadenopathy

lupus-like disorders

respiratory distress syndrome

intercranial hypertension

one major difference between RF and LD is that people infected with RF who have low levels of IL-10 experience a significantly worsening course of infection, sometimes dangerously so. (During Lyme borreliosis IL-10 levels are generally high.) The use of IL-10 modulators during RF is essential, *Withania* being at the top of the list.

Diagnosis

Effective diagnostic testing for Lyme disease was poor in 2005; it's still poor in 2015, and I suspect it will be for some time to come. The reasons are many, complex, and difficult so resolve.

The most important thing to understand about this is that the journal papers are filled with stories, hundreds of them, where hospital admission occurred for serious Lyme infections and despite repeated testing, results continued to come up negative when people did in fact have Lyme disease.

For those who are not hospitalized, test results are generally even more inaccurate since there is often no acute condition forcing a diagnosis. Lee, et al (2014) is succinct . . .

> *The commonly used two-tier serology laboratory test which usually only turns positive during convalescence of the infection is reported to be negative or non-diagnostic in 75% of the "clinically confirmed" cases of early Lyme disease. Blood culture at the stage of bacteremia has met only limited success in specialized laboratories and offers little help to the timely management of patients suffering from early Lyme disease. . . . Conventional polymerase chain reaction (PCR) amplification of the bacterial DNA for detection is not sensitive enough for routine diagnostic purposes because the copies of the target DNA extracted from the very low number of spirochetes in the patient blood samples are often below the limit of detection.*

The only reliable, definitive, diagnostic marker, as has been true all along, is if someone presents with a bull's-eye rash, However, there is a caveat: there are many Lyme rashes that do not show the traditional "bull's-eye" shape during infection – the appearance of the rash is odd enough that Lyme infection is usually missed. These odd-shaped rashes are nearly always misdiagnosed as a variety of other skin diseases. Nevertheless, *if* you have a traditional bull's-eye rash, it is the one definitive marker for a diagnosis of Lyme disease.

However, in the absence of a clear-cut erythema migrans (EM) rash, there is no way to reliably and consistently diagnose Lyme disease. And up to two-thirds of people infected with *Borrelia* have no rash at all. Many never notice the tick either; nymph stage ticks are very small and often missed.

While the tests that are used can sometimes help, and while some unusual and not easily obtained tests are significantly better, tests consistently miss infection with the spirochetes. Many people, formerly pronounced seronegative, upon retesting with more sensitive tests or by better laboratories have been found to have had Lyme infection all along.

There are a number of reasons for the problems with testing. In the first two to four weeks of infection only about half of infected people produce measurable antibodies to Lyme spirochetes. People tested during this period often test negative and are only retested when their health deteriorates significantly. IgM antibodies rise during the third week, peak after four to six weeks and then disappear by week eight – so if you get tested after this, they may not show at all. IgG antibodies, which appear between six weeks and three months of infection, can persist for years or decades after successful treatment, and so when tested, people will be found to be positive for the disease even if they do not have it.

Antibody response can be weak or nonexistent at different stages of the disease in different people. Spirochete levels tend to peak at sixty days after infection and then drop to low levels in the system. The spirochete numbers may be so low that they do not show on even the most sensitive tests; they often cannot be found even with biopsy. Additionally, the bacteria may encyst, making them even more difficult to find.

Antibiotic therapies can cause the motile spirochete levels, already low, to drop by a factor of one thousand in the body, making detection of any remaining spirochetes nearly impossible by any means. As well, testing *after* someone has begun antibiotics will skew the tests, making a negative test much more likely, even if someone is still infected.

Additionally, false positives, false negatives, cross-reactivity, and other problems are common with the tests for this illness. The spirochetes continually alter their genetic makeup, altering their form in such a way that they are invisible to testing (and the immune system). Additionally, there are many different species of the bacteria that can cause infection. The tests are often not specific enough to identify them. The primary diagnostic criteria for determining a Lyme infection have, of necessity, remained individual and symptomatic. The tests are simply used as a backup for individual diagnosis.

ELISA and western blot

The two most common tests used for Lyme borreliosis are the ELISA and western blot. The Centers for Disease Control recommend a two-tiered testing process using both these tests. However there are serious problems with the tests; neither you nor your physician should rely on them as definitive one way or another.

The ELISA test essentially tests blood serum for the presence of antibodies to *Borrelia* organisms. However, a significant number of studies have found, and continue to find, that the ELISA test is not all that effective in diagnosing Lyme disease. In general, some 40 percent of people known to have Lyme (because of EM rash) test negative for Lyme infection with ELISA. To make this statistic worse, studies have found ELISA to be negative in 35 percent of people in whom a skin biopsy found cultivatable spirochetes.

The western blot (or immunoblot) isn't really much better. This test looks for either IgG or IgM (immunoglobulin G or M), two different antibodies that are produced in response to infection; the test works something like this.

Borrelia spirochetes that are being grown in a laboratory are killed and broken apart by washing them in a detergent. This separates the proteins in the outer surface of the borrelial body, it's bacterial membrane, from one another. The proteins are then bonded to a nylon membrane. Proteins of the same molecular size then cluster together in what are called "bands." To test someone for Lyme, some of his or her blood is tested against the *Borrelia*-banded nylon sheet to see how many bands the blood reacts with. The more bands, the more specific the diagnosis.

Note: Results of western blot tests should be reported in full by listing which bands are reactive. However, many labs simply report negative or positive, and *this is highly problematical.*

If you are being tested, you should make sure that you or your doctor gets a complete list of the bands that react with your blood. For example, 41kd bands (which react with the flagella – the motile organs – of the spirochete) are usually the first to react during testing but can also cross-react with other spirochetal organisms such as those that cause syphilis.

Band responses that indicate a positive infection seem to vary considerably depending on the "authoritative" source that is consulted. In 2005, in the first edition, band specificity was considered to be 18kd, 37kd, 39kd, 83kd, 93kd, 23-25kd (which reflects the presence of OspC), 31kd (which reflects OspA), and 34kd (which reflects OspB). (For some reason the CDC eliminated the use of the 31kd and 34kd bands in the reportable diagnosis of Lyme infection even though these bands are highly indicative of Lyme exposure.) Bands other than the 41kd typically appear later in the infection, and many of them many never appear, even during an active infection. For a positive Lyme test (in 2005), the 41kd band and at least one of the others had to be present. Many sources indicated that four bands, at least, were necessary to make a clinical Lyme diagnosis.

Unfortunately, later papers (just as insistently definitive) show some variations on what is considered necessary for a positive test. A relatively recent Chinese paper (Jiang et al., 2010) felt that the following bands should be considered specific:

- For IgG: 58kd, 39kd, 30kd
- For OspC: 17kd, 41kd, 66kd
- For IgM: 58kd
- For OspA: 30kd

A recent Western paper (Evans et al., 2010) considers 20kd, 28kd, and 48kd bands to be specific. And on it goes.

I listed a number of studies in the 2005 edition of this book that found, consistently, that neither the ELISA or the western blot to be very reliable. *There are scores more now.* A recent example:

Ang et al. (2011) took eighty-nine serum samples from people clinically *known* to have Lyme and tested them using eight different ELISA tests (the ones most commonly used by physicians for diagnosis) in combination with five different western immunoblot tests. As they note . . .

The number of IgM- and/or IgG-positive ELISA results in the group of patients suspected of Borrelia infection ranged from 34 to 59%. The percentage of positives in cross-reactivity controls ranged from 0 to 38%. Comparison of immunoblots yielded large differences in inter-test agreement and showed, at best, a moderate agreement between tests. Remarkably, some immunoblots gave positive results in samples that had been tested negative by all eight ELISAs. The percentage of positive blots following a positive ELISA result depended heavily on the choice of ELISA-immunoblot combination. We conclude that the assays used to detect anti-Borrelia antibodies have widely divergent sensitivity and specificity. The choice of ELISA-immunoblot combination severely influences the number of positive results, making the exchange of test results between laboratories with different methodologies hazardous.

"Hazardous" . . . this sums it up about as well as it can be. The tests are not reliable and, even at best, only show about a 60 percent positive infection rate even in groups clinically known to be infected. As Ang and friends continue a bit later in the journal article. . .

Theoretically, the use of recombinant antigens should lead to increased specificity and, possibly, increased sensitivity as well. This does not seem to be true for the currently available ELISAs and immunoblots for the detection of anti-Borrelia antibodies. . . . Therefore, manufacturer claims for the superior performance of assays using recombinant antigens for the detection of Borrelia antibodies must be interpreted with caution.

There is a worldwide assumption, primarily because of the CDC and old-Lyme thinking, that the use of a two-tier testing (ELISA and western immunoblot) is effective in testing for Lyme disease, that such an approach is the gold standard for diagnosis in the absence of a bull's-eye rash. It is in fact this approach that the CDC and nearly all physicians insist upon for a legitimate diagnosis of Lyme. Nevertheless, as the Ang et al., study shows, two-tier testing with these particular approaches is not very effective. As

Donta (2012) comments: "Specific antibodies are not an adequate means to assess the presence or absence of the organism. . . . [consequently] the diagnosis of Lyme disease is based primarily on the clinical picture." In other words, when seeking a diagnosis in Lyme disease, you are dependent on finding a really good diagnostician who knows Lyme disease and its symptom picture very well (there aren't many), and/or, if you are lucky, being one of the 60 percent for whom the tests work.

Borgermans et al. (2014) sum up the state of this approach to testing in their metareview of journal papers and chronic Lyme disease:

> *There is consistent evidence that the two-tier testing lacks sensitivity, cannot distinguish between current and past infection, cannot be used as a marker for treatment, is often dependent on subjectively scored immunoblots, and is considered expensive.*

PCR

PCR testing uses the spirochetal DNA itself and enhances its levels so that it is perceivable to human analysis. The major problem with PCR testing is that the spirochetes are often in very low numbers and are not homogenous in tissues so that DNA cannot, in many instances, be found.

There are a number of different types of PCR tests, and they are becoming more sophisticated all the time. In one recent study (Liveris et al., 2012), researchers compared five diagnostic tests: culture of skin biopsy, culture and nested PCR of skin biopsy, nested PCR, quantitative PCR (qPCR), and a novel qPCR blood-culture test. Oddly enough, this study focused on people with EM (bull's-eye) rash. (I presume because they then knew that everyone did in fact have Lyme.) The study found that those with *multiple* rashes tested most accurately using these five tests – which makes sense as the more EM rashes a person has, the higher the spirochete load. In this study, of 23 people with multiple rashes, 22 tested as infected with Lyme. Of the 42 with one rash, only 24 tested as infected with Lyme.

This gives you a very good idea of the reliability of PCR diagnostic testing. *Of the 42 with one rash, only 24 tested as infected with Lyme.* In other words, the researchers *knew* the people had Lyme, but the most sensitive tests they could find only showed 24 of them as positive for Lyme. And this is the group most easy to diagnose. In those without a bull's-eye rash, which is around two-thirds of those infected, the results are, unfortunately, worse.

In this particular study *five* different diagnostic tests were used on all 52 participants. Of those, 48 (92.3 percent) tested positive *on at least one test*. In other words, to get that high a percentage rate, everyone had to be tested with five tests. Even then around 8 percent showed negative for Lyme when they did indeed have it. Again, these were extremely sensitive tests and *did not* include either ELISA or western blot (which are the normal tests most people use).

A further problem with PCR testing is outlined by Borgermans et al. (2014), "PCR positivity in the absence of culture positivity following antibiotic treatment should be interpreted with caution since *B. burgdorferi* DNA and mRNA can be detected in samples long after spirochetes are no longer viable as assessed by classic microbiological parameters."

So, regrettably, PCR is not a definitive test either, irrespective of the type used.

Biopsy and culture of spirochetes

This is the best of all tests, but unfortunately, it, too, is not very effective. Numbers of spirochetes during infection tend to be rather low; they are hard to find, hard to see, hard to grow . . . and it all takes awhile. Even in instances where the bull's-eye rash is present, direct skin biopsy has often failed to find spirochetes or effectively culture them. So, no, it's not definitive either.

Advanced laboratory Lyme test

I have heard from a few people that the advanced laboratory Lyme test is averaging a 92 percent accuracy rate for diagnosing Lyme infection. The downside is that the test takes two to four months. For long-standing Lyme infections that have refused to be diagnosed through other testing methods, this may be a good choice.

CXCL13

CXCL13 is a chemokine (aka, B-lymphocyte chemoattractant). During Lyme infections of the central nervous system the cerebral spinal fluid often has much higher levels of this chemokine than it normally does. Some people have begun using it as a diagnostic marker for Lyme infection. It is a helpful test in combination with others but is, again, not definitive.

In one study (Wutte et al., 2014) comparing two different ELISAs, immunoblot (IB), and CXCL13 for effectiveness, the researchers found that of 50 people who definitely had neuroborreliosis 29 (58%) were positive when using rELISA-AI testing. This was confirmed by immunoblot in only 19 of them. Testing using flELISA-AI found Lyme in 17 (34 %); it was confirmed by IB in 15. CXCL was positive in 22 of 50 (44%).

These numbers did not, inevitably, cross over. Only 26 percent of the people (about 13 of 50) were found positive for Lyme by all three testing approaches. CXCL13 is a useful test for neurological Lyme but, again, is not definitive and is only indicative, especially when used along with other tests. A negative CXCL13 does not rule out Lyme infection.

CD57

Several early papers (e.g., Stricker, 2001), cited in the first edition of this book, indicated that a low CD57 count could be an indicator of long-term, chronic Lyme infections, thus making it a useful diagnostic marker for the severity of infection. It measures a certain aspect of immune function, so the lower the count, the poorer the immune response to infection. (A later paper [Marques, 2009], did not find an association between CD57+ counts and post-Lyme disease syndrome.) The situation, it turns out, is quite a bit more complex.

High expression of CD57+ NK (natural killer) cells (i.e., CD8+ T cells) is associated with the emergence of various cancers (e.g., renal cell carcinoma, melanoma, certain lymphomas), some that can occur from long-term infections (e.g., chlamydial). However, during autoimmune diseases, as Nielson et al. (2013) comment, "Expanded populations of autoreactive CD57+ T cells are associated with more severe disease – Wegener's granulomatosis, pars planitis, multiple sclerosis, type I diabetes mellitus, Graves' disease, and rheumatoid arthritis (RA), amongst others." Despite this, they go on to note that *some* autoimmune conditions are "consistently associated with reduced frequencies or absolute numbers of circulating CD57+ NK cells and/or impaired NK cell cytotoxicity, suggesting that cytotoxic CD57+ NK cells may play a regulatory role, preventing or suppressing autoimmune disease." They conclude, "Taken together these data are consistent with the hypothesis that immature CD57- NK cells may contribute to autoimmune inflammation and tissue damage whereas more highly differentiated, cytotoxic CD57+ NK cells may fulfill an immunoregulatory role."

The problem, as is usual with borrelial bacteria, is that the immune landscape alters considerably over time, with the type of bacteria, immune status, age, and so on. In consequence, high CD57+ cell counts, for instance, in long-term chlamydial or mycoplasmal infections could actually stimulate the formation of cancers. During RA-type infections (common in Lyme disease), high levels could make the condition worse as well. But in some autoimmune-like conditions, also common in Lyme disease, the more highly activated CD57+ cells could help resolve the condition. So, in some Lyme disease conditions it might be useful to increase CD57+ levels; in others it would be more appropriate to lower them. Thus, absolute levels of CD57+ cells as markers of immune response don't exist in a one-to-one relationship with the state of Lyme infections.

In short, in my opinion, given the increase in understanding of this NK marker, there just isn't enough data to support CD57+ cell levels as a reliable diagnostic for Lyme, chronic Lyme, or post-Lyme disease syndrome.

Future directions

There are a number of other tests that researchers are working to develop; however, none of them, at this point, offer 100 percent diagnostic certainty. One of the best seems to be PCR testing of urine. This makes sense since *Borrelia* tend to colonize the bladder of all vertebrates they infect. I am hopeful that it can emerge as a reliable and common test.

Unfortunately, the lack of truly reliable tests leaves people who are struggling with Lyme infection in a difficult position. Physicians are relying on tests that are not very effective, telling thousands of people that they are not Lyme positive when in fact they are.

I wish I had better news; unfortunately I don't. The best hope for the future, in the absence of a definitive test, is a complex of multiple tests. When five or more tests are used in tandem, diagnostic certainty rises into the eightieth and ninetieth precentiles. It is unlikely that very many physicians will be willing to use a five-test complex; nevertheless it is the only method currently available that has any kind of decent reliability.

Geographical area/symptom diagnosis

In general, if you suffer many of the symptoms on the following list and have been in or live in an area in which Lyme is endemic or increasing in incidence, you should seriously consider Lyme as the reason. In difficult cases the diagnosis is best confirmed by working with someone with deep experience with Lyme disease. An array of symptoms from the following list (this does not mean one or two) and a western blot assay with at minimum two bands, one being 41kd and one other being Lyme specific, is a good beginning for considering a Lyme diagnosis.

Diagnostic symptoms of Lyme borreliosis

Please keep in mind that some people with Lyme present with *none* of these symptoms – see the earlier, more complete list of presenting symptoms. This is merely to help in diagnosis; it is not definitive.

- Erythema migrans (EM) or bull's-eye rash (one-third of those infected)
- Multiple EM lesions (in about one-fifth of those infected)
- Acrodermatitis chronica atrophicans (generally in late stage)
- Borrelial lymphocytoma
- Continual low-grade fever
- High fever, chills, or sweating (generally indicates bacterial coinfections)
- General flu-like symptoms
- Frequent headaches, neck stiffness
- Regular mild to moderate muscle and joint pain
- Severe unremitting headache (generally indicates coinfections)
- Bell's palsy (partial facial paralysis) – usually in children
- Mental confusion or difficulty in thinking
- Disorientation, getting lost, going to wrong places
- Lightheadedness, wooziness
- Mood swings, irritability, depression
- Disturbed sleep
- Fatigue, tiredness, poor stamina
- Blurry vision, or floaters, and/or light sensitivity

- Feeling of pressure in eyes
- Stiffness in joints or back
- Twitching of face or other muscles
- Neck creaks, cracks, stiffness, pain
- Tingling, numbness, burning or stabbing sensations, shooting pains
- Chest pain, heart palpitations
- Shortness of breath, cough
- Buzzing or ringing in ears, sound sensitivity
- Motion sickness, vertigo, poor balance
- Sudden hearing loss
- Tremors
- Weight gain or loss
- Swollen glands (can also be from coinfection)
- Menstrual irregularity
- Irritable bladder or bladder dysfunction
- Upset stomach and/or abdominal pain
- Electrical sensation down the spine

The Lyme vaccine

A Lyme borreliosis vaccine, developed by SmithKline Beecham, arrived in late 1998; the first lawsuit due to damages caused by the vaccine was filed in December 1999. The vaccine was removed from the market in February 2002. The company cited lack of demand.

The primary problem with that vaccine was, apparently, that, in some people, it actually caused borreliosis and/or borreliosis symptoms. These included fatigue, arthritis, and cognitive problems. Case reports showed that from one-tenth to nearly one third of the people vaccinated developed problems. A number of people who had had a previous Lyme infection experienced a reactivation of the disease in spite of previous antibiotic use for the condition. A study at Cornell University found that neurological symptoms such as neuropathy or cognitive impairment occurred in some people within two days to two months following vaccination. Of six patients studied, two developed cognitive impairment, one chronic inflammatory demyelinating polyneuropathy (CIDP), one multifocal motor neuropathy, one had both cognitive impairment and CIDP, and one had cognitive impairment and sensory axonal neuropathy. Those with cognitive impairment had T2 hyperintense white matter lesions, found during MRI scans. Other studies found similar neurological impacts as well as arthritic activation.

Although researchers continue to work toward a vaccine, the unique nature of the *Borrelia* bacteria makes the creation of a reliable vaccine highly problematic. The many papers I reviewed for this updated version showed, in my opinion, little promise in that direction for some time to come, if ever.

Relapsing fever (RF) diagnosis

Relapsing fever is easier to diagnose in that it presents as a malarial-like, continually relapsing illness. That is, you get sick, you get well, you get sick, and so on, with high fever and fatigue every time. Hence *relapsing* fever. The main problem with infection by this group of *Borrelia* is that it is often mistaken for malaria or babesia, both of which have the same symptom picture.

Tests for RF are much more reliable than Lyme because the spirochetes flood the bloodstream (in massive numbers) at regular intervals, something that Lyme spirochetes do not do. This facilitates accurate blood testing; the spirochetes are actually detectable in blood samples. Because of the numbers of spirochetes in the blood, PCR testing has a nearly 100 percent accuracy with RF. ELISA testing for recombinant GlpQ, a protein found in RF spirochetes but *not* in Lyme spirochetes, is also definitive.

Pharmaceutical treatment

Commonly, it's treatment approaches that generate the most virulent animosities between the different Lyme camps. I will deal with this in more depth in the next chapter on post-Lyme disease syndrome and chronic Lyme. What I am going to cover here is the sort of middle-of-the-road recommendations that nearly all non-Lyme-literate physicians use for Lyme treatment.

Most of this material comes from an analysis paper by Girschick, Morbach, and Tappe (2009), which looked at the most up-to-date research on pharmaceutical treatment for Lyme disease from a relatively conservative (but not fanatically so) orientation. In general, from all that I have read and seen in practice, I feel that doxycycline is probably the best initial drug to utilize for Lyme or suspected cases of Lyme. It seems to have fewer failures, which means that people need undergo many fewer antibiotic regimens during treatment. This is important in helping reduce the negative side effects from the drugs. *Please note:* Earlier recommendations (old-Lyme thinking) was for a 5-day course of treatment. This has, in general, been increased to fourteen days and by some to a 14-to-28 day time course (which is what I am looking at here).

General

- Amoxicillin 50mg/kg/day in three divided doses (max dose 1,500 mg/day)
- Doxycycline 4 mg/kg/day in two divided doses (max 200 mg day, after eight years of age)
- Cefuroxime axetil 20-30 mg/kg/day in two divided doses (max 2,000 mg/day)
- Duration for all drugs is 14–28 days

Neuroborreliosis

With lymphocytic meningitis:

- Ceftriaxone, intravenous, 50 mg/kg/day in one dose (max 2,000 mg/day)

   Note: Antitumor necrosis factor alpha treatment after ceftriaxone treatment has, in some instances, reactivated *Borrelia* spirochetes.

With cranial neuritis, facial nerve involvement:

- Cefotaxime, intravenous, 200 mg/kg/day in three divided doses (max 6,000 mg/day)

For encephalomyelitis, late stage:

- Intravenous penicillin G 0.5 million U/kg/day in 4–6 divided doses (max 20 million U/day)

With cardiac complications

- Intravenous penicillin G 0.5 million U/kg/day in 4–6 divided doses (max 20 million U/day)

With eye involvement

- Amoxicillin 50 mg/kg/day in three divided doses (max 1,500 mg/day)

In late stage with uveitis, keratitis:

- Doxycycline 4 mg/kg/day in two divided doses (max 200 mg/day, after eight years of age)

Joint/muscle involvement

- Doxycycline 4 mg/kg/day in two divided doses (max 200 mg/day, after eight years of age)

With antibiotic-refractory/persistent arthritis

- Repeat doxycycline for 30 days, 30 days after initial treatment, or
- Cefotaxime, intravenous, 50 mg/kg/day in one dose (max 2,000 mg/day), or
- Cefotaxime, intravenous, 200 mg/kg/day in three divided doses (max 6,000 mg/day), or
- Intravenous penicillin G 0.5 million U/kg/day in 4-6 divided doses (max 20 million U/day)
- Additional anti-inflammatory therapy

With continuing inflammation, Borrelia *DNA present (or not) in synovial fluid/synovia*

- Intra-articular steroid injection
- Disease-modifying antirheumatic drug therapy
- Arthroscopic synovectomy

Other interventions

A recent paper by Wagh et al. (2015) found that treatment of borrelial infection with antihistaminic drugs produced significant bactericidal effects. *Borrelia*, rather than iron, are highly dependent on manganese. (The bacteria use a *BmtA* transporter to gather manganese from host cells.) Once acquired, the bacteria then create a manganese superoxide dismutase, an enzyme that protects the pathogens from intracellular superoxides. (The bacteria also utilize manganese in a number of other essential functions.)

Wagh et al. explored the impact of a known *BmtA* inhibitor on the bacteria. Specifically, they utilized two forms of a common pharmaceutical used for allergies, loratadine and desloratadine. Loratadine is more popularly known as Claritin; desloratadine (the metabolite of loratadine) as Clarinex.

The study is in vitro – no in vivo work has yet occurred. However, in our work we have found that histamine levels in many people infected with Lyme are extremely high; mast cells are producing and releasing copious amounts of histamine during infection. Plant-based, histamine (mast cell) inhibitors have, sometimes, significantly reduced symptoms.

The strongest pharmaceutical-based effects were found with desloratadine. As the researchers comment, "Desloratidine treatment caused a massive round body formation and also a significant reduction in bacterial pellet size and mass. The findings strongly suggested a loss of structural integrity and destruction of the cell wall after drug treatment. TEM analysis showed that . . . treated spirochetes had massive structural deformities. . . . The data strongly suggest that desloratadine can cause irreversible damage to *B. burgdorferi*, possibly by blocking Mn transporting system that ultimately results in cellular disintegration. . . . Desloratadine treatment not only inhibits BmtA but also kills the bacteria and results in severe structural damage."

Normally, the more severe an environmental insult, the more round bodies the spirochetes form. (Doxycycline, unfortunately, powerfully stimulates round body formation.) Round body formation in response to a drug strongly indicates the chemical (in this instance, an antihistamine for allergies) is bactericidal to the spirochetes. The more promising discovery from this study is that the round bodies that formed had significant structural deformities, something that does not occur with doxycycline. Thus, it seems that the use of desloratadine along with antibiotics in the treatment of Lyme infections could be of real benefit.

- Donta (2007) commented that in his experience (several thousand patients) he found tetracycline, not doxycycline, or a combination of a macrolide antibiotic and a lysosomotropic agent to "appear to yield the best outcomes, including apparent cures or marked, stable improvements in greater than 75% of patients; however these treatments require that they be administered for a number of months to achieve good outcomes, depending on the duration of illness."

- There are mixed reports on the use of tigecycline for borrelial spirochetes. One report, which I tend to give credence to (Brorson et al., 2009 – Lynn Margulis as a coauthor), reported it effective for encysted forms of *Borrelia* indicating that it is very useful in multiantibiotic combinations with (e.g.) doxycycline.
- Meraini et al. (2007) report that a woman with four-limb, intolerable, neuropathic pain from Lyme infection (which did not respond to "conservative" measures) was successfully treated by the use of "concurrent, thoracic, and cervical percutaneous spinal cord stimulation." Progress was slow but steady over eighteen months.
- One study (McCall et al., 2011) with dogs found that a topical application of a combination of fipronil, amitraz, and (S)-methoprene (Certifect) protected dogs from infection by *Borellia*- and *Anaplasma*-carrying ticks.
- A topical application of an azithromycin cream has been found in some studies to protect against tick-transmitted *Borrelia* infection (Knauer et al., 2011).

Treatment failures
I will deal with these in the next chapter.

Antibiotic resistance
Borrelia have not, as yet, seemed to develop much resistance to antibiotics. The relevant frame of reference, however, is that they have only been aggressively treated for a few decades. Most resistant organisms have been experiencing antibiotics over a seventy year period. Major resistance in the more commonly treated pathogenic bacteria did not emerge until the late 1980s and '90s. Although there are some reasons why researchers feel resistance will not be a problem with borrelial organisms (where have I heard this before?), there are already some early signs of resistance – they seem to be increasing in number each year. Although none are apparently (yet) cause for concern, the bacteria do carry resistance mechanisms for a number of antibacterials such as erythromycin. *Borrelia* have, as well, what is called,

an RND-type efflux system that is, as the authors note, "involved in resistance" (Bunkis et al., 2008). In other words, the bacteria have resistance mechanisms; they just aren't yet using them to any degree. It is important to understand that *all* microbial pathogens are capable of resistance, sooner or later.

Antibiotic treatment for relapsing fever *Borrelia*

Oral:

- Chloramphenicol, 500 mg every six hours for 7 days (tick-borne, TBRF) or one 500 mg dose (louse-borne, LBRF)
- Doxycycline, 100 mg every 12 hours for 7 days TBRF, or one 100 mg dose LBRF.
- Erythromycin, 500 mg every 6 hours, 7 days, TBRF, or one 500 mg dose, LBRF.
- Tetracycline, 500 mg every 6 hours, 7 days, TBRF, or one 500 mg dose, LBRF.

Note: Antibacterial use during RF infection can cause Herxheimer reactions that are severe enough to cause death; their use should be closely monitored. The reaction spectrum tends to include tachycardia, hypotension, and (sometimes) disseminated intravascular coagulation.

Herxheimer reactions – Lyme disease

Herxheimer reactions (or Herxing, aka, Jarisch-Herxheimer reactions) are named after the early bacterial researchers Adolph Jarisch and Karl Herxheimer who first described the condition. This reaction occurs during a large die-off of bacterial organisms during the progress of a disease or its treatment.

When antibiotics are given and large numbers of spirochetes die, their bodies fragment. These body parts and associated toxins that they release can cause a temporary worsening of symptoms. These include fever, chills, headache, myalgias, and, sometimes, a resurgence of other, intitial symptoms.

Herxheimer reactions do not occur in all people with Lyme during treatment. In fact, a rather deep analysis of patient experiences showed that only about 15 percent do seem to experience Herxheimer reactions at all, and most of them relatively minor. So . . . a few points: (1) Many people with Lyme believe that their treatment protocols are not working if they do not "herx." This is inaccurate. Having these reactions is not fun; count your blessings if you do not have them and don't worry about it. (2) If you do have Herxheimer reactions they can often be ameliorated by the use of substances that bind the relevant substances that occur during die-off. This is covered in the natural treatment protocols.

Herxheimer reactions – relapsing fever

RF herxheimer reactions are much more common than they are during Lyme infections; approximately 54 percent of the infected report them. That is, during antibiotic treatment, they experience an acute exacerbation of symptoms. The reactions include hypotension, tachycardia, chills, rigors, diaphoresis, and marked elevation of body temperature. It usually begins within one to four hours of ingesting an antibiotic. Symptoms can be so severe that people "feel they are going to die." An opoid partial agonist, meptazinol, has been found to reduce the severity of the reaction. Regrettably, in some instances death has occurred simply from the bacterial die-off. Caution should be exercised during treatment of RF with antibiotics.

CHAPTER TWO

POST-LYME DISEASE SYNDROME AND CHRONIC LYME DISEASE

Participants reported a significant decline in health status with chronic Lyme disease and were often unsatisfied with care in conventional settings. Negative experiences were associated with reports of dismissive, patronizing, and condescending attitudes.
Ali et al., 2014

We should not be debating the existence of persisting or relapsing symptoms. There is ample evidence for their existence. Rather we should be moving forward, discussing the nature of the chronic form of the illness and possible pathophysiologic mechanisms underlying it. . . . Our findings, which were based on careful observations of several thousand patients over the past 20 years, strongly support infection as the probable cause of chronic symptoms. . . . Our findings are consistent with a persisting intracellular localization of the infection.
Donta, 2007

Lyme Borrelia *can survive for years inside the human body without evoking an efficient immune attack by the host.*
Bhattacharjee, et al., 2013

The conflicts between the various camps who either treat or research Lyme tend to become the most vicious, emotional, and irrational when the subset of people for whom conventional medical care does not work are being discussed. As Dubrey et al. (2014) comment, "controversy over the existence of either 'chronic Lyme disease' and/or 'post-Lyme disease syndrome' continues unabated. National medical societies, patient advocacy groups, insurance companies, lawyers, doctors, the private health medical sector and scientific journals have all become embroiled in this bitter controversy." In other words, the rationality capacity of a rabid badger becomes the behavioral norm for many.

Nevertheless, despite the proclamations of the rabid badger group, an extensive analysis of the relevant journal papers is clear: there are a substantial number of people who become infected with borrelial organisms and for whom, after conservative medical treatment, resolution does not occur. Researchers who have examined the issue in depth, and published their results in numerous journal papers, are clear on this (e.g., Borgermans et al., 2014) . . .

> *There is growing and well-documented evidence to the concept of persistent* Bb *infection in both animals and humans. Recent evidence shows* Bb *is able to escape from destruction by the host immune reactions, persist in host tissues, and sustain chronic infection and inflammation, despite aggressive antibiotic challenge. An estimated 20% of patients display recurrent symptoms after antibiotic treatment. A recent study showed that, at six months following antibiotic treatment, 36% of patients reported new-onset fatigue, 20% widespread pain, and 45% neurocognitive difficulties.*

And Margulis et al. (2009) . . .

> *Current medical discussions of two spirochetoses (spirochete-associated infirmities, e.g., Lyme disease, syphilis) omit mention of "round bodies" or state that they have no clinical relevance. . . . We caution that antibiotic treatment may be effective only in the earliest stages of these spirochetoses. Indeed antibiotics such as penicillin and its derivatives induce round body formation and quiescence of symptoms rather than cure. . . . An extensive round body (= cyst) literature exists in Russian, but has remained relatively unknown even to spirochete experts elsewhere.*

I am going to go into this in some depth, for it is this group of people who suffer the most in the Lyme wars.

To begin, there are two primary groups who fall into this category. They are: (1) Those who suffer post-Lyme disease syndrome (PLDS) – this is the group of people who have been successfully treated with antibiotics but, due to bacterial damage to organic structures, still suffer a range of symptoms; and (2) Those who suffer chronic Lyme. These are people who have been treated with multiple courses of antibiotics and despite that are still infected.

To make sure things remain as complicated as possible, PLDS and chronic Lyme are sometimes lumped together, and some people call PLDS chronic Lyme while others call chronic Lyme PLDS. (You didn't think this was going to be easy, did you?)

There are two other, smaller groups that also belong in the PLDS and chronic Lyme disease groupings. The first are those whose immune systems have activated to attack Lyme (or coinfectious) organisms and, as well, are often working to clear freed cellular fragments from the body. Once the organisms (or the fragments) are gone, the immune system attacks similar organic structures throughout the body. This is a type of autoimmune process begun by a Lyme infection. I put these people in the PLDS group because their condition is not due to the presence of any Lyme organisms but solely due to *post*-Lyme disease dynamics in the body.

The second group are those who have borrelial fragments and DNA in their system but no cultivatable spirochetes. They may not be infected with viable bacteria but still suffer symptoms over months or years. This is due to their immune system interacting with the borrelial fragments and DNA. This is similar to the autoimmune-like group except that the immune system is not attacking the body's own organic structures but rather organic remnants of the borrelial organisms. In this case the symptom dynamics are still directly related to the *Borrelia*. (*Of note here as well:* Some papers are finding that those borrelial fragments and/or DNA can, under some circumstances, reconstitute themselves as full-fledged borrelial bacteria.)

I want to be clear here about my own orientation. We have had contact with over twenty-five thousand people with Lyme in the decade from 2005-2015. I have, additionally, reviewed upward of ten thousand peer-reviewed journal papers on Lyme disease, its coinfections, their treatment, and overall outcomes. There is no question in my mind, and none in the literature, that both post-Lyme disease syndrome and chronic Lyme exist. The journal papers, by themselves, leave no doubt for any reader who relies on evidence-based (rather than faith-based) material. The *numbers* of people who experience either (or both) of these conditions may be a legitimate point for discussion but that they exist is not. I personally find the position of many in the conservative medical community on these conditions (i.e., that they do not exist) to be malpractice of the most egregious sort.

Post-Lyme disease syndrome (PLDS)

PLDS refers to a condition that occurs in people who have been successfully treated by antibiotics yet still have symptoms. The reason for their continuing trouble is simple: *the damage the spirochetes did to collagen tissues, primarily in the nervous system, is still present.* The spirochetes are gone, but the damage remains. (Just as the car that hit you is gone, but the dent in your car is still there.)

Hence, some of the symptoms don't go away, and can't, until the damage is healed.

I also include in this group the smaller subset of people whose Lyme infection initiated an autoimmune-like process. Most commonly this comes from spirochete damage to specific body tissues.

When the bacteria break cellular tissue apart, they release many different types of cellular constituents into the surrounding tissues. One of the most damaging is myelin basic protein (MBP). It is released into the regions surrounding the myelin sheaths in the brain as those sheaths are broken down by the bacteria for nutrients. MBP is not supposed to be released in any quantity into the surrounding tissues; the body perceives it as a foreign, potentially damaging substance. Thus, the immune cells, called to the site of the damage, actively begin scavenging MBP for removal from the body. Unfortunately, myelin basic protein is still *in* the cellular surface of the myelin sheaths as well as in oligodendrocytes. The immune system, unfortunately, begins attacking those structures as well. This leads to more degradation in the myelin sheaths and oligodendrocytes, which itself leads to more neural damage.

There really is no question that PLDS exists; there have been a number of large journal reviews and metastudies looking at PLDS. Here is a sample, representative of those studies:

- Post-Lyme borreliosis syndrome: a meta-analysis of reported symptoms (Cairns and Godwin, 2005): "The prevalence of

symptoms was significantly higher in the LB patients for
8 of the 10 symptoms in the three categories listed above.
. . . This meta-analysis provides strong evidence that some
patients with LB have fatigue, musculoskeletal pain, and
neurocognitive difficulties that may last for years despite
antibiotic treatment."

Journal papers exploring outcomes, specifically looking at individuals
or small groups of patients, continually find that there is a subset of those
who are successfully treated with antibiotics (in that the spirochetes are
eliminated) but whose symptoms do not completely resolve. Again, *each
of the following patients were considered by physicians to have been successfully
treated with antibiotics.* What follows is only a representative sampling of the
hundreds of papers that exist. (Just before each quotation, you can insert
the phrase, as the paper's authors often do: "Despite successful antibiotic
treatment. . .")

- Lyme disease: resolution of a serious retinal detachment and
  chorioretinal folds after antibiotic treatment (Ginager et al.,
  2012): "Mild residual chorioretinal folds remained on fluores-
  cein angiogram."
- Neuropsychological profile of children after an episode of
  neuroborreliosis (Zotter et al., 2013): "In the subcategory
  of working memory, children after an episode of LNB
  performed worse than controls."
- Multiple ischemic strokes due to *Borrelia garinii* meningovasculitis (Rey et al., 2010): "The patient is still suffering from
  severe invalidating cognitive disorders."
- Lyme carditis – rare cause of dilated cardiomyopathy and
  rhythm disturbance (Cepelova, 2008): "There is a long-
  lasting persistence of dilated cardiomyopathy with significant systolic dysfunction."
- Borreliosis – simultaneous Lyme carditis and psychiatric
  disorders – case report (Legatowicz-Koprowska et al., 2008):
  "Cardiologic disorders retreated entirely, while cognitive
  deficits did only partly."

- [Extremely Long Title] (Kannian et al., 2007): "Synovitis in patients with antibiotic-refractory Lyme arthritis persists for months to several years after antibiotic therapy."

Again, the problem is that the damage to the body does not always just correct itself after a Lyme infection. The following study, which used MRI to analyze alterations in the brain, reveals alterations that often remain after antibiotic treatment for neuroborreliosis.

- A case of chronic progressive lyme encephalitis as a manifestation of late lyme neuroborreliosis (Verma et al., 2014): "Magnetic resonance imaging (MRI) revealed non-specific white matter changes. . . . Repeat MRI [after two years without treatment] showed worsening white matter changes. . . . [Four years after successful antibiotic treatment] the patient has short-term memory deficits and chronic fatigue, but is otherwise neurologically cognitively, and functionally intact. *Follow up MRI findings remained largely unchanged.* [Emphasis mine.]

This is common. Borgermans et al. (2014) in their metapaper on chronic Lyme disease (which I would define here as PLDS) comment that: "Brain SPECT scans are abnormal in most patients with chronic Lyme disease, and these scans can be used to provide objective evidence in support of the clinical diagnosis."

To correct PLDS and alleviate the symptoms that remain, the damage to the system needs to be repaired. Pharmaceuticals (and conventional allopathic care) are not very effective (or even capable) of doing that. Natural protocols, however, are specific for correcting that kind of damage.

PLDS autoimmune-like dynamics
Autoimmune-like dynamics that persist after successful antibiotic treatment are common in a smallish subset of those with PLDS. (This can usually be rectified through the use of immune and cytokine modulators.) Here are a few representative papers on the dynamic.

- Antineural antibody reactivity in patients with a history of Lyme borreliosis and persistent symptoms (Chandra et al., 2010): "Anti-neural antibody reactivity was found to be significantly higher in the PLS [post-Lyme syndrome] group than in the post-Lyme healthy groups. . . . Immunohistochemical analysis with representative PLS patient sera demonstrated binding of the antibodies to pyramidal neurons in the cerebral cortex and neurons of the DRG."

- Increased IFNa activity and differential antibody response in patients with a history of Lyme disease and persistent cognitive deficits (Jacek et al., 2013): "In conclusion, this study offers further evidence for the existence of an immune-related disease process in patients with persistent symptoms following antibiotic treatment for Lyme disease. It is the first report to demonstrate increased IFNa activity in affected patients, suggesting a potential mechanism contributing to the associated ongoing neuropsychiatric symptoms." *Note: This is an extremely good paper that should be reviewed by anyone treating PLDS in which autoimmune dynamics may play a role.*

- Elevated levels of IL-23 in a subset of patients with post-Lyme disease symptoms following erythema migrans (Strle et al., 2014): "High Th1-associated responses correlated with more effective immune-mediated spirochetal killing, whereas high Th17-associated immune responses, often accompanied by autoanitibodies, correlated with post-Lyme symptoms."

- Persistent joint swelling and *Borrelia*-specific antibodies in *Borrelia* garinii-infected mice after eradication of vegetative spirochetes with antibiotic treatment (Yrjanainen et al., 2006).

Chronic Lyme disease

In examining the evidence for chronic Lyme disease I am going to look at two aspects of the condition: (1) Antibiotic treatment failures; and (2) the presence of persisting borrelial fragments after antibiotic therapy.

Antibiotic failures in the treatment of Lyme borreliosis

From reviewing the literature, there is no doubt that a pool of antibiotic treatment failures exists. Why conservative medical practitioners insist there is not makes no sense as there is *no* journal paper in existence that has studied antibiotic outcomes and that reports a 100 percent success rate in treatment. The most optimistic may report a 99 percent success rate, but that still leaves 1 person out of 100 for whom antibiotics did not work. If there are, conservatively, 300,000 new infections per year, that would mean that there are 3,000 people *per year* for whom antibiotics do not work. Over the past forty years since the disease was recognized, assuming the same infection rate, this suggests the presence of up to 120,000 people who have chronic Lyme disease and who are not treatable by antibiotics. *And this is the most optimistic picture.* So, let's get into specifics:

- Kowalski et al. (2010): "The 2-year treatment failure-free survival rates of patients treated with antibiotics for 10 days, 11-15 days, or 16 days were 99.0%, 98.9%, and 99.2% respectively." The authors conclude that treatment failure after antibiotic therapy is "exceedingly rare." Well, no it isn't. These figures still show that approximately one per hundred of those treated by antibiotics are not cured. Treatment failures, even in this study, are extremely *common*, since at least 1 percent of those treated are not cured *every time antibiotics are used*. This is the most optimistic finding of all studies I have reviewed.
- Girschick et al. (2009): "Some people treated with antibiotics for Lyme arthritis do not experience a resolution of their arthritis even after more than one course of treatment."
- Kadam et al. (2014): "Herein, the authors report a 47-year-old woman, with solitary erythema migrans and positive Lyme disease serology, who presented for medical care 14 days after commencement of doxycycline therapy. . . . By *Borrelia*-specific immunohistochemistry, spirochetes were [still] found in the deep dermis, unassociated with inflammation, and focally in the upper spinous layer, associated with spongiosis."

- Wormser and Schwartz (2009): "In mice that were treated with antibiotic therapy, residual spirochetes could be taken up by ticks during a blood meal and could be transmitted to SCID mice." *Note:* A number of researchers are utilizing what is called *xenodiagnosis*, meaning that they are looking to see if, after "successful" antibiotic treatment, spirochetes can still be taken up by ticks and then transmitted to new hosts.
- Stupica et al. (2011): "Treatment failure was documented in two patients who were culture-positive and none in the culture-negative group."
- Embers et al. (2012): "Small numbers of intact spirochetes were recovered by xenodiagnosis from treated monkeys. These results demonstrate that *B. burgdorferi* can withstand antibiotic treatment, administered post-dissemination, in a primate host. Although *B. burgdorferi* is not known to possess resistance mechanisms and is susceptible to the standard antibiotics (doxycycline, ceftriaxone) in vitro, it appears to become tolerant post-dissemination in the primate host."
- *Note: The following is a significant study, hence the long citation:* Hodzic et al. (2008): "When some of the antibiotic-treated mice were fed on by *Ixodes scapularis* ticks (xenodiagnosis), spirochetes were acquired by the ticks, as determined based upon PCR results, and ticks from those cohorts transmitted spirochetes to naive SCID mice, which became PCR positive but culture negative. Results indicated that following antibiotic treatment, mice remained infected by nondividing but infectious spirochetes, particularly when antibiotic treatment was commenced during the chronic stage [i.e., late stage] of the infection."

The authors go on to note that there was a "resurgence of spirochete burdens in tissues at 12 months," and that "selected ticks that fed upon . . . antibiotic treated mice at 12 months were dissected and examined by fluorescence microscopy for antibody-reactive spirochetes. Immunofluorescent spirochetes were found in ticks that fed upon . . . antibiotic-treated mice. Thus, these results confirmed intact *B. burgdor-*

feri spirochetes and spirochetal DNA in xenodiagnostic ticks.
. . These results indicated that persisting non-cultivatable
B. burgdorferi that resurged at 12 months were transcribing
multiple *B. burgdorferi* genes. . . . These results confirmed that
morphologically intact, antigen-reactive spirochetal forms
were present in cardiac connective tissue of an infected
antibiotic-treated mouse at 12 months after treatment. . . .
Treatment with ceftraixone, and high or low doses of tegecy-
cline resulted in the same outcome: persistence of non-
cultivatable *B. burgdorferi* in tissues of treated mice. . . . The
current study builds upon similar evidence of non-cultivatable
B. burgdorferi persistence in studies involving dogs, mice, and
macques. . . . Transstadial transmission of *B. burgdorferi* DNA
from larvae that fed upon treated mice to nymphs and then
to adults was also demonstrated. . . . The collective conclusion is persistence of non-cultivatable spirochetes following
treatment of mice, macaques, and dogs with various antibiotics. . . . persisting *B. burgdorferi*-specific DNA has [also] been
documented following antibiotic treatment in human Lyme
borreliosis."
- Haupl et al. (1993): "Despite antibiotic therapy, there was
progression to a chronic stage, with multisystem manifestations. The initially significant immune system activation
was followed by a loss of the specific humoral immune
response and a decrease in the cellular immune response to
B. burgdorferi over the course of the disease. 'Trigger finger'
developed, and a portion of the flexor retinaculum obtained
at surgery was cultured. Viable spirochetes were identified.
Ultramorphologically, the spirochetes were situated between
collagen fibers and along fibroblasts, some of which were
deeply invaginated by these organisms."
- Oksi et al. (1999): "A total of 165 patients with disseminated
Lyme borreliosis (diagnosed in 1990–94, all seropositive
except one culture-positive patient) were followed after
antibiotic treatment, and 32 of them were regarded as having
a clinically defined treatment failure."

• Phillips et al. (1998): "47 patients with chronic Lyme disease. All had relapsed after long-term oral and intravenous antibiotics. 23 patients with other chronic illnesses formed the control group. Positive cultures were confirmed by fluorescent antibody immuno-electron microscopy using monoclonal antibody directed against OspA, and Osp A PCR. 43/47 patients (91%) cultured positive. 23/23 controls (100%) cultured negative."

Persisting borrelial fragments after antibiotic treatment

This appears to be a common problem for a subset of those who suffer chronic Lyme disease. There may not be cultivatable spirochetes, but portions of the spirochetes, including their DNA, are still present at various locations in the body and, in consequence, are still stimulating immune responses.

• Boekenstedt et al. (2012): "We observed that *Borrelia burgdorferi* antigens, but not infectious spirochetes, can remain adjacent to cartilage for extended periods after antibiotic treatment. . . . This is the first direct demonstration that inflammatory *B. burgdorferi* components can persist near cartilaginous tissue after treatment for Lyme disease."
• Picha et al. (2014): "Specific DNA was also found in a significant number of patients in later testing periods: 48 patients after treatment, 29 patients after three months, and 6 patients after 6 months."
• Parthasarathy et al. (2013): "These results suggest that spirochetal residues left after bacterial demise, due to treatment or otherwise, may continue to be pathogenic to the central nervous system."
• Boekenstedt et al. (2002): "Nine months after treatment, low levels of spirochete DNA could be detected by real-time PCR in a subset of antibiotic-treated mice."
• Bradley et al. (1994): "Our results show the intra-articular persistence of *B. burgdorferi* nucleic acids in Lyme arthritis and suggest that persistent organisms and their compo-

nents are important in maintaining ongoing immune and inflammatory processes even among some antibiotic-treated patients."

- Iyer et al. (2013): "DNA was detected by *B. burgdorferi*-specific PCR for up to 56 days in aliquots from both ceftriaxone-treated and untreated cultures. . . . The results suggest that *B. burgdorferi* DNA and mRNA ca be detected in samples long after spirochetes are no longer viable as assessed by classic microbiological parameters."

- Hodzic et al. (2013): "We previously demonstrated transmission . . . of *B. burgdorferi* DNA by transplantation of *B. burgdorferi* DNA-positive heart base and tibiotarsus tissue allografts from treated mice into recipient mice, with dissemination of the DNA in the recipient mice. Transtadial transmission of *B. burgdorferi* DNA from larvae that fed upon treated mice to nymphs and then to adults was also demonstrated. . . . earlier studies . . . demonstrated persistence of *B. burgdorferi* DNA in tissues of antibiotic-treated dogs."

A number of studies have revealed that in hosts in which borrelial DNA is found after treatment, noncultivatable spirochetes will eventually begin to emerge. A number of researchers have then found that these noncultivatable spirochetes can become your normal active, cultivatable spirochetes if enough time passes. This paper (Hodzic et al., 2014) is representative; it explores the dynamics in post-ceftriaxone treatment in Lyme positive mice.

Results confirmed previous studies, in which B. burgorferi *could not be cultured from tissues, but low copy numbers of* B. burgorferi *flaB DNA were detectable in tissues at 2, 4, and 8 months after completion of treatment, and the rate of PCR-positive tissues appeared to progressively decline over time. However, there was a resurgence of spirochete flaB DNA at 12 months, with flaB DNA copy levels nearly equivalent to those in saline-treated mice. Despite the continued non-cultivatable state, RNA transcription of multiple* B. burgorferi *genes were detected in host tissues, flaB DNA was acquired by xenodiagnostic ticks, and spirochetal forms*

could be visualized within tick and mouse tissues by immuno-
fluoresence and immunohistochemistry, respectively. A number
of host cytokines were up- or down-regulated in tissues of both
saline- and antibiotic-treated mice in the absence of hisopathol-
ogy, indicating host response to the presence of non-cultivatable
spirochetes, despite the lack of inflammation in tissues.

For a variety of reasons, both post-Lyme disease syndrome and chronic
Lyme after antibiotic treatment exist in a substantial minority of those who
become infected with borrelial organisms. (The involvement of encysted
and other forms of borrelial bacteria in Lyme-persistence will be covered in
their own chapter.) There is no possible doubt that these conditions exist –
nor can any professional group, researcher, or physician with any integrity
or allegiance to evidence-based healing deny the data . . . or the suffering of
the people in question. As Berndtson (2013) admirably sums it up . . .

Based on well-designed post-treatment animal studies and ongo-
ing delineation of Bb's mechanisms for host immune evasion
and persistence, we can reasonably conclude that some, possibly
many, chronic LD patients suffer from persistent infection with
Bb. As inevitably happens in the evolution of scientific ideas,
new research proves that the reality is more complex than we
thought, and the time has now come to move beyond the divisive-
ness of the past into a more reality-based paradigm for research,
education, and patient care. The question is no longer whether
LD can survive an antibiotic challenge in order to become a
persistent infection. High quality studies show not only that it
happens, but they also show how it happens, and why we should
not feel surprised that it happens. Our task in the new era is
to determine which patients suffer from persistent LD, and to
keep pressing for evidence-based wisdom to guide the physicians
called upon to treat them.

There is one other thing necessary to discuss before we get to the next,
even more conservative-physician-upsetting chapter, and that is length of
antibiotic treatment. I am not going to go into tremendous depth on this,

but it does need to be addressed since many physicians have been attacked for long-term antibiotic use.

For some people with chronic Lyme infections, longer durations of antibiotic therapy do seem to help. This may be because of the longer duration (or the use of multiple antibiotics in combination over a longer time period) *or* the suppressive action the antibiotics have on the bacteria *or* the anti-inflammatory actions of the antibiotics – some of them do inhibit the cytokines the bacteria stimulate. A number of studies do show that longer antibiotic regimens reduce symptoms and increase the quality of life for people with chronic Lyme. Here is a sampling . . .

- Clarissou et al. (2009): Efficacy of a long-term antibiotic treatment in patients with chronic Tick Associated Poly-organic Syndrome (TAPOS).

  The authors comment: "Despite a now codified antibiotic treatment for Lyme disease, a significant proportion of patients treated according to recommendations complain of persistent signs and symptoms. . . . This open-label prospective study was made on a group of 100 patients having followed a medical treatment for a chronic TAPOS and to evaluate their evolution under prolonged antibiotic treatment. *The medical management was found to be effective for symptoms.*" [Empasis mine.]

- Stricker (2007): Counterpoint: Long-term antibiotic therapy improves persistent symptoms associated with Lyme disease.

  "In another case, the patient's condition deteriorated despite receipt of repeated courses of antibiotic treatment over a 2-year period. She received 12 months of [regular] intravenous antibiotic treatment, followed by 11 months of oral antibiotics, and her condition improved substantially."

- Delong et al. (2012): Antibiotic retreatment of Lyme disease in patients with persistent symptoms: A biostatistical review of randomized, placebo-controlled, clinical trials.

  "This biostatistical review reveals that retreatment can be beneficial. Primary outcomes originally reported as statistically insignificant were likely underpowered. The positive treatment effects of ceftriaxone are encouraging and consistent with continued infection."

- Berndtson (2013): Review of evidence for immune evasion and persistent infection in Lyme disease.

   "Fallon et al. reviewed published interpretations of the four NIH-sponsored trials [that were evaluating the effects of long-term retreatment in those with persistent symptoms following standard antibiotic protocols]. Their review of the Study and treatment of post-Lyme disease (STOP-LD) trial by Krupp et al. counters prior critiques of this trial and demonstrates that treatment with intravenous ceftriaxone had a statistically significant and clinically meaningful effect on fatigue – the primary outcome measure in this study. They also point out that the Post-Treatment Lyme Encephalopathy trial demonstrated statistically significant and clinically meaningful benefits on pain and physical function.

   "Delong et al. performed a statistical review of these four trials and concluded . . . that ceftriaxone treatment produced clinically meaningful improvements in fatigue and cognitive functioning, and that persistent LD patients with worse baseline pain and physical functioning are likely to experience significant and sustained improvement from such treatment."

My personal opinion is, based on the dynamics of the spirochetes when under assault and hundreds of journal papers that explored it, that long-term antibiotics force the bacteria into, and keep them in, altered morphological forms. These forms have a much-reduced metabolism, they do not reproduce, they are, in essence, rather comatose. This significantly reduces the symptoms that people struggle with. For those with debilitating symptoms, who are *only* using pharmaceutical interventions, long-term antibiotic use may act to restore their quality of life. The downside, of course, is that when antibiotic therapy is withdrawn, the spirochetes may become active again, the symptoms returning.

If you are treating people with Lyme disease, the best journal papers that give a good overview of chronic and post-Lyme disease and the controversies involved are, in my opinion, the following open access journal papers:

- Berndtson, Keith. Review of evidence for immune evasion and persistent infection in Lyme disease, *International Journal of General Medicine* (2013) 6: 291–306.
- Borgermans, L. et al. Relevance of chronic Lyme disease to family medicine as a complex multidimensional chronic disease construct: A systematic review, *International Journal of Family Medicine* (2014) volume 2014.
- Johnson, Lorraine and R. Stricker. The Infectious Diseases of America Lyme guidelines: A cautionary tale about the development of clinical practice guidelines, *Philosophy, Ethics, and Humanities in Medicine* (2010) 5 (9).

CHAPTER THREE

BORRELIAL INFECTION: MORGELLONS, ALZHEIMER'S, AUTISM, AND PANDAS

Morgellons disease is an emerging skin disease characterized by formation of dermal filaments associated with multisystemic symptoms and tick-borne illness. Some clinicians hypothesize that these often colorful derma filaments are textile fibers, either self-implanted by patients or accidentally adhering to lesions, and conclude that patients with this disease have delusions of infestation. . . . [Nevertheless] spirochetes were detected in the dermatological specimens from our study patients.
Middelveen et al., 2013

Chronic spirochetal infection can cause slowly progressive dementia, cortical atrophy and amyloid deposition in the atrophic form of general paresis. There is a significant association between Alzheimer's disease and various types of spirochete.
Miklossy, 2011

These recent historical, geographical and microbiological data should prompt the medical community to realize that cases of persisting post tick-bite syndromes are probably due to multiple pathogens and that these occult infections will require a new approach if not an actual paradigm shift.
Christian Perronne, 2014

I f you think the feelings over chronic Lyme run high, just wait until you enter this playground. For some reason it's becoming somewhat amusing to me (though not to the people with Lyme who are caught in the middle) to see men (it's almost always men) who insist they are completely rational, begin to gibber uncontrollably (often with spittle flying) when something outside their paradigm catches their attention.

Despite this amusement, it is becoming more difficult for me to remain phlegmatic in the face of the continued hostility and dismissive attitudes of reductive physicians toward their patients. Many conventional physicians, the majority of whom have very little or no training in psychotherapy, immediately diagnose their patients as mentally ill when they present symptoms outside that doctor's paradigm.

Such knee-jerk diagnosis has been common toward the Lyme community since the beginning . . . and still is, despite significant amounts of journal data that show most physician ideas about Lyme and its coinfections are outdated, incorrect, or useless. Unfortunately, these kinds of physicians are routinely contacted by the media when any article on Lyme or associated conditions such as Morgellons is being written. Despite numerous journal articles revealing that their orientation is incorrect, inaccurate, and/or groundless, the media still prints their commentaries. It reminds me all too poignantly of something Paul Krugman said in one of his blogs (2000), "If a presidential candidate were to declare that the earth is flat, you would be sure to see a news analysis under the headline 'Shape of planet: Both sides have a point.' After all, the earth isn't perfectly spherical."

In this chapter I am going to touch, briefly, on some of the conditions found to be associated with borrelial infections that regularly cause flying spittle. (Just wear a clear, plastic face shield and you will be okay.) I am not going to go into a lot of depth here, but it makes sense, because of the continuing conflicts, to talk a bit about these conditions.

Morgellons

I first heard about Morgellons in 2006 when the media reported on a strange medical phenomenon occurring in a cluster of people in South Texas. No one knew what was happening, but there were so many people affected, the media couldn't help but report it.

The stories were of odd, multicolored fibers emerging from people's skins: it seemed some sort of outlandish science-fiction story come true. Despite the usual, knee-jerk response of the majority of American physicians to something new ("There is no such thing as AIDS. Your Lyme symptoms are all in your head. You have delusions of parasitosis."), the condition does exist; it is not a delusion. It's now being reported throughout the world. In the United States the largest clusters seem to be in Florida, Texas, and California.

Morgellons, as Middelveen et al. (2014) comment, "is an emerging multisystem illness characterized by skin lesions with unusual filaments embedded in or projecting from epithelial tissue." Associated symptoms such as fatigue, neurological disorders, and joint pain are common. Peripheral neuropathy, decreased body temperature, tachycardia, and abnormal cytokine activity are also regularly reported. Middelveen and Stricker, in an earlier paper (2011) comment that . . .

> [t]he hallmark of Morgellons disease is "mysterious" fibers of unknown etiology, easily visualized with the aid of a 60x hand-held digital microscope, that appear both in nonhealing or slow-healing skin lesions and beneath unbroken skin. The fibers resist extraction, and attempts to remove them may cause shooting pain. Patients with the affliction may experience crawling and stinging sensations from under their skin.

Though a growing number of researchers are finally beginning to examine Morgellons disease (MD) in some depth, the two primary researchers have been Marianne Middelveen and Raphael Stricker. Stricker is a physician and researcher specializing in borrelial infections; Middelveen a microbiologist and medical mycologist specializing in veterinary microbiology. Middelveen's orientation is highly relevant in that there is a disease in cattle very similar to Morgellons – it's called digital dermatitis (DD). DD was first described in 1974 and, since 1993, has been spreading rapidly throughout the US, Europe, and Australia.

Both MD and DD have similarities to another disease, yaws, which is caused by a spirochete *Treponema palladium* subspecies *pertenue*. Similarly to Morgellons and DD, yaws is notable for the presence of skin lesions that ultimately spread over the body. Examination of yaws, MD, and DD lesions have found spirochetes in the affected tissues.

The major Stephen King (SK) factors in Morgellons are: (1) the presence of the dermal filaments that extrude from the skin during infection and, (2) the tremendously freaky feeling of things crawling under the skin trying to get out. The SK factor is exacerbated by the color range of the filaments: white, black, red, blue, purple, and green. Although the anti-Morgellons physicians insist that the filaments extruding from their patents' skins are carpet or other industrial fibers, a forensic analysis of the filaments failed to find a match with any of the fibers listed in the FBI data base or any of the 880 compounds commonly used to manufacture commercial fibers. As Middelveen and Stricker (2011) comment . . .

> Dye-extracting solvents fail to release coloration. The fibers have been shown to be very strong and heat-resistant, so much so that attempts to analyze contents by gas chromatography were not possible. Microscopy of fibers reveals a . . . "metallic-looking" sheen. They may also appear to be coated with minerals, and do not demonstrate a cellular structure. Fibers associated with skin have been shown to emerge or stab through skin and skin lesions, and some appear to have grown from hair follicles. These fibers also flouresce under ultraviolet light.

As analysis of the fibers has deepened, it has been discovered that they are generated by abnormal keratin and collagen expression in epithelial (based) keratinocytes and fibroblasts. (The most specific avenue for plant-based therapies would be finding plants that normalize keratinocyte and fibroblast function in the body. I have not yet been able to find them; however, reduction of the borrelial-initiated cytokines does help.)

DD infections have a lot of similarities to Morgellons, hence the focus of researchers on DD. During DD infections, dermatitis and papillomatous lesions of the skin occur in the region bordering the coronary band in the hooves of hooved animals. The disease is usually found in farm animals such as goats, pigs, and horses, but is most common in cattle. (Which is why it is sometimes called bovine digital dermatitis or BDD.) It's also become an emerging disease in wild animal populations, primarily elk.

Importantly, DD is also characterized by abnormal filament formation. As Middelveen et al. (2013) note, "Lesions demonstrate parakeratotic hyperkeratosis, acanthosis, ulcerated dermal papillae tips, and *elongation of keratinocytes evolving into long keratin fibers*." [Emphasis mine.]

DD emerged into human awareness, primarily farmers and veterinarians, nearly the same time as Lyme disease, around 1974. Both diseases have shown similar growth curves. And while Morgellons did not emerge as a unique entity (in the public mind) until 2006, most striking to me is the tremendously different approaches to the conditions that the physicians and the veterinarians have taken. Human physicians have insisted Morgellons is an illusion, a psychiatric problem with no basis in reality ("delusions of parasitosis"). Veterinarians have instead spent the past twenty years intently focused on figuring out what is causing the problem. It was fairly difficult, I suspect, for the veterinarians to just tell the farmers that their cows had mental problems, that it was all in their heads – hence their closer relationship to reality. Pubmed shows ninety articles on DD since 1992 but only four on Morgellons and those only beginning in 2006.

As soon as DD emerged as a problem among cattle, animal researchers began analyzing the bacterial microbiome associated with the lesions. They quickly discovered that there was a unique grouping of spirochetes always located at the sites of the lesions and the filamentous extrusions. The primary species that seems to be at the root of the disease is a spirochete extremely similar to *T. phagedenis* (common in our bodies) and that is referred to as *T. phagedenis*-like. The next most common is *T. pedis*-like. Others are very similar (or identical) to *Treponema denticola* (which is common in our mouths), *T. vincentii*, *T. brennabolrense*, *T. refringens*, and *T. calligyrum*. (As an aside, in human peridontal disease over sixty different, not-yet-cultivated phylotypes of spirochetes have been identified.) Similarly to borrelial bacteria, infection in hooved animals is accompanied by a large range of spirochetal strains, genotypes, and previously unknown species.

Early research on DD (Demirkan et al., 1999) found that ELISA testing for the infection had "a much higher reactivity to *B. burgdorferi* and the treponemes" than other bacteria. Demirkan (et al, 1998) noted in an earlier study that "immunohistochemical staining demonstrated that spirochetes in skin lesions were identified by polyclonal antisera to *Borrelia burgdorferi, Treponema denicola*, and *Treponema vincentii.*"

In general, when DD occurs researchers have found a collection of bacteria, in which spirochetes predominate, at the site of the lesions. It appears to be a polymicrobial disease complex in which the accumulation of bacteria around a spirochetal core group synergistically acts to produce abnormalities in keratin and collagen expression by the body's keratinocytes and fibroblasts, which results in the extrusion of fibers.

Focused examination of the lesions has found, however, that in the deeper layers *only* treponemal morphotypes exist, lending credence to the belief that the spirochetes are the primary pathogen. During the early stages of the disease, the bacterial colonies show many fewer spirochetes; however, as it progresses treponamal spirochetes begin to dominate the in the lesion tissues. As Krull et al. (2014) comment: "Several key findings include a dramatic increase in *Treponema* sequences as lesions progress, a shift in the *Treponema* spp. between lesion stages, and a nearly complete absence of viral or fungal DNA." Other studies, exploring whether spirochetes were root to the infection, injected the hoof regions of previously healthy calves with material from bovine lesions and also injected pure treponemal spirochetes. The studies found that the lesions that formed were identical to DD in both instances.

DD infections *tend* to be spread so widely in agricultural operations because of unclean conditions (though this should not be taken as foundational since elk are now commonly infected in the wild). In other words, the farm animals excrete and continue to stand in a humid or wet, excretion-filled straw. As is common with spirochetes, the primary species involved in DD tend to take on different morphological forms. They do this not only under stress (see next chapter) but also as part of their infection strategy. They immediately colonize the urinary bladder and GI tract, then shed encysted forms in both urine and feces. These encysted forms then infect the areas around the hooves, again taking on normal spirochetal forms during the infection. Spiral and encysted forms as well as two intermediate forms – spiral forms with spherical bodies and enveloped clusters of granules – are commonly found in the lesions. The organisms, it turns out, are also spread by farm equipment (e.g., hoof trimming equipment).

That animals similar to human beings are experiencing a disease similar to Morgellons should have given pause to the reductive practitioners who have been denying its existence in people. As with Morgellons, DD stimulates the formation of filamentous extrusions from the infected areas. In essence, these are keratin filaments that can reach several centimeters in length giving the infected animals the appearance of "hairy heels."

An analysis of the fibers in Morgellons disease (MD) shows that they are composed of either keratin or collagen. The keratin filaments are derived from keratinocytes, the collagenous from fibroblasts. As Middelveen et al. (2014) note: "Filament formation results from abnormal keratin and collagen expression by epithelial-based keratinocytes and fibroblasts."

Similarly to DD, people with Morgellons produce antibodies reactive to borrelial spirochetes. An analysis by Middelveen et al. (2014) of a number of people suffering from MD found that they were all seroreactive to borellial antigens, none were delusional and had no history of mental illness, and all showed visible spirochetes from staining of dermatological tissues. Borrelial spirochetes were found beneath the callus layer of Morgellons tissue. PCR was positive in the majority of cases. And motile spirochetes were found in half the infected. Cultured spirochetes from one patient were identified as *Borrelia*. As the researchers note . . .

> *The presence of spirochetes in MD dermatological specimens demonstrates that Morgellons lesions are associated with spirochetal infection. . . . spirochetes were readily detectable in dermatological tissue from four MD patients using a combination of [a long list of techniques]. Motile spirochetes were also observed in cultures inoculated with MD dermatological tissue, thus indicating that our specimens contained viable organisms.*

As they continue . . .

> *Unlike BDD which is associated with a variety of treponemal spirochetes, the MD dermatological tissue in this study contained spirochetes that were identified as* Borrelia *by immunofluorescent staining with anti-Borrelia antibodies. Furthermore the MD spirochetes were specifically classified by targeted PCR as* Borrelia burgdorferi.

And conclude . . .

> *Our findings suggest that* Borrelia *spirochetes may be capable of sequestering themselves within karatinocytes and fibroblasts, causing both persistent infection that is refractory to antibiotic therapy and aberrant fiber production by these infected cells in MD patients.*

There is just too much evidence to relegate Morgellons disease to some human tendency toward delusional parasitosis. An intensive review of the literature leaves me wishing that more physicians had both the training and humility of veterinarians. Perhaps if people looked more like puppies . . .

The numbers of those with Morgellons are far fewer than those with other borrelial symptom pictures. In consequence, we have not seen a large number of people with the condition (though we have worked with some). Treatment does present challenges, but MD has been responsive to the same kinds of protocols that are effective in Lyme disease and its coinfections.

The main obstacle to finding help, for most people, is the domination of the conversation by a very vocal and extremely unscientific group of medical professionals. As researchers have noted (Middelveen et al., 2014), this "has stifled scientific research and has prevented appropriate treatment and control strategies from being investigated and implemented. In some cases it has resulted in treatment with ineffective and inappropriate antipsychotic drugs. Some patients have been stigmatized by a diagnosis of mental illness that has resulted in social isolation, loss of employment, loss of custody of children, and a high rate of suicide." This kind of thing is not new in the Lyme world, but it really is time for it to stop.

Alzheimer's disease and borrelial infections

In the past, Lyme infections in the central nervous system and brain have been routinely misdiagnosed as mulitiple sclerosis, Parkinson's disease, Alzheimer's disease (AD), as well as a wide range of psychiatric conditions from bipolar to schizophrenia. The root causes of these conditions have never been known, though there's been a lot of guessing going on.

In the first edition of this book, I noted that some autopsies of Alzheimer's patients had found spirochetes in the brain tissue. As usual this was discounted by the conservative medical establishment. In the decade since, there has been some good research furthering the recognition that, in some instances, Alzheimer's is caused by a borrelial infection of the brain. (*Treponema, Chlamydophyla*, and herpes bacteria and viruses can also cause the condition.) The best work on the connection between *Borrelia* and AD has been done by Judith Miklossy, beginning with her PhD thesis in 2005. As she noted (2011), "Exposure of mammalian neuronal and glial cells and organotypic cultures to spirochetes reproduces the biological and pathological hallmarks of AD." Alzheimer's is accompanied by the emergence of amyloid deposits in the brain. Both normal-looking borrelial spirochetes and their encysted forms have been found in the amyloid deposits in AD patients. Studies have shown that borrelial spirochetes will, in fact, initiate amyloid deposits in the brain of test animals. AD, in this instance, is merely one possible outcome of a decades-long infection with borrelial bacteria. It is a side effect of long-term chronic infection. As Miklossy (2011) notes . . .

> The results show a statistically significant association between spirochetes and AD. When neutral techniques recognizing all types of spirochetes were used, or the highly prevalent periodontal pathogen Treponemas were analyzed, spirochetes were observed in the brain in more than 90% of AD cases. Borrelia burgdorferi was detected in the brain in 25.3% of AD cases analyzed and was 13 times more frequent in AD compared to controls. . . . Importantly, coinfection with several spirochetes occurs in AD. The pathological and biological hallmarks of AD were reproduced in vitro by exposure of mammalial cells to spirochetes.

Miklossy et al. (2004) reported in one study that spirochetes isolated from the brain tissue of people diagnosed with AD could be grown in a growth medium selective for *Borrelia burgdorferi*. Once grown and analyzed, a positive identification for that species occurred.

It appears that a number of "idiopathic" conditions such as Alzheimer's disease are in fact the consequence of long-term bacterial and viral infections.

Lyme and autism

There is a great deal of controversy regarding Lyme and autism. As with Alzheimer's disease, I think there are a number of causes of autism, just as there are with hepatitis. Hepatitis simply means inflammation of the liver; many things cause it. There is some good evidence that a Lyme infection can either contribute to the development of autism or even, in some instances, generate autism itself.

Studies of children diagnosed with autism spectrum disorder (ASD) have found a certain percentage of them to be Lyme positive. As Kuhn and

Bransfield (2014) comment: "The children were [then] treated with anti-biotics and their scores on the ATEC [autism treatment evaluation check-list] improved. Anecdotal data indicated that some of the children achieved previously unattained developmental milestones after antibiotic therapy began."

Probably the best open-source article on this is Bransfield et al. (2007), "The association between tick-borne infections, Lyme borreliosis, and autism-spectrum disorders." In it, the article's authors note that a number of factors indicate a close relationship between autism and borrelial infection (or one of the coinfections). As they comment . . .

> *Support for this hypothesis includes multiple cases of mothers with Lyme disease and children with autism spectrum disorders; fetal neurological abnormalities associated with tick-borne diseases; similarities between tick-borne diseases and autism spectrum disorder regarding symptoms, pathophysiology, immune reactivity, temporal lobe pathology , and brain imaging data; positive reactivity in several studies with autistic spectrum disorder patients for* Borrelial burgdorferi *(22%, 26%, and 20-30%) and 58% for mycoplasma; similar geographic distribution and improvement in autistic symptoms from antibiotic treatment.*

For children with autism spectrum disorders, it makes sense to find an accomplished diagnostician who can sensitively analyze diagnostic tests for Lyme infection to see if Lyme (or mycoplasma) are implicated in the condition. Antibacterial treatment can so significantly improve the condition in some cases that an LD diagnosis should be seriously pursued. It can avoid years of tremendous pain.

PANDAS

PANDAS is another member on the growing list of acronyms plaguing our lives. It is derived from pediatric autoimmune neuropsychiatric disorders associated with streptococcal infections – PANDAS. (It doesn't eat shoots and leaves.) I am not going to go into a lot of depth on this condition. Its importance in this book is because the condition can be and often is mistaken for neuroborreliosis. It almost always occurs in children (generally five to twelve years of age) – hence the "pediatric" part of the name. Onset follows a bacterial infection with *Streptococcus pyogenes*, a Gram-positive bacteria rather than Gram-negative as Lyme bacteria are.

The condition usually begins with a sore throat (strep throat) accompanied by flu-like symptoms. There is then a sudden onset of neurological problems, primarily obsessive-compulsive disorders (OCD) and neurological tic disorders, including Tourette's syndrome. (Stomach pains, emesis, new-onset asthma, sinus infections, severe recurrent ear infections can also occur during the condition.) The cause is the movement of the bacteria into the CNS and brain where they stimulate inflammation. The condition is exacerbated from a cross reaction among immune antibodies and neural tissues.

Hyperactivity, impulsivity, deterioration in handwriting, urinary urgency, separation anxiety, and decline in school performance are the usual, initial signs of PANDAS. Inattention, mood swings, oppositional defiant behavior, personality change, bedtime fears/rituals, and restlessness also occur. Common obsessions are aggression and contamination. Common compulsions are washing, cleaning, and checking rituals.

Besides onset symptoms, there are a number of similarities and differences between neurological Lyme infection and PANDAS. Sore throat is more common in PANDAS for example; it's nearly always present as a presymptom. Specifically, neurological tics and OCD are rare in Lyme infections (though they can occur) but are always present in PANDAS. Hyperactivity, separation anxiety, handwriting alterations, and choreiform movements are more common in PANDAS than LD. (The best open-source journal paper I have found on PANDAS and the distinction between it and LD is Rhee and Cameron, 2012; see bibliography. If you are a clinician or parent, it's invaluable.)

Treatment that we have found useful includes the use of the broad-spectrum systemic herbal antibiotic *Cryptolepis sanguinolenta,* which is specific for this bacterial species. Baikal skullcap (*Scutellaria baicalensis*) to reduce inflammation in the brain and neural structures is essential. Kudzu (*Pueria lobata*) is extremely useful as well for the brain inflammation, which is common in this condition. Chinese senega (*Polygala tenuifolia*) root is also very useful to help regenerate damaged neural structures *if there are seizures.*

Cilantro (*Coriandrum sativum*) is helpful for the extreme environmental sensitivity that sometimes occurs. All taken as tinctures. Omega 3 oils and vitamin D3 can help reverse the brain impacts considerably. Remodulation of the bowel microbiome has also shown very good effects.

Protocol for PANDAS

- Cryptolepis tincture, 1–10 drops 3x daily (up to 30 drops for older children)
- Baikal skullcap tincture, same dosage
- Kudzu tincture, 5–20 drops 3x daily
- Chinese senega root tincture, 10 drops 3x daily (for seizures only)
- Cilantro tincture, 1–5 drops 3x daily (for extreme environmental sensitivity)
- Omega 3 oils (best: fermented cod liver oil), ½ tsp day; otherwise, dosage on label
- Vitamin D3, 2000 IU daily
- Remove all gluten, dairy, sugar (GAP diet is best for PANDAS) until condition improves; add them back *very slowly*.

CHAPTER FOUR

THE ECOLOGICAL REALITY – AND INEVITABILITY – OF LYME AND ITS COINFECTIONS

[Spirochetes] live in marine sediments, deep within soil, commensally in the gut of arthropods, including termites, as well as in vertebrates as obligate parasites. They can also be free-living or host-associated, pathogenic or non-pathogenic, and aerobic or anaerobic. There is also enormous variability in the genome sizes.
Gupta et al., 2013

The role of birds in the ecology and epidemiology of LB is greater than previously understood.
Comstedt et al., 2011

The number of Borrelia *spp. regarded as pathogenic to humans also increased. Distribution areas as well as host and vector ranges of Lyme borreliosis agents turned out to be much wider than previously thought.*
Franke et al., 2013

I've seen patients die of diseases they were not sick enough to have.
Mark DiNubile, 1996

Borrelial organisms are, at root, ecological expressions. They are tightly interwoven into, and their behavior affected by, planetary ecosystems both local and global. Shorthand: Lyme is not "just a disease." It's powerful emergence in our time is a planetary response to human-generated ecological disruption. To successfully work with borrelial organisms means understanding them from an ecological orientation. A shift in viewpoint is essential.

This is necessary, not only at the macroecological level but the micro. For every time the bacteria enter a host organism, they encounter a unique ecological scenario. As we journey through the larger ecosystems that surround us, so, too, do the bacteria, once they are inside a new host, journey through ecological landscapes. *Everyone's body is different*, thus the landscape the bacteria find in every host is always slightly different, the terrain to which they must adapt this time is not the same as that in the last host. So, the bacteria analyze the new host's bodily ecosystem and alter both their physical form and behavior to fit that unique ecology. The Lyme disease in *that* person is not the same as the Lyme disease in *this* one. Nor is it a static process in that individual; it's constantly changing.

Borrelial organisms are engaged in a continual, complex, and very sophisticated conversation with both the larger world outside *and* the smaller world they find inside their host organisms. Our body responds to the bacteria's behavior by altering immune function, and they, in response, *change* their behavior and form depending on the nature of that conversation. They must adapt in this way if they are to be successful at gaining the nutrients they need from our bodies in order to reproduce and, as well, to avoid our immune (or medical) responses.

Understanding the subtleties of this is crucial to creating the kinds of sophisticated treatment protocols that are often necessary for healing, especially in chronic or long-term Lyme infections. This is especially important for those in whom antibiotics do not work, a core group of from 25 to 40 percent of those who are infected. In such circumstances, botanical interventions can be extremely effective – if you understand what the bacteria are doing and which herbs counteract those specific actions. Such herbal interventions run the gamut from a rather simple interventional protocol that can sometimes, immediately, turn the condition around to more extensive sophisticated protocols that can carefully modulate, and correct, the entire range of effects the bacteria cause during infection. This is especially so if the infection has damaged neurological structures in the brain and central nervous system.

This chapter explores the macroecology of the bacteria – the next one the microecology. The picture that emerges is most likely going to be quite different from what you have heard – most of the commonly encountered information about these bacteria has little to do with their reality.

The macroecology of *Borrelia*

Old-Lyme thinking (dominant from the early days when little was known about the organisms) has tended to focus on the *Ixodes* genus of ticks, white-footed mice, and deer as the most important ecological aspects of Lyme disease in the wild. In essence, what you usually hear is that the disease organisms are kept viable in the wild because of their circulation between ticks and white-footed mice and ticks and deer and ticks and . . . *ad repeatum*. Humans, you will regularly be told, are "inadvertent" hosts. This is tremendously oversimplified, and as well . . . it's just plain wrong.

Reservoirs for borrelial organisms

As already mentioned in Chapter One, many genera and species of ticks carry borrelial organisms, including soft ticks. There are many other biting insects and arthropods that carry and transmit the genus as well. White-footed mice are *not* the primary or root reservoirs for the bacteria – many other ground-dwelling mammals, birds, and lizards work equally well in that regard. (The American robin, for instance, is just as competent, and common, a host as the white-footed mouse. . . . You don't have a bird feeder, do you?)

As Rhee and Cameron comment (2012): "The white-footed mouse is a commonly cited *B. burgdorferi* host, but at least ten other wild and domestic mammalian species harbor *B. burgdorferi* including dogs, horses, cows, rabbits, and raccoons." The situation, however, is much more complex than their statement indicates. *All* small, ground-based mammals, as well as birds and lizards, have been found to be reservoirs for the bacteria – squirrels, for example, are intimately involved in transmission cycles (you don't have a bird feeder, do you?). Further, *all* large mammals also act as reservoirs; deer are not unique in this respect. Bear, bison, elk (*all* even- and odd-toed ungulates), *all* carnivores (such as mountain lions), and *all* tested primates have been found to act as reservoirs for the spread of borrelial bacteria. And to make a point here, humans are primates. (Just because someone has a PhD and opposable thumbs doesn't mean they are no longer primates. As Dorian Sagan once put it, "On earth there is no escape, no exit, from global ecology.")

Lyme spirochetes have been found to infect most of our companion and farm animals: dogs, cats, horses, cows, goats, pigs, sheep, and chickens. They don't really seem to like most of them, but they do love to infect dogs and horses. And while infections in both have become a serious problem (and yes, you can treat them with the natural protocols listed in this book – they work just fine), Lyme spirochetes most commonly infect wild hosts. The ticks that carry *Borrelia* spirochetes attach themselves to, and feed from, over three hundred different species of mammals, birds, and reptiles.

Lizards, contrary to old-Lyme thinking, are major reservoirs for the organisms, especially in drier locations (such as Egypt and Texas) where there are fewer small, ground-based mammal species. As Norte et al. (2014) comment: "Our results reinforce the importance of lizards as reservoirs for *B. lusitaniae*, suggesting that *P. algirus*, in particular, acts as a main reservoir for B. *lusitaniae* in Portugal." Birds are also primary reservoirs for borrelial organisms. Further, they act to spread them broadly, most commonly in a north–south–north direction during their annual migrations. Over sixty bird species are known to harbor *Borrelia*-infected ticks.

Borrelia garinii appears to be the most common borrelial species disseminated by birds in Europe – Eurasian blackbirds, song thrushes, and great tits are prominent reservoirs. As Dubska et al. (2009) note that "these birds have the potential to distribute millions of Lyme disease spirochetes between urban areas." (*Urban* is an important word here.) *B. valaisiana*, *B. afzelii*, and *B. burgdorferi* are also common in birds and in the ticks that the birds transmit long distances. As Taragel'ova et al., comment: "We conclude that thrushes are key players in the maintenance of these spirochete species in this region of Central Europe." In fact, *every* tested songbird (sometimes called passerines) has been found to be a reservoir for the bacteria. As Scott et al. (2012) observe. . .

> Our results suggest that songbirds infested with B. burgdorferi-infected ticks have the potential to start new tick populations endemic for Lyme disease. Because songbirds disperse B. burgdorferi-infected ticks outside their anticipated range, health-care providers are advised that people can contract Lyme disease locally without any history of travel.

To repeat: *"Health-care providers are advised that people can contract Lyme disease locally without any history of travel."*

And still other borrelial species have been found in migrating birds. *B. bavariensis* and *B. myamotoi* have been recently discovered in birds, as well as the coinfectious organisms *Rickettsia monacensis, R. sibirica, Anaplasma phagocytophilum, Babesia microti, Coxiella burnetii,* and tick-borne encephalitis virus (TBEV). Most of the coinfectious group can be spread by birds, just as Lyme bacteria are. (You don't have a bird feeder, do you?) Nor are *migratory* birds the only carriers. All types of birds seem hospitable to infection by borrelial organisms. *B. lonestari,* for example, is common in wild turkeys and is spread from them, via ticks, to people in states such as Tennessee.

Borrelial bacteria are also extremely common in seabirds and penguins, the seabirds acting as a major source for the organisms global spread. *B. garinii* spirochetes, isolated from seabirds on islands that contain no mammal species, were found to be identical to the same species of spirochetes found in ticks, mice, and people from both the Northern and Southern Hemispheres.

Because seabirds (and penguins) enjoy living in very cold regions the ticks that infect them are also well adapted to cold. Ticks on these birds can withstand temperatures as low as minus 30 degrees Celsius (minus 22 F). They, similarly to ticks in colder climes such as the American Northeast or Sweden, quest at colder temperatures. They, like all ticks that carry borrelial bacteria, adapt to the climate they are in. The tick life span in these regions is also much longer, up to seven years instead of the more common three in warmer climes.

Birds, because of the long distances they travel, are major players in the wide dissemination of the disease. In the process, they also stimulate the emergence of unique strains and subspecies. During migration, large numbers of many different types of birds tend to congregate around certain geographic locations, usually near large bodies of water. There is considerable horizontal transfer of borrelial bacteria and tick vectors between different types of birds during these stops. This facilitates a lot of genetic intermingling and bacterial innovation. It spreads unique strains and subspecies to new locations as the birds continue their migration. Additionally, latent infections can be reactivated in the birds simply from the stress of migration, furthering global spread of the organisms. In other words, the immune stress of long migrations allows a new bloom of the bacteria, facilitating horizontal transfer during migration stops.

To make matters worse, researchers have found that birds act as selective amplifiers of the bacteria. As Heylen et al. (2014) comment

> Birds were able to host mixed infections of B. garinii and B. valaisiana, as well as mixed infections of genotypes of the same genospecies. We experimentally show that resident songbirds transmit a broad range of Borrelia genotypes, but selectively amplify certain genotypes, and that one bird can transmit simultaneously several genotypes.

And though Lyme borreliosis is (still) considered to mostly be a northern latitude disease, increasing numbers of infections are being found in Australia, northern and southern Africa, Asia, Mexico, the Caribbean, and South America. There is no land mass on this planet where borrelial organisms do not exist nor act to infect people, their companion animals, or wild animal species. The spirochetes have now been found in the Subarctic, Arctic, and Antarctic regions of the planet. Again: there is no place that is free of them, nor is there any place where human infection cannot occur. *Anyone* from *anyplace* can become infected with Lyme disease. There are no Lyme-free zones on this planet.

Borrelia in the cities

It is commonly believed that people get their Lyme infections when they go into wild landscapes – that they don't get them in cities. This is unfortunately untrue. Despite current belief, many, if not most, cities and large towns throughout the world are endemic for Lyme disease.

Cities and large towns produce a great deal of heat. The ticks like this . . . a lot. So-called urban heat islands have been supporting the emergence of large pools of endemic borrelial organisms in their midst. In fact, some studies have found that the risk of contracting borreliosis to be *higher* in cities than in the surrounding suburbs simply due to the increased heat the cities produce. Spirochetes and their ticks have been found to be common in the heavily treed areas, parks, and cemeteries ubiquitous in most cities and towns. Buczek et al. (2014) comment . . .

> Occurrence of pathogen-infected ticks in recreational urban and suburban areas poses a direct threat to human and animal health.

Our study results confirming the presence of I. ricinus *ticks and*
B. burgdorferi *s.l. in urban and suburban habitats correspond*
with the incidence of Lyme borreliosis reported from these areas.
The increase in the incidence of this zoonosis observed over the
last 12 years implies the existence of favorable conditions for
spirochetes and their vectors in the area. . . . Our investigations
suggest that microclimate conditions and pollution within urban
heat islands can affect the abundance and activity of I. ricinus
nymphs and females which more frequently attack humans and
medium- and large-size animals. . . . [There is] a high risk of host
attacks, posed to both residents and domestic and wild animals.

Venclikova et al. (2014) agree: "Our results highlight the need for surveillance of zoonotic tick-borne pathogens even in urban areas." When we take
our dogs for a walk in the city, it is not an innocuous journey. The birds
spread the ticks to the cities, the ticks drop off in parks, treed areas, and
cemeteries, and infect out pets . . . and us.

Lyme infections can occur anywhere. Even in Central Park.

Borrelial islands

Borrelial bacteria are widely spread from north to south to north again by
migrating birds. There has been, until recently, considerably less spread
from east to west to east simply because birds don't tend to migrate in those
directions.

In the first edition of this book, I mentioned that the herbalist Matthew
Wood had found that, under some circumstances, the herb teasel could
act to cure Lyme infections, but that herbalists on the East Coast of the US
did not commonly see that kind of outcome in practice. I speculated at the
time that part of the reason for this was the presence of different genotypes
in the two locations. Recent research has borne this out. An analysis by
Margos et al. (2012) found that until fairly recently large groups of borrelial
bacteria were geographically isolated in North America. As the authors
comment . . .

The spatial distribution of sequence types (STs) and inferred
population boundaries suggest that the current populations are

geographically separated. One major population boundary sepa-
rated western B. burgdorferi *populations transmitted by* Ixodes
pacificus *in California from Eastern populations transmitted by*
I. scapularis; *the other divided Midwestern and Northeastern*
populations.

Their study revealed three distinct geographical concentrations of *B. burg-*
dorferi in the United States, one in California, which is the most geographically isolated, one in the Northeast, and another in the upper Midwest.
(Caveat, in a moment.) Each of these populations possess slight-to-signifi-
cant differences in their core genomic structures. As Margos et al. go on to
say . . .

Populations of infectious agents are shaped by evolutionary and
demographic processes, as well as by population dynamics of their
hosts and (in the case of vector-borne pathogens) arthropod vectors.
These processes can leave signatures in the pathogen's genomes.

Margos et al. develop this further in an earlier paper (2011) . . .

The ecological niche diversity of different species varies in the
degree of specialization (from generalist to specialized strate-
gies) in terms of host and vector adaptation and this influences
the geographic distribution at species and population levels.
. . . The life cycle of the LB group of spirochetes is a dynamic
interplay between bacteria, reservoir hosts and vectors which
is confounded by landscape and climatic factors impacting host
and vector ecology. . . . Recent evidence supports the view that
host associations substantially shape Borrelia *populations by*
impacting their dispersal patterns and geographic distributions.
. . . Consequently, Borrelia *populations are shaped by the dynam-*
ics and demographic processes of host and vector populations,
host and vector immune responses and extrinsic abiotic factors
(e.g., temperature, climate, landscape connectivity) affecting host
and vector populations and contact between them which together
determine R0 for each species and strain of the bacterium.

Borgermans et al. (2014) echo this when they comment that . . .

> [t]he vector model of complexity is a useful model to describe
> case complexity in patients with CLD [chronic Lyme disease].
> [It] proposes that the complexity of an individual patient arises
> out of interactions between different domains: biology, genetics,
> socioeconomics, environment, behaviour, culture, and the health
> system. In a chronic condition such as CLD, these "forces" are not
> easily discerned.

The differences in the LB genomes do, in fact, create differences in bacterial behavior during infection of hosts, including people. These different genomic strains commonly cause a different range of symptoms, and they respond differently to antibiotic and herbal regimens and the ecology of the person they encounter during infection. As only one example, people infected with RST1 strains of *Borrelia* tend to have antibiotic refractory (i.e., resistant) arthritis. Other strains of the bacteria are much less resistant.

Thus: Lyme disease in Wisconsin is not the same as Lyme disease in New Jersey is not the same as Lyme disease in Georgia. As Ostfeld et al. (quoted in Levy, 2013) note: "the California Lyme disease system behaves differently than that in New York." And as Hanincova et al. (2013) observe: "The data revealed that patients from New York and Wisconsin were infected with two distinct, but genetically and phylogenetically closely related, populations of *B. burgdorferi*. Importantly, the data suggest the existence of *B. burgdorferi* lineages with differential capabilities for dissemination in humans." And Rudenko et al. (2011) comment: "Large scale systematic surveys conducted in the northeastern, north-central, mid-Atlantic, and, recently, in the far-western USA reveal striking differences among *B. burgdorferi* genotypes found in different parts of the country." Lyme is not Lyme is not Lyme.

Now the caveat . . .

Mechai et al. (2014) found, in their study of genotypes, that only 17 percent of the genetic types found in Canada and the US are identical; 49 percent occur only in the US, 34 percent only in Canada. As they comment, "These data thus point to a geographic pattern of populations of *B. burgdorferi* in North America that may be more complex than simply comprising Northeast, Midwest, and California groups." And indeed it is more complex.

There are differences in bacterial genomes, no matter how small, or large, the geographic scale you use. As Margos et al. (2011) note: "A pronounced fine-scale phylogeographic population structure was observed where most strains from Mafra [Portugal] clustered separately from the Grandola strains." Other research "showed a population structure that signified restricted movement of strains between geographic regions. This differentiation was pronounced. . . . Chinese and European *B. afzelii* populations also showed high levels of differentiation suggesting very limited movement over these large distances." In other words, the organisms, over time, create "clonal complexes" composed of discrete clusters of unique genomic strains.

Continuing on the larger scale, and thinking in terms of isolated geographic islands of the organisms, there is a fourth primary endemic region in the United States that has been, until recently, genomically distinct. It's in the Southeast. As with the other endemic islands, this group of *Borrelia* is comprised of a unique complex of strains.

Unfortunately, despite a large body of evidence to the contrary, there are still physicians who deny that Lyme is endemic in the American southeast. As Golovchenko et al. (2014) comment . . .

> *Current dogma states that* Ixodes scapularis *is the only vector of the spirochetes in the eastern U.S.;* B. burgdorferi *is antigenically and genetically uniform in North America in contrast to the situation in Europe;* B. burgdorferi *does not occur in wildlife in the southern U.S.A. and thus, humans in the Southeast could not acquire LD. . . . [However] Published data on the prevalence of Lyme disease (LD) spirochetes in vector ticks and vertebrate hosts in the southeastern U.S.A. qualifies this region as a* B. burgdorferi *s.l. endemic area, despite prevailing dogma.*

Whether you are looking at large geogaphic regions or tiny ones – or even the tinier one that is the human body – the borrelial bacteria you will find in each location will differ slightly from the others. This is because they have altered their genomic structure to adapt to those unique locations by varying their outer surface proteins (*osps*). The protein structure of their outer envelope is subtly modulated in response to environmental conditions that surround them. In essence, it is the outcome of a complex conversation between organism and the environment around it. (I will talk in depth about this in the next chapter.) This is, in fact, what makes most strains – the alterations in *osp* structure.

All the different *osp* types are labeled, e.g., *osp*A, *osp*B, *osp*C. And each of those *osp* types have unique strains, each given their own designation as well (and there are thousands if not millions of them, hence the difficulty of creating a workable vaccine). All of these types and strains behave differently, sometimes significantly so, during infections. Genotypes A, I, and K, for instance, disseminate in the body at roughly twice the rate of genotypes B and N. Other genotypes disseminate much slower than B and N do. The various genotypes can also cause widely different symptom pictures. The *ospC* protein strain B, for example, commonly produces the severest Lyme infections worldwide. The *ospC* strain V, on the other hand, is specific for colonizing the urinary bladder; it rarely infects other sites in the body.

> *Infecting this particular site is a unique survival strategy of the bacteria. It allows them to be expressed out of the body in encysted forms onto the ground. They are then taken up by grazing animals, once again take on their normal spirochete form in the GI tract, and thus spread the infection to new hosts. Colonizing the bladder also facilitates the sexual spread of the organisms.*

Each of the endemic islands in the United States tends to have a different complex of strains that are specific to that region. *OspC* strains H, G, and N are common in LD infections in the Northeast and Midwest of the United States. *OspC* strains A, D, E3, F, H, and K are most often found in California – most Californians being infected with *ospC* strain A. The *ospC* strain L has been thought to be very rare and not capable of causing infections in people. (The usual canard.) Nevertheless, *ospC* strain L is extremely common in the southeastern US (as is B and to a lesser extent H, G, and N) and does indeed cause human infections, just as the other strains do. The Southeast is an endemic area containing its own unique complex of borrelial strains; strain L being a major infectious type in that region. People in the South, irrespective of what their doctors say, do get Lyme disease . . . regularly.

Despite my focus here on major endemic areas, please keep in mind that *all* geographic regions, worldwide, have their own unique groupings. *OspC* strains A, B, E, F, and I, for example, are more common in North Dakota. (And of course, to make things more complicated, all of these strains have their own variants.) Depth analysis, no matter the geographic location studied, always finds a complex grouping of strains and variants (often fifty or more) in specific locations, many of them unique. As isolated islands are exposed to each other, more genetic intermingling occurs and still more strains emerge. As Hellgren et al. (2011) comment: "the genetic structure of *Borrelia afzelii* varies with geographic" location. Iyer et al. (2014) explain further . . .

> *The results as a whole make clear that environmental sensing by* B. burgdorferi *directly or indirectly drives an extensive and tightly integrated modulation of cell envelope constituents, chemotaxis/motility machinery, intermediary metabolism and cellular physiology.*

Again: *each* strain type, during infection, creates a unique symptom picture. Each has to be seen as a unique entity and treated as such. There is not a *single* type of Lyme infection – there are thousands upon thousands of them. Nor is there, in an infected individual, a single type of Lyme bacteria. There is, more correctly, a *swarm* of different genotypes, subspecies, variants, strains. These various genotypes are often specific for different parts of the body (it's called organotropism) – *these* for the urinary bladder, those for the joints, and these others over here for the neurological system and brain. And even more specifically – *these* for the amygdala, those for the hippocampus, and those for the peripheral nervous system. As Brisson et al. (2011) note, various "human tissues act as niches that can allow entry to or maintain only a subset of the total pathogen population."

Some strains are highly susceptible to antibiotics, others to our immune system . . . some aren't susceptible to either. This variability is one way the bacteria are able to create long-term infections. They are *very* smart organisms. (Btw, borrelial swarms in humans and their companion animals – dogs, for example – are composed of considerably more strains than wild animal hosts. Our constant exposure to medical chemicals, it appears, stimulates the emergence of significant numbers of variants.)

Ecological fragmentation and depletion

While birds migrate north–south–north, large land mammals tend to migrate east–west–east. And once upon a time there were incredibly large migrations of land-based herd animals east and west, back and forth, throughout the United States. The American bison (buffalo) was one of them.

Extinction events

Initially, somewhere between twenty and forty (or some say sixty) million bison ranged the American continent in what was called the Great Bison Belt. This area included most of the continent – north into Alaska and the Canadian Northwest, southward into Mexico, and throughout most of the rest of the continental United States. The only exceptions were (apparently) the desert Southwest and the extreme Northeast. Herds were so dense and large, commonly numbering more than one million animals, they would take hours to pass a single point. Importantly, massive bison herds were common east of the Mississippi until 1820 or so. They remained present west of the Mississippi until the transcontinental railroad and westward expansion facilitated their near extermination by 1890 (only 600–800 were thought to remain). Massive deer and antelope herds were common as well, also traveling in an east–west–east direction. They, too, were severely reduced by human-caused ecological disruption and hunting. In consequence, the long-standing east–west–east intermingling of the borrelial organisms ceased around 1900. As Margos et al. (2011) note, research "found signatures of ancient population expansions of *B. burgdorferi* likely to date back several thousand, if not millions of years ago. Demographic events in the past 200 years (following the arrival of European settlers) have shaped populations of hosts and vectors by deforestation, dwindling deer and tick populations, and causing severe bottlenecks in *Borrelia* populations."

We don't normally grasp the impact that the loss of such massive numbers of animals in such an extremely short period of time can have on the ecological fabric of a landscape. This can, perhaps, give you a sense of it . . .

In 1813, John James Audubon, traveling by horse from Henderson, Kentucky, to Louisville, described an overflight of passenger pigeons that occurred during the trip. "The pigeons" were, he said, *in greater numbers than I thought I had ever seen them before, and feeling an inclination to count the flocks that might pass within the reach of my eye in one hour, I dismounted, seated myself on an eminence, and began to mark with my pencil, making a dot for every flock that passed. In a short time finding the task which I had undertaken impracticable, as the birds poured in in countless multitudes, I rose, and counting the dots then put down, found that 163 had been made in twenty-one minutes. I traveled on and still met more the farther I proceeded. The air with literally filled with Pigeons; the light of noon-day was obscured as by an eclipse; the dung fell in spots, not unlike melting flakes of snow. . . Whilst waiting for dinner at Young's inn . . . I saw, at my leisure, immense legions still going by, with a front reaching far beyond the Ohio on the west, and the beech-wood forests directly on the east of me. . . . Before sunset I reached Louisville, distant from Hardensburgh fifty-five miles. The Pigeons were still passing in undiminished numbers, and continued to do so for three days in succession. . . . It may not, perhaps, be out of place to attempt an estimate of the number of Pigeons contained in one of those mighty flocks. . . . Let us take a column of one mile in breadth, which is far below the average size, and suppose it is passing over us without interruption for three hours, at the rate mentioned above on one mile in the minute. . . . Allowing two pigeons to the square yard, we have one billion, one hundred and fifteen millions, one hundred and thirty-six thousand pigeons in one flock.*

It's difficult for us to conceive of such numbers in this time of diminished ecosystems, yet such huge overflights were common. Another flock, in 1866, passed into southern Ontario just north of the United States. Observers noted its size as being a mile wide by three hundred miles long; it took fourteen hours for the flock to pass. Estimates put the numbers of birds at over 3.5 billion. By 1900, a mere thirty-four years later, the passenger pigeon was extinct in the wild.

What most of us do not understand is the ecological impact such an extinction event can cause – from just one perspective: the amount of excrement the birds produced during overflights. Tons, literally, of some of the richest fertilizer known fell like rain on the landscapes over which they passed. (To get a minimal experience of this, some contemporary, and amusing, YouTube videos exist of towns where bird flocks have grown so large as to make excretion, umbrellas, and slippery sidewalks common topics.) The removal of those billions of birds, as did the loss of bison and deer herds, caused a severe reduction in the amount of fertilizer Earth received on a continual basis, in turn affecting plant growth and ecosystem health. These are hidden ecological realities that few of us ever consider.

When it comes to *Borrelia*, the near extermination of the buffalo, the severe diminishment of the deer population, and the reduction in numbers of all the large, migrating land mammals significantly inhibited the movement of the bacteria east to west to east. And the bacteria, for a time, became isolated in those four primary zones in the US. Human population pressures were fairly mild, and there wasn't a lot of travel of large land mammals into and out of endemic regions.

This began to change with the development of the interstate highway system during the 1950s and 1960s, the mass purchase of automobiles that accompanied it, and the emergence of inexpensive jet travel in the 1970s. Humans then became the major east–west–east transporters of bacterial and viral pathogens. The recovery of deer herds (and squirrels and . . .) during the 1970s and '80s due to the reduced need to hunt animals for food, created a new east–west–east movement of large (and smaller) land mammals. It reconnected, once again, the separated islands of borrelial organisms. The numbers of infections began to rise.

Ecological fragmentation and human population increases

The damage to wild landscapes, intrusions into forest ecosystems, the cutting of those same forests to make way for suburbs, and the damage to plant diversity and its crucial homeodynamic functions by suburb and agricultural intrusions have all played a major role in stimulating the emergence of stealth pathogens such as Lyme.

Human movement into formerly uninhabited forest landscapes, and the forest fragmentation that co-occurs with it, is a powerful driver of stealth pathogen development and movement into the human species. M. G. Walsh of the Department of Epidemiology and Biostatistics in New York comments that his study (2013) *examined 11 years of surveillance data in New York State to measure the relationship between forest fragmentation and the incidence of human babesiosis. Adjusted Poisson models showed that increasing edges of contact between forested land and developed land, as measured by their shared parameters, was associated with a higher incidence of babesiosis cases, even after controlling for the total developed land area and forest density, and temperature and precipitation. Each 10-km increase in perimeter contact between forested land and developed land per county was associated with a 1.5% increase in babesiosis risk.*

The same is true of borrelial organisms. Tran and Waller (2013) note that "more fragmentation between forests and residential areas results in higher local Lyme disease incidence."

Increases in human population creates the need for more houses, often built in previously unpopulated forest ecosystems. This significantly increases the risk of infections simply from the increased exposure of people to the pathogens. For instance, studies of forest ticks in southern Poland have found that 77 percent carry *Anaplasma*, 60 percent *Babesia*, and only 3 percent *Borrelia*. Coinfection with *Anaplasma* and *Babesia* is common in 50 percent of the ticks. The more that such locations are inhabited by people, the more likely it is that they will get bitten and develop disease.

(Again, the unique grouping of the infectious organisms in that ecological zone determines the kinds of coinfection complex people will develop. Thus in that part of Poland there is a much higher chance of becoming infected with *Babesia* and *Anaplasma* than Lyme. This is something that physicians who treat local populations should understand: they live in a particular ecological habitat, and the grouping of disease organisms in that habitat's ticks are always going to be unique – as is the immune health of that region's people.)

Also crucial to the emergence of these diseases is the reduction of wild predator populations. Mountain lion and wolf depletion, along with the decrease in human hunting for food – as well as issuance of hunting permits for bucks ("Look at that rack, will ya?") and *not* for the young-bearing females – has led to massive increases in deer populations. Depletion of predators, including birds, that feed on ground animals (and ticks) leads to massive increases in mice and other ground animals that carry *borrelia*. And overuse of pesticides has killed off large numbers of the insect predators that feed on tick eggs and larvae.

And finally, the reduction of large, wild mammal populations in undisturbed forest habitats plays its own important role. As fewer larger, wild animal populations are available as hosts for the bacterial diseases that once were (mostly) limited to those populations, the bacteria have had no choice; they have had to jump species in order to find hosts in which to live. Because human beings now live in the habitat formerly occupied by those animals, many of the bacteria have moved into us.

One of the hidden ecological realities here is that large mammals and their herds were once primary hosts for *Borrelia*. The bacteria did not need to infect humans to the degree they do now; there were plenty of buffalo and deer. Despite the increase in deer herds since then, humans are now the major large mammal species that lives and migrates within the great bison belt. We are *not* inadvertent hosts. We are becoming, or already are, primary reservoirs for many of these emerging diseases.

Climate change

Climate change is also a strong driver of increasing infections. Walsh (2013) comments that "[h]igher temperature was also strongly associated with increasing babesiosis risk, wherein each degree Celsius increase was associated with an 18% increase in babesiosis risk." This relationship between temperature and increasing infections occurs with the entire group of stealth pathogens. Sprong et al. note, in their studies of the relationship of temperature and increased infection, that . . .

> [b]etween 1994 and 2009, a threefold increase has been observed in consultations of general practitioners for tick bites and Lyme disease in The Netherlands. . . . Long-term analyses indicated that the length of the annual tick question season increased . . . overall abundance of feeding and reproductive hosts also increased. . . . Population genetic analysis of the collected Borrelia species points to an increase in B. afzelii and B. garinii populations.

Tran and Waller (2013) comment that "results show that Lyme disease incidence has a relatively clear connection with regional landscape fragmentation and temperature." And Danielova et al. (2010) note that "upon analysis of the local climate we consider climate warming to be responsible for the spreading of ticks and tick-transmitted pathogens to higher altitudes." The milder the winters, the farther north (and higher) the ticks go; the more ticks there are, the longer they quest, the more people they bite. Projections based on current warming trends indicate concomitant increases in Lyme disease incidence in a one-to-one relationship. As Simon, et al. (2014) observe, after examining increases related to warming: "We predict a further northern expansion of B. burgdorferi of approximately 250–500 km by 2050 – a rate of 3.5–11 km per year."

Certain areas of Ohio, formerly considered to be nonendemic for Lyme, have shown an increase from 0–5 ticks in the period 1983-2008 to 15 in 2009, to 40 in 2010, to 184 in 2011. Tick population levels have become so high in some areas that researchers in one study, who dragged a white flannel cloth over a sixty foot (20 m) section of ground, found 1,200 ticks attached. In highly endemic areas there may be as many as 60 nymphs (on average) feeding on each mouse or 50 adults on each deer. This is the average. Up to 200 nymphs have been found attached to a mouse, 500 on a single deer.

Other ecological alterations, generally unrecognized as such, have wide-ranging impacts on stealth pathogen increases. Sudden oak death (SOD), is an example. The disease is caused by a pathogen, *Phytophthora ramorum,* that infects oak trees throughout California. Swei et al. (2011) comment that "our data show that SOD has a positive impact on the density of nymphal ticks, which is expected to increase the risk of human exposure to Lyme disease all else being equal."

Ecological manipulation and control of Lyme (not)
Many sources have suggested that the number of Lyme infections can be reduced or even eliminated by altering the (oversimplified) ecological dynamics thought to be at the root of the problem. Unfortunately, this is not likely to be a workable intervention.

Oversimplistically, the story told by most Lyme sources is that nymphs and larvae feed on small animals like white-footed mice. The white-footed mice are (still) thought (by those sources) to be the primary reservoir, and they spread the organism back and forth to the ticks. This keeps the spirochete levels high in tick populations.

Adult ticks, however, have to feed on something bigger before they can lay their eggs, making new generations of ticks. Mostly, we are told, what they feed on is deer. Humans get involved, accidentally, when they take a walk in the woods. And this is a sort-of-their-fault thing since they could just stay home, inside their houses or in the cities, where it is safe. This is sort-of-true, I guess. I mean, we *could* stay inside all the time, or wear hazmat suits when we go outside, or cover ourselves with DEET – the "we're-all-gonna-die" approach to the ecological realities of life. Hysteria of the "I-told-you-nature-was-dangerous" and "we-have-to-defeat-it-at-all-costs" sort.

To get around this, experts insist we could control the size of the mouse population or the deer population or the tick population, allowing us to go outside whenever and however we wish, while at the same time stopping the Lyme epidemic in its tracks. Unfortunately, this is not an accurate representation of the ecological realities – as I hope the previous material has revealed.

What is more true about Lyme bacteria is that *one of* the primary reservoirs in the *Northeast* United States is the white-footed mouse. Ultimately, however, there is no *primary* small-animal reservoir for borrelial spirochetes. Nor are large mammals necessary to spread the bacteria. Madeira, a subtropical island off the coast of Portugal, has no large mammals, yet Lyme spirochetes happily spread through tick attachment to two different species of rats. In other parts of Europe, the hedgehog is the primary "large" mammal that they use; in Japan, it's the red fox. In Europe, as a whole, there are thirty-five known reservoir host species. All are tightly linked together to maintain the disease in the wild.

Reducing deer populations will do nothing to decrease spirochete numbers or transmission to humans. Directly reducing deer populations, in the places it has been tried, causes a short-term reduction in tick numbers with a large rebound shortly thereafter. Reduction of the mouse population in any region simply moves the spirochetes into a new reservoir species (of which there are many). The use of pesticides to kill the ticks does work for a while, but ticks like other insects and arthropods have a tendency to develop resistance to pesticides as time goes by. Populations tend to rebound within two years. (The spirochetes are not going to go away just because we fiddle with a few factors; they have been around for over one hundred million years. They aren't quitters.) The ecological reality of Lyme is very different than old-Lyme thinking would have us believe. It very specifically is *not* tick/mouse/deer oriented. Hanincova et al. (2006) are clear on this . . .

> *Since the reemergence of LB 3 decades ago, the disease has been spreading across the entire northeastern United States and beyond. . . . This expansion is believed to be driven by large-scale reforestation and an explosive growth of deer populations. Deer, however, do not contribute directly to the dispersal of* B. burgdorferi. *. . . If* B. burgdorferi *were host specialized, the strains of this microparasite would migrate differentially, resulting in geographic structuring of this pathogen. Unrestricted cross-species transmission, in contrast, would generate a spatially uniform population structure of* B. burgdorferi *and substantially facilitate its dispersal.*

As they continue . . .

> *Our own data set indicates that several genotypes can infect as many as 5 host species. This suggests that cross-species transmission of* B. burgdorferi *among various mammalian species is common. . . . this study shows a pattern of more relaxed host specificity . . . Therefore, the niche breadth of* B. burgdorferi *is not congruent with host species, [i.e., it is not host specialized]. Furthermore, genotypes 1-5 and 7 can . . . infect many additional, phylogenetically distant host species, covering as many as 3 orders. This indicates that the niche breadth of most* B. burgdorferi *genotypes in the United States is even wider than the taxonomic unit of order. . . . some strains of* B. burgdorferi *are extreme generalists. In view of all ecologic and experimental information available to date, we conclude that host specificity of* B. burgdorferi *ranges from generalism to specialism.*

The bacteria have specific and very sophisticated mechanisms in place to infect a wide range of animals in the wild (discussed in the next chapter). The removal of one host reservoir simply motivates them to move into another. The root of this generalism, the researchers comment, is the consequence of human-generated ecological damage during the mid-to-late nineteenth and early twentieth centuries.

> *The generalist strategy of* B. burgdorferi *is consistent with its uniform population structure across much of the northeastern United States. We may speculate that the generalist strategy of* B. burgdorferi *echoes adaptation to impoverished ecological conditions in the past because of large scale habitat destruction in the northeastern United States in the course of the post-Columbian settlement and during the industrial revolution. We conclude that cross-species transmission is a key property that has allowed LB to spread rapidly across the northeastern United States.*

White-footed mice and deer are not the problem; ecological alterations, including human population growth, are.

Human beings are *not* inadvertent hosts. They are one of a group of large mammal species that exist in the spirochetes macroecological world; they are, in fact, primary reservoirs.

While comforting to think that we can intelligently intervene by interrupting spirochete ecology, it is unlikely to accomplish anything effective. There are just too many other factors in play that are not being taken into account. Unexpected outcomes are inevitable. Our ecological ignorance is one major factor in the emergence of the Lyme epidemic. Extending that ignorance into ecological manipulation when we, as a whole, don't know what we are doing will just continue the process. Here is just one example of the hidden side effects of such intervention. . . .

Researchers have been attempting to utilize an ecological intervention to lower the incidence of dengue fever and malaria organisms in the mosquitoes that transmit the diseases. Their idea has been to infect mosquitos with *Wolbachia* bacteria and release them into the wild. These particular bacteria out-compete both malaria and dengue organisms in the mosquito body, making the mosquitos resistant to infection by those organisms. This, if effective, would lower the incidence of those infections in people. However, researchers found that while the infection with *Wolbachia* reduced both malarial and dengue microorganisms in the mosquitos, it significantly increased West Nile virus (WNV) levels – it stimulated the acquisition and expansion of WNV in the mosquito population. As Dodson et al. (2014) comment, these studies indicate . . .

> *that careful examination of* Wolbachia *is required, since the bacterium influences insect-pathogen interactions in ways that may negatively affect pathogen control efforts. . . . This is the first observation of a* Wolbachia-*induced enhancement of a human pathogen in mosquitoes and suggests that caution should be applied before using* Wolbachia *as part of a vector-borne disease control program.*

There are no simple fixes. And this plays havoc with our tendency to think science can solve any problem we encounter – even those of our own making. Lyme is going to be with us a long time, as are an increasing number of stealth pathogens, resistant bacteria, and emerging viral pathogens. Human disruption of planetary ecosystems is not going to stop – until we hit an ecological limit that forces it. A new approach to our place in the world, to disease, and to our health and healing is essential.

The bacteria are evolving; we should, too.

CHAPTER FIVE

INITIAL INFECTION DYNAMICS, CYTOKINES, ENCYSTED FORMS, AND BIOFILMS: THE MICROECOLOGY OF BORRELIAL INFECTIONS

When B. burgdorferi was discovered and described, it was assumed to be a single species. The use of genome fingerprinting and other methods soon showed that the bacteria were highly diverse and in fact represented a species complex.
Margos et al., 2011

Borrelia burgdorferi are anaerobic heterotrophs that require complex organic food under anoxic conditions. They die if exposed to ambient oxygen. The round bodies, propagules that, until they revert to swimming helices, seem incapable of at least rapid growth by reproduction, form quickly. Within less than an hour, under adverse conditions round bodies develop in large population numbers when the spirochete's needs are not met. They survive for extended periods of time. They revert to helical swimmer populations that grow vigorously when food, salt, temperature, acidity, media viscosity and other conditions become adequate.
Margulis et al., 2009

Again, as I mentioned earlier, this chapter is much more technical than other chapters in the book. You don't need to read this section if you simply are wanting to learn about natural treatment protocols for Lyme disease. This chapter (and the next) is primarily for clinicians and those with a not-to-be-denied desire to understand more of the technical aspects of what the spirochetes do while living inside other organisms, including their tick facilitators.

The micro-ecology of *Borrelia*

Borrelial organisms, when they enter a new host, encounter a unique ecological environment. They are extremely adept at adapting to a wide variety of such environments, whether in a tick, a human being, or any of the three hundred different animal species they can use as hosts. Their capacity to subtly shift their genomic structure in response to their analysis of the interior landscape in each different host is part of what makes them so hard to treat during infections. Understanding what they do during infection and how they alter themselves in response to the host environment is crucial, I think, for creating successful treatment interventions in a large minority of those who are infected.

The uniqueness of *Borrelia*

Borrelial organisms are unique in the microbial world. They possess features unusual to bacteria (prokaryotes), features that are more often associated with what are called eukaryotes (more complex, nonbacterial life-forms such as ticks and people). Unlike nearly all other bacteria, they have, as researchers Saier and Paulsen (2001) comment, "linear chromosomes, a cytoskeleton, and periplasmic flagelli that confer rapid motility and unusual chemotactic properties." As Brisson et al. (2012) confirm: "The genome of *B. burgdorferi* is one of the most, if not the most, complex of any bacterium." *Borrelia* are so unusual, in fact, that they were initially classified with protozoa, not bacteria. They are also unique in that they possess the largest number of genetic units of replication (DNA replicons) of any bacteria known, making them by far the most complex in this respect. As Pulzova and Bhide (2014) comment . . .

> Borrelia *are unique among bacteria in their ability to express a wide variety of lipoproteins on their surface, which play an essential role in pathogenesis. . . . Vast diversity in the expressed*

surface proteome of Borrelia *in different niches and multifunc-*
tionality of proteins are the major strategies of Borrelia *to avoid*
the destructive effect of the immune system.

They are also among the extremely low number of organisms that do not require iron in order to live (they use manganese instead). Too, they have no close relatives, the closest probably being *Treponema* spirochetes, the same genus that causes syphilis and a number of dental diseases. But even those only show about a 40 percent similarity to the genome of Lyme spirochetes.

While heretical in many respects, Lyme *Borrelia* organisms can (and possibly should) be thought of as an intermediate life-form between bacteria and more complex parasites, having the qualities of both. While this is outside conventional thinking, it automatically engenders a better understanding of the organism's behavior during infection. For Lyme spirochetes act like nothing so much as an exceptionally intelligent protozoal parasite. *Borrelia* organisms are parasitic and must be thought of as such, because of the way their metabolism is structured. They are capable of only minimal metabolism, and all nucleotides, amino acids, fatty acids, and enzyme cofactors must be scavenged from their hosts – in other words, us.

Spirochetes are difficult organisms for researchers to work with, which is why, even at this late point, so little (bacterially speaking) is known about them. They are what are called obligate fastidious organisms, meaning that don't live freely in the wild but have to live *inside* other organisms (obligate), and they are real particular about what they eat (fastidious). The syphilis spirochete, even after sixty years of focused research still cannot be grown in a laboratory. Thus, special, and difficult-to-manage, growth mediums are necessary to grow Lyme *Borrelia* in laboratories.

Spirochetes are not your any old bacteria that will grow on any old piece of toast at the drop of a hat. Borrelial spirochetes are also very thin, and this makes them difficult to see under magnification without unusual lighting or specific and expensive kinds of microscopes. And, finally, they grow very slowly. Unlike many bacteria that produce a new generation every twenty minutes, Lyme spirochetes do so every eight to twelve hours. These three factors alone (and there are others) have made it very hard to do research on spirochetes (compared to other bacteria), and the Lyme spirochete is no exception.

Even though incredibly tiny, Lyme spirochetes resemble nothing so much as a corkscrew-shaped worm. This is, in fact, what they act like when they enter living tissues. They literally "screw" or "worm" their way through tissues to the sites they wish to colonize.

Like other mobile bacteria, spirochetes have wiggling tails called flagella. Their flagella, however, are different than the external flagella of bacteria such as *E. coli* (which radiate outward). Borrelial flagella traverse the length of the spirochete body, and they are *inside* the outer protein coat. Further, they have two "motors," one in the front, one in the rear, which increases their motile power. This kind of mobility allows them to colonize highly viscous mediums, such as the collagenous tissues around the knees or the aqueous humor of the eye. As Berndtson (2013) observes . . .

> Bb *motility is designed for swimming through liquid environ-ments such as blood, lymph, and CSF, and for squirming and tunneling through viscoelastic gel environments like the ECM [extracellular matrix] and other connective tissues. . . . Advanced imaging techniques make it clear that* Bb *is no ordinary bacte-rium. It has motility prowess heretofore unseen in the microbial world. It is built to infiltrate, evade, and persist.*

And Lyme spirochetes are *fast*, the fastest of all the spirochetes. They move much more quickly than the white blood cells our bodies create to kill them, upward of two orders of magnitude faster than neutrophils, the fastest white blood cell of all.

Once in their new host, Lyme spirochetes continually alter their structure in order to evade host immune responses and to enhance their colonization of different parts of the body. They are, in essence, continually experiment-ing with genomic alterations to find those that maximize survival in host tissues. Researchers have described their capacity in this regard as "nearly inexhaustible" and have noted, importantly, that these alterations occur only in vivo, never in vitro making much of the data collected on the spiro-chetes during in vitro studies to be nearly useless.

Thus the structure of the Lyme spirochetes is constantly in flux. Research-ers have found that when they recovered infectious spirochetes from inten-tionally infected mice (and other animals, including humans), the spirochetes they get out are not the same as the ones that went in. In one study, from a single spirochete type 1,400 clones were isolated from the bladder, heart, joint, ear, and skin of long-term Lyme-infected mice. As researchers Qiu et al. (2004) note: "Frequent recombination implies a potential for rapid adaptive evolution and a possible polygenic basis of *B. burgdorferi* pathogenicity." And different genomic combinations decidedly do create different symptom pictures in the people infected with Lyme spirochetes.

Borrelial spirochetes have a large number of tremendously complex and sophisticated behaviors. Some of the most important of them occur within and in concert with the ticks that transmit them. There has been a lot of fairly simplistic information published about the ticks that transmit Lyme bacteria. Most of it, unfortunately, is either incorrect (old-Lyme thinking) or so oversimplified that it is incredibly misleading or even useless.

About those ticks

While borrelial organisms are transmitted in many ways . . .

> *Again, ticks are **not** the only transmitters of Lyme disease.*
> *That is old-Lyme thinking; it's incorrect.*

. . . and by many arthropods, the most common vector is the hard tick, most commonly members of the *Ixodes* genera.

> *I am being oversimplistic here for a reason,*
> *and that's because . . .*

A deeper look at this particular genus of tick gives a good picture of the processes involved during arthropod transmission. It shows just how important the ticks (or other arthropods) are during infection and the life cycle of the bacteria.

Most of the oversimplistic information on the tick transmitters of Lyme has been repeated *ad nauseam*, so much so that it has become incredibly tiresome to read; it's tremendously clichéd. Nevertheless, repetition, to some extent, can't be avoided (as much as I would like to). Hence . . .

Ixodes ticks have three stages of growth: larvae, nymph, and adult. The adult ticks lay their eggs in the early spring, and the larvae hatch from them in early summer. It takes about a month for the eggs to hatch once the temperature warms enough. Most sources will, incorrectly, tell you that the new larvae are not infected with Lyme bacteria and that they cannot transmit Lyme disease. In other words, they assert that transovarial transmission (which means *Borrelia*-infection is transmitted from adults through their eggs, into the tick babies) does not occur.

It does occur, of course; things are never as simple as old-Lyme thinking makes out. (As Rudenko et al., 2011, phlegmatically observe, "Data generated during the last decade demand reevaluation of the previously held concepts about LB around the world.") The rates tend to be rather low when compared to transovarial transmission in mosquitoes, for instance. But the exact rates of transovarial transmission, in fact, depend on the *species* of *Borrelia* you are talking about.

If you are looking at *Borrelia burgdorferi* s.s., on average, only about 1 percent of the newly hatched larvae tend to be infected. Nevertheless, even this is relatively inaccurate; some studies have found up to a fourth of the larvae carry *Borrelia* at birth. There are other factors in play here, including geographical location, type of tick, which variant of *Bbss* is involved, and so on. In contrast, the rates of transovarial transmission for *B. miyamotoi* are often extremely high. Some studies (e.g., Tappe et al., 2014) have also begun to document an increase in transovarial transmission among all types of *Borrelia* since 2005. (No one really knows why.) And to make matters more complicated, most ticks are generally infected with multiple borrelial species. The species are often compartmentalized in different parts of the tick body, and each possesses different degrees of transovarial transmission.

Thus, some larvae, in contrast to received wisdom, are infective as soon as they emerge from the egg. They will pass the infection on to whichever host they first feed upon. Infections from larvae are, in fact, more common than old-Lyme thinking would have you believe.

Unfortunately, larval ticks are tiny, about the size of the point of a pin or the period at the end of this sentence. Impossible to see, really. (You don't have a bird feeder, do you?) Soon after they hatch, the larvae begin questing for animals to feed on (peak larval activity in the Northern Hemisphere generally occurs in August). Because they are so tiny, larvae tend to infect smaller animals, animals closer to the ground, such as mice. Still, they do bite and transmit the disease to people.

Uninfected larvae become infected when they feed on an infected host. As soon as they attach, the larval ticks release various salival chemicals into the animal's bloodstream. These chemicals have a multitude of different functions (discussed more comprehensively in a moment); some of them act much like pheromones. They stimulate any spirochetes already in the animal to rapidly migrate to the larval feeding site where they then infect the newly hatched larvae. In this way, the infection passes into new generations of uninfected ticks.

Interestingly, two of the chemicals that stimulate spirochete transfer to new larvae are the host's neuroendocrine stress hormones epinephrine and norepinephrine. When the host body releases these chemicals into the bloodstream in response to a tick bite, they are immediately bound by the spirochetes to their exterior membrane. This stimulates the upregulation in the exterior membrane of the membrane protein *ospA*. This is essential for bacterial entry and survival in the larval tick because . . .

Ticks contain a special receptor (TROSPA, an acronym for "tick receptor *ospA*") that is coded for proteins on the outer surface membrane (aka, skin) of the spirochetes' bodies. Spirochetes primarily (but not exclusively) express *ospA* when inside a tick. (In humans, early on, it tends to be primarily, but not exclusively, *ospC*.) The outer surface protein (*ospA*) attaches to TROSPA receptors in the tick gut allowing colonization in the tick midgut to occur. (This is the preferred, but not exclusive, colonization site of the bacteria in ticks.)

A good analogy for the chemo-attraction between *ospA* and TROSPA is the attraction between a piece of iron and a magnet. The iron filings are powerfully pulled toward the magnet, and when contact is made, they stick to it. Once attached to the tick gut tissues, smaller numbers of spirochetes often go on to infect other sites within the tick: the hypodermis, central ganglion, salivary glands, ovaries, and connective tissues. When the newly infected tick bites another animal, the spirochetes swarm from the midgut to the salivary glands and thence into the blood, passing the infection on to a new host. (As with many things Lyme, it is a bit more complicated than this picture makes it seem. There are always *some* borrelial organisms already present in the salivary glands; they flow into the new host's bloodstream as soon as the tick bites a new host.)

Most people think (old-Lyme ratiocination) that each of these three tick stages feed only once. This is both true and untrue. What is *true* is that each of these stages only feeds *to completion* once during their stage of growth – completion meaning feeding until they are completely full (engorged). What is *not* true is that they feed only once. Recent research has found that it is extremely common for ticks to disengage from a host before they feed to completion. These "fed" ticks, once they attach to a new host, can transmit Lyme organisms in as little as ten minutes

as little as ten minutes

not the 24 to 48 hours that most sources cite. Most ticks are partially fed, not unfed, when they bite a new host.

As well, even the very old, very early Lyme studies found that *unfed* ticks themselves quite often transmit borrelial bacteria in less than 24 hours. (From 8 to 16 hours, not 24.) Deeper analysis has shown that transmission in less than 24 hours occurs 83 percent of the time; that 24-hour figure is just not accurate. Nevertheless, the CDC and nearly every other source endlessly repeats it. (The accurate figures are concealed in open-source, peer-reviewed journal papers easily available on the web at Pubmed and Google Scholar, where the CDC can't seem to find them.)

Another important transmission factor is cofeeding. In other words, it is extremely common for host animals to have both larvae and nymphs feeding on them at the same time (and occasionally adult ticks as well). Cofeeding by the different developmental stages has been found to reduce the time necessary for the spirochetes to infect a new host – as well as the time necessary for them to infect uninfected larvae.

When they're finished feeding (about 72 hours for full engorgement), the larval tick drops to the ground wherever the host animal happens to be. The larvae then spend their time absorbing the blood meal. Soon afterwards they begin their molt – altering form to the next stage of tick development, aka the nymph. The molting process takes about thirty-five days on average. The newly formed nymphs hibernate during the winter, beginning their activity the next spring. (Still oversimplistic, sometimes they wake up and seek blood meals if the temperature warms enough. Yes, even in Connecticut.)

The number of nymphs infected by *Borrelia* depends on many things, from what kind of winter they experience to the density of mice and other small mammals in that area in that particular year. Infection rates have been found to run anywhere from 3 to 100 percent, depending on the study. Generally, in endemic areas, at least half of all nymphs are infected by the beginning of their feeding season. More become infected when they feed on infected animals.

The nymph is bigger than the larvae but still horribly small, about the size of the head of a pin. They are usually very hard to see when not engorged with a blood meal. Nymphs begin their activity as soon as it is warm enough (by May latest) and are very active throughout the summer. They will feed on pretty much anything they can, from mice to people. The nymphs are highly infective, and so by the time the larvae hatch and begin *their* peak activity in August, most animals in a Lyme endemic area will be infected, many with nymphs attached. This overlap in the tick cycle ensures that many if not most larvae will be infected before they molt.

Nymphs feed longer than larvae, four or five days. (They, too, usually feed more than once before they become engorged.) When they are done feeding, they drop off and begin their molt into adult ticks. (It's kind of a caterpillar and butterfly sort of thing.) This takes a bit longer than the larval molt, about forty-two days on average.

The adult ticks emerge from molt in October or early November, and they immediately begin looking for a meal themselves. They are larger than the larval- and nymph-stage ticks. They look about the same as any old tick you might have seen. Similarly to larvae and nymphs, they climb to the top of grass stalks or other plants and wait, their upper legs stretched out, for a passing animal to brush against them so they can hitch a ride.

Lyme ticks, of whatever species, are not very mobile, they have been found to be able to move on their own only about nine feet (3 m) from where they hatch or drop off after feeding. They basically just sit there until something with blood comes along. The animal they are feeding on is who moves them to new locations. Still, mice don't travel all that much. They tend to remain within an area of about one hundred by one hundred feet (30 m square). Deer, on the other hand, maintain a home range of several miles (4 km). Birds and people (and their companion animals) spread them much farther. There is no place on the globe they do not take them.

Adult ticks are more discriminatory in their feeding habits than larvae and nymphs. They tend to focus their feedings on animals larger than, say, a woodchuck or small dog, preferring larger animals such as buffalo, deer, horses, dogs, and people. They also feed much longer – seven or eight days. (And yes, they, too engage in multiple feedings.) Once they are full, they drop off the host animal and get ready to overwinter. Then, in the spring, they lay their eggs and die, starting the cycle all over again.

Any adult ticks that do not find a host to feed on during the fall will over-winter, seeking a new host in the spring. Both fall-fed and spring-fed adult ticks lay their eggs in the spring, anywhere from two to three thousand of them. Then they die. If winters are especially warm, as they increasingly are, they may emerge from hibernation and feed at any time. (So, yes, it is possible to get a Lyme infection in December or February.)

The eggs they lay take about a month to hatch. Lucky for us, there is an exceptionally large egg and larval mortality rate. Both are fed upon by a number of predatory insects and arthropods, such as ants, spiders, and wasps. Birds eat a great many of the ticks as well, often before they lay their eggs. (Yuck)

Importantly – and something that old-Lyme thinking has not understood – each of the different tick developmental stages stimulate differences in spirochete genome structures. In essence, they facilitate strain and subspe-cies development – each in a different way. As Iyer et al. (2014) note, "The results show clearly that spirochetes exhibit unique expression profiles during each tick stage . . . importantly, none of these profiles resembles that exhibited by *in vitro* grown organisms." (The fact that test-tube-grown spirochetes are very different than tick-grown spirochetes means that much of the old-Lyme research was deeply flawed. It had little to do with reality. This is part of the reason why what doctors "know" about Lyme is so often incorrect.)

Ticks that transmit Lyme spirochetes do live in warmer climates such as the American South, the American West Coast, South America, and north-ern Africa and southern Europe. Their growth patterns differ from ticks that are limited by colder winters such as those from the American North-east. Their life cycles can run anywhere from two to six years. And unfed ticks, no matter where they live, are remarkably patient, some of them can live up to seven years without a meal.

The usual picture we are given about both ticks and Lyme disease is greatly oversimplified. Ticks are highly adaptable, and there are a lot of them. As Durland Fish (1993) comments . . .

> With Ixodes dammini, *the birth rate clearly exceeds the death*
> *rate over most of its range. Populations of* I. dammini *seem to be*
> *increasing in density in areas where they are already established,*
> *and there is considerable evidence that the range of this species*
> *is expanding both in the Northeast and upper Midwest . . .*
> *Nowhere does there seem to be a trend for a population decline*
> *of this species. It is likely that this situation will continue for the*
> *immediate future, as* I. dammini *has all the characteristics of*
> *an invading species.*

Tick/*Borrelia* interactions

Ticks and borrelial bacteria have been working together for perhaps a
hundred million years, perhaps more. Both organisms benefit from the relationship. The ticks offer a supportive, nurturing home for the bacteria and,
because they feed on so many different types of animals, are exceptionally
good at transferring the bacteria to other life-forms. (And this occurs not
only through biting but also by the extremely hardy borrelial biofilms and
encysted forms expressed in tick feces. This spreads the organisms everywhere a tick poops, and like most life-forms, ticks poop a lot.)

Ticks are also incredibly good at assisting bacterial movement into
new hosts; tick saliva is in fact essential to the ability of the spirochetes to
successfully infect other organisms. As Kern, et al (2011) comment, "*Borrelia*
pathogens specifically use the tick saliva to facilitate their transmission to
the host." Further, passage of the spirochetes *through* tick bodies enhances
the infectivity of the bacteria; it makes them more virulent. And what's
more, tick saliva stimulates the numbers and growth of spirochetes, helping
them reproduce. *Borrelia* receive many, and multiple benefits from the ticks.
In exchange, the spirochetes facilitate tick survival and behavior. As Herrmann et al. (2015) comment . . .

> *[The spirochetal] parasite can modify the phenotype of its*
> *host by changing the host perception of the environment and/*
> *or behaviour in order to complete its transmission cycle . . .*
> *For vector-borne pathogens . . . manipulation usually consists*

of modifying vector behavior so that the number of bitten hosts
(and thereby infected hosts) is increased using strategies such as
higher biting rates, shortened blood meals, a longer lifespan, etc.

Ticks, especially larvae and nymphs, are extremely sensitive to dessication, i.e., loss of water from their tissues. Ticks don't drink water (nearly all the water taken up in a blood meal is regurgitated back into the host as they feed – total yuck). Instead, they gain water by crawling under the leaf litter where it is more humid. The water from the air is then directly absorbed into their bodies.

When ticks crawl to the top of vegetation and wait for a passing animal, they lose water to the atmosphere. They begin to dry out. They lose even more water as they breathe. This limits the amount of time they can remain in a questing position; they have to return periodically to the leaf litter in order to rehydrate. Ticks infected with borrelial spirochetes are much less prone to dehydration. This allows them to quest longer, which in turn makes them better adapted to finding new hosts.

The blood meal that most ticks take is mostly composed of proteins. It is stored in their body as fats – similarly to how we store sugars as fats. The fats in ticks are stored in the epithelial cells of the midgut and in the fat body (a diffuse organ found throughout the tick). The stored fat declines between feedings (even more is used during the molting process). The longer between feedings, the lower the fat reserves.

Ticks experiencing dry conditions consume fat stores about twice as quickly as those in more humid conditions. The more the ticks have to move up and down grass stalks to rehydrate, the more fat stores they use.

Borrelia increase the fat reserves of the ticks by at least 12 percent, and the spirochetes use very little of that fat for their own needs. A single tick can support a population of around 3,500 spirochetes. Yet, the borrelial community inside it only uses about 0.10 percent of the tick's fat reserves, even at full capacity. The extra fat stores that the spirochetes generate is used by the tick to enhance its functioning, helping it survive adverse conditions and more easily find new hosts.

Borrelia-infected ticks can move more quickly, can climb higher, are more tolerant to tick repellants, can take in larger blood meals, have more fat stores, and stay more hydrated than uninfected ticks. Their life span also increases; they can last much longer without a blood meal than uninfected ticks – up to seven years.

And to add insult to injury, the borrelial bacteria (and coinfectious bacteria such as *Ehrlichia* and *Anaplasma*) create and systemically release a kind of antifreeze (made from glycoproteins), which helps the ticks remain active during freezing temperatures. (This means that tick bites can sometimes occur in winter, and yes, the bacteria have no mercy. They don't even care about Christmas.)

Spirochete transfer to a new host

When a tick carrying Lyme spirochetes attaches itself to an animal and bites into the skin, a complex series of events immediately begins, much of it oriented around the unique nature of tick saliva. (Needle inoculation of lab animals produces significantly different kinds of infections than tick infections do. The studies done with needle-infected lab animals that have been conducted in the past tend to be relatively useless in understanding borrelial infections in people.)

When a warm-blooded mammal walks by (or even birds or reptiles, the ticks don't really care), the questing tick grabs hold and begins to seek its preferred attachment site (with rodents, it's often near the ears). When it finds that spot, the tick begins to saw through the outer layer of the skin so that it can reach the blood vessels that lie just below the surface. Once penetration occurs, the tick secretes a milky cement that hardens around the penetration site, holding the tick in place. It's composed of a unique combination of glycosylated proteins, which are very similar in their makeup to collagen and keratin – two of the major components of vertebrate skin. This holds the tick firmly in place and acts as a kind of gasket that prevents loss of blood from the host or leakage of tick saliva from the point of entry. The entire process takes less than ten minutes.

Under the point of attachment, a tiny pit is gouged out of the skin and fills with blood. Ticks are a kind of pool feeder. Once the pit fills, they drink at their leisure. As the tick (larva, nymph, or adult) feeds, its body swells (engorges) to hold all the blood it is taking in. Larvae and nymphs ingest 10 to 20 times their unfed weights, adults 100 to 120 times. Once fully engorged, the ticks detach from the host and fall to the ground. They then digest the blood meal and begin the molting process. The cement core is left behind, embedded in the skin. (A lot of tick excrement is left behind as well. When any of this enters the wound – think scratching – it carries borrelial biofilms and encysted forms into the body. These have different infectious dynamics than the motile spirochetes do.)

During feeding, the tick alternates between taking blood and releasing saliva (and the blood's water content) back into the wound. Tick saliva is filled with a complex blend of powerful, pharmacologically active molecules (120 are known, only a few of which have been studied in depth). These molecules spread rapidly throughout the host body via the lymph and bloodstream, affecting a wide range of biological processes. They have especially potent effects on the three main host immune defenses against blood-feeding organisms. These are: (1) hemostasis (blood coagulation, platelet aggregation, and vasoconstriction); (2) inflammation (the swelling, redness, and heat that accompanies cellular damage); and (3) immunity (innate and acquired).

Antihemostatic compounds inhibit platelet adenosine phosphate (ADP), prostaglandin and prostacyclin receptors, and thrombin. Anti-inflammatory compounds inhibit anaphylatoxins, histamine, and bradykinin. (Salival compounds specifically downregulate "alarmins" in skin keratinocytes, that is, mediators that mobilize and activate antigen-presenting cells.) Anti-immune response compounds inhibit the alternative pathway of the complement system. They also inhibit the TLR-2 (toll-like receptor) innate immune response, which is specific for recognizing pathogen-associated microbial patterns (PAMPs) and then upregulating an immune response. A number of salival compounds bind CD4+ T immune-cell receptors, inhibiting their activation and proliferation.

The salival compounds downregulate (or inhibit) the activity of neutrophils, macrophages, natural killer (NK) cells, dendritic cells, splenic T lymphocytes, and B lymphocytes. They do the same with many cytokines, chemokines, and other immune cells, such as interleukin 2 (IL-2), IL-6, IL-8, monocyte chemoattractant protein-1 (MCP-1), macrophages, nitric oxide, interferon alpha (IFN-a), IFN-$beta$, IFN-$gamma$, immunoglobulin G (IgG), STAT-1, ERK 1/2, NF-kB, TNF-a, and a number of antimicrobial peptides (defensins, cathelicidin, psoriasin, and RNase7). The anti-inflammatory Th2 cytokine IL-10 is upregulated.

Tick saliva contains compounds known as "evasins," which bind to and neutralize chemokines that recruit cells from the innate immune system that are intended to counteract parasites. Evasin-1 binds CCL3, CCL4, CCL18; evasin-3 binds CXCL8 and CXCL1; and evasin-4 binds CCL5 and CCL11. As Radolf et al. (2012) comment . . .

> *The host factors in tick saliva that enhance survival of B. burgdorferi . . . include the molecules that can impede various mammalian responses, including the generation of reactive oxygen species, activation of complement, release of antimicrobial peptides, chemotaxis of neutrophils, and antibody-mediated killing, dendritic cell-mediated priming of T cells, and keratinocyte-mediated release of cytokines and antimicrobial peptides.*

The salival immune-inhibiting molecules have a potent, and broad, impact on host immune defense. To get a very brief idea: IgG plays an important role in host defense responses to infection. It protects tissues from bacteria, viruses, and toxins. IgG neutralizes bacterial toxins, activates the complement immune response, and enhances phagocytosis (white blood cell activity against disease organisms). And this is only one part of the immune response that is inactivated or inhibited by tick saliva. Simply counteracting salival inhibition factors can prevent or significantly reduce spirochetes' ability to infect a new host. For example, studies have found that if the levels of interleukin-2 and interferon gamma in lab mice are kept high, the rate of *Borrelia* infection drops precipitously. (*Astragalus*, an immune-potentiating herb, is very effective at keeping these levels high, which is why those in endemic regions should take the herb as a regular part of their diet.)

Tick saliva inactivates one of our most potent innate immunities to disease – the alternative complement system. When we are born, we have what is called *innate* immunity. (Over time we also *acquire* immunity to diseases with which we have been infected.) The complement system is an especially important part of our innate immune capability. It can be activated through any of three pathways: the classical complement pathway, the lectin pathway, or the alternative complement pathway. Each pathway is useful for dealing with different kinds of microbes. The alternative complement pathway is the part of our innate immunity that can deal with stealth bacteria such as *Borrelia*. In fact, if the alternative pathway remains uninhibited, Lyme spirochetes cannot gain a foothold in our bodies. The complement system kills them immediately. Lyme spirochetes take advantage of alternative complement-inhibiting factors in tick saliva to seek out immunoprotected sites in the host body where they can then take root and reproduce.

If the new host already has low or impaired immune function, the salival compounds have an even greater impact and infection is much easier for the bacteria. (The severity of the infection also tends to be much worse.) *Infection efficiency and severity of symptoms are directly proportional to host immune strength or weakness – this is why enhancing immune function is essential during Lyme infections.* In addition, a healthy host immune defense also stimulates antibodies to tick saliva and inhibits future tick attachment. Anti-tick-saliva antibodies in those with the healthiest immune systems stimulate tick rejection before lengthy feeding can take place. The stronger the immune response, the less able a tick is to attach and feed. The higher the immune function, the lower the rate of Lyme infection in those who are exposed to an infected tick.

Spirochete transformation

Spirochetes tend to exist in a kind of hibernating state in unfed ticks. But as soon as a tick readies itself to feed, it begins to produce significant amounts of salival compounds in order to alter the blood host's biological responses. This shift alerts the spirochetes in the tick, awakening them from their hibernation. They begin to ready themselves for movement into a new host. Then, as the tick begins to feed, blood flows into the tick midgut. This begins a cascade of alterations in both the spirochetes' form and behavior.

Ticks are ambient temperature organisms, that is, the temperature of their bodies is the same as the temperature in the region in which they live. Mammal hosts are warm-blooded. The spirochete must be able to move from an ambient temperature environment to one where the temperature is generally higher and doesn't significantly fluctuate. As well, when in ticks, the spirochetes primarily sequester themselves in the tick's midgut where the pH is extremely alkaline (about 9.5).

So, when blood enters a feeding tick's midgut, two things immediately occur: temperature increase and a pH decrease (from 9.5 to around 7.4). The dramatic increase in temperature and the alteration of pH are essential environmental cues for the spirochetes; the cues initiate a regulatory cascade in the spirochete that change its nature considerably. First, they begin to rapidly multiply, increasing their numbers three to four times. They then migrate from the tick midgut to the salivary glands. Once there, they engage in a sophisticated analysis of the blood meal the tick is taking and start to alter their genetic structure, creating new forms of themselves. (A caveat here: a few spirochetes are already in the salivary glands. These are the most infective and enter the new host immediately upon tick feeding.)

Through blood meal analysis, the spirochetes are able to identify the host animal supplying the blood. They alter their genomic structure so they can enter into and live within that new host, avoiding its immune responses. To accomplish this, they clip out segments of their genome and weave other segments in. Each spirochete possesses up to twelve linear and twelve circular plasmids – twenty-four extra segments of DNA that are available at any one time. These are extrachromosomal DNA molecules that may, in total, equal half the length of their central linear chromosome. Each of these different DNA strands contains information about the different mammals that tick hosts might feed on. Further, these extra genetic segments are in constant rearrangement, depending on environmental cues. They act, as Berndtson (2013) has commented, as portable incubators "for genetic innovation that allows *Bb* to accomplish immune evasion feats not witnessed elsewhere in the animal kingdom." The bacteria literally innovate new plasmid arrangements in order to facilitate their adaptation to a constantly changing environmental field.

Spirochetes are unusual in that they have an inner protein coat and an outer protein coat. You can visualize this two-coat arrangement as something like a hand wearing a thin latex glove. The skin of your hand is the inner coat, the glove the outer. It is this outside coat that comes into contact with the host organisms the spirochete lives within. The spirochetes maintain an informational database about each animal species they can infect that specifically indicates how their outer protein coat must be restructured in order to survive. The protein coats are referred to by the initials *osp* (for outer surface protein); there are six primary types, from *ospA* to *F*.

Outer surface protein dynamics

While in the tick, many of the spirochetes' outer surface protein coats are type A (*ospA*). After they encounter a blood meal, some, but not all, of the spirochetes downregulate *ospA* and begin to upregulate *ospC*. This change occurs in a minority of the spirochetes, less than half. Others upregulate, for example, *ospE*, or *ospF*. And there are still other proteins that are upregulated to the outer protein coat, such as *vlsE* (variable major protein-like sequence E) and *erp* (a similar *ospE/F* protein). In addition, the exact structure of these various protein coats are altered minutely each time they are expressed. In essence, gene conversion is used to create novel variants, allowing thousands of variants to be created from a small pool of genes. These spirochetal variants during infection, again, act as a bacterial swarm of similar but different organisms. This facilitates infection in widely varying hosts as well as multiple niches within those hosts.

Once inside the new host, recombination continues to occur every time the bacteria replicate. *VlsE* recombination, for instance, is crucial for persistence in an *immunocompetent* host. During mammalian infection a number of what are called *vls* "silent cassettes" are transferred into the central *vlsE* core. This alters its amino acid sequences. "Thus," as Norris (2012) comments, "antibodies directed against previous versions of *vlsE* will not be effective in eliminating organisms expressing the new variants of *vlsE*. This process keeps the spirochete one step ahead of the immune response and hence contributes to immune evastion." These alterations in *vls* structure continue, actually accelerating the longer infection persists. Over time, it gets harder and harder for the immune cells to find the spirochetal variants. (Though, in most cases, they eventually do.) As Berndtson (2013) wryly observes . . .

> *The net effect for the host is production of B-cells and plasma cells whose antibodies seek surface epitopes that are not easy to find, and whose clonal populations accumulate in lymph nodes and bone marrow where one can imagine crosstalk aimed at figuring out which way the suspects went.*

Importantly, the *degree* of antigenic variation that occurs in the spirochetes is much higher in *immunocompetent* animals than it is in the immunodeficient. In other words, the immune system itself *drives* innovation in the recombination events that occur. As Berndtson notes, "the sicker the host's immune system, the less *Bb* needs to rely on antigenic switching."

Still, the healthier the immune system is, the faster it will ultimately figure out how it's being hustled, and the sooner you get well. Importantly, in those with *very* healthy immune function, during infection there will often be few or no symptoms; and the body will clear the infection fairly quickly. (Once the immune system figures it out and clears a Lyme infection, future infection *with those strains* of *Borrelia* is rare; infection with other strains can still occur.)

The *ospC* protein, induced during the blood meal, is specific for preventing early elimination of the bacteria from the injection site as well as promoting its dissemination in the body. Once *ospC* is induced and expressed in the exterior membrane, it binds a unique tick salivary protein (Salp15) to itself. In other words, the spirochete coats its exterior membrane with that particular salivary protein – like putting on a coat during inclement weather. By coating its exterior surface with Salp15, the spirochete inhibits the complement pathway of the innate immune system. This protects the spirochete from antibody-mediated killing long enough for it to find sequestered niches that are, themselves, protected from immune attack. There it can begin its own unique diminishment of immune responses.

All the spirochetal surface proteins are highly synergistic with each other. Other surface proteins (*ospA, ospE, vlsE*) act to *protect ospC*-deficient *forms* from elimination by the immune system. Increased expression of those proteins allows *ospC*-deficient forms to widely disseminate in the host. In other words, there is not just one spirochetal form (*ospC*) injected into new hosts. There is a whole range of types, all of which do specific things, all of which are synergistic with each other.

Other substances, such as decorin-binding proteins (Dbp A and B), are upregulated as well. These proteins, also called adhesins, bind decorin (as well as other glycosaminoglycans), a small proteoglycan associated with collagen fibrils in all connective tissues. It is common in the extracellular matrix of articular cartilage that covers the bone in movable joints. Decorin is primarily composed of a glycosaminoglycan chain made of chondroitin/dermatan sulfate attached to a core protein. Decorin interacts with type I and II collagens throughout the body. (The spirochetes have other kinds of proteins that are able to bind both type IV and VI collagens.) Decorin binding aids the spirochetes in colonizing collagen sites in the new host, most importantly in the skin during the initial infection stage. (Without the decorin-binding proteins [Dpbs], the spirochetes cannot disseminate in the new host.) They also help the bacteria hide from the host immune system by, again, covering their surfaces with something the immune system does not recognize as a threat. As with most of their proteins, the spirochetes also generate subtle variations in Dpb structure. *Each of these strains has a tropism for different tissues.* Some have more affinity for heart tissues, others joints, others neurological structures.

Another glycoprotein the spirochetes bind is complement factor H (CFH), one of the most important regulators in the alternative pathway of the complement immune response. It is synthesized mainly in the liver and is an essential compound for eliminating the spirochetes from the body. By binding CFH, the spirochetes inhibit the ability of this part of the immune system from affecting them, enabling the spread of the pathogens throughout the body. It gives them a sort of "hall pass," allowing the bacteria free passage through the body. CFH primarily binds to *ospE* on the bacterial membrane.

And remember: *Borrelia* can bind multiple types of cells to its surface membrane . . . just in case. More than any other bacteria, this one believes in redundancy.

Plasminogen (as well as its activator urokinase) binding factors *(ErpA, ErpC, ErpP, CspA,* and the enzyme enolase) are also upregulated. Plasminogen is an inactive substance that circulates in the blood. It is converted at need to plasmin (by its activator urokinase). Plasmin is an enzyme that digests fibrin (helping reduce blood clots), but it is also specific for degrading large glycoproteins and many extracellular matrix (ECM) components. When plasmin is on the surface of the bacteria, it facilitates its movement from the blood through the endothelial junctions into the ECM, then facilitates the degradation of ECM components. Once in the ECM, the pathogens escape the notice of many immune cells and the antibodies that are monitoring the lymph and blood.

A different borrelial protein binds fibronectin as well as glycosaminoglycan (GAG), which like fibronectin is common on cell surfaces. GAG binding from these kinds of proteins allows colonization of joint tissues within as little as sixty minutes postinfection (as well as skin and neural tissues).

Fibronectin is common in the extracellular matrix (EM) between cells in these locations. By binding both GAG and fibronectin, *Borrelia* can easily colonize *anyplace* these substances occur. The bacteria then release (or stimulate the release of) various cytokines that cause both fibronectin and GAG to degrade, gaining the bacteria the nutrients they need to survive.

Some 154 genes are known to be altered when the spirochetes encounter a tick's blood meal. Seventy-five genes are upregulated, 79 are downregulated. As Zuckert (2013) succinctly observes . . .

> As the Lyme disease spirochete Borrelia burgdorferi *shuttles back and forth between arthropod vector and vertebrate host, it encounters vastly different and hostile environments. Major mechanisms contributing to the success of this pathogen throughout this complex transmission cycle are phase and antigenic variation of abundant and serotype-defining surface lipoproteins. These peripherally membrane-anchored virulence factors mediate niche-specific interactions with vector/host factors and protect the spirochete from the perils of the mammalian immune response.*

To enhance survivability, not all the spirochetes alter themselves in the same manner. Instead, a swarm of similar but antigenically different strains are generated, all released into the new host during tick feeding. (I am not sure this can be repeated too many times.) This ensures that many will avoid the new host's immune response, find sequestered locations in which to locate themselves, and survive to reproduce.

Lyme borreliosis: the disease

To reiterate, it is important to realize that *Borrelia* are parasites. They cannot make many of the nutrients they need to survive, so they scavenge them from their hosts. As Brisson et al. (2012) reveal . . .

> B. burgdorferi *lacks the capacity to synthesize amino acids, nucleotides, fatty acids, and enzyme cofactors. . . . Instead B.* burgdorferi *is an accomplished importer and scavenger that has at least 52 genes encoding transporters and/or binding proteins*

of carbohydrates, peptides, and amino acids. Additionally, energy is derived by glycolysis [the breaking down of sugars] and the fermentation of sugars to lactic acid, as the genes encoding the components necessary for the citric acid cycle and oxidative phosphorylation are missing.

The simplest way to get a grasp on the various symptoms the spirochetes cause is to understand that they get most of their nutrients from collagen and collagen-like substances. They seek them out in the host's body, attach to them, then degrade them, making them into a kind of soup from which they can feed. Wherever the spirochetes degrade tissues is where symptoms arise. In the joints, arthritis; in the heart, Lyme carditis; in the brain, neurological problems.

While the spirochetes can live in many places in the body, *Borrelia* have a preference for the joints, the aqueous humor of the eye (which is why so many people with Lyme disease report "floaters" as a symptom), heart tissue, the meninges of the brain, and various collagenous sites in the body (such as the skin and knees). In the brain, the spirochetes adhere to endothelial and epithelium cells, differentiated neural cells, brain cells, and glial cells. They tend to live deeper within tissues than other kinds of bacteria.

Initial stages of infection

Because ticks feed on blood, the spirochetes initially flow into the bloodstream (and the lymph) where they immediately begin moving throughout the body. Once inside the bloodstream or lymph channels, they attach themselves to the blood vessel walls and the various organs through which the blood and lymph flows (e.g., lymph nodes, heart, spleen, and liver).

They are nearly always found in capillaries, postcapillary venules, and larger veins rather than arteries, because of the shear forces involved. As Coburn et al. (2013) note: "In the case of vascular adhesion, the process being studied is subject to tremendous shear forces of circulating blood and is akin to a spider trying to gain a foothold on the [interior] wall of a garden hose with the tap turned on full." The bacteria *adhere* to the blood vessel walls. To resist the shear force they have to have tremendous adhesive capacity . . . this is provided by the bacterial *adhesins* on the surface of the spirochete body.

Once attached (or tethered as the case may be) to the vessel wall, the spirochete begins to slowly drag itself (or crawl) along the surface until it reaches its preferred location, either a particular endothelial cell or the attachment points (aka, junctions) between the endothelial cells (ECs). EC junctions tend to be a borrelial bacterium's primary adhesion site. Nevertheless, they also attach to and penetrate into endothelial cells themselves.

When attaching to a cell (rather than a junction), the bacteria stimulate their engulfment by the cell. In essence, they co-opt the normal processes that cells utilize to take substances inside themselves. As they move inside the cell, they cause the cell to create a protected compartment, a vacuole, in which the bacteria can safely reproduce. Some forty-eight hours after initial infection, the vacuoles will be filled with dozens of new spirochetes. These are then released back into the extracellular space that surrounds the cell.

Intracellular sequestering of the bacteria protects them from both immune and antibacterial assaults. Inside a cell, for example, spirochetes can resist, for a minimum of fourteen days, exposure to ceftriaxone. But the blood vessels' endothelial cells are not the only targets. Intracellular *Borrelia* have also been found in macrophages, keratinocytes, neurons, and glial cells.

The bacteria that locate to the EC junctions, instead of penetrating cells, penetrate the junctions, gaining deeper access to the body's tissues. They release (or stimulate the release of) cytokines, which cause the EC junctions to loosen, creating a doorway deeper into the body. Once the junctions open, the bacteria move through them into the extracellular matrix or ECM (which exists between cells in the body). This is a difficult niche for immune cells to penetrate and gives the bacteria protected spaces in which to live – niches in which their preferred food sources are abundant. As Berndtson (2013) comments . . .

> Bb *contains the most redundant set of chemotaxis-related genes found among eubacteria. Once inside an animal host,* Bb *uses chemoreceptor arrays at its cell poles to follow chemoattractant trails to reach specific host cells or tissue compartments. . . . Once a favorable target is reached,* Bb *uses adhesions to target molecules including glycosaminoglycans (GAGs), decorin, and fibronectin. The ECM is a mesh-like superstructure that consists of interstitial tissue, basement membranes, collagen [the most*

abundant ECM proteins], and polysaccharide gels, and it appears
to be Bb's most favored destination in mammalian hosts. The
ECM is rich with GAGs, decorin, and fibronectin. . . . Bb [has a]
predeliction for ECM tissue because it contains ample nutrition,
pathway support, environmental cues, and less immune cell and
antibody traffic than blood or lymph.

GAGs that the pathogens have an affinity for also include laminin, integrins, chondroitin sulfate, dermatan sulfate, keratin sulfate, and heparin and heparin sulfate (which is why pharmaceutical heparin can help during Lyme infections, it gives a non-self-binding substance for the bacteria to attach to).

Aggrecan is another proteoglycan common in the ECM and cartilage, particularly the articular cartilage of joints. *Borrelia* release the enzyme aggrecanase, which breaks down aggrecan into its component parts to gain nutrients. (The use of aggrecanase inhibitors can prevent this, they include, in no particular order: *Polygonum cuspidatum*; *Aralia cordata*; *Camellia sinensis*; *Cimicifuga heracleifolia*; a blend of *Clematis mandshurica*, *Tricosanthes kirilowii*, and *Prunella vulgaria*; the TCM formulation SiMiaoFang, which is composed of *Pellodendri Chinese cortex*, *Atractylodis rhizoma*, *Coicis semen*, and *Achyranthis bidentatae radix*; a blend of *Aralia cordata* and *Cimifuga heracleifolia*; and the supplements curcumin, EGCG, luteolin, chondroitin sulfate, and glucosamine.)

The bacteria can also attach to and degrade (via the enzyme hyaluronidase) hyaluronic acid (aka, hyaluronan). Hyaluronic acid (HA) is a glycosaminoglycan that is widely distributed throughout connective, epithelial, and neural tissues. It is a major component of the synovial fluid that surrounds the joints, increasing its viscosity and lubricating actions. HA aggregates are root to the resilience of cartilage (making it rubbery). It is also a major component of the extracellular matrix. HA, through a number of mechanisms, inhibits the actions of plasmin (which the Lyme bacteria also generate). HA's breakdown, as with other glycosaminoglycans, is the root of many symptoms that Lyme causes. (The use of hyaluronic acid as a supplement can help immensely; it adds back in what the spirochetes are taking out . . . and no, it won't feed the spirochetes. They are feeding themselves just fine on your body's tissues.)

During inflammatory diseases, such as various forms of arthritis (and Lyme), the use of a hyaluronidase inhibitor can reduce or even prevent the breakdown of cartilage (and synovial fluids). This increases the amount of cartilage (and fluid) in and around the joints, helping counteract, even reverse, the pathology. Some useful inhibitors are *Echinacea angustifolia* (large continuing doses), *Areca catechu*, *Lycopus lucidus*, *Scutellaria baicalensis*, *Withania somnifera*, the herbal blend *Triphala guggulu*, any plants containing rosmarinic acid – such as lemon balm and rosemary and the supplements quercetin, curcumin, and tannic acid.

HA is a major component of the skin and is integral to skin repair. HA contributes to tissue dynamics, cell movement and proliferation, and the generation of new cellular tissues. It is an essential element of granulation, that is, the new cellular tissue that slowly takes the place of the clotted blood (scab) that first forms over a wound. The more HA, the faster and better new tissue forms. Inhibiting hyaluronidase increases the amount of HA present in the skin/wound area. This is beneficial in Lyme infections because it helps the body naturally repair the collagenous structures damaged by the bacteria.

In many types of cancer, hyaluronidase (HYL) plays a major role in metastasis. It degrades the extracellular matrix and allows cancer cells to escape the main tumor mass. HYL also degrades other cellular structures, allowing the cancer cells to also penetrate them. It also plays a role in the formation of the new blood vessels that cancerous tumors need to survive. HYL inhibition then produces a particular kind of anticancer, or antitumor action. (Hyaluronidase is also found in some snake venoms. It increases the lethality of the venom, in part by allowing it to penetrate more easily into the body. This is why *E. angustifolia* is useful in treating some types of snake bite.)

Many bacteria, including *Borrelia*, create and release hyaluronidase in order to loosen the connective tissue matrix (in this case the EC junctions) and facilitate their penetration into new areas of the body – similarly to the way cancerous tumors do. Part of what echinacea does is to strengthen the structure of the mucus and skin membranes of the body by stopping their structural breakdown through HYL inhibition, while at the same time counteracting the HYL release by bacteria. This stops the bacterial movement into the body.

Borrelia are adept at seeking, and finding, cartilage and other collagenous substances and breaking them down. Radolf et al. (2012) explicate further . . .

> *To disseminate,* B. burgdorferi *penetrates the matrix between cells and enters capillary beds. The spirochete circumvents its inability to produce enzymes that are capable of digesting extra-cellular matrix components by appropriating host proteases such as plasminogen and its activator urokinase.* B. burgdorferi *also induces multiple host matrix metalloproteinases (MMPs), the major class of host proteases involved in the degradation of extracellular matrix components, from both phagocytic and non-phagocytic cells. Entry into capillaries provides* B. burg-dorferi *with access to the bloodstream [so it can continue to spread throughout the body].*

Loosening the EC junctions and penetrating into the ECM only takes about ten minutes after the initial tick bite. From that location, the spirochetes begin to spread through the skin giving rise (in those who have it) to the bull's-eye rash. You can actually track the spirochetes movement through the skin by watching the expanding zone of the rash. Over time, they begin penetrating deeper into the body. Ultimately, they have the ability to infect and damage any part of the body. This is because GAGs and collagen are present throughout the body. Muller (2012) observes . . .

> Borrelia *are capable of breaking down soluble and insoluble ground substance within the extracellular matrix. They activate metalloproteinases, cause collagen to dissolve and can colonize as microcolonies in collagen fibres. They inhibit regeneration of collagen promoted by fibronectin, and hence delay the healing process or prevent it completely. . . . The persistence of* Bb *in human ligaments was described as early as 1993. In primates,* Borrelia *have been detected in the connective tissue of the aorta, the atria, and the ventricles of the heart.*

Additionally, and not commonly part of Lyme disease thinking, spon-taneous ruptures of tendons and ligaments (collagen-heavy structures) may occur during Lyme infections. Ruptures of the tendons in the fingers, quadriceps, Achilles, and epicondylitis humeri (tennis elbow) have all been reported; spontaneous vertebrate dislocations (your back goes out) are not uncommon once the disks have been damaged. Very little physical stress is necessary for these types of Lyme-dependent ruptures to occur.

Once they spread throughout the body, finding various collagen-rich niches, the bacteria settle down to the business of breaking the collagen structures apart in order to feed and reproduce. (At each site they do this, a kind of lesion or unhealed wound forms.) To accomplish the tissue break-down, they carefully modulate the production and release of cytokines and other chemical molecules such as chemokines. (A chemokine, btw, is a cytokine with strong chemotactic actions. Really, just a cytokine by any other name. To irritate purists, I am just going to call them all cytokines.)

Note: Unfortunately, cytokine taxonomists (the offspring of asexual reproduction between plant taxonomists) are now present in the cytokine world and are happily renaming many cytokines, leading to tremendous, as usual, confusion. Hence, IL-8 is now, sometimes, CXCL8. ICAM-1 is also CD54; CXCL1 can be Gro1 or Gro*a*; MCP-1 is now CCL2; RANTES is now CCL5; MAPKs are now, sometimes, MEKs; MAPK1 is sometimes ERK1. The linguistic alterations are not consistent; I am just going with whatever journal paper I am sourcing in identifying which cytokine is present.

The cytokine profile

Borrelia stimulate cytokine production through two mechanisms: (1) direct action (they actually create the cytokine); and (2) indirect action, by stim-ulating, in specific ways, the body's own natural cytokine responses to infection.

As the spirochetes begin breaking down collagenous structures, many of those structural fragments, released in free form into the body, stimu-late cytokine release. Fibronectin breakdown, for instance, stimulates the release of ICAM-1, IL-6, CXCL1, CCL1, CCL2, and CCL5.

Some of these breakdown products, as well as fragments of killed spiro-chetes, can, from time to time, create a sort of autoimmune dynamic where the body's immune system begins to attack similar structures in the body. In short, the bacteria initiate a cytokine cascade, which is the main cause of tissue breakdown, which is itself the root of the many symptoms Lyme disease causes. They also utilize redundant mechanisms to accomplish this; it is not a simple linear process of cytokine generation (though I will sort of treat it as if it is).

A closer view

As soon as the spirochetes attach to the vascular endothelial cell surface and begin to crawl along them, the endothelial cells, through their innate pattern recognition system (PAMPs), sense the presence of flagellin, a protein that all bacteria with flagella possess. (Many pathogenic bacteria possess flagella, and over a long evolutionary time, living organisms inserted pattern recognition processes for them into their genome. This was passed down from one generation to the next, distressingly – for neo-Darwinists – a rather Lamarckian process, i.e., inheritance of acquired characteristics. The immune response then became *innate*, basically meaning we are now born with it.)

Flagellin is potently inflammatory; it stimulates the release of NF-*k*B from the endothelial cells (which is intended to begin the bacterial killing process). Normally NF-*k*B is sequestered in the cell by a group of closely related inhibitors, lumped together as I*k*B (inhibitor of *k*B). Flagellin activates a signaling process from the surface of the cell, which activates an enzyme (I*k*B kinase), which degrades I*k*B, releasing NF-*k*B from its sequestered sites. The freed NF-*k*B molecules then enter the nucleus of the cell, activating genes that generate a number of physiological responses, including inflammatory and immune responses, apoptosis of infected cells, and cellular proliferation. (The three most potent I*k*B inhibitors I know of are *Salvia miltiorrhiza*, *Cordyceps*, and *Uncaria rhynchophylla*.)

Rather than being negatively affected by it, *Borrelia*, instead, utilize the NF-*k*B response to enhance inflammation and immune cell proliferation at infection sites. They co-opt this response and use it to help them break down the tissues they want to feed from. Inhibiting NF-*k*B (by the use of I*k*B of NF-*k*B inhibitors) will shut down many of the inflammatory processes the bacteria initiate; this will reduce or eliminate many of the symptoms of Lyme infection – and, as well, inhibit the bacterial scavenging of our cellular nutrients. (NF-*k*B inhibitors include *Astragalus* spp., *Bidens* spp., *Chelidonium majus*, *Cordyceps*, EGCG [green tea], *Eupatorium perfoliatum* [boneset], *Forsythia suspensa*, *Glycyrrhiza* spp., *Houttuynia* spp., luteolin, *Olea europaea*,

Paeonia lactiflora, Polygonum cusipidatum, Polygala tenuifolia [Chinese senega] root, *Pueraria lobata, Punica granatum, Salvia miltiorrhiza* root, *Schisandra chinensis, Scutellaria baicalensis* root, *Withania somnifera,* and *Zingiber officinalis.*)

Very early in the infection process, the bacteria stimulate the release of specific types of kinases (such as I*k*B kinase). Kinases are enzymes that are used in the body to regulate cellular function and activity – essentially, and very simplistically, they turn cellular actions on and off. Protein kinases, which the borrelial bacteria appear to really like, are a subset of the kinase family, and regulate, well, proteins. A subset of those are mitogen-activated protein kinases, aka MAPKs. Three important subsets of MAPKs are ERKs, c-Jun N-terminal kinases (JNK), and p38 kinases. (As usual, terms are in a bit of flux due to taxonomitis – ERKs are sometimes referred to as classical MAPKs, sometimes as a special subset of MAPKs.) In essence, each of these subsets represents a specific *pathway* of kinase activation. Various ERKs, JNK, and p38 MAPK are primary pathways the bacteria utilize once they are in a new host. Activation of any of these pathways begins a cascade of processes in the body's biological functioning. Often the effects are complex; the subtle bacterial manipulation of these pathways often creates unique and very sophisticated effects in the body. Modulation of ERK5, for example, strongly affects the integrity of endothelial barriers. Other modulated ERKs strongly affect cardiac functioning, the integrity of neural structures in the brain, and endothelial formation throughout the body.

Borrelial bacteria have been at this for hundreds of millions of years; they are very good at it. It is useful to recognize that these bacteria are very intelligent, that they possess complex communication capabilities and are highly sophisticated tool makers . . . and users. What they do in the body is *more* sophisticated than any human scientists can accomplish, in any field.

Inhibition of ERK, JNK, and p38 MAPK can help reduce, even eliminate, the borrelial cytokine cascade and its effects. (ERK inhibitors include *Chelidonium majus, Cordyceps,* EGCG [green tea], *Olea europaea, Polygonum cusipidatum, Pueraria lobata, Scutellaria baicalensis* root. Among the JNK inhibitors are *Cordyceps, Polygonum cusipidatum, Scutellaria baicalensis* root. Some good p38 MAPK inhibitors are *Cordyceps,* EGCG [green tea], *Olea europaea, Polygonum cusipidatum, Scutellaria baicalensis* root, and a blend of *Aralia cordata* and *Cimifuga heracleifolia.*)

During infection, *Borrelia* commonly stimulate ERK, JNK, p38, and NF-*k*B in sort of that order. Flagellin upregulation of NF-*k*B and the stimulation of these kinase pathways are generally followed by the upregulation of interferon-alpha (IFN-*a*), Interleukin-10 (IL-10), IL-8, IL-1*B*, IL-6, tumor necrosis factor alpha (TNF-*a*), and metalloproteinases (MMPs). Again, sort of in that order. (Levels of these cytokines increase a minimum of ten times as soon as the body's cells are exposed to *Borrelia*.)

To reiterate however: *the bacteria utilize multiple, redundant processes to generate this cytokine cascade.* The listed, linear, order of emergence outlined above does occur. So, too, does simultaneous emergence; so, too, does emergence in a different order (MMPs right after IL-8, for example). They utilize multiple, redundant processes in order to facilitate infection and circumvent the immune response. They are very good at what they do.

And, of course, there are other, more specialized cytokines that emerge as the cascade continues. Still, these are the primary upstream cytokines Lyme infection stimulates. Interrupting their emergence, inhibiting them, is one of the most effective strategies for treating Lyme infections, especially in people for whom antibiotics have not worked. It can turn the condition around, generally within a few months, sometimes within weeks.

A bit of depth on the cytokines
Each of the cytokines the spirochetes initiate has a range of different, synergistic, and profound effects on and in the body.

IFN-alpha (a type one interferon) is a potently antiviral cytokine that possesses a number of strongly impactful effects in the body when upregulated. Abnormal expression of the cytokine (as it is during Lyme infection) contributes to tissue inflammation and organ damage throughout the body. IFN-a levels are often high in autoimmune conditions, such as lupus, rheumatoid arthritis, idiopathic inflammatory myopathies, Sjogren's syndrome, and multiple sclerosis – all conditions associated with Lyme disease. Fever, fatigue (from the cytokine's impacts on mitochondrial functioning), and leukopenia are common with high IFN-a levels. (Simply injecting people with IFN-a pharmaceuticals will create a lupus-like disease syndrome.) Many of the impacts of IFN-a come from its stimulation of indoleamine 2,3-dioxygenase (IDO – discussed in a moment).

Reducing IFN-a can reduce the cytokine cascade the bacteria initiate. There hasn't been a lot of work done on herbs or supplements that can reduce abnormal IFN-a levels, still, *Polygonum cuspidatum, Salvia miltiorrhiza, Scutellaria baicalensis,* and curcumin will all do so. However, inhibiting IDO is just as effective, and there are quite a number of natural IDO inhibitors.

Increased levels of IFN-a stimulate the production of indoleamine 2,3 dioxygenase (IDO). During neuroborreliosis, IDO levels in the brain significantly increase (as do levels of TNF-a, IL-1b, and IL-2). (Lyme bacteria also stimulate dendritic cells to produce IDO.) IDO is an enzyme that breaks apart (catalyzes) the amino acid L-tryptophan, reducing the amount of tryptophan in the body. There are a number of wide-ranging effects from this, all of which have deleterious effects in the body. This is especially true in the brain.

Among its many effects, IDO is a potent inhibitor of T cells (it also induces apoptosis of competent T cells) and it degrades tryptophan. The amounts of IDO produced and the degree of tryptophan degradation are specific indicators for the progression, and seriousness, of CNS Lyme infection. (Tryptophan supplementation can help reverse this.)

L-tryptophan, when degraded, becomes L-kynurenine, which then degrades further into three intermediary compounds. All are highly neuroactive in the brain: 3-hydroxykynurenine (3-HK), quinolinic acid (QUIN), and kynurenic acid (KYNA).

High QUIN levels in the brain will cause an overstimulation of neurons, produce excitotoxic lesions, degradation of brain tissue, high levels of reactive oxygen species in the brain, and, sometimes, seizures. The precursor to QUIN, 3-HK, is highly neurodestructive as well, causing cellular disintegration, primarily through the generation of free radicals. Neurons are particularly vulnerable to its actions.

KYNA, on the other hand, is neuroprotective and ameliorates the impacts of QUIN and 3-HK. Unfortunately, the amount of KYNA depends on healthy neuron function, which, during CNS Lyme infection, is severely inhibited. Compromised cellular energy metabolism (specifically, inhibited mitochondrial function – also common during Lyme infections) will also reduce KYNA levels significantly. (Supporting mitochondrial function is crucially important during Lyme infections.)

During CNS Lyme infection, 3-HK and QUIN levels tend to be high and KYNA levels low. Upon microglial and astrocyte activation 3-HK and QUIN levels can increase one hundred to one thousand times; this is especially true if there is the kind of macrophage infiltration that occurs during Lyme infection in the CNS. The number and seriousness of seizures, convulsions, and brain malfunction that people experience are directly proportional to the level of IDO generated in the brain (and its subsequent generation of QUIN and 3-HK).

During chronic neuroborreliosis QUIN levels in the CSF are consistently elevated (35 nmols), while during acute episodes these levels increase even more, to nearly ten times chronic levels (325 nmols). Levels in the brain are substantially higher than those in the CSF. Tests of the impact of QUIN on the brain have found that levels from 40 to 80 nmols produce little neuronal loss in the hippocampus, while 120 nmols can produce over 90 percent neuronal loss. However, when QUIN levels increase in the presence of reactive oxygen species (ROS), the ROS significantly potentiate the effects of QUIN. The addition of ROS to QUIN causes 80 percent neuronal loss in the hippocampus at 80 nmols. The levels of QUIN generally found in acute neuroborreliosis approach the low end of those found in neurological AIDS infections and AIDS dementia. (Hippocampal damage is very common during neuroborreliosis.)

Macrophages and polymorphonuclear leukocytes, human immune cells, routinely produce ROS during bacterial infections. They are potent bactericidal agents. Lyme spirochetes have been found to be exceptionally potent stimulators of ROS production, more so than other spirochetes (e.g., those that cause syphilis and leptospirosis). Additionally, *Borrelia burdorferi sensu lato* are exceptionally sensitive to alterations in oxygen levels during infection, and they actively begin to alter their gene expression and antigenic profiles to escape its effects. They do this through a specific transcriptional activator – the *Borrelia* oxidative stress response regulator or BosR.

When Lyme spirochetes invade the CNS and brain they cause a potent stimulation of QUIN by macrophages *and* significant ROS production. These two substances act synergistically to damage the CNS. In many respects, QUIN is considered a *pro*-oxidant rather than an antioxidant. It potentiates the effects of free radicals and other reactive oxygen species on tissues, especially the brain. QUIN also induces the production of nuclear factor-kappa B (NF-*k*B). NF-*k*B, in high levels in the brain, can increase inflammatory dynamics, exacerbating neuronal death.

QUIN impacts on the brain and brain function have been found to be severe. This includes such things as neurotransmitter interference, damage to the synaptic connections, brain atrophy, cerebral volume loss, and neuronal death. Strongly impacted are the hippocampus, the striatum, limbic cortex, neocortex, and amygdala. The main problems associated with these are memory and recall deficits and confusion.

Impairment of performance on memory-related tasks is consistent with elevated QUIN levels. Without specific therapies designed to protect the brain from QUIN impacts and to stimulate regeneration of damaged areas, the damage is unlikely to correct. Antibiotics alone can do nothing to either protect or help regenerate areas susceptible to the neurotoxic effects of QUIN. (The most potent herbs and supplements for protecting the brain from the effects of QUIN and reducing its levels are *Sida cordifolia, Uncaria rhynchophylla, Angelica sinensis, Scutellaria baicalensis,* melatonin, and selenium.)

Additionally, QUIN levels tend to be exacerbated in older people, a natural consequence of aging. This correlates with the more severe impacts of neuroborreliosis in older people and the tendency among them for long-term problems in memory and other cognitive functions.

IDO stimulation also has the regrettable ability to significantly inhibit serotonin and melatonin production in the brain. Melatonin, besides its potent sleep regulatory actions, is also an incredibly strong antioxidant (as is tryptophan), more powerful than many other similarly acting molecules. It is specific for deactivating the oxidants that 3-HK and QUIN create. During neuroborreliosis infections, however, melatonin levels can fall very low in the brain.

Keeping melatonin levels high will help protect neural function in the brain. Thus, increasing melatonin levels by using plants such as *Scutellaria baicalensis,* which are very high in melatonin (or even direct melatonin supplementation), can reduce the brain's vulnerability to Lyme infection and symptom picture. It can significantly help with reducing seizures; it's highly protective of the brain's neural structures. It also helps reverse the sleep disturbances common during Lyme infection.

IDO inhibitors can help reduce neuroborreliosis symptoms immensely (as well as helping reduce TNF-a levels). They help protect brain tissues and reduce symptom severity and postinfection complications. The most potent inhibitors of IDO are *Scutellaria baicalensis, Polygonum cuspidatum, Isatis* spp., and, most especially, *Crinum latifolium.*

The high levels of IDO also lower tryptophan levels in the body. Tryptophan is an essential amino acid that cannot be synthesized by the body; it has to come from outside sources. During Lyme infections, tryptophan levels can fall, and supplementation should occur. (This will *not* feed the bacteria, making the disease worse but will, in fact, help repair CNS damage.) Studies have found that exogenous tryptophan can help restore healthy T cell function and responses as well as protect brain tissues, enhance sleep, and overall well-being.

IL-8, aka CXCL8, is produced by macrophages and epithelial cells, airway smooth muscle cells, and endothelial cells. Because of the constant contact between the bacteria and the endothelial cells, IL-8 is ubiquitous during Lyme infections. IL-8 *induces* the migration of neutrophils (and some other cells) to wherever it is released. This is part of the reason that massive quantities of neutrophils are often located at the lesion sites of borrelial infection. In essence, IL-8 brings inflammatory cells to its location, stimulating the breakdown of the nearby cells. Endothelial cells are particularly sensitive to IL-8-stimulated damage. High IL-8 levels are one of the primary causes of systemic inflammation during Lyme disease. Reducing its presence has been found to significantly reduce inflammation (and cellular damage) during infection. Some of the herbs and supplements that inhibit IL-8 are: *Cordyceps,* EGCG, *Isatis* spp., NAC, *Polygonum cuspidatum, Punica granatum.* Doxycycline and minocycline are also effective in lowering IL-8 levels; their actions are dose dependant.

IL-1beta (stimulated by borrelial bacteria) is produced by activated macrophages and is processed into its active form by caspase 1 (something *Borrelia* also upregulate). IL-1beta is another primary cytokine expressed during Lyme disease. It stimulates cell proliferation, differentiation, and apoptosis. It's a common source of both chronic and acute inflammation in many conditions. IL-1beta induces the upregulation of COX2 in the central nervous system (another source of damage to neural structures). The cytokine is intimately involved in the increased sensitivity to pain that many people with Lyme often experience. Its levels are often high in a number of conditions, such as recurrent pericarditis, heart failure, and rheumatoid arthritis – all problems that can occur during Lyme infections. And it is what causes the sudden hearing loss that sometimes happens during Lyme infections. IL-1b inhibitors include *Cordyceps* spp., *Eupatorium perfoliatum*, *Polygala tenuifolia* (Chinese senega) root, *Polygonum cuspidatum*, *Pueraria lobata*, *Salvia miltiorrhiza*, and *Scutellaria baicalensis*.

IL-6 is also an inflammatory cytokine (in this situation). The cytokine is generally released by macrophages in response to bacterial infection. It also has major impacts on neurological function. IL-6 easily crosses the blood-brain barrier and stimulates the production of PGE2 in the hypothalamus, altering the body's temperature regulation processes. (This is root to the temperature problems that some people with Lyme experience.) It's one of the cytokines that potently affects the pituitary/adrenal/hypothalamus axis. IL-6 overexpression can damage, and cause the degeneration of, neurons in the peripheral and central nervous systems. Elevated levels of this cytokine are common in Alzheimer's, multiple sclerosis, lupus, meningoencephalitis, depression, cognitive decline (with brain fog), stroke, seizures, impaired hippocampal function, subacute sclerosing panencephalitis, and progressive hearing loss – all conditions associated with Lyme infection.

Constant overexpression of IL-6 in the CNS can lead to neuroanatomical and neurophysiological alterations in the CNS. The cytokine is especially damaging to hippocampal tissues, structure, and function; astrocytes and microglia. It is especially damaging to the endothelial cell junctions in the brain vasculature. In response, the cerebellum can experience progressive atrophy and loss of granular layer neurons accompanied by spongiosis, marked axonal dystrophy, and demyelination throughout the cerebellum. These changes are generally accompanied by perivascular accumulation of mononuclear cells.

Reducing or modulating IL-6 levels will reduce many of the neurological symptoms of Lyme infection. Some useful herbs for this are *Andrographis paniculata*, *Isatis* spp., *Pueraria lobata*, *Salvia miltiorrhiza*, and *Scutellaria baicalensis*. Both doxycycline and minocycline can be of use in lowering IL-6 levels. Again, the drugs' effects are dose dependent.

TNF-alpha is another cytokine intimately involved in Lyme-initiated inflammation processes in the body. It is produced by a wide range of cells including macrophages, lymphocytes, NK cells, neutrophils, mast cells, eosinophils, and, most importantly, neurons. It, too, tends to be elevated in many chronic conditions, such as Alzheimer's, depression, inflammatory bowel disease, and cancer. It is often synergistic with IL-1 and IL-6, having similar effects on the hypothalamic/pituitary/adrenal axis, as well as appetite, body temperature (fever), liver function, and insulin resistance. It is a potent chemoattractant for neutrophils and stimulates the expression of adhesions on endothelial cells. (This facilitates neutrophil attachment to endothelial cells.) Heat, swelling, pain, and redness are all common inflammation signs associated with increased TNF-a. The cytokine also stimulates higher levels of IL-10. During septic shock, high TNF-a levels are common. Some of its more damaging effects occur in the brain and CNS. Reducing TNF-a levels can sometimes help reduce many of the symptoms of Lyme, especially in the CNS. (For example, the use of a pharmaceutical TNF-a inhibitor suppressed Jarisch-Herxheimer reactions in people infected with the relapsing fever spriochete *Borrelia recurrentis* who were being treated with penicillin.) Some useful inhibitors are *Andrographis paniculata*, *Cannabis* spp., *Cordyceps* spp., *Eupatorium perfoliatum* (boneset), *Glycyrrhiza* spp. (licorice), *Houttuynia* spp., *Panax ginseng*, *Polygala tenuifolia* (Chinese senega) root, *Pueraria lobata* (kudzu), *Sambucus* spp. (elder), *Scutellaria baicalensis*, *Tanacetum parthenium* (feverfew), *Salvia miltiorrhiza*, and *Zingiber officinalis* (ginger). Both doxycycline and minocycline can be of use in lowering TNF-a levels; again, the effects are dose dependent.

Matrixmetalloproteinases (MMPs) are, more accurately, metal dependent proteases (hence the *metallo*). They are a group of enzymes that are specific for degrading extracellular matrix (ECM) components and collagen. MMPs are sometimes referred to as collagenases, in other words, enzymes that degrade collagen. They are involved in a number of other functions, including cell proliferation, migration, adhesion, and differentiation. They help angiogenesis (new blood vessel formation) by breaking apart the ECM, which allows passage through it for new vessels. Bone development, wound healing, learning, and memory are also dependent on healthy MMP function. During Lyme disease their major impacts are on collagen and ECM degradation *in every location where symptoms occur, from skin, to joint, to heart, to brain*. Malfunctions in MMP expression and behavior are linked to a wide range of pathologies, from arthritis, to neurological problems, to cerebral hemorrhage, to cancer and its metastasis, to vertebral disc problems, to atrial fibrillation and aortic aneurisms, to septic shock. They are especially damaging to the brain and CNS.

MMPs, due to their action on the ECM, facilitate the penetration of the spirochetes through extracellular matrix component barriers and subsequent degradation of the ECM. The type of MMPs that the spirochetes stimulate differs depending on a number of factors, including host immune strength, genospecies and strain type, and whether or not there are preexisting inflammatory conditions already present. (If, for example, you already have arthritic inflammation in any of your joints, the spirochetes take advantage of it, stimulating it even further for their own purposes.)

The most common Lyme-stimulated MMPs are MMP-1, -3, and -9. (MMP-2, -8, -13, and -19 are sometimes present as well). The spirochetes stimulate the monocytes and primary human chondrocytes (mature cartilage cells) in the synovial fluid to release MMP-1 and -3. The neutrophils that are called to locations of spirochete invasion release large quantities of MMP-9. Production of MMP-9 and 130 kDa gelatinase (aka MMP130) in the nervous system occur through borrelial impacts on astrocytes and microglia. During neuroborreliosis, MMP-3 is common in the spinal fluid. The MMPs in the CNS break down the myelin sheaths that surround the nerves, which is why the disease so closely resembles multiple sclerosis and other, similar, nervous system diseases.

MMPs are highly synergistic with, and need, plasminogen. The combination of these two compounds causes the most damage in infected sites. As already noted, the Lyme spirochetes possess a plasminogen-binding factor on their outer membrane. Plasminogen, in consequence, binds to their outer protein coats, which raises plasminogen concentrations wherever spirochetes are located. Once MMPs are stimulated, they synergistically interact with the plasminogen, causing significant glycosaminoglycan (GAG) and hydroxyproline release from affected structures. If the collagen being scavenged is in the joints, cartilage damage occurs. If in the heart, heart disease. If in the brain, neurological pathology. Once the GAGs are released, the spirochetes release *Borrelia* glycosaminoglycan binding protein (Bgbp). This binds GAGs to the spirochetes' protein surfaces, allowing them to more easily ingest them as a nutrient source.

MMP production, especially MMP-1 and -3, is stimulated through a unique group of Lyme-initiated pathways, all involving mitogen-activated protein kinases (MAPKs): the c-Jun N-terminal kinase (JNK), p38 mitogen-activated protein (p38), and extracellular signal-regulated kinase 1/2

(ERK 1/2). MMP-9 production occurs both through the JNK pathway and another, the protein kinase C-delta pathway.

While there are a number of herbs that can reduce the autoinflammatory conditions stimulated by MMP-1 and -3 (e.g., curcumin), the only herb that specifically blocks MMP-1 and -3 induction through these three particular pathways is *Polygonum cuspidatum*. Resveratrol (one of the plant's constituents) is also directly active in reducing MMP-9 levels through both the JNK and protein kinase C-delta pathways; it specifically inhibits MMP-9 gene transcription. Rhein, another constituent in the herb, inhibits the JNK pathway for all three MMPs: -1, -3, and -9. *Polygonum cuspidatum's* constituents also, rather easily, cross the blood-brain barrier where they exert actions on the central nervous system: antimicrobial, antiinflammatory, as protectants against oxidative and microbial damage, and as calming agents. The herb specifically protects the brain from inflammatory damage, microbial endotoxins, and bacterial infections. After more than a decade of use, we have found this one herb to be foundational for stopping the damage that *Borrelia* cause, especially in the nervous system. Once the inflammation is stopped, rebuilding the damaged neural structures can occur, restoring function and quality of life. Often times, the body's natural repair mechanisms can accomplish this on their own; other times, herbs that facilitate the rebuilding of nerve sheaths and other damaged neural structures are necessary.

Some additional MMP-9 inhibitors are *Cordyceps*, EGCG, NAC, *Olea europaea*, *Punica granatum*, *Salvia miltiorrhiza*, and *Scutellaria baicalensis*. *Cordyceps* is also a MMP-3 inhibitor; *Punica granatum* inhibits MMP-1 and -3.

Inhibiting MMP production stops most of the breakdown of collagenous structures in the body, inhibits GAG releases, and will often halt the development of the disease. If the bacteria cannot breakdown collagen, they cannot feed. If they cannot feed, they cannot reproduce and spread.

IL-10, Th1, and Th2 function in Lyme disease

IL-10 is an important cytokine for many of the stealth pathogens in the Lyme-group. Normally, IL-10 is part of the Th2 response to infection. It's usually upregulated *after* infections have been controlled by Th1 cytokines. (It's also known as human cytokine synthesis inhibitory factor; it's primarily an anti-inflammatory cytokine.) It's main purpose is to downregulate the Th1 inflammation that occurred while fighting the infection. However,

A BRIEF LOOK AT TH1 AND TH2

One of the primary strategies of the Lyme-group of microbes is their ability to shift human immune responses from a Th1 dynamic to Th2. T helper cells (abbreviated Th) are a specific form of T cell (named such because they mature in the thymus and tonsils . . . you didn't have your tonsils out, did you?). T cells are white blood cells that become active during certain kinds of infections; there are a number of different kinds, among them T helper cells. Th cells, well, they help other white blood cells do their job. (They are also known, just to make us grouchy, as CD+4 T cells – because they have a CD4 glycoprotein on their cellular surface. And CD? It means "cluster of differentiation." Knowing this doesn't add anything useful, does it?) Once stimulated, Th cells rapidly reproduce and begin generating a range of cytokines to help deal with infections. Th1 cells usually stimulate highly inflammatory, very active cytokines. There are, of course, a number of different kinds of Th cells, not just Th1 and Th2. There's Th3, and Th9 and Th17, and so on. Each subgroup has evolved to deal with different kinds of infections. (Th17 cells are apparently upregulated as an intermediary process facilitating Th1 and Th2 immune shifting; the bacteria also modulate this immune response to some extent.) Th1 cells are specific for intracellular infections; that is, infections from microbes that hide inside other cells (as most of the Lyme-group do). It's not surprising then that, long ago, most of this bacterial group learned

to subvert Th1 responses, shifting them to a mostly Th2 dynamic. (Th2 responses are normally intended to deal with intestinal parasites such as nematodes; they also are specific for reducing upregulated and overactive Th1 responses.) The shift from Th1 to Th2 facilitates infection by the Lyme-group of stealth pathogens and strongly inhibits an effective immune response. A polarized Th2 response is also common in many autoimmune diseases such as lupus and systemic sclerosis. This is part of why so many of the Lyme-group of infections appear to be an autoimmune disorder. (Generally, with this group of infections, it is not an "auto" immune disorder; it is specifically created and modulated by the bacteria . . . it can be reversed.) Unsurprisingly, each Th group initiates different cytokine profiles. Th1 cells tend to generate IFN-gamma, IL-12, and TNF-a; Th2 tends to produce IL-4, IL-5, IL-10, and IL-13. Inhibiting IL-10 can force the infection away from the Th2 dynamic and back into Th1, which is necessary for the immune system to be able to clear the infection. (*Caveat*: In long-term, chronic Lyme infections, the Th1/Th2/Th17 dynamic becomes very strange. Th17 is used to modulate a combination of very high Th1 and Th2 responses. So, very high IFN-gamma levels can occur, but they do nothing to stop the infection, which they would do in earlier stages. This is why astragalus, which can stimulate IFN-gamma production, will sometimes make chronic infections worse.)

many stealth pathogens (such as *Borrelia*) carefully modulate the entire cyto-kine profile and Th1/Th2 dynamic. This makes the immune response inef-fective, allowing continued spirochete feeding and reproduction. Borrelial stimulation of IL-10 production is an intimate part of the bacterial strategy.

Tick salival proteins begin the process, shifting the human immune response into a Th2 dynamic. During infection, the *Borrelia* modulate the system to keep it that way (primarily by utilizing the ERK 1/2 and p38 pathways). As Jarefors et al. (2006) comment: "We have found that the spontaneous cytokine secretion in patients with a history of chronic LB is Th2-dominated."

Some conditions associated with Lyme disease, such as cutaneous marginal zone B-cell lymphomas, can only occur in the long-term Th2 environment that *Borrelia* stimulate. Suppression of Th2 dynamics have been found to lower spirochete load. In fact suppression of other Th2 cyto-kines (IL-4 and -5) prior to tick attachment results in significantly decreased spirochete burdens in the joints, bladder, heart, CNS, and skin. (*Astragalus* and *Glycyrrhiza*, aka licorice, will both lower IL-4 and -5; *Tanacetum parthe-nium* will lower IL-4.)

During the very early stages of Lyme infection, the body upregulates IFN-gamma, a very potent Th1 cytokine. But during many Lyme infec-tions, the bacteria counter it fairly quickly. As Binder et al. (2012) note . . .

> The first immune response almost clears the infection. However, approximately one week post infection, the bacterial popu-lation recovers and reaches an even larger size before entering the chronic phase. . . . The mathematical model predicts that Borrelia *recovers from the strong initial immune response by the regrowth of an immune-resistant sub-population of the bacteria. The chronic phase appears as an equilibrium of bacterial growth and adaptive immunity.*

IL-10 upregulation is part of how they accomplish the downregulation of IFN-Gamma and other Th1 responses. By keeping IL-10 high, they keep a long-term, chronic infection ongoing.

IL-10-deficient mice (meaning they can't make it) have much lower infec-tion levels and clear the disease much more quickly than IL-10-functional mice. Persisting symptoms have been continually linked to a decreased expression of Th1 immune responses. As Chung et al. (2013) comment . . .

> Our previous studies indicate that virulant Bb can potently enhance IL-10 production by macrophages and that blocking IL-10 production significantly enhances bacterial clearance. . . . skin-associated APC types, such as macrophages and dendritic cells are potent producers of IL-10 in response to Bb, which may act in autocrine fashion to suppress APC responses critical for efficient Bb clearance. . . . both APCs rapidly produce IL-10 upon exposure to Bb [and] these levels inversely correlate with the production of many of Lyme-relevant proinflammatory cytokines and chemokines.

Remodulating (or decreasing) the IL-10 and Th2 response will reduce many of the Lyme symptoms and help eliminate the organisms from the body. A number of herbs are excellent for this. They include: *Glycyrrhiza* (downregulates IL-10, acting primarily as an immune modulator and tonic), standardized *Silybum marianum*, aka milk thistle, seed (silymarin inhibits IL-10 overexpression and helps support endothelial health), *Cannabis sativa* (ibid), *Scutellaria baicalensis* (downregulates IL-10 and Treg), plants containing scopoletin (an IL-10/Th2 downregulator) such as noni, manaca, passion flower (*Passiflora* spp.), stevia, *Artemisia* spp. (especially *A. scopria* and *A. capillaris*), nettle leaf (*Urtica dioca*), and black haw (*Viburnum prunifolium*). However, the best is by far *Withania somnifera*, aka ashwagandha, which very specifically *modulates* IL-10 expression (it doesn't simply downregulate it).

However . . . a note . . .

In late-stage or long-term Lyme infection (sometimes called "chronic" Lyme), the cytokine profile alters. Th1 cytokines can begin to proliferate, for example, at the sites of lesions in the synovial tissue and CNS. During late-stage conditions, enhancing Th1 responses can make the conditions worse. Hence . . . if you take *Astragalus* long term if you live in an endemic area, you will keep your Th1 immune function extremely robust. This can reduce the likelihood of Lyme infection; if you do become infected, the symptom picture will often be mild. However . . . taking *Astragalus* or any immune herb that *stimulates* Th1 activity can sometimes make the condition worse. The problem, of course, is how to tell a long-term (mostly) Th1 semidominant, autoimmune-like process in chronic Lyme and simply a later stage of a Th2 dominant Lyme infection. Essentially, if you take *Astragalus* and you feel worse, you are in the late stages. (This is often the only way to tell.) *Astragalus can* modulate Th1/Th2 dynamics, but it does not do so for all people, in some it simply aggravates the Th1 late-stage dynamics.

Other cytokines

Borrelia do stimulate many other cytokines, but the majority of them are downstream. We have found that interrupting or modulating the ones already mentioned will do the most to reduce or eliminate symptoms during Lyme infection. In our experience, constantly suppressing the Lyme-driven cytokine cascade can lead, in nearly all situations, to one of three outcomes: (1) remission of the disease; (2) a complete cessation of symptoms, or; (3) at the least, a considerable reduction in symptoms.

Here is a list of the other downstream cytokines often found to be present during Lyme infections: IL-7, IL-9, IL-12, IL-17, IL-18, IL-22, IL-23, CCL2, CCL3, CCL4, CCl5, CCL20, CXCL1, CXCL2, CXCL5, CXCL9, CXCL10, CXCL13, G-CSF, COX-2, PGE-2, PGD(2), TGF-beta, and MCP-1.

Immune evasion: encysted (atypical) forms and biofilms

I have already talked a bit about the ability of spirochetes to find protected niches in which to hide from our immune responses. *Borrelia* have a plethora of such responses, most of them driven when hostile (or adverse) events occur in their environment. As Berndtson (2013) notes, the bacteria, "when confronted with certain tissue-specific antibodies, seek cover in more defensive locations within that tissue region and in the process, inflammation resolves at least temporarily." So, one of the things that occurs is that, in the face of a robust immune response, the bacteria quickly translocate to harder-to-find niches, reduce their activity, and the infectious condition appears to resolve. Once the hostile environmental factors (in this case, human antibody response) reduce their activity, the bacteria emerge and become active once more.

Antibiotics are another source of negative environmental pressure. One of the reasons that long-term antibiotic use can alleviate some cases of Lyme disease is that the bacteria, in response to the constant presence of antibiotics, become niche-bound and reduce their activity. As well, some kinds of antibiotics (e.g., doxycycline and minocycline) will directly reduce levels of some of the cytokines that have been released. Once the antibiotics are stopped, the bacteria become active once more, and cytokine levels rise again.

Still, the capacities of the spirochetes go far beyond this. They can alter their form considerably, making themselves more capable of withstanding both antibiotics and immune responses. Two of their primary strategies for this are encysted forms and biofilms.

Encysted and atypical forms

A number of imaging techniques have found that spirochetes, including *Borrelia*, can take on a variety of forms when confronted with adverse conditions. (Nevertheless, adverse conditions are not essential to this: borrelial organisms *always* create *some* encysted forms during infection; it is one of the techniques they use to ensure continued infection in a new host.) Adverse events include such things as our natural immune response and/ or the use of antibiotics. Doxycycline, for example, will reduce spirochetal forms by 90 percent but it *immediately doubles* the numbers of round body (atypical) forms. The transition into an encysted form, btw, takes virtually no metabolic activity. It appears to be an autonomic genomic response to adverse environmental events.

Atypical forms that have, so far, been observed include cystic, rolled, knob-shaped, looped, ring-shaped, globular, spherical, and granular. (Despite being sometimes referred to as cell-wall-deficient forms, *they are not* deficient. They do in fact have cell walls. The term "L-forms," another strange misnomer, is not because they are in the shape of an L but because they were first noticed at the Lister institute – hence L or Lister forms.) The atypical forms of spirochetes are more properly generalized under the inclusive term "round bodies." That term encompasses, as Brorson et al. (2009) note, "coccoid bodies, globular bodies, spherical bodies, granules, cysts, L-forms, sphaeroplasts, or vesicles." Or as Merilainen et al. (2015) describe it . . .

> *Previously, the spherical round bodies (RBs) of* B. burgdor-feri *have been ambiguously named in various ways. These terms include cell wall deficient (CWD) and L-forms, sphero-*

plasts, protoplasta, propagules, and even cysts. Nonetheless, all of these labels describe the same spherical structures. This terminology is confusing and makes presumptions about the biochemical and morphological characteristics of B. burgdorferi RBs, such as a lack of cell wall (CWD, spheroplasts, and protoplasts), or that these forms are encysted within a capsulated outer membrane (cysts).

Simplistically (and more accurately), it makes sense to think of borrelial bacteria as having three primary forms: (1) normal spirochetal forms; (2) round bodies; and (3) blebs – aka granules. (Biofilm communities might, and probably should, be considered a fourth form.) An important point to keep in mind, however, is that many of these "round body" forms are in fact unique atypical forms of the bacteria, each designed to endure hostile assaults. They are, all of them, able to generate new, motile spirochetes once the hostile assault ceases. And while many of these forms have been seen during in-depth analysis of Lyme-infected tissue, their *functions*, for the most part, are unknown. What is being discovered, however, confronts many of the underlying beliefs about the nature of bacteria present in old-Lyme thinking (see discussion of granular forms, below).

The physical alteration, from normal spirochetal forms to round bodies, is also very fast. As Berndtson (2013) comments, "Atypical forms were seen within 1 hour of exposure to environmental stress." In these infections, he continues . . .

[l]arge colony-like aggregates formed that were anti-Bb positive. Extracellular and intracellular ring-shaped spherical forms stained positive for OspA antibody. Blebs were seen emerging from coiled as well as rolled spirochete forms. When atypical forms were transferred from stressed neuronal cultures to the friendly BSK2 medium, typical spiral forms of Bb were eventually recovered.

The longer the hostile environment lasts, the more atypical forms that emerge. They continue to increase for every hour of environmental pressure that is put on them. By the end of one week, the majority of the spirochetes in a pharmaceutically treated Lyme infection will show atypical morphology.

Blebs, btw, are protrusions or bulges of the membrane of a cell extruding through a weak spot in the cell wall – a sort of cellular hernia. Often generated through what is referred to as a "budding" process, blebs emerge from and then separate from the cell, taking some of the cellular cytoplasm or other cellular contents with them. Borrelial blebs (which may more properly be considered to be *granules*) have been found to contain spirochetal surface proteins and both linear and circular DNA. Merilainen et al. comment that borrelial "blebs were revealed to be an intermediate stage between the spirochete and the round body." Miklossy et al. (2008) describe the granular forms that the spirochetes take on . . .

> *Minute granules are liberated from the periplasmic sheath through budding and extrusion . . . These spore-like minute granules may pass the 0.2 um "China" filter* [making them almost submicroscopic] *and can grow into young spirochetes. The newly formed spirochetes are delicate L or metacyclic forms [i.e., round bodies].*

In other words, similarly to some plants that can spread from any tiny root parts that break off and are left in the soil, spirochetes, when they granulate, extrude tiny parts of themselves that will, when environmental conditions improve, produce new spirochetes. As Miklossy et al. continue . . .

> *These various atypical forms were suggested to be part of a complex developmental cycle, a form of resistance to adverse conditions, and a source for reproduction under more favorable conditions.*

The concept "a complex developmental cycle" is important here. Old-Lyme thinking has tended to view borrelial bacteria through the lens of "normal" bacteria, but they aren't. It is probably more accurate to think of these "atypical" forms as a typical elements in the spirochetes' evasion and survival strategies *as well as* unique forms of spirochete reproduction that can take place during hostile environmental assaults. (*Note:* Round body, or encysted forms, are also known as persister cells. Persister cells are metabolically inert; they are antibiotic-tolerant (as opposed to resistant). During infection about 1 percent of all bacterial cells are persisters. There are more of them in biofilms, the longer the biofilm exists, the more of them there are. Environmental stress or insult stimulates significant numbers of persisters to form; once the insult is removed they take on normal forms and begin to reproduce once more.)

Analysis of cyst form formation has shown that when environmental conditions turn hostile, the spirochete ceases its worm-like behavior and rolls up into a tight ball inside the outer membrane sheath. The sheath then shrinks tightly around the rolled spirochete. Borrelial spirochetes, as Merilainen et al. describe it, "have an elastic outer wall which expands and allows the folding of the protoplasmic cylinder within the cell. This leads to the transformation of the spirochetal corkscrew morphology to a spherical shape."

In this form, the bacteria are almost completely metabolically inert, essentially in a hibernating state, similar to plant seeds. And like plant seeds, they continue to monitor their external environment, seeking the moment it becomes nonhostile once more. When conditions improve, they emerge from their cystic forms and begin spreading throughout the body again.

Various genera and species of spirochetes can survive up to three years in encysted forms, returning to spiral forms when conditions improve. As Brorson et al. (2009) comment: "*Borrelia vincentii* RBs that had remained in their 'granular' form for 31 months converted to helical motile spirochetes when transferred to fresh medium under conditions favorable for growth." Old-Lyme-thinking physicians commonly insist that these forms of *Borrelia* have no clinical relevance (where have I heard that before?); nevertheless, as Brorson et al. – a group that, significantly, includes Lynn Margulis – note . . .

> *Anglophone medical discussion of spirochetoses . . . omit mention of "round bodies" or state that they have no clinical relevance. Yet evidence abounds not only that RBs are viable but also that they may locomote, grow, and reproduce.*

In other words, the wide variety of forms the bacteria take on persist and are viable. They are *not* irrelevant.

Antibiotics have mixed impacts on RB forms. Doxycycline, as mentioned, will reduce spirochete loads by ~90 percent, but the antibiotic causes a doubling of the number of RBs that are produced. And more, doxycycline is not effective against RBs – it can't kill them. Amoxicillin will reduce spirochete load by ~85 to 90 percent *and* RB forms by ~68 percent. Motronidazole will lower RB levels by ~80 percent and spirochetal forms by ~90 percent. Tigecycline and tinidazole will lower both spirochetal and RB forms by ~80 to 90 percent. (Thus one of the better combinations of antibiotics could be doxycycline and tinidazole.)

Because of the concern over atypical forms, including cysts (which sometimes rises to hysterical levels on Internet sites), it is important to note here that other bacteria besides spirochetes encyst or create spore-like forms, so do protozoa, and other microorganisms. As Merilainen et al. (2015) note . . .

> B. burdorferi *sensu lato is pleomorphic being able to change its morphology as a response to environmental conditions. . . . Today it is well known that many Gram-negative and Gram-positive bacteria can spontaneously or by stimulation change their morphology both in vitro and in vivo.*

The important point here is that atypical forms have been around for a very long time. They did not just suddenly show up with Lyme bacteria. Our bodies have been dealing with them for a very long evolutionary time. Thus, the human immune system, when healthy, is very good at killing encysted forms. Neutrophil extracellular traps (NETs), which are formed by neutrophils as part of their sophisticated immune strategy (discussed in a bit of depth below), trap round bodies within them and kill them just fine. (Supporting healthy immune function, again, is essential when dealing with stealth pathogens.)

And crucially, plants have been infected by these atypical forms for millions of years. Plants can't call the doctor or go to the hospital, they have to make their own medicines, and they are very good at it. They have been treating encysted forms for far longer than the human species has existed and they do so effectively. The hysteria over encysted forms (and biofilms), promoted by some in the Lyme world, is *not* an emotional necessity.

NETs

Neutrophils freely circulate in the blood vessels and are called to sites of inflammation during microbial infections. For a very long time, neutrophils were viewed through a fairly simplistic (i.e., stupid) lens as being nothing more than dumb suicide killers of pathogens. Specifically, they simply enveloped (phagocytosed) pathogens and killed them. However, this view, in the past decade or so, has come under increasing scrutiny; it is in fact wrong. Neutrophils orchestrate an extremely complex response to microbial pathogens. Among them is the recently discovered capacity to create neutrophil extracellular traps or NETs for trapping and killing microbes.

NETs are formed by neutrophils on contact with many microbes (including a large variety of protozoa), as well as activated platelets, and a number of inflammatory stimuli. Once stimulated in this way, a major alteration in the structure of the neutrophil cells occurs. The cells begin to unwind and then extrude their DNA as well as histones (and a few other substances) to form a kind of net or spiderweb or cage that traps pathogens within it. In essence, the DNA is unspooled and used, along with the histones, to create a web work to entrap pathogens. NETs are able to trap nearly all types of pathogens, including those too large to phagocytose, among them Gram-negative and -positive bacteria, viruses, protozoa, and yeasts.

To generate NET formation, a number of enzymes, held in special granules in the neutrophils, at the moment of contact with a pathogen, are released. Neutrophil elastase (NE) and myeloperoxidase (MPO) are two of the most crucial. They break apart the DNA-histone formation and initiate their extrusion into the extracellular space. Once the NET forms, a number of compounds – NE, MPO, cathepsin G, proteinase 3, lactoferrin, calprotectin, and numerous antimicrobial peptides – are also released into the extracellular space. These act to kill the pathogens held inside the NETs. The histones integrated into the NET webs disintegrate the pathogen cell wall membranes, making them more susceptible to these microbial killing compounds.

A vital immune system enhances the ability of neutrophils to form NETs, ultimately clearing the *Borrelia*, no matter the form, from the body.

Biofilms

The twentieth century's early bacterial work was terribly flawed, for many reasons. One simple one is that scientists were working with acute bacterial infections, *not* chronic (something they still know little about). During acute bacterial infections, as Berndtson (2013) notes, "the microbes responsible involve a single species that disseminated in a planktonic, free-floating fashion. In chronic infections," on the other hand, "infectious microbes are found in biofilms – complex polymicrobial communities embedded within an exopolymeric gel."

In other words, the bacteria make cities (this is especially common with mouth/dental pathogens, which is where the most research has occurred – dental plaque is a biofilm). Some biofilm communities, such as those at the bottom of oceans, actually make insulated cables and run electricity through them to heat their cities. (Yes, it's true.) Bacteria are quite different than we have been led to believe. As James Shapiro (2006), at the University of Chicago, reveals . . .

> Forty years experience as a bacterial geneticist have taught me that bacteria possess many cognitive, computational and evolutionary capabilities unimaginable in the first six decades of the twentieth century. Analysis of cellular processes such as metabolism, regulation of protein synthesis, and DNA repair established that bacteria continually monitor their external and internal environments and compute functional outputs based on information provided by their sensory apparatus. . . . My own work on transposable elements revealed multiple widespread bacterial systems for mobilizing and engineering DNA molecules. Examination of colony development and organization led me to appreciate how extensive multicellular collaboration is among the majority of bacterial species. [Studies] show that bacteria utilize sophisticated mechanisms for intercellular communication and even have the ability to commandeer the basic cell biology of "higher" plants and animals to meet their own basic needs. This remarkable series of observations requires us to revise basic ideas about biological information processing and recognize that even the smallest cells are sentient beings.

"Sentient beings." A revolutionary recognition that contradicts *everything* that most people, and most scientists, currently believe about bacteria. Shapiro concludes his twenty-three page paper with this remarkable statement:

> The take-home lesson of more than half a century of molecular microbiology is to recognize that bacterial information processing is far more powerful than human technology. . . . These small cells are incredibly sophisticated at coordinating processes involving millions of individual events and at making them precise and reliable. In addition, the astonishing versatility and mastery bacteria display in managing the biosphere's geochemical and thermodynamic transformations indicates that we have a great deal to learn about chemistry, physics, and evolution from our small, but very intelligent, prokaryotic relatives.

Biofilms are closely knit bacterial communities similar in nature and structure to our cities. And like our cities, they provide bacteria protection from hostile outside forces. This is why bacteria *in* biofilms are much less susceptible to antibiotics than bacteria *outside* biofilms. Despite antibiotic treatment (for example, with doxycycline, amoxicillin, metronidazole, or tigecyceline), viable borrelial organisms are still detectable in biofilms 70 to 85 percent of the time. As Sapi et al. (2011) note, "only tinidazole reduced viable organisms by ~90%." McAuliffe et al. (2006) take this further, commenting that . . .

> [u]nattached bacteria can be cleared by antibiotics and phagocytes and are normally susceptible to antibiotics. However, adherent biofilm cells are resistant to antibiotics, antibodies, and phagocytes. In addition, biofilms can cause host damage as phagocytes are attracted but phagocytosis is frustrated, and phagocytic enzymes are released which damage surrounding tissue and exacerbate infection. As well as enabling chronic infection of hosts, biofilms may cause bouts of acute infection when planktonic cells are periodically released from the biofilm.

(Btw, that last sentence is important.)

During the initial stages of borrelial infection, a small percentage of the bacteria (about 2 percent) immediately form biofilm aggregates (just as a certain percentage encyst, create multiple strains, sequester themselves in hard-to-locate niches, or become intracellular).

Borrelial biofilms include a complex mix of microbes (including other bacteria) that continually alter the structure of the colony (just as we remodel our cities over time). The extracellular matrix of the biofilm (the city itself) is composed of sulfated and nonsulfated forms of polysaccharide, including alginate. This forms a viscous gum, which, additionally, provides the bacteria with nutrients. (They don't have to leave home to eat.) Calcium is often mixed with the alginate to form a dense outer shell. (Think crab or lobster – or dental plaque.) Biofilm fragments often break off from the main core and disseminate to other parts of the body, much like cancer when it metastasizes.

> *Something to keep in mind is that aggressively breaking up pathogenic biofilms will release bacteria, bacterial fragments, and biofilm fragments into the body, sometimes in large numbers. This can cause a massive worsening of symptoms. And further . . .*

It is important to keep in mind that there are *healthy* biofilms in our bodies that are crucial to us remaining healthy. As Xing et al. (2005) comment . . .

> Lactobacillus *and* Bifidobacterium *are main components of the anaerobic bacterial biofilm in the intestinal tract, which, as an important part of the intestinal mucosal barrier, could prevent adhesion of transient pathogens to the surface of epithelial cells and mucin associated with the intestinal wall and limit the overgrowth of aerobic gram-negative enteric bacilli (mainly* Enterobacteria) *in the intestinal tract. The structural and functional damage of the intestinal mucosal barrier may increase its permeability to macromolecules and bacteria, thus contributing to the elevation of plasma endotoxin and [bacterial translocation] to multiple organs.*

An overly exuberant attempt to "break up biofilms" in an attempt to more effectively treat a Lyme infection will also break up these types of biofilms leading not to better health but to more problems, especially in gut permeability. The important thing to remember, again, is that plants have been dealing with biofilms for millions of years; they are pretty good at it. A number of the herbs listed (in a moment) for treating biofilms are already part of suggested Lyme protocols. They will, indeed, *slowly* break up the borrelial biofilms and, over time, help eliminate them.

One of the main factors leading to biofilm formation is quorum sensing. In essence, when enough bacteria exist in somewhat close proximity they can tell that a "quorum" is present, that is, enough to form a multimicrobial colony. As Berndtson (2013) puts it: "Quorum sensing refers to the ability of taxonomically diverse microbes to detect cell density thresholds and release diffusible signals that in turn, induce changes in gene expression involving other species in the vicinity." Bacteria, when they sense a quorum is present, release autoinducer molecules (specific kinds of pheromones) that begin the process of biofilm formation.

The ability to create biofilms is one of the primary strategies that *Borrelia* utilize to create long-term, chronic conditions. Nevertheless, it is important to remember that plants have been dealing with this particular bacterial strategy for hundreds of millions of years. There are many herbs (and supplements) that are effective for breaking up biofilms or inhibiting quorum sensing. The main ones to utilize in Lyme infections are, in my opinion, *Andrographis paniculata, Houttuynia cordata, Polygonum cuspidatum, Rhodiola* spp., *Scutellaria baicalensis*, apigenin, and the supplements N-acetyl cysteine (NAC) and resveratrol.

Others include *Achillea millefolium, Achyranthes aspera, Aegle marmelos, Boesenbergia rotunda, Capparis spinosa, Cassia siamea, Chelidonium majus, Coccina grandis, Dendrophtheoe falcata, Dolichos lablab, Embelia ribes, Emblica officinalis, Epimedium brevicornum, Glycyrrhiza* spp., *Juniperus* spp., *Lonicera* spp., *malus pumila, Melaleuca alternifolia, Mentha piperata, Nigella sativa, Paeonia lactiflora, Piper sarmentosum, Plectranthus barbatus, P. ecklonii, Rhodomyrtus tomentosa, Rosmarinus officinalis, Salvadora persica, Sclerocarya birrea* (bark decoction), *Zingiber*, the compound Chinese formulation Baifuqing, berberine-containing plants, the Chinese formulation TanReQing, and the supplements piperine, royal jelly, and curcumin. There are a lot of them.

Biofilms are *not* the problem they have been made out to be . . . except for protocols that *only* use antibiotics to treat the infection.

CHAPTER SIX

A CLOSER LOOK AT NEUROBORRELIOSIS

The group of bacterial species represented by Lyme disease pathogens has one of the most complex and variable genomic architectures among prokaryotes. [The bacteria show] frequent recombination within and limited gene flow among geographic populations. . . . The coexistence of a large number of genomic groups within local B. burgdorferi s.l. populations may be driven by immune-mediated diversifying selection targeting major antigen loci as well as adaption to multiple host species.
Qiu and Martin, 2014

Borrelia burgdorferi *can also persist in the brain in chronic neuroborreliosis and, in analogy to* Treponema pallidum, *may cause dementia, cortical atrophy, and amyloid deposition.*
Miklossy et al., 2008

As mentioned earlier, the most significant problems we have seen from Lyme infections over the years is neurological. The subtle bacterial manipulations that occur in the brain and central nervous system (CNS) are rarely amenable to pharmaceuticals. Understanding the complex dynamics that occur in the brain during neuroborreliosis gives a clearer picture of the symptoms that often occur; it also helps in designing effective interventive protocols.

Neuroborreliosis
I am not going to go into much depth on the skin and arthritic dynamics of Lyme infection (as I did in the first edition of this book), though there will be some depth on the intervention protocols for symptom alleviation of

Lyme arthritis and a few skin problems in the treatment section. We have found over the past decade that dermatoborreliosis and Lyme arthritis are more amenable to fairly simple treatment interventions. (Yes, I know, not always, but usually.) Neuroborreliosis, on the other hand, tends to be more difficult; most of the people who have contacted us over the years are struggling with unremitting neurological impairments of one sort or another. A deeper look at neuroborrcliosis will also highlight both dermatoborreliosis and Lyme arthritis because the spirochete strategies are similar in all three pathologies (as they are for all areas of the body they infect).

The meninges

Before the spirochetes find their way into the brain, they have to pass through the meninges, the three membranes that surround and protect the brain and spinal cord. (The membranes are, respectively, the dura mater, the arachnoid, and the pia mater.) Once they enter the meninges, the first symptom they cause is often meningitis.

Meningitis means an inflammation of any or all of these membranes. One of its symptoms is meningismus (stiff neck), another is headache. Lymphocytic meningitis (meaning it comes from lymphocytes), another aspect of Lyme infection in the CNS, comes from dense collections of lymphocytes (white blood cells) accumulating in the meninges as they try to fight the infection. (This can occur in the brain as well.)

The dura mater ("tough mother" – you had to say it didn't you?) is a thick, tough membrane that adheres to the skull (in the spinal cord it is separated from the bone by the epidural space, which contains fat and blood vessels). It contains the larger blood vessels that split into capillaries in the pia mater and feed the brain.

The arachnoid ("spider-like") is attached to the dura mater and lies between the pia and the dura.

The subarachnoid space lies between the arachnoid and the pia mater; it's filled with cerebral spinal fluid – which is sometimes tapped and examined for the presence of spirochetes. There aren't very many of the bacteria most times and they are hard to find – such testing is not a useful diagnostic for the most part. There is a blood-spinal fluid barrier, similar to the blood-brain barrier,

and the spirochetes break it down, too. Ninety percent of people
with neuroborreliosis have impaired blood/CSF barrier function.

Unlike the pia mater, the meningeal layer closest to the brain, the arachnoid layer, doesn't follow the convolutions of the brain; it looks somewhat like a loosely fitting sack. There are a large number of very fine filaments that flow from the arachnoid, through the arachnoid space, blending into the tissue of the pia. (Because of this, the pia mater and the arachnoid are sometimes referred to as one unit, the leptomeninges, literally meaning "thin meninges" – researchers know big words.) These thin filaments (trabeculae) are dense collagenous tissues, which are often infected, and broken down, by spirochetes during neuroborreliosis. It's the most commonly infected part of the meninges.

The pia mater ("tender mother") adheres to the brain and spinal cord (nervous system tissue). It's very thin and bonds tightly to the surface of the brain, following all its contours. The blood vessels that feed the brain flow through the pia mater and into the brain. Generally, spirochetes can degrade the endothelial junctions in any of these blood vessels and pass through them into the underlying structures, in this case, the brain.

Movement through the blood-brain barrier
Shortly after tick bite, spirochetes enter the new host (unfortunately, this time, it's us). During the process, the bacteria are hidden from the immune response by tick salivary protein Salp15 (with which they have covered their body). Protected, they begin circulating through the body in both the blood and lymph, which they access from the tick penetration site.

The lymph system quickly takes them to the closest lymph nodes (and ultimately into the spleen, liver, heart, and bone marrow). The spirochetes immediately begin to accumulate in the lymph nodes' cortical regions. There they stimulate, as Hastey et al. (2014) comment, a "rapid and strong tissue enlargement, a loss of demarcation between B cell follicles and T cell zones, and an unusually large accumulation of B cells." In other words, they alter the normal lymph node cell structure while at the same time promoting the migration of naive B cells from the bone marrow into the nodes.

During this initial period of infection, the bacteria are still stimulating a Th1 immune response. Thus the increase in Th1 cytokines (such as

IFN-gamma) and B cell production, their migration and localization in the lymph nodes.

The lymph nodes *may* (but will not always) enlarge, sometimes considerably (think golf ball size or larger), during this process.

The borrelial-induced alterations in the node architecture, along with altered production of important cytokines (such as CCR7, CXCL13, and the B cell survival factor – BAFF) inhibit the capacity of the body's B cells to fight the infection.

At the same time that the immune responses in the nodes are altered, the bacteria use the bloodstream to carry them deeper into the body. At this early stage, they generally locate in just four other areas: skin, joints, heart, and the neurological structures in the periphery and brain. (Though, of course, they can infect any place in the body where collagenous tissues exist, which is pretty much everywhere.) Although they can cause severe disruption in any of these areas (e.g., the heart), the brain and central nervous system are often the most significantly damaged.

Because the blood circulates incredibly quickly through the body, it takes very little time for the blood-borne spirochetes to travel into the regions surrounding the brain. It is here that they encounter the blood-brain barrier (BBB).

Because of my predilection for four-year-old thinking, I have always visualized the BBB as something like a shield that surrounds the brain so that no blood can get into it; a barrier at the brain that keeps blood out. Blood-brain *barrier*. Nevertheless, this is not what it means; otherwise our brains would never get any blood.

(Still, four-year-old thinking is often accurate: hot dogs really were once made from dogs – in nineteenth century New York during the bratwurst wars. A newspaper columnist created the term after his investigation found that there was a reason one company's sausages were so cheap . . . all the stray dogs in that area had disappeared and had been used in the manufacturing process. Reportedly the hot dogs were really good: my mind is a junkyard of useless facts.)

What is actually true, in the case of the BBB, is that the cellular structure of the blood vessels that feed the brain are different than most other blood vessels in the body. (There are other organ–blood barriers here and there throughout the body; most are somewhat similar to the one in the brain.)

The blood vessels in the brain (aka cerebral microvessels) are lined with endothelial cells (aka microvascular endothelial cells) just like those in the rest of the body. However, the junctions between microvascular endothelial cells are, perhaps, a thousand times stronger than those in the body's other blood vessels. There is an extremely high "transendothelial electrical resistance," or TEER rate, (2000 Ω cm^2) in these particular junctions. (This is a measure of the strength of the bond between the cells.) The resistance in normal endothelial cell junctions is much less, generally ranging from 3 to 33 Ω cm^2. This is where the "barrier" concept comes from. It is very hard for anything to get past these, much stronger, junctions.

The endothelial structures underlying the brain's microvascular blood vessels include pericytes (similar to the smooth muscle cells that surround endothelial structures in the rest of the body), astrocytes (a form of immune cell), and a basal membrane. All are part of the endothelial structures at the BBB. All work together to make the brain's microvascular as strong and impenetrable to outside pathogens as possible.

To allow nutrients to cross the BBB (and to allow wastes out), these endothelial cells possess a number of efflux/influx transporters specific for the purpose. (Efflux takes things out; influx takes things in.) You can think of these as small portals in the cells that open and close to let things in and out whenever they receive a physiological signal to do so. Some of these efflux transporters are specific for removing xenobiotics (non-self molecules and pathogens). They very rapidly eject foreign bodies that are trying to cross the endothelial cells, keeping them out of the endothelial region.

Pathogens use a number of mechanisms to circumvent this, allowing them to gain entry into the brain. They may hide inside some of the cells that are commonly allowed to cross that barrier, such as phagocytes (aka the Trojan horse approach). (The borrelial bacteria are the Greeks in this process, sneaking in to wreak havoc on the innocent Trojans, i.e. our brain cells, just trying to lead safe and happy lives.) The bacteria may also directly infect the BBB's endothelial cells, forcing the cells to take a spirochete-filled vacuole into their interior. The primary method the bacteria use, however, is damaging the endothelial junctions in the vessel walls, allowing them to penetrate through them – just as they do in the rest of the body. Due to the difference in EC junction architecture at the BBB, they utilize somewhat different processes than they do elsewhere.

It's important to not lose sight of the fact that the exterior membranes of all borrelial spirochetes are very complex. They have many, many molecules they can express at any time on the exterior of those membranes, and they change the composition and nature of those molecules continually. Many of these alterations are designed to facilitate their movement into as many niches in the body as possible, including the brain. As Pulzova et al. (2011) comment: "*Borrelia* regulate the expression of their surface proteins during various stages of dissemination in the host. Therefore, the surface protein arsenal of *Borrelia* is different during the BBB translocation from that in the early stages of dissemination out of the peripheral vasculature."

Spirochetes cross the BBB, accessing the nervous system, in anywhere from twelve hours to one month after tick bite (generally within seven to fourteen days). How long depends on many factors, from the bacterial variant in question to the health of the individual's immune system to whether the BBB is already compromised (as it often is in the elderly), and so on. The spirochetes that infect the brain almost always have remodulated their exterior membrane to present *ospA* rather than *ospC* proteins on their surfaces. This allows them to adhere to the unique structural proteins (especially CD40) that are found on the brain's microvascular endothelial cells (BMECs).

BMECs express a number of unique surface glycoproteins: cerebral cell adhesion molecule, the BBB-specific anion transporter-1, a number of CXC chemokines, and so on. One of the unique BMEC proteins is cluster of differentiation 40 (CD40). The uploaded spirochetal *ospA* membrane protein has a specific tropism for this particular molecule. Once the spirochetes locate CD40 on the BMEC surface, they strongly adhere to it, then begin to crawl along the endothelial surface to get to the junction sites.

When CD40 proteins are touched by pathogens, they begin to produce a number of cytokines as part of the cell's innate immune response. These cytokines play important roles in the development of neuroborreliosis. The primary cytokines activated are: TNF-a, IL-1, VCAM-1, PECAM, ICAM-1, and MMP3 and -9.

(As an aside: chronic activation of the CD40 protein receptors is intimately involved in amyloid-beta-induced activation of microglia in the brain. This is the initial event that occurs prior to the emergence of Alzheimer's disease; it's a root cause of the condition. That borrelial bacteria continually stimulate this protein during long-term brain infection ties the spirochetes even more closely to the generation of Alzheimer's disease.)

The CD40 cytokine activation is potent: IL-1 increases 130-fold, TNF-a 100-fold, VCAM-1 155-fold, PECAM 106-fold, ICAM-1 100-fold, and MMP3 and -9 are increased 160-fold. Although the cytokines can themselves be inhibited, *blocking CD40 expression has been found to impede the upregulation of these cytokines* thus protecting the brain structures from inflammatory damage. Inhibiting both CD40 *and* the upregulated cytokine cascade is even more effective. (Hint: *Polygonum cusipidatum*.)

At the same time that the cytokines are stimulated, the bacteria also alter the TEER levels three- to fourfold via alterations in the calcium signaling in the BMECs. This significantly weakens the bond between endothelial cells at the junctions. As that weakens, the inflammatory cytokines can more easily degrade the junctions between the BMECs, allowing the spirochetes access to the extracellular matrix underneath them.

Via chemotactic compounds, the spirochetes attract plasminogen to the surface *ospA* proteins, convert it to plasmin, then bind it tightly to their surfaces. The plasmin upregulates large quantities of MMPs, especially MMP-9. The CD40-activated cytokines and the massive amounts of MMP-9 degrade foundational elements of the extracellular matrix, allowing an enhanced penetration across various endothelial matrix molecules such as collagen I, laminin, and collagen IV.

The inflammation in the EC matrix also break the matrix molecules into their constituent parts, allowing the bacteria access to essential nutrients. As the EC matrix degrades, the bacteria gain access to the brain itself. Once inside the brain, the *ospA* protein on the spirochetal surface binds to the brain's neural structures, beginning the neuroinflammatory processes that lead to the many symptoms of neuroborreliosis.

It is important to note, again, that the bacteria utilize redundancy during the infection process. Inhibiting *ospA* expression will not stop the penetration of the bacteria into the brain, it will only reduce it by ~70 percent; there are other mechanisms in play here. The *ospC* associated protein vsp1 (for variable small protein 1) is also specific for BMEC adhesion. The spirochetes release this protein into the blood; it then flows to the BMECs. The proteins adhere to the surface of the BMECs where they are soon internalized as intracellular pathogen fragments. These fragments degrade the brain microvascular endothelial cells themselves via the generation of inflammatory cytokines, making the BBB still more porous. (Think Swiss cheese.) Some of the spirochetes, expressing vsp1 on their exterior surface, will also be internalized, taken inside the BMECs themselves. This causes a long-term infection of the BMECs; it creates a protected niche from which the bacteria can still access the brain.

No matter the infectious strategy, the cytokine cascade that occurs is identical, which is why *Polygonum cuspidatum* is always useful. The herb strongly protects endothelial structures (and junctions), including those in the brain, from this kind of damage.

Polygonum cuspidatum, and many of its individual constituents (such as resveratrol), are not only angiogenesis adaptogens (i.e., controlling the under- and overexpression of blood vessels) but calcium channel adaptogens. That is, they modulate calcium channel signaling, raising it if it is depressed, decreasing it if it is too high. Thus they very specifically protect TEER strength, inhibiting the capacity of the spirochetes to degrade it. The herb also inhibits *every one* of the upregulated cytokines: TNF-a, IL-1, VCAM-1, PECAM, ICAM-1, and MMP-3 and MMP-9. It also acts, strongly, to *downregulate* CD40 expression on endothelial cells. It's no wonder then that the use of the herb *tightens* endothelial junctions and protects endothelial structures from degradation. In many studies (and our own practice), it has been found to be specific for enhancing the BBB, strongly increasing TEER strength and protecting brain structures from pathogenic assault.

Infection dynamics in the brain

Once the spirochetes degrade the BBB's endothelial cell junctions, they move into the brain itself where they seek out and attach to a wide variety of the brain's neural structures. (They also, simultaneously, spread widely throughout the body's peripheral nervous system.) As Garcia-Monco and Benach (2013) describe it . . .

> B. burgdorferi *disseminate to the brain, brainstem and cerebellum, spinal cord, and the meninges. Peripheral neuroborreliosis was documented through nerve conduction studies. . . . Conduction velocities were recorded on motor nerves of the extremities*

at various stages of the infection, and axonal multifocal neurop-
athies of the arms and legs were confirmed along with evidence
of denervation. B. burgdorferi was detected in the tissues of the
peripheral nervous system. . . . The histopathologic and immu-
nohistochemical features of early and late neuroborreliosis of the
peripheral nervous system showed that neuritis involving multi-
ple nerves was the most consistent manifestation with immune
cell infiltration.

(Neuritis simply means inflammation of the nerves. That inflammation is primarily caused by the cytokines that the bacteria upregulate during infection.)

Importantly, the authors comment that cerebral inflammation (microgliosis) is more severe in the immunodeficient. "This finding," they note, "emphasizes the role of the immune response in the development and severity" of the disease. (Again, supporting immune function is essential.) Other important factors in the degree and form of neural damage are the *type* of borrelial organism, the length of an undiagnosed infection, and improper pharmaceutical treatment.

The longer the spirochetes are in the body prior to treatment, the more adjusted they become to the specific immune situation in that host and the more antigenic variation they will have created in their offspring. Journal studies consistently show that improper antibiotic treatment (e.g., wrong antibiotic, too short a dosing period) stimulates both antigenic variation and the development of persistent forms in the bacteria. A number of studies have found that treatment that occurs later than seven days postinfection has more relapse and more bacterial resistance to treatment than treatment within that first week. (Treatment within the first week almost never happens.)

Micro- and macrogliosis

Glial cells are non-neural cells that are scattered throughout the brain; there are a number of different types. Those most commonly activated (or damaged) during neuroborreliosis tend to be the microglia, astrocytes, and oligodendrocytes. (Gliosis, btw, simply refers to the activation of glial cells in response to CNS damage or pathogen entry.)

Glial cells surround neurons, holding them in place, forming an integral element in the structural strength of the brain. They also help regulate the internal environment of the brain, especially the fluid that surrounds neurons and synapses. These brain cells modify the migration of neurons in the brain and supply nutrients and oxygen to neural structures. The oligodendrocytes, by forming myelin, insulate neurons from one another, allowing them to function. Glial cells also play essential roles in assisting neurons in forming synaptic connections. They are especially active in the hippocampus and cerebellum (two of the regions most commonly damaged during neuroborreliosis). And finally, the glia act similarly to white blood cells in attacking, destroying, and removing pathogens from the brain. They are essential partners to the neural cells in the brain. Many of the problems that occur from borrelial infection in the brain and CNS come from the activation of glial cells as immune responders.

Normally, the first response to infection in the brain is the movement of microglia to wherever the spirochetes have attached themselves to neural structures. This usually occurs within a few hours of brain penetration. Somewhat later oligodendrocyte precursor cells become activated (three to five days) and finally the astrocytes (five days and onward). Sustained gliosis (no matter the cause) inhibits the normal regeneration of damaged neurons leading to chronic debilitating CNS conditions such as multiple sclerosis, ALS, Parkinson's disease, and so on.

Microglia are specialized macrophages, making up 10 to 15 percent of the cells in the brain, and are scattered throughout the brain and spinal cord. They are much smaller than regular glial cells (hence the *micro*), are highly mobile, and tend to congregate at areas of infection or damage. They are essential players in the inflammation that occurs during Lyme infection in the CNS.

As soon as they detect foreign bodies (or the damage those bodies cause), they become activated to fight it; they are constantly monitoring the brain for plaques, pathogens, and damaged neurons. Microglia are tremendously sensitive to even the tiniest pathological alterations in the CNS; they are highly responsive to, and strongly activated by, any damage to neurons. As well as the normal, everyday microglia, there are some specialized types located in the perivascular spaces of the brain (i.e., perivascular microglia). Both MRI scans and brain autopsy in long-term Lyme sufferers consistently finds spirochete-initiated lesions throughout the perivascular spaces, much of it caused by chronic microglial activation.

The sustained activation of microglia is what is referred to as microgliosis. This is one of the main causes of neuronal damage in the brain during neuroborreliosis. Microglia activation causes the upregulation of a number of cytokines: IL-1, IL-6, IL-8, TGF-beta, TNF-a, PGE-2, IFN-gamma, MCP-1, M-CSF, MIP-1a, MIP-1b, CCR3, CCR5, CXCR4, CX3CR1, and MMP-1, -2, -3, and -9. These cytokines stimulate inflammation in the brain and lead to neuronal damage and neuronal death over time. They also activate astrocytes, which increases the inflammation in the brain.

Microglia also synthesize amyloid precursor protein when activated. Over time this causes the buildup of amyloid plaques in the brain leading to the development of Alzheimer's disease. Chronic activation of microglial cells is integral to a number of conditions: schizophrenia, Alzheimer's, Parkinson's disease, and, importantly during borrelial infections, cardiovascular diseases – especially myocardial infarction.

Macroglia, in contrast to microglia, are much larger; the most abundant are astrocytes. Astrocytes are star-shaped cells (hence their name), and vastly outnumber the neurons in the brain. They are essential to the maintenance of the BBB, having very close associations with endothelia and fibroblasts. They are intimately involved in many metabolic interactions with neurons. Their close association with the brain's endothelia results in the induction of many of the BBB properties, including the incredibly tight EC junctions and the actions of the various endothelial transporters, which move things back and forth across the ECs.

Astrocyte overactivity inhibits axon regeneration after (and during) infection, stimulates and secretes a number neurotoxic cytokines, and releases excitotoxic glutamate, all of which have severe impacts on neural functioning. (Sustained astrocyte activation is one of the main causes of ALS or amyotrophic lateral sclerosis.)

As spirochetes continue their movement into the brain tissue, astrocytes become strongly activated to fight the infection. They, too, begin to produce a range of cytokines to deal with the problem: IL-6, IL-8, IL-10, TNF-a, CCL2, CCL3, CCL4, CXCL1, and MMP-9 are primary. (IL-8 is commonly found in the CSF of people with neuroborreliosis; it is sometimes used as a marker of infection.) CXCL1 and IL-8 have the additional ability to act as neutrophil chemoattractants. (Neutrophils are a leukocyte, aka white blood cell.) Once these cytokines are expressed, neutrophils from the body begin flooding the bloodstream, heading for the brain. They then move across the BBB into the brain to fight the infection.

Unfortunately, during borrelial infections, as the neutrophils move through the endothelial layers they take on a particularly neurotoxic phenotype. This is not uncommon, a particularly cytolytic phenotype of the Th1 cytokine IFN-gamma is produced in late neuroborreliosis infections. *Note:* The herb *Capparis spinosa*, roots, leaves, or fruits, can help correct the form of this neurotoxic cytokine.)

The neurotoxic neutrophils increase the release of proteases (MMPs), inflammatory cytokines, chemokines, and NETs (neutrophil extracellular traps). As these activated immune cells penetrate the brain tissue, because of the alterations that have occurred, they begin causing neuronal death. Thus, through a variety of mechanisms, the various areas in which the spirochetes congregate in the brain all experience neuronal loss. This includes the hippocampus.

Hippocampal damage is especially serious as it interferes with the ability to extract meaning from the surrounding sea of sensory inputs within which we are immersed. (Inhibiting MMPs, especially MMP-9, can often significantly reduce inflammatory impacts on the brain. Some good inhibitors are *Cordyceps, Olea europaea, Polygonum cuspidatum, Punica granatum, Salvia miltiorrhiza, Scutellaria baicalensis*, and the supplements EGCG and NAC.)

Oligodendrocytes, discussed in more depth in a bit, are the third important glial cell that is affected during borrelial infection of the brain.

Continued activation of these cells creates what are known as glial scars in the brain. And like any scar, they may inhibit normal function, even after healing has occurred. (Inhibition of TGF-beta, btw, has been found to reduce glial scarring. Some useful inhibitors are *Artemisia* spp., *Astragalus* spp., *Cordyceps, Ginkgo biloba, Magnolia officinalis, Paeonia lactiflora, Schisandra chinensis, Salvia miltorrhiza, Scutellaria baicalensis,* and *S. barbata*.)

Generally, the bacterial invasion of the brain and the gliosis it stimulates give rise to a spectrum of common symptoms which differentiate into location-specific symptoms as the disease progresses. Cranial neuritis (inflammation of brain neurons), meningitis (inflammation of the meninges of the brain, often leading to severe or constant headache), and radiculoneuritis (inflammation at the root of a nerve in the spine just after it exits from the spinal cord) are the most common early symptoms. As time progresses, chronic conditions arise, most commonly radiculo-neuropathy (constant inflammation in the nerve roots causing pain and loss of function to varying degrees in the parts of the body that those nerves serve), encephalopathy (brain inflammation) accompanied by impairment of various cognitive processes including memory loss, and leukoencephalitis (i.e., brain inflammation caused by the movement of neurotoxic leukocytes into the brain). Infected regions of the brain begin to degrade, leading to area-specific functional damage.

In about 11 percent of Lyme infections, most often children, a partial facial paralysis (Bell's palsy) occurs. Two-thirds of those affected only experience it on one side of the face. Numbness or tingling in the extremities, "crawling" sensations, facial weakness, and radiating nerve pain are very common as well.

Encephalopathy is often accompanied by memory problems and depression. Sleepiness in the daytime and wakefulness at night are common. Extreme irritability, fatigue, headaches, disorganization, and continual mild incoherence occur as well. Nerve pain is often present.

Medical testing continually finds measurable deficits in: memory, new learning, retrieval of information, attention and concentration, perceptual-motor skills, and problem solving. (In other words, while the infection is in their heads, it's not all in their heads.)

Despite most people's strenuous efforts to overcome these deficits, they are generally unsuccessful in doing so; the spirochete infection of the CNS has too many impacts on cognition. Children tend to have significantly fewer cognitive problems (e.g., memory and thinking) than adults – most likely because the older we become, the less vital our neurological structures and immune function are. In adults, the ability to think and solve problems can be severe. (This incapacity has to be taken into account when treating people who have Lyme infections; they may not be able to follow a treatment regimen without help.)

During early stages of the infection, those who are infected *know* something is wrong, yet proper medical diagnosis rarely occurs. ("You're fine. Perhaps some antidepressants?") Brain scans are generally useless as, during the early stages of infection, they rarely show any of the soon-to-be-evident neural damage. *Brain scans are rarely clinically useful until the damage is exten-sive enough for them to perceive it*; by then things are much worse. Comments such as this one from Binalsheikh et al. (2012) regarding a boy presenting with Alice in Wonderland syndrome are common: "Cranial magnetic reso-nance imaging produced normal results." (Reliance on machines, unfor-tunately, degrades most healers' capacity for perceptual, and diagnostic, acuity. Useful corollary: automobile prevalence and leg strength decline from the failure to walk every day.)

Brain cell alterations

Although they can infect any areas of the meninges cluster, the spirochetes mostly tend to invade the subarachnoid space – simply because of all the collag-enous filaments that connect the arachnoid to the pia mater. (The inflamma-tion in those filaments is the most common cause of the headaches and stiff neck that accompany infection.) The leptomeninges, nerve roots, and dorsal root ganglia are where the spirochetes tend to cluster most strongly during early neuroborreliosis. (In the peripheral nervous system, they localize to the endoneurium and the connective tissues of peripheral nerves.)

One of the reasons why Bell's palsy occurs so often with Lyme infections is that when people, usually children, are bitten on the neck, the spirochetes are injected close to the site of the long facial nerve. The spirochetes move quickly to the connective tissue in this nerve, cause inflammation, which swells the nerve, and it seizes up, causing facial paralysis.

The spirochetes that occur in the CNS are, again, antigenetically differ-ent than those that infect the rest of the body. Those in the CNS tend to be neurotropic, that is, attracted to neural cells.

Once the spirochetes are well established in the meninges, they will often penetrate the brain, adhering to a number of the brain's cells, specifi-cally endothelia, neurons, and various glial cells (neuroglia).

Inside the brain, the spirochetes use their potent chemotactic abilities to seek out a particular kind of substance in the brain, glycosphingolipids. The bacteria are primarily interested in one form of it: galactocerebroside (aka galactosylceramide). It's a common molecule in neural cells throughout the brain (including astrocytes and microglia) and is especially available on the plasma membrane of neurons, oligodendrocytes, and the myelin sheaths that surround nerves.

Once attached to the neural structures, the spirochetes begin to break them down into their constituent parts in order to access the underlying nutrients that make up the more complex molecules. As the breakdown occurs, each infected region of the brain generates different and unique neurological problems; each producing different symptoms. (To some extent, diagnosis of the affected regions can occur simply through an analysis of the symptoms that emerge. For example, extreme emotional lability is commonly due to infection of the amygdala.)

The myelin sheaths in the brain wrap around the axons of neurons – think electrical wire and its insulated cable – and serve a similar purpose, that is, keeping the electricity *in* that particular wire. (Axons, btw, are white, hence the "white matter" of the brain.) Myelin also increases the speed at which nerve impulses travel along the axons, making the signals more efficient. Every so often, along the axon, there are sheath gaps called the nodes of Ranvier. It is here that oligodendrocytes are located. Oligodendrocytes wrap around the axon and extrude their plasma membrane lengthwise along the axon, creating the myelin sheath that covers them.

The spirochetes, once inside the brain, immediately find and bind to the galactocerebroside molecules on the surface of the oligodendrocytes' plasma membranes. (This is one of their favorite places to gain nutrients.) They then begin their usual cytokine-initiated processes, degrading both the oligodendrocytes and the myelin sheaths. (The flow of energy along the axons is immediately affected; brain function begins to degrade; early symptoms of neuroborreliosis begin.) As the myelin is broken apart for its nutrients, many of the cellular components are released into the extracellular spaces in the brain, where they most definitely should not be.

The spirochete-initiated cytokines and the free-floating cellular fragments stimulate an immune response by the body. Over time, this can become an autoimmune-*like* condition. This is because, as the myelin sheaths (and oligodendrocytes) degrade, they release myelin basic protein (MBP) from their cells. The constant presence of free MBP stimulates the immune system to create antibodies to MBP in an attempt to remove it from the region. Unfortunately, MBP is still a component of the membranes of both oligodendrocytes and myelin sheaths. The immune antibodies, regrettably, may, sometimes, begin to attack MBP in both those locations, increasing the breakdown of the sheaths. As Ramesh et al. (2012) comment;

"Astroglial and neuronal proteins, anti-myelin antibodies, and cells secreting antibodies to myelin basic protein have been detected in the cerebral spinal fluid (CSF) of patients with LNB."

The spirochete-generated cytokines, immune-response cytokines, and the MBP antibodies, over time, cause massive damage to the cellular structures of the brain, which leads to the range of problems that occur during neuroborreliosis. As more nerve cells are demyelinated, the same kinds of symptoms appear as those in multiple sclerosis, cerebral palsy, ALS, and Parkinson's disease.

Studies have found that as soon as the spirochetes attach to oligodendrocytes, they immediately induce the production of CCL2 (aka MCP-1), IL-6, IL-8, IL-10, and caspase-3 in those cells. (Again, IL-10 is an anti-inflammatory cytokine designed to reduce Th1 responses. This is why the spirochetes tend to keep its levels high.) Due to their location, the oligodendrocytes in brain tissue adjacent to the subarachnoid space are especially vulnerable to damage.

The spirochete-induced expression of IL-8 induces the expression of matrix metalloproteinases MMP-2 and -9 and the proapoptotic protein Bim, which leads to death of neurons, normally, within twenty-four hours of induction. Anti-apoptic Bcl-2 molecules are strongly downregulated, pro-apoptic molecules such as Bim, Bax, and NOXA-1 are strongly increased. (Modulating Bcl/Bax expression can sometimes be of immense help in reducing symptoms, in this instance upregulating Bcl-2 and downregulating Bax – the opposite of what is needed during a mycoplasma infection. (Some useful herbs for this are *Scutellaria baicalensis*, *Olea europaea*, and *Rhodiola* spp.)

The cellular production of CCL2 is especially high when oligodendrocytes are stimulated by *Borrelia*. The CCL2 itself recruits monocytes, T cells, and microglia to the affected areas of the CNS during acute neuroinflammation, often making the problems more acute. High CCL2 is a common marker for many neurodegenerative conditions, including LNB. As Ramesh et al. (2012) note . . .

> *CCL2 is implicated in mediating oligodendrocyte/white matter damage indirectly by mediating the influx of immune cells such as T cells and macrophages, resulting in cytotoxic damage of the myelin sheaths of axons, followed by phagocytosis of myelin debris, culminating in demyelination and axonal damage.*

Studies have found that reducing the levels of these inflammatory cyto-kines prevents oligodendrocyte deaths, thus protecting neural structures in the brain. Dexamethasone (for example) can help and has been found to protect neural cells during infection specifically by lowering CCL2 (though at high doses it can make the cell death worse – dosage moderation is essential). It can be a helpful adjunct as can any substance (such as *Polygonum cuspidatum*) that lowers CCL2 and any of the other cytokines that occur in the brain during infection. Some herbs that can lower CCL2 (MCP-1) levels are *Coptis chinensis, Lonicera japonica, Polygonum cuspidatum, Salvia miltiorrhiza (strongly so), Scutellaria baicalensis, Sophora flavescens,* and *Tanacetum parthenium.*

Borrelial spirochetes stimulate the production of CCL2 via an ERK/JNK/p38/NFkB pathway. Inhibiting this pathway can significantly reduce CCL2 presence and the damage it can cause. As Parthasarathy and Philipp (2014) comment; "Inhibition of the ERK pathway in the presence of *B. burgdorferi* markedly reduced inflammation, followed by the JNK, p38, and NF-kB pathway inhibition." (ERK inhibition also reduces caspase-3 and p53 levels, which also have roles in the problems that occur during neuroborreliosis.) *Polygonum cuspidatum* is the most specific for inhibiting this exact pathway. Some of the other herbs (and supplements) specific for this are *Chelidonium majus, Cordyceps* spp., *Pueria lobata, Scutellaria baicalensis,* and EGCG.

Studies have also found that cellular *fragments* of killed *Borrelia* will induce the same inflammatory cytokines that live spirochetes do. Successful antibiotic treatment, which kills the spirochetes, will produce these fragments, which then continue to cause damage to brain structures until, and if, they are scavenged by the immune system. This is why during and after the use of antibiotics symptoms can become much worse. The use of effective anti-inflammatories is essential during and after antibiotic treatment.

Cellular fragments are not the only problem: blebs, biofilms, and round body (encysted) forms are extremely common in the brain and CNS during infection. As Miklossy et al. (2008) comment (in a particularly fine article) . . .

> Atypical cystic, granular forms, and colony-like aggregation of spirochetes into large masses enclosing cystic forms were also observed following 1 week infection of primary neurons and

astrocytes with Borrelia *spirochetes. . . . Following one week exposure of the cells to* Borrelia burgdorferi, *it is difficult to find spirochetes that have preserved the typical spiral form. . . . Atypical forms, including ring-shaped, uni- or multi-spirochetal cystic and granular forms also occurred free floating in the medium of primary neuronal and glial cell cultures.*

As their research found, all these forms easily recovered the typical spirochetal form whenever adverse conditions improved.

This study is particularly elegant in that, while much of it was concerned with in vitro work, they also examined postmortem brain specimens from three people (in their eighties) who had been diagnosed with long-term neurological Lyme infections. As they note . . .

Identical atypical and cystic forms were observed in the cerebral cortex of the three patients with pathologically confirmed chronic Lyme neuroborreliosis. . . . OspA immunoreactive colony-like agglomeration of spirochetes [can be] seen in panel A. In such "colonies" or agglomerates of spirochetes, atypical, stretched filamentous forms, as well as numerous ring-shaped forms and spherules are frequently present. . . . Rolled spirochetes forming large rings in the cerebral cortex and in the cytoplasm of an epithelial cell of the choroid plexus are seen in panels G and H. . . . The atypical and cystic spirochetes observed in the brain of the patient from which ADB1 strain was cultivated were identical to those induced when the spirochetes of this strain were cultivated under various harmful conditions or when primary astrocytes or neurons were infected by these spirochetes.

As the article continues . . .

The intracellular localization of filamentous, ring-shaped, cystic and granular forms suggests that such intracellular Borrelia *spirochetes can be protected from the immune system. [The presence of these forms, intracellularly, in the patients' brains] indicated that* Borrelia burgdorferi *can form resistant cystic forms, which may persist in the brain. . . . The results also showed that atypical* Borrelia *forms may be present in the absence of typical coiled forms, indicating that detection of atypical forms in infected tissues may be of diagnostic value. . . . That* Borrelia burgdorferi *was successfully cultivated from the brains of the three patients with Lyme neuroborreliosis in BSK-II medium where pleomorphic and cystic forms were observed in the brain suggests that at least part of the persisting spirochetes are viable. . . . The accumulation of immunocompetent HLA-DR positive microglia and reactive astrocytes in the cerebral cortex of these patients clearly indicates the presence of chronic inflammation . . . The response elicited by the major membrane lipoproteins of* Treponema pallidum *and* Borrelia burgdorferi *was analogous to that observed with whole bacteria. The vegetative and cystic forms including the vesicular blebs and free vesicular structures of* Borrelia burgdorferi *all contain the biologically active spirochetal surface proteins indicating that they all elicit inflammatory responses including complement activation.*

In later stages of neuroborreliosis, because the damage is extensive enough, MRI scans finally do reveal a range of problems in the brain. Matera et al. (2014), in examining MRI scans of a *Borrelia*-infected twenty-six-year-old man presenting with epilepsy, found that . . .

[b]rain MRI revealed hyperintense lesions in T2 and FLAIR sequences, with a bright appearance in diffusion-weighted images, not enhancing after gadolinium administration, and involving the right temporal cortex, the left temporal pole, insula and hippocampus, as well as the periventricular white matter, semi-oval centers and corpus callosum. . . . Ischemic lesions were found in the vascular territory of the middle cerebral artery.

Farshad-Amacker et al. (2013), scanning a *Borrelia*-infected twenty-eight-year-old woman, found . . .

> [m]ild hyperintense lesions on T2w. TSE images were visible in
> the pons. Furthermore, strong bilateral T2w hyperintense signal
> alterations and post contrast enhancement of hte vestibular
> nerves within the auditory canal was noted.

The authors continue, noting that . . .

> [a] retrospective study of 66 patients revealed that positive neuro-
> imaging findings on MRI of patients with neuroborreliosis are
> relatively unusual and the authors concluded that findings are
> usually focal lesions in the white matter of the brain or nerve-root
> or meningeal enhancement.

Long-term infection is generally accompanied by, as Miklossy (2012) notes, "diffuse cortical atrophy with frontotemporal predominance, severe neuron loss, and microglial and astrocytic proliferation." Brain biopsies regularly show nonspecific perivascular or vasculitic lymphocytic inflammation. Postmortem analysis commonly finds lymphocytic perineuritis with multisegmental axonal injury of nerve roots, spinal ganglia, and distal nerve segments.

Ramesh et al. (2009) comment that "[t]he influx of immune cells from the periphery into the CNS is reflected in the cellular composition of the inflammatory lesions that were identified in the brain, spinal cord, dorsal root nerves and DRG of infected animals." Hildenbrand et al. (2009) note that "[a]pproximately half of the patients with LNB demonstrate nonspecific abnormal imaging findings predominantly within the frontal cortex white matter arcuate fibers. Despite successful clinical resolution with antibiotic management, white matter involvement often persists on MR imaging."

Hypoperfusion (decreased blood flow) with accompanying cerebral atrophy of the frontal subcortical and cortical structures is common. This will partially reverse upon antibiotic therapy but has been found to be present, though at much lower levels, in those with post-Lyme disease syndrome or those who have been treated successfully with antibiotics.

Most of the damage to the neural system, especially in older people, will not easily correct, even if antibiotic therapy is successful. As Tan et al. (2010) note: "The patients of late stage with center nerve damage were not improved [by antibiotics]." Specific interventives are generally needed to restore neural and brain function (e.g., *Ginkgo biloba* for hypoperfusion or *Hericium erinaceus* to stimulate neural regrowth/regeneration).

It should be clearly understood that coinfection with other stealth pathogens can make the damage worse. As Grab et al. (2007) note: *"Anaplasma phagocytophilum-Borrelia burgdorferi* coinfection enhances chemokine, cytokine, and matrix metalloproteonase expression by human brain microvascular endothelial cells." Coinfection with the malarial parasite *Plasmodium berghei* (similar to *Babesia* spp in its effects) and borrelial spirochetes likewise showed increased problems. As Normark et al. (2014) comment, "Co-infected mice further showed an increased inflammatory response through IL-1B and TNF-*a*, as well as inability to downregulate the same through IL-10."

The damage to neural structures in the brain can be extensive. Nevertheless, it can be reversed. The main treatment interventions are protecting endothelial structures, protecting neural structures (primarily by reducing inflammation dynamics), and regeneration of neural structures. There are many plants that can accomplish all of these. They are detailed in the extended repertory in the protocol chapter. Depending on the damage, restoration of the CNS can take anywhere from six months to three years.

Some comments on relapsing fever infections

RF borrelial bacteria are powerfully focused on endothelial cells, much more so than Lyme bacteria. It is their primary niche, from which they emerge to flood the bloodstream every seven days or so. Their increased numbers and their continual flooding of the bloodstream means that their impacts on both the spleen and liver are generally much greater than Lyme *Borrelia*. Their impacts on brain endothelia are also more pronounced. They tend to adhere to them much more strongly than they do other brain cells.

RF spirochetes are closely associated with red blood cells, aka RBCs (hence anemia in some cases). Some of the RF species (i.e., *B. hispanica, B. duttonii,* and *B. coriaceae,* but not *B. crocidurae, B. hermsii, B. recurrentis*) induce what are called erythrocyte rosettes, in essence RBC aggregates. The more they do this, the worse the symptoms, the more organ invasiveness, hemorrhaging, and microemboli formation and the poorer the immune response.

The bacteria bind to a specific substance on RBC surfaces, a subset of glycosphingolipids, i.e., neolactotetraosylceraminde. (*B. burgdorferi,* on the other hand, does not have the capacity to bind this GSL.) Neolactotetraosyl-ceramide exists throughout the body, on neutrophils, the brain, the stomach, semen, and the GI tract.

Because of these impacts, protecting endothelial integrity *(Polygonum cuspidatum)*, RBC integrity *(Sida acuta)*, the spleen *(Salvia miltiorrhiza)*, and liver *(Silybum marianum)* during the treatment of RF infections is crucial.

CHAPTER SEVEN

ON THE NATURAL HEALING OF BORRELIAL INFECTIONS

Extracting the secrets from a pathogen that has honed its ways through eons of evolution sometimes may require subtle tools that minimally disrupt subtle and sometimes covert mechanisms. The Borrelia surface has been metaphorically likened to a "rainforest," where lipoproteins may form different layers of the canopy.
Wolfram Zuckert, 2013

A range of persistent misconceptions in family medicine exists, ranging from the reliability of available diagnostic tools, the signs and symptoms of nervous system involvement, the importance of coinfections, the appropriate choice and duration of antimicrobial therapy, the importance of Jarisch-Herxheimer reaction after the commencement of treatment with antibiotics, the curability of the infection, and the cause of symptoms that may persist in some patients after treatment. Lyme literate family physicians seem to be rare.
Borgermans et al., 2014

The advantages of natural compounds are fewer side effects in comparison to orthodox medical drugs, and the production of synergistic effects for a more positive treatment outcome.
Kaio Kitazato et al., 2007

I f you are familiar with the first edition of this book, you will notice some alterations in the protocol that is outlined in the next chapter. The past decade has taught us a lot about the *Borrelia* and the subtleties of treatment that are most effective for healing; our understanding has deepened considerably.

Firstly, after a decade of experience, *Smilax* spp. don't really seem to help Herxheimer reactions all that much. Nor does it, despite its reputation as an antispirochetal herb, work – at all from what we have seen – as an antibacterial for borrelial bacteria. (The theory was good on this one, but like many theories, the gods laughed.) That herb has, in consequence, been removed entirely from the protocol.

Secondly, I have gone back and forth about *Andrographis* over the years. As I suspected, even in the first edition, the herb is not as specific as I would have liked as an antibacterial for Lyme *Borrelia*. It *is*, however, specific for a related spirochete, *Leptospira*, and, as well, is commonly used in traditional practice in Africa to treat borrelial relapsing fever infections. In our experience, it seems to be effective as an antibacterial for about 60 percent of those who use it. It has, as well, a number of other, very useful actions that make it a good herb, still, for treating borrelial infections. (Specifically: it reduces some of the primary cytokines active during infection; it is very good at slowly breaking up biofilms and interfering with quorum sensing; it is very active against intracellular bacteria, e.g., chlamydia.) We have seen very good results in preventing Lyme infection if *Andrographis* tincture is applied to the tick bite as soon as the tick is removed.

For all these reasons, and a few others, we still consider it useful (sometimes tremendously so) during borrelial infections. *However,* it also has one particularly uncomfortable side effect that occurs in about one percent of those taking it: it can cause a really nasty case of hives. *Please read the side effects and contraindications on this herb before using it.*

Third, I am *mildly*, that is *mildly*, altering my stance on *Astragalus*. It can, *sometimes*, be useful during chronic Lyme. However, experience has found that for some people it does in fact exacerbate the condition. Rather than acting as a immune-modulating herb, it can, for some, stimulate the exact cytokines that are present during chronic neuroborreliosis, thus making the condition worse. I would not worry about its presence in small quantities in herbal mixtures. It is worth trying as an adjunct to any protocol just to see if it helps. However, if symptoms worsen when it is added, it should be discontinued.

Fourth, please note: when the first edition was written there were no easily accessible sources in the United States for *Polygonum cuspidatum*. Because of that, the primary form of the herb I suggested for use was resveratrol. While some resveratrol is made from grapes, the herb that contains the most of any plant known is the root of *Polygonum cuspidatum* (Japanese knotweed). Many of the resveratrol formulations in the United States are in actuality just knotweed root standardized for a certain percentage of resveratrol content. Because the herb is now widely available (there are some very good organic growers), that is what I now recommend for use. I think it works much better than resveratrol tablets. Nevertheless, if you wish to use the knotweed-based resveratrol tablets, they will still be effective.

A word, well, a rant actually

A repeat, but I keep getting these questions . . .

*The herbs and supplements in this book are **not** the only ones in the world that will help.* During the past decade, I have received hundreds of emails and Facebook messages asking why I don't recommend this or that herb, or if this other herb can be added, or that one deleted. So . . . again . . . *these are not the only herbs in the world that will help.* This is just a starting place, a reference point, a place to begin.

For some people, the protocol as outlined in this book (and in the first edition, as rudimentary as it was) will completely clear up the infection and symptoms they are struggling with. For others, the protocol will have to be adjusted to meet their unique circumstance. To reiterate: From feedback over the past decade we have found that ~75 percent of people experienced what they consider a "cure" from using the protocol, another 15 percent needed to continue with a reduced form of the protocol – generally minimal doses of knotweed and cat's claw to keep any symptoms from returning, 5 percent experienced some relief, and the remaining 5 percent found the protocol useless. Nearly everyone we have heard from who used the protocol moderated it in some fashion, *that is: they added stuff.*

Please use the protocols outlined herein *only* as a starting place, a guideline. Add anything you feel will help you and delete anything that you feel is not useful. Bacteria, when they enter a human body, find a very unique ecosystem in that particular person. Thus the disease is always slightly different every time it occurs. This means that a pharmaceutical or herb that works for one person may not work or work as well for another. There is no one-size-fits-all treatment that works for all people in all times and places.

Also: *there is no one thing that always has to happen first, be treated first, or that you must always do or must never do in order to get well.* There is no one herb that will always work for everyone; there is no one protocol that contains the solutions to all the infectious organisms that exist or all the forms of infection that the Lyme-group can cause.

**There is no one-size-fits-all treatment
that will work for all people in all times and places.**

Anyone who says there is, is either trying to sell you something, has powerful self-image needs involved, or doesn't really understand the borrelial group of infectious organisms. *There is not and never has been one single way to health such that in all times and in all places and with all people it will always work.* Life, and disease, and the journey to wellness are much more complex and challenging than that. Each treatment intervention, as treatment progresses, will become unique to each person. It has to do so for healing to occur.

Thus the protocols in this book should solely be considered as a foundational place to begin. For most people they will help considerably, for some they will clear the infection completely. Nearly everyone (practitioners and the infected alike), however, will find that they will need to add this or subtract that. *Please do so.* Please trust your own feeling sense and pay attention to what your body is telling you. *You* are the best judge of whether something is working for you or not, whether you need to add something else or not, whether you are getting better . . . or not.

Dosages, the rant continues

I will often suggest a dosage or a *range* of dosages for the herbs and supplements that can help. If you have a very healthy immune system, or a very mild case, you will probably need smaller doses; if your immune system is severely depleted or if you are very ill, you may need to use larger doses. If you are *very* sensitive to outside substances, as some people with Lyme and these coinfections are, then you might need to use very tiny doses, that is from one to five drops of tincture at a time. (This is true for about 1 percent of the people with these infections.) I have seen six-foot-five-inch, 280-pound men be unable to take more than five drops of a tincture and a tiny, 95-pound woman need a tablespoon at a time. *Dosages need to be adjusted for each person's individual ecology.*

Dosages need to be adjusted for each person's individual ecology

Also: I have received several hundred queries about the use of bulk, powdered herbs versus capsules versus tinctures. (People often want an equivalency chart – I don't have one.) The most common query is how to figure the milligram dosage for comparable amounts of powdered herbs to that present in resveratrol tablets. (I don't have one, and no, please don't send me one because . . .)

The thing to understand about all this is that dosages are made up, created out of the blue, generally based on typical dosages used in clinical practice in various cultures around the world, usually over millennia, *and an intuitive sense of the herb and its proper dose for specific conditions.* There is generally a range of dosing for most herbs; there is no one dose that is "the right one" for any of them.

I generally break down herbs into three categories: food, medicinal, and toxic grades. Food-grade herbs (e.g., hawthorn, knotweed root, astragalus) can be taken by the ounce, sometimes by the pound (e.g., dandelion and burdock root), just as apples, asparagus, and potatoes are. Medicinal herbs are stronger but still rarely cause severe side effects; they can be taken by the milligram to the ounce. Toxic herbs tend to be poisonous in large doses (there aren't very many of them despite the hype in the media) but are often extremely useful for internal use in tiny or homeopathic doses – think one to three drops of a tincture (e.g., arnica, poison hemlock leaf) or an essential oil (e.g., peppermint, eucalyptus).

Many of the herbs used for Lyme are food grade, some are medicinal grade, thus there is a very wide dosage range that can be explored for treatment. Still, the understanding that the dosage for individual plants can legitimately vary over a wide range tends to be uncommon in herbal – and medical – practice.

Contemporary American herbalists (in contrast to those in the nineteenth century) tend to use small, infrequent doses, due primarily to fear of malpractice accusations from the medical community (who generally know little or nothing about herbal medicines – remember they were *never* trained in them, so why would we, or they, expect to know anything about them?). Herbalists in the UK tend to use much larger doses; they have had a continual herbal thread in their national health care since Henry VIII; they aren't so afraid. Herbalists in China tend to use very large doses, many grams, sometimes throughout the day. It is not unusual to see dosages in China that range from five to fifteen grams (that latter figure being approximately half an ounce). The Chinese know herbs work. They aren't scared of them; they just want to find out what works best.

The lack of understanding of the variability of dosing ranges in the United States is fostered by the (highly inaccurate) paradigm of pharmaceutical dispensing that American physicians use. There is a common belief that there is a single accurate dose (discovered through reductive, analytical science) for every pharmaceutical. It isn't true; it never has been. Drug doses need to be adjusted for age, weight, health, sex, and side-effect emergence. That few physicians do so is one of the reasons that *properly* prescribed pharmaceuticals (that is, according to the drug guidebooks given out by pharmaceutical companies) are, at minimum, the fourth leading cause of death in the United States and why some three million people a year are hospitalized (or permanently disabled) from using them. (Herbs, in contrast, are very safe; they do not produce those kinds of outcomes.)

So, please understand that the dosages listed are, again, just a starting place. You may not need very high doses or you may. (Please don't email me any more about how one tablespoon of knotweed root is not the same as four tablets of resveratrol.) This is why I generally suggest that you begin with smaller doses and work up over time. This allows you to determine *if* there are any side effects you will experience with that particular herb. Starting slow allows your body to find the right dose: the one *it* needs.

A few other points

Here are responses to the most common treatment questions we get:

1. Yes, you *can* combine all the herbs together in the liquid of your choice. You do not have to take them separately.
2. Yes, these herbs can be taken along with antibiotics.
3. No, the bacteria do not develop resistance to the herbs. (This is because of the complexity and number of the

compounds in the plants, and should, despite that, bacteria develop resistance, the plants, which are living beings, create responses to the resistance. The goldenseal you grow this year is not the same as the herb you grew last year.)

4. Yes, you can take these herbs along with protocols suggested by other practitioners.

5. No, except with a very few herbs (such as the 1:1 form of eleutherococcus tincture), you do not need to pulse the herbs; in fact, I have continually heard from people struggling with the Lyme-group of infections that they were getting better, were told to pulse by their personal practitioner, and, once they did, relapsed. (Pulsing is an herban myth, a zombie idea that no matter how often the myth is killed it keeps coming back to life. Yes, you may need to alter dose and herbal combinations, deleting this and adding that, but pulsing, for the most part, no.)

6. Yes, it is common for about half the people who use an herbal protocol, when they begin to get better, to be so excited about being themselves again that they do too much, overexert themselves, and relapse. This is extremely common (and very understandable; it's tiring being sick for so long). So, please be very careful once your strength and joy begin to return. It may seem as if you can immediately begin exerting yourself as you used to do; however, your body has been under a long-term stress, its reserves are low. It will take, if you have been ill for a long time, at least a year to rebuild. (I never pay attention to this advice either. I think it's called living in . . . well, something, I can't remember.)

Part of the function of serious chronic illnesses is to increase personal awareness (I know from personal experience). There is the life you had before Lyme; there is the life you have after. It is very rarely possible to go back to being unaware of the impacts of stress on your system, the kind of self-caretaking your body (and spirit) needs, or the

dangers of overextending yourself and your energy. Ignorance may be bliss (however short that bliss may be), but
awareness is empowering . . . and health enabling.

7. And, finally, *please be conscious of how you respond to the medicines you are taking. If something disagrees with you, if you feel
something is not right in how you are responding to a medicine,*
stop taking it. Remember: You will always know yourself
better than any outside physician.

Regarding antibacterials for Lyme disease

Despite the ten years since the first edition of this book, there has been very
little, virtually no, research on plants that are directly active as antibacterials against borrelial organisms. While there has been some, most of it is
not very useful. But before looking at them, here are some essentials to
keep in mind regarding herbal and pharmaceutical antibacterial treatment
of borrelial infections.

First, the population of people using herbs for Lyme disease are nearly
always those for whom antibiotics did not work. That is, the spirochetes
were resistant for one or more of a variety of reasons (e.g., they were in
round body forms or sequestered in niches antibiotics could not reach).

This population of people, when they began to work with us, were
already nonresponsive to antibacterials in the treatment of Lyme disease.
Because of this *and* the lack of powerful, specific herbal antibiotics for Lyme
infections, we never were able to rely on antibacterials as *the* fundamental
approach to healing Lyme; we had to find another way to health.

A decent percentage of the people with Lyme that we have had contact
with (some twenty-five thousand over ten years) have used *Andrographis* as
an antibacterial; some used pharmaceutical antibiotics (there is no problem with doing so). Nevertheless, we have seen symptoms disappear and
health return without the use of any antibacterial substances. Antibiotics
don't appear to be essential, though, again, they can help. (This is obvious
given that approximately half of those who use pharmaceutical antibiotics
experience a cessation of infection.)

Second, herbal (or other natural) antibiotics, to work for any systemic
bacterial disease, have to spread comprehensively throughout the body.
One of the reasons that *Polygonum cuspidatum* root is so effective during

Lyme is that it is *very* systemic; it crosses the blood-brain barrier as well as the GI tract barrier, which all herbs do not do (e.g., very little goldenseal crosses the GI tract membrane). Knotweed also reaches difficult to reach areas throughout the body (the joints, for example).

Antibacterial herbs, to be effective, need to do the same thing. This is one of the reasons why *Cryptolepis* is so good for treating MRSA and babesiosis; it spreads everywhere. So, the antibacterial challenge in treating Lyme disease is twofold; finding herbs (or supplements) that are specifically antibacterial for borrelial spirochetes – including *every* variant the bacteria generate – *and* that are extremely systemic. This is not an easy challenge to meet. Scores if not hundreds of herbs would need to be tested to find the ones that fit into that grouping; there just isn't much interest (or money) in it yet. (*Andrographis*, btw, is a pretty good systemic herb; it crosses the BBB and reaches many of the niches in which the bacteria hide.)

Third, it is also important to understand that in vitro (test-tube) studies often do not translate to effective treatment in living organisms, including us. During petri dish testing, the herbs make direct contact, easily, with the pathogen, something that rarely occurs in vivo (in the body). While in vitro testing is a good place to begin, the essential next step is finding out if the herb will work as well in a human body – most of the time it doesn't. So, it is rarely legitimate to extrapolate from in vitro studies alone. Sometimes, if there is a very long history (millennia) of use of that plant, it is possible to cross-correlate the in vitro work with that history of use. Patterns emerge that really do have something to do with the real world.

Because of the lack of antibacterial plant studies on borrelial organisms, people in the Lyme world who seek antispirochetal plants tend look to plants effective for *Leptospira* spirochetes, which are loosely related to *Borrelia*. There has been some good research on this, and when correlated with historical use, highly useful plants do turn up (e.g., *Andrographis*).

Although some people also look toward herbs historically used for syphilis, I haven't seen that approach work very well in practice. The better choice has been looking at lab research on (and history of use for) oral pathogens in the same genus as syphilis, (e.g., *Treponema denticola* and *T. vincenti*). (Researchers around the world have done some good work on the antibacterial effects of traditional chewing sticks, taken from local plants, on oral pathogens.)

Some of the herbs that traditional use and laboratory analysis (in vitro, in vivo) show as useful for *Leptospira* bacteria include *Andrographis paniculata, Bupleurum chinensis, Eclipta alba, Garcinia mangostana, Justica adhatoda (Adhatoda vasica), Phyllanthus amarus, Plantago asiatica, Pogostemon cablin, Polygonum cuspidatum* (mildly so), *Salvia miltiorrhiza, Scorzonera hispanica, Senecio scandens,* and *Taraxacum officinalis.* Of these, the only one we have clinical experienec with is *Andrographis.* This does not mean the others won't work.

Of note: *Justica adhatoda* (in vitro, leaf extracts, ethanol extracts) has been found to be directly antispirochetal for *Leptospira,* severely damaging the cellular structure of the bacteria. *Eclipta alba* (in vitro, leaves, water and ethanol extracts) is active against four serogroups of *Leptospira,* showing a broad range of action against this genus. *Garcinia mangostana,* because it is also active against *Treponema* (see below), appears to have a broad activity against spirochetes in multiple genera and should be considered for use with *Borrelia.* Because both *Salvia miltiorrhiza* and *Salvia officinalis* contain similar (though different) constituents and each is active against a different spirochete (see below), it seems that this genus could be an effective choice for treating *Borrelia.*

Some of the herbs that traditional use and laboratory analysis (in vitro) show as useful for *Treponema* bacteria include *Cinnamum verum* (which is most likely why some people find cinnamon oil useful as an antibacterial for Lyme infections), eucalyptus, *Garcinia mangostana, Ginkgo biloba, Mentha arvensis, Ocimum* spp. (including *O. sanctum*), *Polygonum cuspidatum* (mildly so), *Salvia miltiorrhiza, Salvia officinalis, Syzygium aromaticum,* and *Thymus vulgaris.*

As to *Borrelia* antispirochetals : There has only been one study that focused on treating *Borrelia* with herbal medicines in people (that I can find). Unsurprisingly it is from China:

- Bai-Hu-Tang: Hang et al. (2005) used a combination of antibiotics and TCM for treating Lyme infections. Twenty-one people used antibiotics alone, eighteen the combined treatment. The researchers found that the use of the Chinese herb formula Bai-Hu-Tang in combination with antibiotics over twenty-one days was highly effective in treating Lyme. They note that "the cure rate and total effective rate in the

TCM combined with western medicine group was significantly higher than that in the western medicine alone group and that the course of the disease in the former group was apparently shortened more than that of the western medicine alone group."

Bai-Hu-Tang contains gypsum (sometimes *Dendrobium moniliforme* replaces this), *Anemarrhena asphodeliodes*, *Glycyrrhiza*, and *Oryza sativa*. Bai-Hu-Tang has been used in China for several thousand years for acute infections accompanied by systemic inflammation. Studies have found it effective in treating sepsis as well, as it modulates many of the cytokines involved in septic conditions.

The study did not explore any direct antibacterial action of the herbs against the Lyme bacteria; nevertheless, since it is one of the very rare human studies (and it was effective), I have included it here.

• Antihistamines: As noted in Chapter Two, the allergy (antihistamine) medication desloratadine (aka Clarinex) has shown some powerful bactericidal actions (in vitro) against borrelial bacteria. We have found in our work that histamine levels (from mast cell activation) are extremely high in many people with Lyme and that reducing those levels can significantly help the symptom picture and the progression of the disease.

There are a significant number of herbs that are specific for lowering histamine levels. (Unfortunately, no testing has occurred for those that are *BmtA*, manganese transport, inhibitors.) Herbs (and there are scores more not listed here) that can significantly lower histamine levels include *Agaricus blazei*, *Ailanthus altissima*, *Angelica sinensis*, *Camellia sinensis*, *Cichorium intybus*, *Cinnamum verum*, *Cordyceps militaris*, *Eleutherococcus senticosus*, *Forsythia koreana*, *Ganoderma lucidum*, *Houttuynia cordata*, *Ginkgo biloba*, *Glycyrrhiza glabra*, *Isodon japonicus*, *Lycopus lucidus*, *Magnolia officinalis*, *Mentha arvensis*, *Morus alba*, *Olea europaea*, *Oryza sativa*, *Paeonia suffruticosa*, *Perilla frutescens*, *Plumbago zeylanica*, *Polygonum cuspidatum*, *Polygonum tinctorium*, *Prunella vulgaris*, *Rehman-*

nia glutinosa, Rhodiola sacra, Salvia miltiorrhiza, Salvia plebeia, Schizonepeta tenifolia, Silybum marianum, Sinomenium acutum, Solanum lyratum, Sophora flavescens, Syzygium aromaticum, and chaga, chlorella, lavender essential oil, propolis, pycnogenol, and spirulina.

(Part of the reason for the effectiveness of Bai-Hu-Tang may be that both Oryza sativa and Glycyrrhiza reduce histamine levels. Additionally, Glycyrrhiza is a fairly potent synergist, increasing the effectiveness of both pharmaceuticals and herbs when used in combination.)

The following studies are all in vitro (test tube/petri dish); they explore natural substances possessing antibacterial activity for Lyme Borrelia:

- Grapefruit seed extract (GSE): The brand tested is an organic form from Germany (Citrosept brand only) that does not contain nonplant chemicals (please see my depth commentary on this in the second edition of Herbal Antibiotics, Storey publishing, 2013). Many GSE products contain artificial chemical compounds that I would not suggest taking internally. However, this product (Citrosept) is organic and was found in vitro to be active against Borrelia, both round body and motile forms. The problem with this is that GSE is not very systemic; it doesn't cross the GI tract membrane very well or get into the bloodstream in large quantities. It is, however, very good for treating borrelial infections in the GI tract.
- Cistus creticus leaf (pink rock-rose, hoary rock-rose): Both the essential oil and the ethanolic extract of the leaves of this plant are antimicrobial for borrelial spirochetes. Please note: Despite assertions to the contrary on the Internet, the tea of this plant has not been found to be active against the bacteria – the antiborrelial constituents don't extract well in water. However, a substantial number of people using the herbal tea have consistently reported considerable pain relief from its use.

Unfortunately, this species is difficult to find for sale, either essential oil or leaves (though the seeds are common and easy to grow). Internet sources for the genus (2015) show that the essential oil of *C. ladanifer, C. labdanum,* and *C. icanus* are available. No studies have occurred on the substitutability of any of these for *C. creticus.* Nor do I have any real data on the pharmacokinetics of the herb, that is, how systemic it is. And again, this study is in vitro only, not in vivo.

- *Dipsacus sylvestris* (teasel) root: This study, again in vitro, is highly problematical. To quote (Liebold et al. 2011): "The hydroethanolic extract showed *no* growth inhibition [against *Bbss* spirochetes]." (A hydroethanolic extract is the normal water/alcohol tincture you will find for sale in stores.) What the study did find is that an ethyl acetate extract of a polar fraction did exhibit "significant growth inhibiting activity." This is not something anyone is likely to be able to make themselves or that anyone can currently purchase. The components in the ethyl acetate fraction of the plant would, however, be accessible if the root powder is taken internally rather than as a tincture. Thus, the whole root, as a powder, might be a useful antibacterial adjunct in the treatment of Lyme infections.

- Lactoferrin: Lactoferrin is a protein found in human and cow milk (and easily findable as a supplement). There is one paper (via Google Scholar) by Dylan Haenel (no date but presumably published in later 2012 or early 2013) in the form of a journal paper (but it isn't) that discusses some minimal experimental work using lactoferrin as an anti-microbial against borrelial biofilms. (An earlier form of the same material contains subtle differences in content that I consider revealing – Haenel is part of the Lyme disease research group at the University of New Haven.) The title of the paper is misleading: "Antimicrobial effects of lactoferrin and cannabidiol on *Borrelia burgdorferi.*" I don't seem to see cannabidiol in the paper at all; though allicin is mentioned (it did not work very well).

In this paper, Haenel reports that lactoferrin inhibited borrelial biofilms by ~15 percent. That is not very good: there are a number of herbs (and pharmaceuticals) that are much better at it (see the relevant chapter in this book, or the protocol repertory). In contrast, another paper, Lusitani et al. (2002), found, as they note, "*B. burgdorferi* had limited susceptibility to killing by lysozyme and were not killed by azurocidin, proteinase 3, or lactoferrin."

There isn't enough data (or empirical use) to support lactoferrin as a borrelial antibacterial, though no harm in using it; it has a lot of useful effects all on its own.

- Samento and Banderol: There is one paper, also from the Lyme disease research group at New Haven, which looks at the effect of these herbs separately and in combination on borrelial bacteria. It, too, appears to be a peerreviewed journal article (but is not); it appeared in the *Townsend Letter* (July 2010) and is primarily available on the Nutrimedix website (the makers of Samento and Banderol) and the New Haven site. *Because this paper is being used as justification for asserting that Samento and Banderol are antiborrelial antibiotics, I am responding in depth to its findings.*

The paper describes an in vitro study of Samento and Banderol, alone and in combination, and notes that they "eliminated both the spirochetal and round-body forms." It also notes that borrelial biofilms treated by Samento were "significantly smaller" while the Banderol-treated colonies retained the same size; however, more than 90 percent of the Banderol treated biofilm bacteria were dead.

There are a lot of problems with the study itself (besides the other problems that bother me and which are discussed in a bit).

1. There is no indication of the *Otoba* (Banderol) species used.
2. The paper was never published in a reputable journal (but presents itself, in structure and form, as if it is a journal paper).

3. There are no follow-up studies that have been
   published anywhere, including on the Internet (as of
   summer 2015).

4. They used doxycycline as a comparative. Numerous
   study papers have already found that doxycycline is
   a very strong stimulant of round body formation;
   it's not news. There are other pharmaceuticals that
   are much better at preventing it. Using doxycycline,
   given what is known about it, inflates the apparent
   effectiveness of the herbs in relation to round body
   formation.

5. The herbs did not eliminate the spirochetes *or* the
   round bodies *or* the biofilms. They were about
   comparable to doxycycline at killing motile forms.
   (However, I do not find the paper rigorous enough
   to accept those results at this time.) The only thing
   the herbs did differently was fail to stimulate round
   body formation. This is commonly true of herbs;
   they don't tend to drive the bacteria into alternate
   forms the way pharmaceuticals do.

6. Scientifically, the paper is very vague; it doesn't
   rise to the standard of a journal article (for a lot of
   reasons).

I am not saying here that Banderol and Samento do not work; my concerns
lie in other areas. (The research *may in fact be accurate*.) After thirty-five years
in the medicinal herbal field, I have come to be considerably more rigorous in
my analysis of the effectiveness of herbal medicines that are being promoted
by a single company, herbs that quite often cannot be found anywhere else.

I don't have any problem in using or promoting herbs that have no or
little scientific study of their use (*Lomatium* is a case in point). But in that
case, I rely on the plant's history of use over long time lines as well as use
by contemporary practitioners. When herbs are extremely rare and hard to
find, with no or little history of use, with no or very little scientific study,
and when they are touted for use by a vulnerable population at high prices
by a single company, well. . . I have problems.

Some relevant points . . .

Samento is a TOA-free cat's claw; I have a lot of problems with this concept (which I go into in depth in the monograph on cat's claw). In short, there is no reason to remove the TOA from cat's claw. In fact, many of the plant's crucial medicinal effects come from those very same TOA components. The plant has been used for millennia in South America in its whole form and has apparently worked just fine all that time. Removing the TOA merely created a form of the herb that was unique; saying that the TOAs would produce adverse effects created a market niche that leveraged vulnerable people into using the product.

Banderol (probably) comes from one of eight species of *Otoba* trees in South America, most likely *Otoba parvifolia* (or perhaps *O. novogranatensis*). There is a bit of research on these plants, not much, and none that has been repeated. All of it is in vitro. There are a few papers (not many) that list the plant among those found in indigenous practice. Tellingly, these plants are not and never were *major* botanicals for those groups – otherwise they would show up throughout the ethnobotanical record (I did look, in depth). Again, this plant may be incredibly good as an antispirochetal, but I have a number of serious concerns; they are:

1. The herb is not available to the general public, except from Nutrimedix, as far as I can determine.

2. There is no information on the species used (listing the exact species is just basic to reputable science, especially when promoting an herb no one else manufactures).

3. The herbal tincture is very expensive, which is unfortunately common when herbs no one else is using become a primary recommendation in a protocol.

4. The hype on the website bothers me tremendously: "Nutramedix utilizes a proprietary extraction and enhancement process that makes the product more effective than any other *Otoba sp.* product that is available." (As far as I can determine, at this time there are no other *Otoba* products available.)

5. There is almost no presence of this plant in either the scientific or ethnobotanical world, virtually no journal papers

and very few mentions in any explorations of traditional indigenous use in the region.

6. It is not clear from the website who the principal shareholders in Nutrimedix are. A clear problem arises in my mind if those who recommend a product also have ownership positions in the company that makes it. Conflicts of interest should be clearly revealed. I don't know that there are, but . . . I don't know that there aren't either.

That being said, *Uncaria tomentosa* (cat's claw), in its whole state, is a very good herb for treating Lyme infections. *Otoba parvifolia* bark (or resin, which is what some indigenous people use) may be a very useful herb as well. I just don't see it from the material that currently exists. Further, the marketing leverage and hype around it makes me extremely uncomfortable. (I am very sensitive to the vulnerable among the Lyme community being taken advantage of, whether by the medical system *or* those in the herbal world. It's ethically and morally wrong.)

Sooner or later, researchers will begin to actively explore plant antibacterials for borrelial bacteria. Until then, the herbs found effective for *Treponema* and *Leptospira* are a good place to begin.

Because we have seen that *Andrographis* does work as an antibacterial for Lyme spirochetes (albeit only for about 60 percent of people using it), it is still the herb we recommend if you wish to pursue an antibacterial approach. Bai-Hu-Tang also seems like a potentially useful adjunct to Lyme infection. (It is somewhat difficult to find though Amazon.com does have it listed.)

Some comments on muscle testing

The Western herbal tradition, because of its suppression by reductive medicalists early in the twentieth century, lost its connection to centuries of empirical diagnostic methodology. (For a good overview of this, see Barbara Griggs, *Green Pharmacy*, Healing Arts Press, 1991.) Significant elements of that methodology remained somewhat in place in the allopathic medical community until just after World War II, when it began to be displaced by machine and laboratory diagnosis (increasingly so as the decades have progressed). Training of young doctors in human-human medical diagnostics by physician mentors has become, in our time, nearly nonexistent, even within the allopathic medical community. (See, for example, Lara Goitein, "Training Young Doctors," *London Review of Books*, June 4, 2015.) In consequence, as the neoherbal movement developed, many Western herbalists turned to Chinese and Ayurvedic diagnostics in an attempt to correct the problem. My own work on depth diagnosis and Kathleen Maier's work in Virginia on the development of herbal diagnostic techniques that only partially rely on allopathic approaches are also attempts to address the problem.

One of the more common diagnostic approaches that many Western herbalists have been using the past few decades is muscle testing, aka kinesiology, aka ART (autonomic reflex testing). After forty years of exposure to the technique, seeing the outcomes it produces in practice, I think that while it can sometimes be tremendously effective, more commonly it is often only minimally useful and often does more harm than good. (I realize this is heretical within the herbal community, bear with me.)

Muscle testing works something like this. The practitioner asks you to resist their pulling on your arm; this gives them a sense of the strength of your resistance to their pull. They then put the medicinal substance in your hand, and pull again to see if the degree of resistance has changed. If the hand resistance weakens the herb is contraindicated; if it remains the same or gets stronger, then it is a good herb for the condition. (The stronger the resistance, the better the herb.)

We have seen, more times than I care to remember, instances where people are getting considerably better on herbal protocols (not just those in this book), and for some reason known only to the gods, they go to a practitioner who muscle tests them, insists that some of the herbs are useless, insists that they be discontinued, and the person begins to relapse, sometimes seriously so. (Other times, and incredibly commonly, the people are told they have "parasites," which must be eradicated before they can be healed from [*insert any random condition*]. "Parasites" is rarely defined – though black walnut and wormwood are commonly prescribed – and no cognizance is taken of the fact that all of us have commensal, helpful parasites, if we did not we would not be alive.)

From long-term analysis, it seems to us that there are two primary problems with muscle testing as a definitive diagnostic technique. The first (should this be Buhner's diagnostic axiom #1?) is . . .

A tool, diagnostic or otherwise, is only as good as its user.

For some reason this fundamental understanding has been lost. It makes no difference whether the practitioner is an MD or an herbalist with 20 years of training. (As a people, we in the West have regrettably been trained to think that an advanced degree or licensure is a reliable substitute for fundamental skill sets.) As most of us have found, often to our dismay, it is the perceptual acuity and sensitivity of the practitioner that is the most essential element in any healing and diagnostic process. No scientist, physician, herbalist, or naturopath is exempt from this axiom.

When it comes to muscle testing, there are a multitude of factors that can affect outcomes – few of which are ever taken into account by its proponents.

Here are some of them:

1. Is the muscle response to the herb or the company or person that produced it? Many herbs are poorly produced; you might say that the people growing the plant put a lot of disrespect into the process. Some herbs glow with health; others are quite the opposite. While the aesthetic dimensions of herbal medicines are generally neglected by reductionists, it does play an essential role in the vitality of the medicines.

2. Is the response to the supplement actually to the primary compound in it or other constituents in the supplement?

3. Is the response to the herb or to the practitioner doing the testing? (Some practitioners are not pleasant people or may possess activated unconscious aspects of their personality that make them unsafe in a healing environment.)

4. Is the response to the herb or the room in which the testing is occurring? (The aesthetic dimensions of the healing environment play essential roles in healing and well being.)

5. Is the response indicative of secondary gain or does the person really want to get well? (The lack of understanding among herbalists and naturopaths of secondary gain in disease complexes is egregious; some people have diseases because of the attention they get from having them. They

do not want to get well and will resent any attempts to truly heal them.) Sometimes a banana is just a banana; sometimes it's not.

6. Human beings are complex aggregates of a multitude of consciousness modules (discussed in depth in my book *Plant Intelligence and the Imaginal Realm*, Inner Traditions, 2013). Each conscious module has its own agenda, in other words, which part of the person being tested is controlling the physiological response?

The secondary problem with muscle testing is even more complex. It rests in a more accurate understanding of bacteria and what they do in the body. To quote Lynn Margulis (Margulis et al., 2009) . . .

> *Spirochetes need to be re-evaluated. Is the situation better described as an obligate and ancient symbiosis where the bionts (spirochetes and humans) are integrated at the behavioral, metabolic, and genetic level?*

Bacteria are highly intelligent, spirochetes extremely so. When the spirochetes establish a long-term infection in a human body, they begin to modulate large segments of the body's physiology in order to control their habitat, making it suitable for them. They modulate, as Margulis noted, the *behavior* of the human organism at very deep and subtle levels. So the question arises:

> *Who is controlling the resistance response to the muscle testing, the person or the bacteria?*

It is not beyond the realm of possibility that an herb that is definitely antispirochetal for the bacteria would stimulate a response from the bacteria. That is, the bacteria *weaken* the muscle testing response in order to avoid the herb. Is that any more difficult a conception than the recognition of their subtle immune system remodulations that circumvent effective clearance of the bacteria from our systems?

Muscle testing, just like ELISA, can be useful, but like ELISA it is rarely diagnostically definitive. In the end, as it always does, it depends on the perceptual acuity of the practitioner and not the technique itself. (Again, some practitioners really are very good at muscle testing; it's just that many others are not.)

Natural treatment of borrelial infections

Again, we have found this combined approach extremely effective for the majority of people who use it. The approach entails:

1. Protecting endothelial structures.
2. The use of cytokine remodulators.
3. Protecting collagenous structures.
4. Using immune-modulating herbs to restructure the immune response.
5. Using herbs/supplements to protect and restore damaged physiological structures.
6. The use of herbs/supplements for reducing specific symptoms.
7. Antispirochetals.

CHAPTER EIGHT

THE CORE PROTOCOL AND EXTENDED REPERTORY

These natural active compounds, which contain more character-istics of high chemical diversity and biochemical specificity than standard combinatorial chemistry, offer major opportunities for finding novel lead structures that are active against a wide range of assay targets. In addition, natural products that are biolog-ically active in assays are generally small molecules with drug-like properties. Namely, they are capable of being absorbed and metabolized by the body.

Kaio Kitazato et al., 2007

We've used the approach outlined in this section for over a decade in the treatment of borrelial infections; it works very well, even for people who are experiencing severe neuroborreliosis.

Treatment rationale

The intervention rationale, using a natural protocol, for borrelial infections, whether Lyme or relapsing *Borrelia*, entails: (1) Protecting endothelial struc-tures; (2) cytokine remodulators; (3) protecting collagenous structures; (4) immune modulating herbs to restructure the immune response; (5) herbs/ supplements to protect and restore damaged physiological structures; (6) herbs/supplements for reducing specific symptoms; (7) Antispirochetals (primarily *Andrographis*).

- *Protecting endothelial structures.* Because *Borrelia* orient the majority of their infection of the body around their penetra-tion through endothelial cells and junctions, it is imperative those cells be protected. The bacterial assault on endothelial

structures, especially in the brain and heart, is the root of
the most damaging symptoms that occur during infection.
Thus, protecting endothelial cells and junctions protects
the brain and heart from damage. This is *the* foundation of
successful treatment of Lyme infections. The best herb for
this is *Polygonum cuspidatum* root. (EGCG is also useful and a
very strong protector of endothelial structures.) Protecting
endothelial cells from borrelial damage stops the bacteria's
movement deeper into the body. Over time, this denies them
access to the nutrients they need to survive and replicate.
It is one of the main ways to eliminate the infection. At the
very least, it will significantly diminish symptoms, considerably reducing the amount of damage the organisms can do
to the body.

- *Cytokine remodulators.* Herbs that are specific for interfering
with the cytokine cascade that the organisms initiate will
stop most of the inflammation in the body and interfere with
the pathogens' abilities to find and enter target cells, gather
nutrients, and reproduce. This, in and of itself, is essentially
antispirochetal; if the bacteria can't feed and reproduce, they
can't survive in the body. Though there are a number of
these we recommend (see the extended protocol/repertory),
the best *general* cytokine remodulators to use during Lyme
infection are *Scutellaria baicalensis* and *Salvia miltiorrhiza*.

- *Restoring collagenous structures.* Most of the damage the body
experiences during infection occurs because the bacteria
break down collagenous structures for food. The more they
are broken own, the more severe the symptoms become.
Restoring the body's collagenous structures helps reverse or
decrease many of the organisms' impacts on the body. There
are a number of things that can help, from a gelatin supplement to selenium to bone broth soup. Kudzu (*Pueria lobata*)
is also very helpful for this.

- *Immune remodulation and support.* The healthier the immune
system, as scores of researchers have commented, the fewer
the Lyme symptoms and the less damage that occurs in the

body. Cadavid (2006) is typical. He notes that "little if any tissue injury occurs in immunocompetent animals . . . in contrast, impairment of specific antibody production results in significant tissue injury." Thus, keeping immune function vital is essential if you live in Lyme-endemic areas; restoring it if it is diminished is important in the successful treatment of Lyme disease.

Borrelial bacteria also very specifically restructure the architecture and response of the immune system to meet their own needs. Counteracting this pathogen-initiated restructuring restores immune integrity and supports the clearance of the organisms from the body.

We have found *Astragalus* excellent at keeping immune function vital if you live in an endemic area. Other herbs that are exceptionally good for remodulating immune function are *Cordyceps, Eleutherococcus, Rhodiola, Scutellaria baicalensis, Uncaria tomentosa* (cat's claw), and *Withania somnifera* (ashwagandha).

- *Herbs/supplements to protect and restore damaged physiological structures.* Borrelial organisms can massively damage a number of the body's organs, including the brain, parts of the lymph system, joints, and the heart. Supporting and strengthening those systems while stimulating the regrowth of damaged tissues (e.g., neural structures) reduces the symptom picture and helps restore the body to health. *Uncaria rhynchophylla* (Chinese cat's claw) and *Hericium erinaceus* (lion's mane), as examples, are both good for protecting and regenerating neural structures on the brain.

- *Specific symptom treatment.* These bacteria can create a rather broad range of symptoms. Every symptom that is reduced will increase quality of life and add motive force to the healing process.

The most important thing during initial treatment is to reduce the most severe symptom as quickly as possible. This helps restore quality of life and feelings of joy (in people who have often been long without it), which in and of

CYTOKINE REMODULATORS

Here's an overview of the most effective cytokine remodulators for the major cytokines that borrelial bacteria activate. As you can see *Scutellaria baicalensis* and *Salvia miltiorrhiza* (as well as *Polygonum cuspidatum* and *Cordyceps*) are common throughout the list.

- IL-6 Inhibitors: *Andrographis paniculata, Isatis* spp., *Pueraria lobata, Salvia miltiorrhiza, Scutellaria baicalensis,* and melatonin.
- IL-8 inhibitors: *Cordyceps,* EGCG, *Isatis spp,* NAC, *Polygonum cuspidatum,* and *Punica granatum.*
- CCL2 inhibitors: *Coptis chinensis, Lonicera japonica, Polygonum cuspidatum, Salvia miltiorrhiza (strongly so), Scutellaria baicalensis, Sophora flavescens,* and *Tanacetum parthenium.*
- ERK/JNK/p38/NFkB pathway inhibitors: *Chelidonium majus, Cordyceps, Polygonum cuspidatum, Pueria lobata, Scutellaria baicalensis* root, and EGCG.
- ERK inhibitors: *Chelidonium majus, Cordyceps,* EGCG (green tea), *Olea europaea, Polygonum cuspidatum, Pueraria lobata,* and *Scutellaria baicalensis.*
- JNK inhibitors: *Cordyceps, Polygonum cuspidatum,* and *Scutellaria baicalensis.*
- P38 MAPK inhibitors: *Cordyceps,* EGCG (green tea), *Olea europaea, Polygonum cuspidatum,* and *Scutellaria baicalensis.*
- CD40 expression inhibitior: *Polygonum cuspidatum*
- TGF-beta inhibitors: *Artemisia* spp., *Astragalus* spp., *Cordyceps, Ginkgo biloba, Magnolia officinalis, Paeonia lactiflora, Schisandra chinensis, Salvia miltorrhiza, Scutellaria baicalensis,* and *S. barbata.*
- TNF-a inhibitors: *Andrographis paniculata, Cannabis* spp., *Capparis spinosa, Cordyceps, Eupatorium perfoliatum, Glycyrrhiza, Houttuynia cordata, Panax ginseng, Polygala tenuifolia, Pueraria lobata, Sambucus* spp., *Scutellaria baicalensis, Tanacetum parthenium,*

Salvia miltiorrhiza, Zingiber officinalis, and melatonin.
- IL-1*b* inhibitors: *Cordyceps, Eupatorium perfoliatum, Polygala tenuifolia, Polygonum cuspidatum, Pueraria lobata, Salvia miltiorrhiza, Scutellaria baicalensis,* and melatonin.
- IDO inhibitors: *Isatis, Polygonum cuspidatum, Scutellaria baicalensis,* and, most especially, *Crinum latifolium.*
- IFN-*a* inhibitors: *Polygonum cuspidatum, Salvia miltiorrhiza,* and curcumin.
- NF-*k*B inhibitors: *Astragalus, Bidens spp, Chelidonium majus, Cordyceps,* EGCG (green tea), *Eupatorium perfoliatum, Forsythia suspensa, Glycyrrhiza, Houttuynia cordata,* luteolin, *Olea europaea, Paeonia lactiflora, Polygonum cuspidatum, Polygala tenuifolia, Pueraria lobata, Punica granatum, Salvia miltiorrhiza, Schisandra chinensis, Scutellaria baicalensis, Withania somnifera,* and *Zingiber officinalis.*
- MMP-9 inhibitors: *Cordyceps, Olea europaea, Polygonum cuspidatum, Punica granatum, Salvia miltiorrhiza, Scutellaria baicalensis,* and the supplements EGCG and NAC.
- Hyaluronidase inhibitors (reduces/prevents the breakdown of cartilage and collagenous tissues: *Echinacea angustifolia* (large continuing doses), *Areca catechu, Lycopus* spp., *Scutellaria baicalensis, Withania somnifera,* the herbal blend *Triphala guggulu,* any plants containing rosmarinic acid (e.g. lemon balm and rosemary) and the supplements quercetin, curcumin, and tannic acid.
- Aggrecanase inhibitors (protects collagenous tissues from breakdown): *Aralia cordata; Camellia sinensis* (EGCG); *Cimicifuga heracleifolia;* a blend of *Clematis mandshurica, Polygonum cuspidatum, Prunella vulgaria, and Tricosanthes kirilowii.* The TCM formulation SiMiaoFang, which is composed of *Pellodendri Chinese cortex, Atractylodis rhizoma, Coicis semen, and Achyranthis bidentatae radix,* and the supplements curcumin, EGCG, luteolin, chondroitin sulfate, and glucosamine.

itself produces powerfully beneficial effects on the healing process. It also increases belief in the medicines and in the possibility of truly getting well. *General:* Tryptophan supplementation is a good place to begin.

- *Antispirochetals.* These can often help reduce the numbers of spirochetes in the body and assist the healing process. *Andrographis* is, in our experience, the most effective one at present. (There will eventually be others.)
- *Also:* Antitick repellants can help reduce the incidence of infection. The recipe for a natural, 99 percent effective blend against the ticks that carry *Borrelia* is included in the recipe section at the end of this chapter.

Again, there are thousands of plants that can be, and are, used in the treatment of disease. While throughout this book I have included many plants that are active for the damage that borrelial organisms cause, the following list contains the ones that, based on use, analysis of the organisms and the herbs, exhaustive journal research, and the experiences of both practitioners and those with the infection, I think are the most effective. (This includes a very few that *may* be very good, which we have not yet used, and which I think show promise.) This does not mean there are not others, not listed herein, that are just as effective.

Core protocol
Please check the known side effects on these herbs (in the materia medica chapter) before you use them.

Answers to the most commonly asked questions: (1) yes, take all of these; (2) yes, you can combine them; (3) alter the protocol as you find necessary; (4) the dosages are just guidelines, alter as needed; (5) no, you don't have to pulse; (6) use the extended protocol/repertory to modulate the protocol for your particular symptom picture; (7) yes, it works.

Note: Children's dosages *must* be adjusted for their age and weight. To adjust the dose divide their weight by 160 (if they weigh forty pounds, you would give them one-quarter the adult dose, which these dosages are). And, as with adults, the protocol must be adjusted to their specific circumstances, and symptom picture/response to the herbs over time.

Endothelial protection

Polygonum cuspidatum root, powder, tincture, or tablets.

- Powder: 1 teaspoon to 1 tbl of the root powder 3x daily. Start at the lower dose and work up, or . . .
- Tincture: ¼ to 1 tsp 3-6x daily, or . . .
- Tablets: These are normally labeled as *resveratrol* on the bottle. They are in fact knotweed root standardized for resveratrol content. (*Note:* Don't use grape resveratrol; it won't work very well.) Some comments on tablet dosages below:

    For the first edition of this book, the only reliable source I could find for a standardized knotweed tablet was Source Naturals brand. Those tablets contain 500 mg per tablet. However, a point of confusion arose (hundreds of emails), and that came from the directions on the bottle. They list a serving *size* of *two* tablets, thus the *one gram* (1,000 mg) on the label. (They get that from multiplying 500 times 2.) Each *serving* contains 8 percent total resveratrols (there is more than one kind), giving 80 mg total resveratrols with 20 mg of resveratrol itself. There is, as well, 5 mg of red wine extract (don't worry about this). This dosage works pretty well. If you get a different brand, it just needs to be in that range.

    The Source Naturals brand worked just fine for most people, however . . .

    Some people found that the Source Naturals resveratrol produced a number of unpleasant side effects for them. After switching to another brand (e.g., Paradise Herbs), the side effects disappeared.

Cytokine remodulation

Combined tinctures, equal parts, of *Salvia miltiorrhiza* and *Scutellaria baicalensis*: 1 tsp 3x daily.

Collagen protection

Great lakes gelatin powder, I prefer the pork but any variety will work, and it works very well: 1 tbl, once a day.

Vitamin C: 1,000–3,000 mg daily. I generally use an effervescent powder.

Selenium: 200 mcg daily.

Other supplements can also help immensely: See the expanded protocol/repertory below. Of these, the bone broth soup, *Echinacea angustifolia* tincture, and the herbal infusion combination are probably the strongest.

Immune remodulation

Note: If you are using tinctures, they can all be combined into a single formulation, you just have to increase the dose of the combination appropriately. The *Withania*, however, is best as a powder. (Homeopathic bio-salts, e.g. Bioplasma, dosage as per bottle label, can also be of help.)

1. *Uncaria tomentosa* bark.
   • Powder: 1 tsp 3x daily, or . . .
   • Tincture: ¼ to ½ tsp 3x daily, or . . .
   • Tablets/capsules: 1–4 500 mg tablets/capsules 3x day.
2. *Cordyceps* mycelium.
   • Powder: 1 tsp–1 tbl 3x day, or . . .
   • Tincture: ½–1 tsp 3x day)
3. *Withania somnifera.*
   • Powder: ½ tsp in a.m., 1 tsp p.m. before bed.
4. *Eleutherococcus senticosus* (1:5 formulation *not* the 1:1)
   • Tincture: ½ tsp 3x daily.
5. *Glycyrrhiza.*
   • Tincture: ¼ tsp 3x daily.

Antispirochetal

Andrographis capsules: *Begin with a small dose and work up.* I would recommend 600 mg (one capsule of a 1,200 mg formulation, for example) 3x daily to begin with, for one week. Then, if there are no side effects, increase the dose to two capsules 3x daily. *Please check the side effects on this herb:* Unpleasant allergic reactions can occur.

Neuroborreliosis

If you have neuroborreliosis, it is crucial to add to the core protocol:
Uncaria rhynchophylla.
   • Tincture: ½ –1 tsp 3–6x daily, depending on severity of brain infection.

AN EXAMPLE OF A USEFUL NEUROBORRELIOSIS PROTOCOL

(To be modified as necessary, please read Core Protocol section)

- *Polygonum cudpidatum* tincture, ½ tsp 3–6x daily
- *Salvia miltiorrhiza/Scutellaria baicalensis*, combined tincture, 1 tsp 3x daily.
- *Cordyceps/Eleutherococcus/Uncaria tomentosa* combined tincture, equal parts of each, 1.5 tsp 3x day
- *Glycyrrhiza* tincture, ¼ tsp 3x day

- *Uncaria rhynchophylla* tincture, ½–1 tsp 3–6x daily.
- *Withania somnifera.* Powder: ½ tsp in am, 1 tsp pm before bed.
- *Andrographis*, 1–2 600 mg capsules 3–6x daily.
- Tryptophan, 1500 mg 3x daily.
- Great lakes gelatin powder, 1 tbl in the morning in juice or water.
- Vitamin C, 1,000–3,000 mg daily.
- Selenium, 200 mcg daily.

The expanded protocol/repertory

An herbal *repertory* is a mechanism for increasing the sophistication of a protocol for specific disease complexes. Each section of the repertory is designed to address a specific symptom dynamic. So, for instance, if you have Lyme disease with severe anxiety, use the core protocol and *also* take vervain (*Verbena officinalis*).

1.1 To prevent infection

- In endemic areas: 1,000 mg *Astragalus* daily throughout the year.
- For duration of tick season: 3,000 mg *Astragalus* daily.
- Liberal use of natural tick repellant before going outdoors.
- At tick bite: Remove tick, liberally apply *Andrographis* tincture to bite site, cover with a moistened glob of bentonite clay, cover that with thin cotton, and leave on for twelve to twenty-four hours. (From reports, this seems to prevent active infection nearly every time.)
- At tick bite: Homeopathic ledum 1M 3x daily for three days. (From reports, this also seems to work for some people.)
- At appearance of rash: Homeopathic apis 30C 3x daily for three days, and begin core protocol.

1.2 Expanded collagen support protocol

You can add the following to the collagen support protocol if desired; this full protocol does help considerably; the more damaged your collagen structure are, the more likely you are to need as many of these are you can tolerate taking:

- Vitamin B complex: Daily, should include B-5, B-6, B-12, and folic acid.
- Vitamin E: 400–800 IU daily.
- Zinc: 25–50 mg 1x daily.
- Copper: 2–3mg daily (unless you have a known copper toxicity problem).
- Hyaluronic acid: 1 tbl daily (this can really help a lot).
- Bone broth soup: Bones of beef, best but stinky; chicken, pork, elk, bison will all work as well. (Check online for recipes.)
- Strong infusion of nettle, horsetail, oatstraw, parsley: Add 1 tablespoon of each to a quart of hot water, simmer for four hours; drink one quart each day.
- *Echinacea angustifolia* (**not** *E. purpurea*) tincture: 1 tsp 3-6x daily
- Propolis, royal jelly, bee pollen: 1 tsp of each, 1x daily (WS organics royal jelly mix contains all three, 1 tbl 1x daily.)
- Pine pollen tincture: ¼ tsp 2x daily.
- Cod liver oil (or its fermented form, if you can take the taste):1 tsp 2x daily.
- *Pueria lobata* tincture: ½ tsp 3x daily.

1.3 For neuroborreliosis

Core protocol plus . . .

  A. Specific:

   1. *Uncaria rhynchophylla* tincture: ½ to 1 teaspoon 3–6x daily, depending on severity of brain infection. (*Note:* absolutely crucial during neuroborreliosis.)
   2. Tryptophan, 1,500 mg 3x daily. (*Note:* will lower brain inflammation, decrease a number of psychological/physiological symptoms.)

B. With severe brain/CNS involvement, add:
   1. *Scutellaria baicalensis*, tincture, can increase current dose, plus . . .
   2. *Chelidonium majus* (greater celandine), tincture: ¼ tsp 3x daily, plus . . .
   3. *Pueria lobata* (kudzu) root, tincture, ¼ tsp 3–4x daily.
   4. NAC may also help: 2000 mg, 2x daily, as will . . .
   5. *Leonurus cardiaca* (motherwort) fresh plant tincture: ¼ to ½ tsp to 6x daily.
C. For Bell's palsy, add:
   1. Specific: *Stephania* tincture (either species): ½ tsp tincture 3x daily.
   2. Specific: *Pueria lobata* (kudzu) tincture, ½ tsp 3x daily.
   3. If recalcitrant: acupuncture.
   4. Supportive: Vitamin B-12, 1,000 mcg daily (lower to 500 as symptoms resolve).
D. To reduce borrelial neurotoxins (e.g., quinolinic acid), add:
   1. *Sida cordifolia* tincture: 5–40 drops to 3x day, and/or . . .
   2. *Angelica sinensis* tincture: ¼–½ tsp 3x day, and/or . . .
   3. Melatonin, 3–9 mg daily.
   4. The selenium already in the collagen protocol will help with this.
E. Brain "feels toxic," add:
   1. *Centella asiatica*: 500 mg 2x daily or ¼ tsp tincture 2x daily. (*Note:* may cause headaches)
F. Low brain energy, add:
   1. Acetyl-L-carnatine: 500 mg 2x daily (*Note:* contraindicated if seizures are present.)
G. Brain "pressure," add:
   1. *Pueria lobata* (kudzu): ¼–½ tsp of tincture 3x daily.
H. For remyelination of neurons, add:
   1. *Salvia miltiorrhiza*, can increase dosage by 2–3x, and/or . . .
   2. *Uncaria rhynchophylla*, can increase current dosage, and/or . . .
   3. *Withania somnifera*, can increase current dosage, and/or. . .
   4. *Eupatorium perfoliatum* (boneset), hot tea 3–4x daily.

I. With tremors, add:

1. *Sida acuta* (or equivalent species): 5–40 drops 3x daily, and/ or . . .

2. *Scutellaria baicalensis*: can increase current dosage, and/ or . . .

3. *Mucuna pruriens* (L-dopa precursor): 500 mg 1x day in morning, and/or . . .

4. Gabapentin (by prescription), as prescribed.

J. Memory/cognitive dysfunction, trouble finding words, brain fog, add:

1. Phosphatidyl-serine: 100 mg 3x daily, and/or . . .

2. *Ginkgo biloba*, standardized: 150 mg 2x daily, and/or . . .

3. *Centella asiatica* (gotu kola): 500 mg 2x daily, or tincture ¼ tsp 2x daily (may cause headaches), and/or . . .

4. Taurine: 125 mg, 3x daily.

5. Some of the following may also be of use: Phosphatidyl-choline, 500 mg 3x daily; *Cordyceps* powder, 1 tsp - 1tbl 3x day; *Pueria lobata* (kudzu root), 500–1000 mg 3x daily or ¼–½ tsp tincture 3x daily; *Polygala senega* (Chinese senega root) tincture, 30 drops 3x daily; *Hericium erinaceus* (lion's mane) 1 tsp powder 3x daily or ¼–½ tsp tincture 3x daily; quercetin, 1,200 mg daily; pycnogenol (from french martime pine bark only) 100 mg 1x daily; Vitamin D-3, 5,000–10,000 IU daily; *Bacopa monniera* (especially for short-term memory help) 500 mg 2x daily; homeopathic Kali Phos, 30C, 4 pellets 3x daily.

K. With hypoperfusion of the brain, add:

1. *Ginkgo biloba* tincture (standardized): ¼ tsp 3x daily, or standardized capsules: 125 mg 3x daily.

L. With neural pain, add:

1. *Chelidonium majus* (greater celandine), tincture; ¼ tsp 3x daily, and/or . . .

2. *Pueria lobata* (kudzu) root tincture: ½ tsp 3–4x daily, and/ or . . .

3. *Melissa officinalis* (lemon balm) tincture, ½ tsp 3–4x daily, and/or . . .

4. Homeopathic Kali Phos: 30C 4 pellets 4x daily.

M. With "buzzing" or "electric feeling" in nerves, add:

1. *Sida acuta* (or equivalent species), tincture, 5–40 drops 3x daily.

N. With epilepsy/seizures, add:

1. *Uncaria rhynchophylla*: increase dose up to 1 tbl 6x daily depending on severity of seizures, and also take . . .
2. *Gastroida elata* tincture: ¼–½ tsp 3-6x daily.
3. *Salvia miltiorrhiza* may also be of help: increase dose to 1 tbl, depending on severity of seizures, 3–6x daily, and/or . . .
4. Cannabis oil or equivalent, variable dosages, and/or . . .
5. *Cryptolepis sanguinolenta* tincture may also be of help: ½ tsp 3–6x daily, and/or . . .
7. Taurine sometimes helps: 125 mg 3x daily.
8. Frankincense essential oil, applied topically, daily, to the temples and base of skull may help alleviate severity of seizures.

O. With left temporal strokes, add:

1. *Salvia miltiorrhiza*, increase dose: up to 1 tsp 6x daily, and/or . . .
2. *Uncaria rhynchophylla*, increase dose: up to 1 tsp 6x daily, and/or . . .
3. *Ginkgo biloba* tincture (standardized): 1 tsp 3–6x daily, or standardized capsules: 600 mg 3x daily.

P. With subarachnoid hemorrhage, add:

1. Melatonin: 3–9 mg daily

Q. With bouts of unrestrained rage, add:

1. *Uncaria rhyncyophylla*: increase dose, up to 1 tsp 6x daily, and/or . . .
2. *Cryptolepis sanguinolenta* tincture: ½ tsp 3–6x daily, and/or . . .
3. Tryptophan, 1,000–1,500 mg 3x daily.

R. With behaviorial outrage in children, add:

1. Dimethyl glycine, 125–375 mg 2x daily, and/or . . .
2. *Uncaria rhynchophylla*, ¼–½ tsp 3x daily.
3. Trytophan, 1,000–1,500 mg 3x daily.

S. With feeling that brain is on fire, add:

1. Homeopathic gelsenium, 30C 4 pellets 4x daily

T. With OCD, add:

1. Inositol, 600 mg 2x daily, and/or . . .
2. Vitamin D-3, 5,000–10,000 IU daily, and/or . . .
3. Cod liver oil, 1 tsp 2x daily, and/or . . .
4. Dimethyl glycine, 125–375 mg 2x daily, and/or . . .
5. Zeolite, liquid: 15 drops 3–4x daily, or powder 2 heaping tsp daily or 3 capsules 3x daily.

U. To restore neuronal structures, add neural regrowth stimulants:

1. *Polygala senega* (Chinese senega root) tincture, 30 drops 3x daily, and/or . . .
2. *Hericium erinaceus* (lion's mane) powder, 3–8 grams daily or 1 tsp tincture 3–4x daily.

V. Limbs feel heavy, add:

1. *Centella asiatica* (gotu kola) , 500 mg or ¼ tsp tincture 2x daily.

W. Swallowing difficulty, add:

1. *Ailanthus altissima* tincture, 5–10 drops to 4x daily.

1.4 With anxiety/ hysteria/extreme fear

A. General, add:

1. *Pulsatilla* (pasque flower) tincture, 10 drops each hour as long as necessary, and/or . . .
2. *Leonurus cardiaca* (motherwort) fresh plant tincture, ¼–½ tsp to 6x daily, and/or . . .
3. *Corallorhiza maculata* (coral root), or equivalent species, 30 drops (full dropper) to 6x daily, and/or . . .
4. *Scutellaria baicalensis* tincture, ¼–½ tsp 3x daily, and/or . . .
5. *Verbena officinalis* (vervain) tincture, 30 drops to 6x daily, and/or . . .
6. *Uncaria rhynchophylla* tincture, 30 drops to 6x daily, and/or. . .
7. Tryptophan, 1,000–1,500 mg 3x daily.
8. *Sambucus* (elder) flower tea throughout the day may also be of help.

1.5 With unconsolable anxiety

A. General, add:

1. Homeopathic aconite 30C 4 pellets dissoved in half cup water, sipped throughout day.

1.6 With sleep disturbance/insomnia

A. General, add:

1. Melatonin liquid, manufacturers directions, one hour before bed, and/or. . .

2. *Withania somnifera* (ashwagandha) tincture, ½ tsp one hour before bed; or powder or capsules, 1 gram an hour before bed, and/or . . .

3. *Scutellaria baicalensis* tincture, ½–1 tsp 3x daily, and/or . . .

4. *Leonurus cardiaca* (motherwort) fresh plant tincture, ¼ *ounce* (yes, that is right) in liquid just before bed (if the melatonin does not help), and/or . . .

5. Suan zao rhen tang tablets/pellets, plum flower brand (5 tablets just before bed), and/or . . .

6. Te xiao zao ren an mian pian (sleepeace) tablets/pellets, 5 tablets just before bed, and/or . . .

7. Glycine, 125–375 mg daily, and/or . . .

8. Tryptophan, 1000 mg just before bed, and/or . . .

9. Gabapentin (prescription), as prescribed.

B. For bolting awake in middle of night, add

1. Phosphatidyl serine (100 mg 3x daily), and/or . . .

2. *Withania somnifera* (ashwagandha), ½ tsp tincture one hour before bed; or powder or capsules, 1 gram an hour before bed, and/or . . .

3. *Schisandra chinensis* tincture, ½ tsp just before bed.

4. Cannabis, various formulations.

1.7 Depression

A. General:

1. core protocol, plus . . .

2. *Eleutherococcus,* 1:1 formulation, ¼–½ tsp 3x daily, and/or . . .

3. Melatonin, 3–9 mg day, and/or . . .
4. *Mucuna pruriens*, 500 mg 1x daily in morning, and/or . . .
5. *Leonurus cardiaca* (motherwort) fresh plant tincture, ¼–1tsp as often as needed, and/or. . .
6. *Corallorhiza maculata* (or equivalent), ½–1 tsp to 6x daily, and/or . . .
7. SAMe, 200 mg 1–2x daily, and/or . . .
8. Tryptophan, 1,000–1,500 mg 3x daily.
9. Kratom (*Mitragyna speciosa*) powder, ½ tsp mixed in warm water, 1–3x daily (may cause jitteriness).

1.8 For relapsing fever borreliosis

A. Red blood cell protection, add:
1. *Sida acuta* (or equivalent species), tincture, 5–40 drops 3x daily

B. Spleen/lymph node protection, add:
1. *Salvia miltiorrhiza* (if you are not already taking it), ½ tsp 3x daily. *Note:* can be increased to 1 tsp 6x day if spleen damage is severe.

C. Liver protection, add:
1. *Silybum marianum* (milk thistle seed), standardized, 1,200 mg 3x daily.

D. For additional endothelial protection, if necessary, add:
1. EGCG (green tea catechins) capsules: Try to get a supplement with at least 80 percent polyphenols and 50 percent or so of EGCG. A supplement with the natural green tea flavonoids would be even better. Dosage range is 400–800 mg daily. For greater effectiveness in treating *Rickettsiae*-generated endothelial cell damage, take it with 1200 mg quercetin daily – both at the same time, in the morning. *Note:* there is about 100 mg EGCG in a cup of green tea. I would imagine that drinking green tea itself throughout the day would be a good approach and it produces better bioavailability.

E. For Herxheimer reactions:
    1. *Note:* These can be extremely severe during relapsing fever episodes, see the listing for Herxheimer reactions in this repertory (page 234).

F. For septic shock:
    1. You can read an in-depth look at the dynamics of sepsis and septic shock in *Natural Treatments for Lyme Coinfections: Anaplasma, Babesia, and Ehrlichia* (Healing Arts Press, 2015). The protocol for sepsis is assertive, large doses are necessary to turn the condition around. The following protocol should be followed until the cytokine storm stabilizes. The core protocol *except for the Japanese knotweed root* should be *discontinued* and this intervention used instead.
    2. Tincture combination of *Angelica sinensis* and *Astragalus* spp.: equal parts, 1 tbl each hour.
    3. Tincture of *Salvia miltiorrhiza*, 1 tbl each hour.
    4. Tincture of *Pueraria lobata* (kudzu) and *Cordyceps* spp, equal parts, 1 tbl each hour.
    5. Tincture of *Glycyrrhiza* spp (licorice) and *Scutellaria baicalensis*: equal parts, 1 tbl each hour.

1.9 Low libido

A. General, add:
    1. *Pinus* (Pine pollen) tincture: ¼–½ tsp 3x daily (must be held in mouth for one minute then swallowed, do not put in water) and/or . . .
    2. *Withania somnifera* (ashwagandha) powder: ½ tsp in a.m., 1 tsp p.m. before bed, and/or . . .
    3. Maca (*Lepidium meyenii*) powder: 1 tsp 2–3x daily.

1.10 Fever

A. General, add:
    1. *Eupatorium perfoliatum* (boneset): hot tea as often as needed.
    2. *Sambucus* (elder) flower: hot tea, as often as needed.
    3. *Mentha piperata* (peppermint): hot tea, as often as needed.

4. *Corallorhiza maculata* (coral root), or equivalent species: 30 drops (full dropper) to each hour depending on severity, and/or . . .

5. *Achillea millefolium* (yarrow): hot tea, as often as needed, or tincture, 10–30 drops as often as needed.

6. *Cryptolepis sanguinolenta* tincture: ½–1 tsp 3–4x daily.

B. If severe, add:

1. Wash with cool cloth or in tub until fever lowers, and/or. . .

2. Dosages of above may be increased if very severe.

1.11 Eye involvement

A. Specific: *Stephania* tincture (either species): ½ tsp tincture 3x daily.

1. *Stephania* eyewash can also help: see materia medica for preparation.

B. Supportive:

1. Vitamin C: 1,000 mg 3x daily (effervescent salts), and . . .

2. Zinc: 25–50 mg once daily, and . . .

3. Lutein: 50 mg 3x daily, and . . .

4. Bilberry: 500 mg 2x daily, and/or. . .

5. *Schisandra chinensis*: tincture, ¼–½ tsp 3x daily.

C. Floaters:

1. *Stephania* tincture (either species): ½ tsp tincture 3x daily, and/or

2. Chlorella: 1 tbl 3x daily, and/or . . .

3. Zeolite, liquid: 15 drops 3–4x daily, or powder 2 heaping teaspoons daily or 3 capsules 3x daily.

D. Photosensitivity:

1. Melatonin: 3-9 mg daily, and . . .

2. *Leonarus cardiaca*: ½ tsp 3–6x daily, and/or . . .

3. *Hericium erinaceus* tincture: ¼–½ tsp 3x daily, and/or . . .

4. Lichi berries: eat throughout the day.

1.12 Pain

A. General, add:

1. Bryonia homeopathic 30C: 4 pellets 4x daily, and/or. . .

2. Arnica homeopathic: same dosage, and/or . . .

3. Hypericum homeopathic: same dosage, and/or . . .

4. *Corydalis* tincture: ⅛–¼ tsp 3-4 x daily (contraindicated in liver disease), and/or . . .

5. *Monotropa uniflora* (Indian pipe) tincture: ¼–½ tsp hourly or as needed, and/or . . .

6. *Corallorhiza maculata* (coral root): or equivalent species, ½–1 tsp to 6x daily, and/or . . .

7. *Verbena officinalis* (vervain) tincture: ¼–1 tsp as needed, and/or . . .

8. *Leonurus cardiaca* (motherwort) fresh plant tincture: 1 tsp–½ ounce (yes, ounce) in water, as needed, and/or . . .

9. *Pedicularis* (lousewort) tincture: 1 tsp– ½ ounce (yes, ounce) in water, as needed, and/or . . .

10. Gabapentin (prescription): as prescribed.

B. If severe, add:

1. *Angelica* tincture is useful for pain, especially when combined with *Salvia miltiorrhiza* tincture, 1 tbl of the combination (equal parts) every fifteen minutes, reducing dosage and frequency as the pain lessens.

1.13 To lower histamines

A. General (this helps bring inflammation down/lower allergic responses/help response to protocol), add:

1. *Petasites hybridus* (butterbur): 50mg 3x daily, and/or. . .

2. Inositol: 600 mg 2x daily, and/or . . .

3. Any of the following may be of help: *Agaricus blazei, Ailanthus altissima, Angelica sinensis, Camellia sinensis, Cichorium intybus, Cinnamum verum, Cordyceps militaris, Eleutherococcus senticosus, Forsythia koreana, Ganoderma lucidum, Houttuynia cordata, Ginkgo biloba, Glycyrrhiza glabra, Isodon japonicus, Lycopus lucidus, Magnolia officinalis, Mentha arvensis, Morus alba, Olea europaea, Oryza sativa, Paeonia suffruticosa, Perilla frutescens, Plumbago zeylanica, Polygonum cuspidatum, Polygonum tinctorium, Prunella vulgaris, Rehmannia glutinosa, Rhodiola sacra, Salvia miltiorrhiza, Salvia plebeia, Schizonepeta*

tenifolia, Silybum marianum, Sinomenium acutum, Solanum lyratum, Sophora flavescens, Syzygium aromaticum, and chaga, chlorella, lavender essential oil, propolis, pycnogenol, and spirulina.

1.14 Lyme arthritis

A. General:

1. Entire collagen support protocol, and . . .
2. *Boswellia serrata*: ¼–½ tsp 2x daily, or 500 mg 2x daily, and . . .
3. *Apium graveolens* (celery seed) tincture: ¼–½ tsp 3x daily (very effective), and/or . . .
4. Arthritis tea daily (really does help, see end of chapter for recipe), and/or . .
5. Cod liver oil: 1 tsp 2x daily (really does help), and/or . . .
6. Cannabinoid oil: topically and internally, variable dosing, and/or. . .
7. *Dipsacus sylvestris* (teasel) root: 10 drops to 1 tsp 3x daily, and/or . . .
8. *Harpagophytum procumbens* (devil's claw): 1000–2000 mg, 3x daily.

B. With pain:

1. Curcumin/bromelain combination: 400–500 mg, 3x daily, and/or . . .
2. Capsaicin (in lemon water drink, see end of chapter for recipe), and/or . . .
3. Turmeric powder: ½–1 tsp 3x daily, and/or . . .
4. *Salix alba* (white willow) bark tincture (works very well for some) ½ tsp 3x daily, and/or . . .
5. Cannabinoid oil: topically and internally, variable dosing, and/or. . .
6. *Valeriana officinalis/Passiflora incarnata/Piscidia* spp. (valerian/passion flower/Jamaican dogwood) tincture combination, equal parts, ¼–½ tsp 3–6x daily, and/or. . .
7. *Monotropa uniflora* (Indian pipe) tincture: ¼–½ tsp hourly or as needed, and/or . . .

8. *Corallorhiza maculata* (coral root) or equivalent, ½–1 tsp to
   6x daily, and/or . . .

9. Homeopathic chamomilla 30C 4 pellets 4–5x daily, and/
   or . . .

10. Homeopathic hypericum: same dose, and/or . . .

11. Homeopathic arnica: same dose, and/or . . .

12. Homeopathis arsenicum: same dose, and/or . . .

13. Homeopathic rhus tox: same dose.

1.15 Skin involvement

A. General:

1. Core protocol

B. With dry skin, add:

1. Hyaluronic acid: 1 tbl daily, and/or . . .

2. *Arctium lappa* (burdock) root powder: 1 tsp 3x daily, and/
   or . . .

3. Coconut oil: topically, liberally, and . . .

4. Coconut oil: internally, 1 tsp–1tbl 3x daily, and/or . . .

5. Cod liver oil: 1 tsp 2x daily.

C. With loss of elasticity, add:

1. Strong infusion of nettle, horsetail, oatstraw, parsley: (Add
   1 tbl of each to a quart of hot water, simmer for 4 hours.
   Drink one quart each day.)

2. Great lakes gelatin powder, I prefer the pork but any
   variety will work, and it works very well: 1 tbl, once
   a day.

3. Vitamin C salts: to bowel tolerance.

C. With psoriasis, add:

1. Homeopathic rhus tox 30C: 4 pellets 6x daily for two
   weeks, repeat as necessary.

D. With excessive sweating, add:

1. *Sambucus* (elder) leaf tincture, 1–5 drops 3x daily.

1.16 Morgellons

A. General:

1. Core protocol (does help), plus . . .

2. *Sida acuta* (or equivalent species): tincture, 5–40 drops 3–4x day, and/or . . .

3. *Cryptolepis sanguinolenta* tincture, ½–1 tsp 3–4x day, and/or . . .

4. Artemisinin: 100 mg, 3–4x daily, plus. . .

5. Borax (20 mule team): internally and topically. Internally: 2 tsp in quart of water, mix well, take 1 tsp–1 tbl 3x daily (alternate: ⅛ tsp in 20 ounces of water once a day). Topically: Put the mix in spray bottle and spray affected areas. Use borax as well when you wash your clothes. (This last one does help many people.)

6. Topical application of *Andrographis* tincture to lesion/fiber extrusion sites. Pour tincture into a bowl; use cotton balls for direct application.

1.17 Muscle twitches, tingling/crawling sensations/ numbness in extremities

A. General:

1. Vitamin B-12: 1,000 mcg daily (lower to 500 as symptoms resolve), and/or . . .

2. Vitamin B-6: 100 mg 2x daily (lower to 50 as symptoms resolve), and/or . . .

3. Folic acid: 400 mcg daily, and/or. . .

4. Magnesium: 200–400 mg to 3x daily, and/or. . .

5. *Sida acuta* tincture: 5–40 drops 3x daily, and/or . . .

6. Gabapentin (prescription): as prescribed.

B. With numbness, add:

1. *Polygonum cuspidatum* (knotweed root) tincture: ½ tsp 6–10x day. (*Note:* especially useful for carpal tunnel- and lateral epicondylitis-type problems.)

2. *Ginkgo biloba* tincture (standardized), 1 tsp 3–6x daily, or standardized capsules: 600 mg 3x day.

3. *Zingiber officinalis* (ginger) root: 2 ounces fresh juice, squeeze of lime, pinch of cayenne, honey to taste, in 8–10 ounces hot water, 3–4 cups daily.

1.18 Lyme carditis

A. With angina, add:

1. *Polygonum cuspidatum* (knotweed root) tincture: ½ tsp 3–6x daily, and/or . . .
2. *Salvia miltiorrhiza* tincture: ½ tsp 3–6x daily, and/or . . .
2. *Astragalus*: 1,000 to 4,000 mg, 3–4x daily, and/or . . .
3. *Stephania* tincture (either species): ½ tsp tincture 3x daily, and/or . . .
4. *Crataegus oxyacantha* (hawthorn) 120–900 mg 3x daily, and/or . . .
5. *Amni visnaga* (khella): 250–300 mg daily, and/or . . .
6. L-Carnitine, 500 mg 3x day.

B. With arrhythmia, add:

1. *Stephania* tincture (either species): ½ tsp tincture 3x daily, and/or
2. *Crataegus oxyacantha* (hawthorn): 120–900 mg 3x daily, and/or . . .
3. Taurine: 125–375 mg 3x day, and/or . . .
4. *Leonurus cardiaca* (motherwort): fresh plant tincture, ¼ tsp 4x day.

C. With palpitations, add:

1. *Polygonum cuspidatum* (knotweed root) tincture: ½ tsp 3–6x daily, and/or . . .
2. *Astragalus*: 1,000–4,000 mg, 3–4x daily, and/or . . .
3. Liquid chlorophyll: 1 tbl in 20 ounces water, once day, and/or . . .
4. Cataplex E, standard process: dose as on bottle.
5. *Urtica dioca* (nettle) leaf tea strong infusion: ¼ cup herb in quart of hot water, let stand overnight, drink throughout day.
6. (Check potassium levels and electrolytes.)

D. With shortness of breath, add:

1. *Polygonum cuspidatum* (knotweed root) tincture: ½ tsp 3–6x daily, and/or . . .
2. *Astragalus*: 1,000–4,000 mg, 3–4x daily, and/or . . .

3. Liquid chlorophyll: 1 tbl in 20 ounces of water, once daily, and/or . . .

4. *Cordyceps* powder: 1 tsp–1tbl 3x daily, and/or . . .

5. *Ailanthus altissima* tincture: 10 drops–½ tsp 4x daily.

E. With hypotension:

1. *Glycyrrhiza* (licorice) tincture: 1 tsp to 6x daily depending on severity of condition (*Note:* do not take for more than 60 days in this form), and/or . . .

2. Caffeine: variable dosing, and/or . . .

3. If nothing else works, yohimbine as supplement: begin with dosing on bottle and increase as needed. (Please note warnings on label and use caution.)

F. With hypertension:

1. Specific: *Uncaria rhynchophylla* tincture: ½ tsp to 6x day.

2. *Crataegus oxyacantha* (hawthorn): 120–900 mg 3x daily, and/or . . .

3. *Leonurus cardiaca* (motherwort): 30 drops–1 tsp to 6x daily, and/or . . .

4. *Mimosa pudica* tincture: 20–60 drops daily. (*Note:* May also be of benefit in depression, anxiety, headaches, and damaged nervous structures.)

G. With poor circulation (cold extremeties), add:

1. *Zingiber officinalis* (ginger) root: 2 ounces fresh juice, squeeze of lime, pinch of cayenne, honey to taste, in 8–10 ounces hot water, 3–4 cups daily.

1.19 Headaches

A. General:

1. The core protocol should help immensely, however . . .

B. With migraine-like, add

1. *Verbena officinalis* (vervain) tincture: ¼–1 tsp as needed, and/or . . .

2. Cannabis or CBD: variable dosages, and/or . . .

3. *Pueria lobata* (kudzu): ½ tsp 3–4x daily, (will also help prevent), and/or . . .

4. *Scutellaria baicalensis* tincture: ½ tsp 6x daily in addition to core protocol dose, and/or. . .

5. Lithium orotate: 5–20 mg daily.

C. With headache at back of head:

1. *Verbena officinalis* (vervain) tincture: ¼–1 tsp as needed.

D. At front of head:

1. *Silybum marianum* (milk thistle seed): standardized, 1,200 mg every 3 hours, and/or . . .

2. *Rumex crispus* (yellow dock) root tincture: 1 tsp in water at bedtime, and/or . . .

3. Castor oil packs topically on liver region.

1.20 Fatigue

A. General:

1. The core protocol should help immensely, however . . .

B. For chronic, add:

1. *Eleutherococcus* tincture: 1:5 formulation as a tonic, ½ tsp 3–6x day. (*Note:* if it is severe or acute onset use the 1:1 or 2:1 formulation, pulse every ten days. When it becomes less severe, convert to the 1:5 formulation.)

2. Chronic fatigue formula: see recipe at end of this chapter, ¼ cup of the powder, blended in juice or water in morning and again just before bed.

C. For adrenal fatigue, add:

1. *Pinus* (Pine pollen) tincture: ¼–½ tsp 3x daily (must be held in mouth for one minute then swallowed, do not put in water), and/or . . .

2. *Glycyrrhiza* (licorice) tincture: ¼–½ tsp 3x daily (not to exceed 30 days), and/or . . .

3. Vitamin C effervescent powder: to bowel tolerance, and/or . . .

4. Maca (*Lepidium meyenii*) powder: 1 tsp 2–3x daily, and/or . . .

5. *Rhodiola* tincture, 10–40 drops 2–4x daily, and/or . . .

6. *Codonopsis pilosula* tincture: ¼ tsp 4x daily.

D. For thyroid fatigue, add:
1. *Juglans nigra* (black walnut hull) tincture: 5–10 drops 2x daily, and/or . . .
2. Selenium: 200 mcg daily, and/or . . .
3. Kelp: 500 mg every other day, and/or . . .
4. *Rhodiola* tincture: 10–40 drops 2-4x daily.

E. For mitochondrial fatigue
1. *Leonurus cardiaca* (motherwort) fresh plant tincture, ½-1 tsp 3x daily, and/or . . .
2. NADH: 10–20 mg 2x daily
3. D-ribose: 1 scoop 2x daily, best if combined with apple cider vinegar or effervescent magnesium)
4. L-arginine: 1,000 mg 3x daily.
5. Also of use: L-carnitine (500 mg 3x day), Alpha lipoic acid (200–600 mg daily), Coenzyme Q10 (60–150mg daily).

1.21 Muscle weakness

A. General:
1. *Pinus* (pine pollen) tincture, *Aralia naudicaulis, Panax quin-quefolius* (American ginseng), combination tincture: equal parts of each, full dropper of the tincture 3x daily for six months (take by mouth, do not put in water), and/or . . .
2. L-carnitine: 1,000 mg 3x daily, and/or . . .
3. Taurine, 500–1,000 mg 3x daily, and/or . . .
4. Homeopathic lycopodium 30C: 4 pellets 4x daily.

1.22 Swollen lymph nodes/sluggish lymph

A. General, add:
1. *Ceanothus* (red root) tincture: ¼–1 tsp 3x daily, and/or . . .
2. *Salvia miltiorrhiza* tincture: 1 tsp 3x daily, and/or . . .
3. *Phytolacca* (poke) root tincture: 5–10 drops 2x day, and/or . . .
4. *Galium aparine* (cleavers) tincture: (especially for nodules and cysts), ½ tsp 3x daily.

1.23 For Herxheimer reactions

A. General, add:

1. Zeolite, liquid: 15 drops 3–4x daily, or powder 2 heaping tsp daily or 3 capsules 3x daily (*Note*: do not accidentally breathe in), and/or . . .

2. Activated charcoal: 2 capsules, 1–2x daily, and/or . . .

3. Chlorella: 1 tbl 3x daily, and/or . . .

4. Green clay (internally): 1 tbl in cup of water, drink at bedtime, and/or . . .

5. Fruit pectin: 1 tsp in water at bedtime, and/or . . .

6. Increase *Ceanothus* (red root) and *Salvia* dosage, and/or . . .

7. Epsom salt baths: daily, and/or . . .

8. Castor oil packs on liver, daily, and/or. . .

B. With Herxheimer reactions in GI tract, add:

1. Zeolite: same dosage as above, and/or . . .

2. Activated charcoal: 2 capsules, 1–2x daily, and/or . . .

3. Chlorella: 1 tbl 3x daily, and/or . . .

4. Food-grade diatomaceous earth (don't breathe in): 1 tbl in half-cup water, at bedtime.

1.24 Multiple chemical sensitivity

A. General, add:

1. *Hericium erinaceus* (lion's mane) tincture: ¼–½ tsp 3x daily, and/or . . .

2. Homeopathic nux vomica 30C: 4 pellets 4x daily or as needed, and/or . . .

3. Melatonin: 3–9 mg daily.

1.25 Digestive

A. General:

1. Digestive bitters: 5 drops fifteen minutes before a meal, and/or . . .

2. Raw fermented foods as general intake daily.

3. Digestive enzymes in food, i.e., regular consumption of papaya, pineapple, and so on.

4. Betaine HCL (with or without pepsin): 500–1,000 mg just before meals.

B. Constipation:

1. Vitamin C: to bowel tolerance
2. Magnesium: to bowel tolerance
3. *Rumex crispus/Arctium lappa/Althaea* (yellow dock/burdock root/marshmallow root) powders: equal parts of each, 1 heaping tsp in water, just before bed.

C. Diarrhea:

1. Blackberry root strong infusion: (¼ ounce herb in one quart of hot water, cover and steep overnight), strain, and then drink throughout the day.

D. Nausea:

1. Homeopathic nux vomica 30C: 4 pellets every hour, and/or . . .
2. *Mentha piperata* (peppermint) essential oil: ONE drop only, on tongue, followed by 6 ounces water.
3. *Moringa oleifera*: 1 tsp powder in water 3x daily.

E. Leaky gut:

1. *Salvia miltiorrhiza* tincture: 1 tsp 3x daily.
2. *Althaea officinalis* (marshmallow) root: 1 tsp–1 tbl powder in liquid, 3x daily.
3. Tumeric milk: 3x daily, see recipe section below.
4. Glutamine: 500 mg 2x daily.

F. IBS/Crohn's:

1. Fresh juice of piece of green cabbage the size of a medium carrot (the core of the protocol), four fresh plantain leaves (if you can find them – look in the yard, the plant really does help heal the mucosa and lower inflammation), one medium beet, four stalks celery, three carrots. Daily in a.m. and again just before bed.

1.26 Liver pain, just under rib cage

A. General:

1. *Salvia miltiorrhiza* tincture: 1 tsp 3x daily, and/or . . .

2. *Ceanothus* (red root) tincture: ¼–1 tsp 3x daily, and/or . . .

3. *Schisandra chinensis*, tincture: ¼–½ tsp 3x daily.

B. Specific:

1. *Silybum marianum* (milk thistle seed): standardized, 1,200 mg every four hours.

1.27 For candida overgrowth from antibiotics

A. General:

1. Caprylic acid: ~2163 mg, 2 capsules 3x daily.

2. Undecenoic acid (suggested: Thorne Research Formula SF722): 50 mg, 2 gel caps 3x daily.

3. *Chapparo amargosa*/desert willow tincture combination: equal parts, ½ tsp 4x daily for 30 days, can be repeated.

4. *Phellodendron* (or other berberine plant) tincture: ½ tsp 4x daily for 30 days, can be repeated,

B. To restore bowel flora/fauna:

1. PB8, probiotic acidophilus capsules: 2 capsules daily.

1.28 To maintain bowel health while on antibiotics

A. General:

1. Probiotic 8 (PB8) or equivalent: 2 capsules daily.

1.29 For breaking up biofilms

A. General (if you must):

1. The core protocol will do it by itself, however . . .

2. Any of the following will also do so: *Andrographis paniculata, Houttuynia cordata, Polygonum cuspidatum, Rhodiola spp, Scutellaria baicalensis*, apigenin, and the supplement N-acetyl cysteine (NAC) and resveratrol.

3. Also effective are: *Achillea millefolium, Achyranthes aspera, Aegle marmelos, Boesenbergia rotunda, Capparis spinosa, Cassia siamea, Chelidonium majus, Coccina grandis, Dendrophtheoe falcata, Dolichos lablab, Embelia ribes, Emblica officinalis, Epimedium brevicornum, Glycyrrhiza spp, Juniperus spp, Lonicera spp, malus pumila, Melaleuca alternifolia, Mentha piperata, Nigella sativa, Paeonia lactiflora, Piper sarmentosum, Plectranthus*

barbatus, *P. ecklonii*, *Rhodomyrtus tomentosa*, *Rosmarinus offi-cinalis*, *Salvadora persica*, *Sclerocarya birrea* (bark decoction), *Zingiber*, the compound Chinese formulation Baifuqing, berberine-containing plants, the Chinese formulation TanReQing, and the supplements piperine, royal jelly, and curcumin.

Recipes

The following are some of the need-to-be-prepared formulations suggested in the extended protocol/repertory.

Natural tick repellent

This blend is ~99 percent effective for the major tick species that carry *Borrelia*. (Really)

To make: Take ½ teaspoon *each* of the essential oils of *Rhododendron tomentosum* (formerly: *Ledum palustre*, aka Labrador tea, and no *Rhoden-dron anthopogon* will not work, don't use it), *Tagetes minuta*, *Chamaecy-paris nootkatensis*, *Artemisia absinthium*, *Myrica gale* (aka, bog myrtle), *Juniperus virginia*, *Eucalyptus citriodora* (aka, lemon eucalyptus), and *Origanum majorana* (aka, marjoram – note: *Origanum vulgare*, aka oregano, will work it is just not quite as strong.

Add the essential oils (1 tsp total volume) to 8 (that is, eight) ounces pure grain alcohol (95 percent alcohol) or as close to that as you can get. (Some local governments do not think you should have access to that percentage of alcohol because of your past behavior in college – getting naked and dancing on top of a cop car is no way to go through life. Son, I am disappoint.) Blend well and keep in a tightly capped brown bottle out of the sun.

These oils range in effectiveness from 50 to 95 percent in repelling ticks (it also works fairly well on black flies). The combination runs around 99 percent effective.

To use: I use a 1 ounce brown herb bottle with a spritzer/spray attachment. Apply *liberally* and often during tick season, especially before you go outdoors.

Accessibility and cost of the oils: All these oils are findable on the Internet. Just access Google, type in the oil name, and hit the shopping function. Nearly all the oils are inexpensive, and they will make many, many batches of the repellant. *However: Ledum palustre* essential oil is very expensive (as you will find). It is, nevertheless, essential to the mixture. It has the highest repellant rate, 95 percent, of all of them, so don't scrimp. (*Epitaph on Tombstone*: I skipped the expensive one.) Total, you will be looking at around $125 (2015 dollars) for a season or two's protection for you and your family. Pretty cheap really.

Arthritis tea

This tea combination will help with inflammation and pain considerably and it tastes pretty nice.

Ingredients: 1 pound dried, cut and sifted (i.e., not whole or powdered) each of: nettles, horsetail, dandelion leaf, peppermint leaf, celery seed, tumeric, devil's claw, and meadowsweet.

Directions: Combine all ingredients and mix well. Add 1 cup of the mixed herbs to ½ gallon of nearly boiling water and allow to steep covered overnight. Drink 3–4 cups daily.

Side effects: Will increase urine expression–don't drink right before bed.

Capsaicin/lemon hot water tea

Ingredients: ½–1 lemon, juiced; cayenne pepper powder, one pinch.

Directions: add juice of lemon and cayenne pepper to 6–8 ounces hot water, drink as often as needed.

Turmeric milk

This can often help leaky gut if taken over time.

Ingredients:

1. can of coconut milk with 1 cup of water added (some people just use organic milk).
2. 1–2 tsp powdered turmeric.
3. 1 tsp powdered cinnamon.
4. wildflower organic honey or maple syrup to taste.
5. ⅛ tsp black pepper (will help the turmeric move through the bowel wall).
6. Pinch of cayenne pepper.

To make:

1. Blend in blender until smooth, then . . .
2. Heat on stove until hot but do not boil, then . . .

To use:

1. Drink as soon as heated, once a day for 30 days.

Chronic fatigue formula

This is *very* specific for reversing chronic fatigue, especially if it is long term. *Note:* all the herbs *must* be *powdered.*

To make:

1. Take two parts (for example, 4 ounces) *each* of: spirulina, milk thistle seed, licorice, *Astragalus*, turmeric, dandelion root, and nettle leaf, and . . .
2. One part each (for example, 2 ounces) *each* of: chlorella, burdock root, ashwagandha, eleutherococcus, bladder-wrack, and dried wheatgrass juice.
3. Mix them well in a *very* large bowl.

Dosage:

1. I normally take ¼ cup of the powder, blended in a blender in water or juice in the morning and late afternoon. The dose can be adjusted up or down as necessary.

CHLAMYDIA

Infection with C. trachomatis *is among the most frequent causes of sexually transmitted diseases (STD). Infections of the upper inner eyelid eventually leading to scarring blindness (trachoma) are worldwide among the most frequently occurring ocular infections with nearly 140 million infected and 500 million at risk.* C. pneumonia *is a common agent of respiratory disease with sero-positivity as high as 30-45% in adults and association with chronic diseases like arteriosclerosis or lung cancer.*
Mehlitz and Rudel, 2013

Most chlamydial infections are asymptomatic and thus go undiagnosed and untreated, which can lead to chronic inflammation and irreversible tissue and organ pathology.
Daniel Rockey, 2011

Despite aggressive control efforts, C. trachomatis *infections have continued to constitute a serious public health risk.*
Frohlich et al., 2014

Chlamydiae bacteria, while not generally considered to be part of the Lyme coinfection family, do belong with them. They have a lot in common with the Lyme-group of organisms (as you will see); many people with Lyme, it turns out, are also infected with *Chlamydiae.* Unknown to most physicians, they are, like the rest of the Lyme-group, endemic within various tick species, the same ones that carry Lyme and its many coinfections. The bacteria have also been found in houseflies, fleas, lice, and mites (similarly to other members of the Lyme-group). Chlamydial spread is not limited to sex, ingestion, or inhalation.

Like most of the Lyme-group, the *Chlamydiae* are relatively new to medical science (even though the diseases they cause are not), and research on them is, like the rest of the Lyme-group, still somewhat thin.

Chlamydiae are unusual microorganisms. Initially believed to be viruses, they have now been reclassified as Gram-negative bacteria. (They appear to possess attributes of both bacteria and viruses.) Their exterior cell wall is atypical for Gram-negative bacteria; it is much more rigid, in consequence they're hardier. The *Chlamydiae* are, like the other coinfections of Lyme disease, obligate intracellular bacteria. In other words, they can't live free in the wild; they are obligated to live inside other organisms (hence obligate). They tend to reside *inside* host cells (hence intracellular) from which they extract the nutrients they need to live and create offspring. And like the other Lyme coinfections, they are stealth pathogens; they are very good at hiding from the immune system. The symptoms they create, just like Lyme disease, depend on which part of the body they infect.

There are nine species of the *Chlamydiae* genus known so far; though similarly to the other coinfections, more are being discovered yearly. (There are also three closely related genera of organisms, each containing numerous species.) DNA analysis by microbial taxonomists – yes, there is, unfortunately, such a thing – has thrown the family tree, along with the rest of the world, into disarray; considerable restructuring of the genus is occurring.

At present, these are considered the nine primary chlamydial species: *Chlamydia trachomatis, C. pneumonia, C. muridarum, C. suis, C. abortus, C. pecorum, C. psittaci, C. felis,* and *C. caviae.* Of these *C. trachomatis, C. pneumonia, C. abortus, C. pecorum, C. psittaci* and (rarely) *C. felis* infect people. (More will inevitably be found as the organisms are better understood.) The most common infectious species are *C. trachomatis* and *C. pneumonia.* Both are considered serious public health problems. (As usual, many of our companion animals, such as cats and dogs, are commonly infected with chlamydial bacteria, e.g., *C. felis,* and they do spread to us.)

As with other stealth pathogens, each chlamydial species creates numerous subspecies (serovars, serotypes) of themselves. *Chlamydia trachomatis* presently has nineteen (and counting). Each serotype causes slightly or very different disease symptoms. All the chlamydial strains promiscuously share genetic material with each other. One ocular strain of *C. trachomatis,* for example, contains genetic code from *C. abortus.* As with other stealth pathogens, understanding these organisms is not as simple as many physicians would like.

Historical interrelationships

Chlamydiae are ancient organisms and have played an extensive role in the evolution of other life-forms. They were common infectious organisms in early plant forms (e.g., algae) and were instrumental in the development of early land plants. Over fifty-five chlamydial genes have been found in plant genera throughout the world, including ADP/ATP translocase genes. (ATP is adenosine triphosphate, ADP, adenosine diphosphate. The tri- and the di- refer to the presence of either three or two phosphate molecules.)

Chlamydiae like many parasitic microbes scavenge ATP from host cells in order to gain energy. (In consequence, during infection ATP levels may be very low. This often causes extreme fatigue.) ATP is a molecule that stores the energy most organisms use to power their cells. In essence it's a kind of battery, a storage molecule for *potential* energy. The breaking off of one of the phosphate molecules from ATP (creating ADP) generates energy. ADP is then converted back into ATP by mitochondria, which are former free-living bacteria that are now incorporated into most cells. They use the glucose and fats in the food we eat as the source of energy to do this. Plants, unlike us, use sunlight to access the energy needed to convert ADP to ATP.

Translocase genes are crucial in this process. They enable the transport of adenosine triphosphate (ATP) across the mitochondrial membrane in exchange for adenosine diphosphate (ADP). These translocase genes originated in chlamydial organisms and were first transferred during infection, often by viruses, into early plant forms. This allowed the emergence of the first land plants. Ultimately, the genes were incorporated into larger life forms such as us.

Many intracellular bacteria, such as Rocky Mountain spotted fever and the other *Rickettsiae* bacteria, also utilize that gene. This allows them to parasitize energy (ATP) from host cells. *Anaplasma phagocytophilum*, another coinfection of Lyme, utilizes ancient chlamydial proteins, again acquired by genetic transfer, in its creation of the vacuole (invasome) that it utilizes to infect neutrophils. *Chlamydiae* proteins and genes appear, then, to be root to many if not most of the stealth pathogens that accompany Lyme infections.

Genetic analysis has found that amoeba-infecting chlamydial bacteria are the oldest in the genus, followed by plant-infecting, then animal-infecting – the newest being the human-infecting species. *Chlamydiae* jumped into people long ago from a domestic animal partner (cats really are evil), altering their genome in the process, enabling them to utilize humans as a primary reservoir. In essence, the bacteria successfully altered their genome to make infection of succeeding evolutionarily innovated life-forms possible. They are some of the most successful bacteria on Earth.

Life cycle

Once a new host has been inoculated with the organisms, they tend to exist in three primary forms: the minimally metabolically active infectious extracellular elemental bodies (EBs); highly metabolically active reticulate bodies (RBs); and minimally metabolically active aberrant bodies (ABs).

EBs are the form of bacteria that are usually transferred to new hosts. These are an extremely hardy spore or seed form of the organism. Like seeds, they seek out the best soil in which to grow. Their preferred cells (soil) are the epithelial cells that line mucosal surfaces in the body (e.g. vagina/cervix, colon/rectum, lungs/bronchi, eyelid/eye). Still, they can also infect endothelial cells, monocytes, macrophages, and smooth muscle cells (and most likely others). Neither the EB nor AB form of the organism is susceptible to pharmaceutical antibiotics. (This is why antibiotic treatment has to occur long enough to cover the entire reproductive cycle of the organism.)

Once inside the body, EBs travel to their preferred cellular site, adhere to the host cell, and then alter that cell's functioning to enable bacterial replication. To facilitate replication, EBs generate a vacuole or invasome, which the host cell ingests, allowing the bacteria access to the interior of the cell. The creation of vacuoles and their ingestion are a common process used by cells to kill off bacterial invaders. However, stealth pathogens in the Lyme-group co-opt this process for their own purposes, allowing them access to cellular nutrients. Like other members of the Lyme group, chlamydial bacteria are parasites.

Once internalized the EBs shut down the mechanisms the host cell uses to kill invading bacteria. This includes cell suicide, aka apoptosis. The bacteria then move the vacuole close to the cell nucleus and begin modulating the interior mechanisms of the host cell, forcing it to provide the nutrients they need to reproduce. As they do so, they begin differentiating into the more metabolically active RBs, usually within 8 to 12 hours post-infection. Once expressed, the RBs begin splitting in two (binary fission, aka taxonomist sex), creating more bacterial organisms. When the vacuole is filled with RBs (18–30 hours), the bacteria begin altering their form, becoming EBs once more. They then exit the cell (48–72 hours) by either causing the vacuole to be extruded out through the cellular membrane or by destroying the cell (lysis). Once out of the cell, the newly created EBs use chemotactic compounds to find new cells in which to continue the cycle. Throughout the process, the *Chlamydiae* strongly modulate the host's immune defenses and responses to keep the body from killing them off. They also hijack immune responses to enable their acquisition of nutrients.

While many people do clear the infection on their own, extremely large numbers of people (at minimum one hundred million in the US) remain asymptomatically infected. The asymptomatically infected fall into three groups: (1) those with an infection that never damages the body or causes symptoms; (2) those with an infection that continues to damage the body but causes no symptoms until years or decades later; and (3) those in whom the organisms have altered their structure, taking on the aberrant AB form of the organism. Minimally metabolically active, these ABs damage the host body through continual, low-level inflammatory processes.

The AB form is a unique state that allows the bacteria to survive over long time lines in the face of adverse conditions that could otherwise kill off the bacteria. (Sound familiar?) Some of the stressors that have been found to induce ABs are antibiotics, the generation of gamma interferon (IFN-y) by the host's immune system, viral infection of the bacteria, heat shock, tryptophan depletion in host cells, iron deprivation, exposure to cigarette smoke, extracellular adenosine, and coinfection with herpes simplex or porcine epidemic diarrhea viruses.

During the AB state, the bacteria are viable but noninfectious, bacterial metabolism slows, RB division and differentiation into EBs stops. This state is a form of bacterial hibernation that protects them from environmental impacts that could kill them. (This is similar to the encysted state that Lyme spirochetes take on when stressed. It is a survival strategy of many microorganisms.) The ABs continually monitor their environment for the presence of stressors, maintaining that state as long as the stressor is present. However, once the stressor is removed, even after decades, the bacteria readily convert to the infectious EB form once more. As Bonner et al. (2014) sum up. . .

RBs are replicative bodies that exhibit high metabolic activity and are associated with acute disease: they parasitically exhaust the cellular resources and eventually cause lysis of the host cell in concert with the formation of EBs. The released EBs are infectious entities that find and infect new cell hosts. In the persistant [AB] mode, metabolic activity of the pathogen is greatly altered. . . . Persistence is a sophisticated survival mode, whereby a state of reversible quiescence is implemented.

A less well known persistence mechanism is chlamydial infection of the GI tract. Every species of this genus, once inoculation occurs, immediately infects the GI tract. Although they have been found throughout that organ, they prefer the cecum. Interestingly, they rarely cause disease there; they infect the cecum's outer mucosal layer in a fairly tolerant, human-friendly fashion. This shields them from the effects of antibiotics and gives them a protected niche in which to reproduce. Here, they create a pool of related but different bacterial serotypes, which are then released back into the system – often after "successful" treatment with antibiotics or an "effective" immune response. (No, your reinfection did not come from your partner. The cecum did it. In the library. With the candlestick.)

Chlamydial infection of the cecum (or GI tract) is a successful element in their spread within your own body and into other hosts. EB forms of the bacteria are continually "shed" into the feces of infected animals (including you). They are then expressed out of the body (in poop), spreading the infection to other organisms. The presence of the EBs in feces is also a major factor in autoinoculation of the vagina and eyes. (EBs get on your fingers – even though you can't see them – then one thing leads to another.) *C. trachomatis* infections tend to be more common in women because of the nearness of the anal sphincter to the vagina.

The generation of ABs and the release of bacterial serotypes from the GI tract are the two main strategies the bacteria use to create persistent infections. Because the ABs are still minimally biologically active, they continue to stimulate low levels of inflammation in the body via immune system activation. This can often contribute to the development of immune-mediated pathology (such as scarring) in the affected tissues.

Most animals, from amoeba to mammals, can serve as hosts for the various, different chlamydial strains. The bacteria are commonly found infecting amoeba in water treatment plants, for instance, and are very common in domestic farm animals and pets. All serve as reservoirs for human infection.

Infection specifics

In 2012 the Centers for Disease Control and Prevention (CDC) in the United States received 1,422,976 reports of chlamydial infections from the fifty states and Washington, DC. This is the largest number of cases of any disease *ever* reported to the CDC. Most of the infections were caused by *Chlamydia trachomatis* and *C. pneumonia*. The other (primary) human infectious forms, *C. abortus* and *C. psittaci,* cause many fewer infections.

The overall rate of infections for women is 643.3 per 100,000, more than twice that of men (262.6 per 100,000). The rate for men from 2008 to 2012, however, increased 25 percent. (It still seems to be increasing.) The incidence of infection for both sexes is certainly much higher. Up to 90 percent of cervical infections in women and 60 percent of urethral infections in men are asymptomatic. At minimum, researchers speculate there are 3 to 5 million new infections per year.

In general, all chlamydial organisms can and will infect similar tissues, creating similar conditions. While *C. trachomatis* is thought to be primarily genital and *C. pneumonia* primarily respiratory, they are not limited in their choices. Heart and vascular disease, arthritis, lymphomas, and neurological disease are common problems from both; both can infect the genital and respiratory tracts.

Evidence is emerging that chlamydial organisms may be a major source of neurological disorders. For example, of 180 patients with acute neuroinfection, *C. pneumoniae* was found in nervous system lesions in 67 percent of the patients, *C. trachomatis* in 24 percent, and *C. psittaci* in 9 percent. (Serous and purulent meningitides and meningoenchphalitides were commonly present.)

Chlamydial organisms are also the most common pathogens causing reactive arthritis (ReA). Viable *C. trachomatis* bacteria, for example, are regularly found in synovial tissues of those with ReA. In many women with the condition, there are often no signs of genitourinary infection. Chlamydial and borrelial bacteria (split about half and half) have also been found to be present in 30 percent of patients with early undifferentiated oligoarthritis.

Chlamydia trachomatis

Chlamydia trachomatis at present has nineteen known serovars or str.
of the bacteria. The various *Chlamydia* bacteria and their strains regular.
exchange DNA with each other, creating new varieties or strains, which
can more effectively survive immune assault. They do this by altering
their external membrane proteins through DNA rearrangement. When the
membrane proteins change, the immune system has much more trouble
recognizing them. The current strains or serovars are labeled A–L. Each
causes slightly or very different types of infections.

Serovars A, B, Ba, and C cause trachoma of the eye. The bacteria infect the
thin membrane that covers the inner surface of the eyelid and white part of
the eyeball (the conjunctiva). It causes an inflammation that can, over time,
create severe scarring leading to blindness. The World Health Organization
estimates that there are 40 million active infections worldwide and 1.3 million
people that have become blind from the disease. The main route of infection is thought to be autoinoculation from rubbing the eye after touching the
genitals or rectum; the common housefly also plays a large part, especially in
Africa, in spreading the disease. (Why do flies like poop anyway?)

Serotypes L1, L2, L2', L2a, L2B, and L3 cause lymphogranuloma
venereum (LGV). LGV is, usually, an infection of the lymph nodes and
lymphatic system. The bacteria get into the lymphatic channels, travel to
the lymph nodes and infect their immune cells, the monocytes and macrophages. The lymph nodes in the groin may enlarge tremendously, as can
the nodes around the rectum. Symptoms include drainage from the skin
via the lymph nodes in the groin and/or rectum, painful bowel movements,
swelling of the labia, painless sores on the genitals, and blood or pus from
the rectum. (Words fail me.)

Serovars D, Da, E, F, G, H, I, Ia, J, Ja, and K infect the reproductive tracts
of men and women worldwide. Estimates are that in approximately 75
percent of women and 50 percent of men, the infection is asymptomatic.
These strains are the most common form of STDs worldwide.

In women genital infection may cause a range of clinical manifestations:
acute urethral syndrome, urethritis, bartholinitis, cervicitis, endometriosis, salpingo-oophoritis, pelvic inflammatory disease, perihepatitis, reactive
arthritis, infertility, ectopic pregnancy, chronic pelvic pain, and misce
riage. In two-thirds of cases of tubal-factor pregnancy and in one-thir

.ic pregnancy, the cause is a chlamydial infection. (The bacteria infect .ated and nonciliated epithelial cells in the Fallopian tubes, damaging the .ubal integrity, eventually blocking the tubes themselves.) Infection during pregnancy can cause preterm labor, premature rupture of the amniotic membranes, low birth weight, neonatal death, and postpartum endometriosis. Infection can be transmitted to the infant during birth. Birth-acquired infection can result, for babies, in chlamydial conjunctivitis, nasopharyngeal infection, and chlamydial pneumonia.

In men *C. trachomatis* can cause urethritis, epididymitis, epidiymo-orchitis, prostatitis, seminal vasculitis, and infertility. There is reduced sperm motility, reduced sperm counts, increased sperm abnormalities, reduction in semen density, and more sperm presenting with fragmented DNA. In epididymitis, partial or complete obstruction of the tubules can occur.

Prostate secretions are often filled with chlamydial organisms. As Redgrove and McLaughlin note (2014): "Miniature *C. trachomatis* forms have been observed in total ejaculate and expressed prostate secretions from patients with chronic chlamydial prostatitis." Coinfection with mycoplasma increases the severity of the problems – threefold more sperm cells experience fragmented DNA than during single infection. There are approximately six hundred thousand cases of epididymitis recorded each year in the population of 150 million males in the US. The symptoms include pain, nodules, edema, urinary difficulties, fever, and urethral discharge.

C. trachomatis can infect mobile monocytes and be carried to joint tissues where they tend to persist as ABs and induce arthritic inflammation. Studies have found a 50 to 80 percent incidence of *C. trachomatis* infection in those with reactive arthritis. The bacteria can also infect the nervous system causing a wide range of moderate to severe neurological problems. Meningoencephalitis is the most common though multiple sclerosis, Alzheimer's disease, schizophrenia, autism, vegetative states, and a range of psychiatric disorders can also occur.

Prevalence is highest among young women fifteen to twenty-four years of age and among men twenty to twenty-four years of age. Recurrent or persistent infection occurs in 10 to 15 percent of those who have been antibiotically treated for the organism. Atypical RBs have been found in cases of reactive arthritis (Reiter's syndrome), in chronic prostatitis after antibiotic treatment, and in the female reproductive tract. Researchers (Frolich et al., 2014) note that aberrant and mixed forms during chronic infection is common. . .

> TEM studies have visualized atypical pleomorphic RBs and aberrant C. trachomatis forms in individuals with chronic infections, in Fallopian tube tissues , and in the synovium of reactive arthritis patients. . . . . chlamydial infection in the human endocervix could result in a variety of inclusion types, containing normal forms, a mixture of relatively "normal" forms, and this varies between patients.

Chlamydia pneumonia

C. pneumonia are primarily respiratory pathogens, infecting lung tissue and the bronchi. However the bacteria can disseminate via infected macrophages deeper into lung, arterial, and joint tissues. (The bacteria were first discovered by researchers in 1985 in Finland where they were causing widespread epidemics of pneumonia in military barracks. Like most of the Lyme-group it is relatively new to science.)

Ten percent of community-acquired pneumonias are attributable to the organisms as are 5 percent of incidences of bronchitis; 50 to 80 percent of adults have been found to have antibodies to the bacteria. As Huston et al. (2014) comment: "Of the nine species of the genus, C. pneumoniae is arguably the most successful pathogen. In humans, serological studies show that almost all of the world's population is, or had been, infected with C. pneumoniae." Infections of the respiratory tract are the most common; infection can be both endemic and epidemic. While acute infections do occur, most infections present as a range of chronic disease conditions.

Generally, infections are asymptopmatic, at most presenting as mild upper tract infections that self-resolve. However, low-level, asymptomatic infections over years and decades can develop into severe compromises of the respiratory system. (Chronic infection with AB forms produce the same outcome.)

Some infections are more acute, again producing a wide range of respiratory problems. These range from upper respiratory conditions such as pharyngitis, sinusitis, and otitis to acute bronchitis, exacerbation of chronic bronchitis, asthma, pneumonia, and chronic obstructive pulmonary disease (COPD). The organism can persist for months after initial infection, and despite antimicrobial therapy, persistent lung infections have been reported. Long-term mild infection with the bacteria has been linked to the development of lung cancer.

Most of this group of stealth pathogens, because they stop cellular death (apoptosis), keep cells alive in aberrational forms, sometimes for decades. This ultimately jump-starts the emergence of certain cancers (most commonly lymphomas), which are, in essence, cells that cannot die.

Besides respiratory problems, *C. pneumonia* can cause a range of disease conditions if they migrate deeper into the body. Besides the lungs, the bacteria can infect the liver, heart, brain, eyes, and vascular cells. The primary diseases that occur are of the vascular system and include acute myocardial infarction, chronic coronary heart disease, stroke, atherosclerosis, acute coronary events, and increased intima-media thickness in children. *C. pneumonia*, all forms of the bacteria, have been found in atherosclertic plaques. Both atheromas and aneurysms of abdominal aorta are commonly infected with the bacteria. Patients with acute myocardial infection and chronic heart disease more frequently (68%) than controls (17%) were found to have anti-*C. pneumonia* antibodies.

Atheromas are an accumulation of degenerate material in the inner layer of artery walls. The accumulation is mostly composed of white blood cells (macrophages) both living and dead, various fats, calcium, and fibrous connective tissue. Their formation causes a form of arteriosclerosis called atherosclerosis. It is caused by a low-level inflammation in the artery walls that stimulates the movement of while blood cells, over years, to the area. As the material builds up, the artery walls begin to bulge, becoming bulbar or sausage-like in appearance. This is what leads to the majority of vascular problems from infection.

C. pneumonia bacteria are also linked to the development of arthritis and diabetes. Similarly to *C. trachomatis*, *C. pneumonia* can also infect the nervous system, causing the same range of moderate to severe neurological problems. (Meningoencephalitis, multiple sclerosis, Alzheimer's disease, schizophrenia, autism, vegetative states, and a range of psychiatric disorders.) They tend to be chronic conditions that develop from years-long infections.

Many of the Lyme-group of coinfections are now being implicated in such diseases as Alzheimer's, ALS, giant-cell arteritis, and multiple sclerosis

(MS); diseases that, until now, had no known cause. Vasculitis, for example, often occurs in the brain during MS. There is a sudden death of oligondendrocytes followed by an inflammation-caused removal of the myelin sheath around the nerves. *Chlamydia pneumonia* have been found in the brain lesions that accompany the disease, as have a number of other Lyme-group bacteria, which points to stealth pathogens being primary causes of the condition. Of them mycoplasmal species appear to be the most commonly found, followed by chlamydial, then borrelial.

Chlamydia abortus

Though all mammals are susceptible, *C. abortus* generally infects ruminants. It's a common problem in zoos and farms and among those who keep horses, rabbits, goats, and sheep.

C. abortus is transmitted to people via intake of, or contamination by, feces, urine, or other secretions during close contact with the infected animals. Contact with aborted fetuses, placenta, and vaginal discharges also spread the infection. Aerosol ingestion can also occur during habitat cleaning. Infection generally presents as malaise, flu like signs, mild dry cough, or dyspnoea, which can progress to more severe respiratory disease. Pregnant women may experience abortion (hence *abortus*) accompanied by severe complications, sometimes fatal. These chlamydial organisms, like the others, can sometimes cause arthritis, pneumonitis, conjunctivitis, vesiculitis, and epididymitis.

C. abortus genital infections are common among women who work with domestic farm animals. Rates can be as high as 40 percent in countries heavily dependent on animal farming. The bacteria also infect the nervous system, causing the same kinds of trouble the other species do.

Chlamydia psittaci

C. psittaci primarily infects birds; however, those who work with domestic fowl (pet birds included) are often infected by the organisms – infection rates run from 30 to 96 percent in staff at wildlife bird centers, workers at chicken and turkey farms, and those who handle parrots, racing pigeons, and other birds in pet shops, zoos, and birding clubs. The bacteria shed EBs in fecal matter where, despite hand washing, they are either orally ingested or breathed in with fecal, urine, or other secretion aerosols during habitat cleaning (i.e., you sweep, breathe in the dust, and get sick). As with other bacteria in this group, the organism has developed a number of serovars, each with slightly different impacts during infection.

The bacteria generally infect the lungs and can cause severe respiratory distress with systemic organ involvement leading to serious disease and death. It is also a common source of nongastrointestinal extranodal MALT (mucosa-associated lymphoid tissue) B-cell lymphomas, specifically lung, thyroid, salivary gland, ocular adnexia (OAL), and skin. Autoimmune precursor lesions (e.g., in Hashimoto's thyroiditis and Sjögren syndrome) have been found to contain *C. psittaci* DNA. The bacteria are also implicated as a causative factor in myoepithelial sialoadenitis (MESA).

(In one study, treatment of OAL with doxycycline [100mg bid] for three weeks [then repeated if necessary] generated a 61 percent cure rate. The antibiotic failures were successfully treated with chemotherapy and radiation.)

C. psittaci is also a source of genital infections, producing impacts similar to *C. trachomatis*. Rates can be as high as 50 percent in countries dependent on fowl farming. The bacteria can also infect the nervous system causing the exact same range of symptoms as the others.

Chlamydia pecorum

C. pecorum, like *abortus* and *psittaci*, are transferred into humans from domestic farm animals, cattle, sheep, goats, and pigs. The normal route of infection is inhalation of bacteria-laden fecal- and urine-contaminated dust when mucking out barns. The most common problem is respiratory infection, but the bacteria can also cause abortion, conjunctivitis, encelphalomyelitis, enteritis, pheumonia, and polyarthritis, in essence, much the same as the others. This particular bacteria is a relatively uncommon source of human infection, reported most often (at present) in Poland.

Diagnosis

Due to the nature of the bacteria, successful diagnosis of chlamydial infections is often difficult. As Puolakkainen (2013) comments: "Despite considerable efforts, persistent infections are difficult to diagnose, and no widely accepted serological criteria for persistent infection exist at present."

The most accurate tests for these four organisms are nucleic acid amplification tests (NAAT) of which PCR (polymerase chain reaction) is an example. There are many fewer false negatives due to the sensitivity of the tests. Unfortunately, researchers have found that some clinical isolates have become very good at deleting the target sequence used by the diagnostic kits. As researcher Daniel Rockey (2011) notes . . .

> This can lead to false negatives. Studies have reported an apparent clonal expansion of C. trachomatis isolates carrying this deletion. It is possible that the inability to detect infections caused by strains carrying the deleted plasmid has contributed to the rapid expansion of variant strains in patient populations.

ELISA, or enzyme-linked immunosorbent assay, is a quick test, not as sensitive or reliable as NAAT, and can produce many more false negatives.

DFA, or direct fluorescent antibody test, is similar to ELISA in its effectiveness.

Cell culture is a test conducted by growing the bacteria in a lab, then staining them and viewing them on a fluorescent light microscope. It's expensive and takes a minimum of forty-eight hours to conduct. However, despite its effectiveness in many infections, it is problematical in chlamydial infections. Researchers commonly observe (Campbell and Rosenfeld, 2014) that, as they note, there are times, postinfection, when "the organism can no longer be cultured from the lungs (but pathology persists and the organism can be detected by PCR)."

There are, however, often vast differences in what testing reveals depending on the laboratory used. There is no standard for laboratory testing to which testing labs have to adhere.

Note: Invasive diagnostic procedures and tests within the reproductive tract have been found to exacerbate *C. trachomatis* infection.

Medical treatment

There are a number of important things to keep in mind when using antibiotics to treat chlamydial organisms. It requires, as Marrazzo and Suchland (2014) comment, "special consideration." They continue . . .

> The infectious form of the organism, the extracellular elementary body, is metabolically inert and resistant to killing. Thus antibi-

otics must target the sequestered intracellular and intravacuolar
phases of the life cycle of this pathogen. For this reason, antibiot-
ics with good intracellular penetration must be used. Antibiotic
concentrations must be present throughout the entire 36-48 hour
life cycle of the organism.

The main antibiotics for treating chlamydial infections are tetracyclines and azithromycin. Azithromycin is generally considered to be the standard drug for treating *Chlamydia*, usually administered as a single-dose therapy (One gram orally). Recent studies using NAAT to analyze results have, however, found doxycycline to be more effective, 94.8 percent for the doxycycline versus 77.4 percent for azithromycin. Rifalazil (again single dose) has also shown good results in clinical practice.

A deeper look at doxycycline and asithromycin, however, has found that they don't do well in the low-oxygen environment of the female genital tract. As well, genital oxygen levels decrease even further during inflammatory processes. Researchers (Shima et al., 2011) found that *C. trachomatis* was more resistant to those two antibiotics when infection was in the female genital tract than it was to moxifloxacin and rifampin. The use of a multidrug resistance protein (MDR-1) restored the activity of doxycycline. The authors note: "We suggest careful consideration of tissue-specific characteristics, including oxygen availability, when testing antimicrobial activities of antibiotics against intracellular bacteria."

While there is concern about these organisms developing resistance to antibiotics, it hasn't yet been found in clinical practice. A number of studies have found that the bacteria do develop resistance to fluoroquinolones and rifamin. Four clinical isolates have been found to be resistant to macrolides.

Because the organisms can develop a resistant AB form when confronted by antibiotics, there is legitimate concern about the use of antibiotics too early during infection, especially since half of all *C. trachomatis* infections are cleared by the immune system within one year. As Marrazzo and Suchland comment . . .

Some investigators have hypothesized that high rates of rein-
fection are due in part to antibiotic therapy being provided,
on average, earlier in the course of infection than would have

been the case had screening programs not been in place. This "arrested immunity hypothesis" suggests that early antibiotic treatment effectively attenuates the optimal development of protective immunity, leaving individuals as susceptible as before to reinfection with the same or a new serovar. Population-based surveillance data certainly support high rates of reinfection. The most relevant animal date are from the murine [mouse] model, which show that when primary chlamydial infection resolves in the absence of antibiotic therapy, the animals show evidence of immunity against subsequent challenge. Geisler and colleagues evaluated whether spontaneous resolution of chlamydial infection in humans was associated with decreased infection . . . Of the women who experienced spontaneous resolution, reinfection was less frequent relative to those women who had persistent infection detected at follow-up (19.5% versus 4.5%).

Some practitioners are suggesting allowing sufficient time for the body to develop an immune response before using antibiotics in order to reduce instances of reinfection.

Chlamydial bacteria are also often present with other microbial pathogens; up to 60 percent of individuals with gonorrhea are coinfected with *Chlamydia*. B-lactam antibiotics are generally used to treat gonorrhea, but their use induces persistent AB forms of chlamydia and may exacerbate disease in the genital tract. It is crucial to discover what coinfections are present when treating chlamydial organisms in order to minimize the development of persistent forms.

Corticosteroid treatments for those experiencing exacerbations of asthma and chronic obstructive pulmonary disease from *C. pneumonia* infection may, under some circumstances, reactivate AB forms of the bacteria causing them to convert to the more infective EB forms.

CHAPTER TEN

CHLAMYDIA INFECTION: A DEEPER LOOK

Persistence appears to be a mechanism that allows the Chlamydiae to "ride out" hostile conditions and maintain long-term infection within a host cell.
Schoborg, 2011

Unresolved genital, ocular, and respiratory infections that fail to respond to antibiotic treatment are extensively documented.
Sandoz and Rockey, 2010

This chapter is more technical than the overview chapter and is primarily for practitioners or those who wish a deeper look at the bacterially scavenged nutrient loads and the cytokine cascade the bacteria initiate. Understanding what they do during infection supports the creation of a protocol that will specifically inhibit their behavior and protect the body's tissues and organs.

Initial infection strategies

The *Chlamydiae* possess an enzyme, sphingomyelinase (SMase), on their cellular surface that is integral to their infection of host cells. Once the bacteria touch the exterior of a host cell, this compound catalyzes (or breaks apart) sphingomyelin (SM, aka ceramide phosphorylcholine), a lipid contained on the surface of the host cell membrane. (Sphingomyelinases, by the way, are particularly damaging to the coronary artery's endothelial cells; they are integral to the chlamydial generation of atheromas.) This causes the sphingomyelin to separate into its constituent parts, ceramide and phosphorylcholine.

Because ceramide in the intracelluar space between cells is highly bioactive, the bacteria carefully control its production. Too much free ceramide causes cellular death and calls macrophages to the location, stimulating them to engulf the infected cell. The bacterial SMase – because of the ceramide release – induces the formation of the invasome vesicle in which the bacteria will hide from the immune system. Its exterior is created from the SM in the plasma membrane of the host cell. At the same time, ceramide stimulates the formation of microscopic invaginations, or entry portals, in the host cell membrane. This allows the invasome entry to the interior of the host cell.

The levels of ceramide during this initial phase of infection remain low in order to delay cell death. It is later, after bacterial replication, that its levels increase, causing cell death, thus allowing the newly formed EBs to escape the cell and find new host cells to infect.

Ceramide can cause a variety of problems when it's released into the extracellular space in any quantity – as it is when the chlamydial bacteria exit a cell. The compound is heavily involved in cellular functioning. Besides apoptosis, it affects cellular growth, arrest, differentiation, senescence, migration, and adhesion. Ceramide malfunction or excess extracellular ceramide has been linked to a number of chronic problems: cancer, neurodegeneration, diabetes, and various inflammatory states. Excess ceramide, for example, can, over time, cause insulin resistance. (It upregulates SOCS-3 expression, which inhibits the insulin signal transduction pathway, thus creating diabetes.) As researchers Tuula et al. (2014) comment, "by increasing the cellular levels of ceramide in the affected host tissues the presence of *C. pneumoniae* could perturb the metabolic state of cells and tissues and thus contribute to the pathophysiology of the secondary disorders connected to *Chlamydia* infection."

Once the bacteria have created an invasome and accessed the interior of the cell, the invasome moves near to the nucleus, the endoplasmic reticulum (ER), and the Golgi bodies. They then begin altering cellular function in order to gain needed nutrients so they can reproduce and spread. (This includes additional SM, which is essential to reproduction.) As researcher Guangming Zhong (2009) comments . . .

> *After an EB induces its own entry into a non phagocytic epithelial cell, the EB-containing vacuole diverges from the default endocytic pathway (which would lead to the destruction of the microbes) and intercepts the ER/Golgi secretory pathway.*

The default endocytic pathway is what our cells utilize to engulf and destroy bacteria that are attacking them. Fascinating (to me), is that the bacteria *only* stop the cell from engulfing the chlamydial invasome. They do not stop the cell from processing other microbial pathogens, *including* dead *Chlamydiae* and chlamydial detrititus released when EBs burst out of nearby infected cells.

Golgi bodies (aka Golgi apparatus, Golgi structures) are essential to the survival of *Chlamydiae* during infection. In mammalian cells, they are usually located close to the nucleus, near the endoplasmic reticulum (ER) exit sites. The Golgi structures receive various proteins from the ER, then package those proteins (and various lipids) for transport to different structures inside the cell (or for expression outside the cell into the extracellular space).

The Golgi bodies are a stacked series of sort of flattish plates connected together by microtubules. They can be visualized, loosely, as something like an open, multilevel parking structure, each level performing different functions. (The microtubules can be envisioned as the concrete pillars that support the parking structure.) Each "plate" in a Golgi stack contains various enzymes that are responsible for modifying proteins to fulfill cellular functions. The separation of these plates allows for consecutive-step processing of compounds by the different group of enzymes in each plate. Once altered, the compounds are sent to the next plate through the microtubules. If the microtubules are depolymerized (as they are by many bacteria), the Golgi structures fragment, becoming individual stacks. Upon fragmentation, which happens toward the end of host cell infection, their function is degraded, and cellular health is significantly affected.

During infection, these bacteria co-opt the transportation processes in the cell, diverting the Golgi products (including SM) to the invasome for chlamydial use. This begins an escalating process of host cell malfunction. As Zhong (2009) observes . . .

> The availability, from the mammalian cell cytoplasm, of numerous metabolites not normally found in the external environment has provided selective pressure for chlamydiae to evolve a unique capacity to utilize host metabolic intermediates. . . . The expansion of the inclusion in the cytoplasm and the alteration of host signaling pathways during parasite acquisition of nutrients are

> *inevitably destructive to the infected cells. Indeed, infected cells often display altered metabolic, immunological, and cell biological characteristics.*

At early stages of the infection, the Golgi retain their integrity, the bacterial vacuole nearby simply alters where the Golgi proteins and lipids go. Without explaining too much here what the following processes mean, chlamydial bacteria co-opt GBF1, a regulator of vesicle trafficking, in order to acquire more SM. This increases the *size* of the bacterial invasome and its *stability*. The bacteria use another pathway, CERT, to acquire SM for *replication*. (Protecting these pathways will inhibit SM acquisition and reduce or eliminate bacterial load. I know of no herbs for this at this time.) The bacteria also utilize a Rab14-mediated transport for SM interception. Fifty percent of the SM produced by the Golgi bodies is hijacked by the bacteria. Unfortunately (for us), as the infection progresses, the Golgi progressively fragment.

There are two important points to keep in mind, (1) the bacteria hijack the Golgi bodies in order to acquire SM (and other products); and (2) eventually the *Chlamydiae* force the Golgi to fragment. *Interrupting either or both of these processes will inhibit SM acquisition and reduce or eliminate the bacterial infection.* Without SM the bacteria cannot reproduce.

The primary herb (so far) for inhibiting SM acquisition is *Mallotus philippinensis* (fruit) – a common herb in Ayurvedic medicine. There are a good number of plants that will protect Golgi body integrity and function while inhibiting their fragmentation and damage. These include any of the berberine-containing plants, *Scutellaria baicalensis*, *Salvia miltiorrhiza*, *Terminalia chebula*, and HCMO5, a water extract of eight herbs (*Atractylodes macrocephala*, *Gastrodia elata*, *Citrus unshiu*, *Poria cocos*, *Crataegus pinnatifida*, *Siegesbeckia pubescens*, and *Coptidis japonica*).

Altering immune response and function

Similarly to the rest of the Lyme-group of intracellular pathogens, *Chlamydiae* initiate a cascade of cytokines during infection; they hijack immune responses and function. Cytokines are small cellular messaging molecules that facilitate bacterial infection and the acquisition of nutrients from host cells. One of the main impacts is the bacterial shifting of immune response from Th1 to Th2 dominant. (Again, a common strategy of the Lyme-group

– please see the short discussion of this in Chapter Five.) Briefly, Th1im-
mune responses are designed to deal with intracellular bacteria; Th2 are not.
This switch circumvents the healthy immune response and, as researchers
comment, "hosts can remain chronically infected despite chemotherapy."
As Wizel et al. (2008) continue . . .

> Numerous studies have shown that type 1 cytokine-secreting
> CD4+ T (Th1) cells inhibit Chlamydia replication mostly via
> the secretion of IFN-y [i.e., gamma] and by stimulating the
> protective function of other immune and inflammatory cells.

By altering immune response to Th2, the bacteria stop the more effective Th1 interventions. An integral element of this shift is, similarly to other
Lyme-group organisms, the stimulation of interleukin-10 (IL-10). IL-10 is
normally activated *after* a healthy Th1 response. The antibacterial actions
of Th1 stimulate a healthy cascade of inflammatory cytokines, which kills
bacteria. IL-10, once the infection is successfully stopped, halts that process.
An adaptive strategy of most stealth pathogens is to initiate this cytokine
early during infection to keep Th1 responses dormant.

IL-10 also strongly suppresses apoptosis or cellular death, an important
Th1 strategy to kill infected cells. By inhibiting apoptosis, the bacteria keep
infected cells alive, allowing nutrient acquisition and reproduction. Reducing IL-10 levels will, in and of itself, restore healthy apoptosis in affected
cells, thus limiting infection. A number of herbs are excellent at reducing
IL-10 levels throughout the body. These include: *Glycyrrhiza* (downregulates IL-10, acting primarily as an immune modulator and tonic), standardized *Silybum marianum* (silymarin inhibits IL-10 overexpression and helps
support endothelial health), *Cannabis sativa* (ibid), *Scutellaria baicalensis*
(downregulates IL-10 and Treg), and *Andrographis paniculata*, which lowers
IL-10 expression, as do plants containing scopoletin (an IL-10/Th2 downregulator), such as noni, manaca, passion flower (*Passiflora* spp.), stevia,
Artemisia spp (especially *A. scopria* and *A. capillaris*), nettle leaf (*Urtica dioca*),
and black haw (*Viburnum prunifolium*). However, the best is by far *Withania
somifera,* aka ashwagandha, which very specifically *modulates* IL-10 expression (not simply downregulating it). *Withania* is also moderately protective
of Golgi structures.

Modulation of gamma interferon (IFN-y) is a crucial strategy of the *Chlamydiae* (as it is for many in the Lyme-group). So, it makes sense to discuss it a bit here in order to understand both its role in eliminating *Chlamydiae* and its contribution to problems from long-term chronic infections.

IFN-y plays an important role in eliminating the bacteria during infection. It is, as many researchers comment, a "critical mediator in immunity to *Chlamydia*." People with poor immune function, who cannot mount a strong IFN-y response, are more susceptible to chlamydial infection, have more difficulty clearing it, and suffer more serious damage during chronic stages of the disease. A strong and healthy IFN-y response has been found to protect living organisms from infection by chlamydial organisms. So, again, *a healthy immune system is essential in preventing, treating, and recovering from the Lyme-group of organisms.*

IFN-y inhibits the bacteria through a number of mechanisms. First, it mediates the activation of inducible nitric oxide synthase (iNOS), which stimulates the production of nitric oxide (NO), which itself inhibits bacterial growth (one of its main functions); second, it enhances the mechanisms that increase major histocompatibility complex-1 (MHC-I) and MHC-II-dependent presentation of the bacterial antigens to T cells so that the immune system recognizes and can then kill them; third, IFN-y activates indolamine 2,3-dioxyenase (IDO), which reduces the levels of *Chlamydiae*-essential tryptophan in cells (one of the primary anti-bacterial actions of the immune system); and fourth, IFN-y activation ultimately depletes intracellular iron, which the bacteria need for reproduction. In consequence, the *Chlamydiae* have developed specific strategies to inhibit IFN-y, as well as IDO and MHC production and activation.

Most *Chlamydiae* cannot synthesize tryptophan (which they need as a nutrient and for reproduction). This is why the reduction of tryptophan in the cell by IFN-y can limit infection. However . . . some of the *C. trachomatis* serovars encode genes for tryptophan production. Interestingly, these serovars are able to obtain IDO, which they use to synthesize tryptophan, from the vaginal microbiome. In other words, the other microorganisms in the genital tract in women work synergistically with the chlamydial bacteria, giving them the IDO they need to continue the infection. This is especially true if the microbiome of the reproductive tract has been disturbed – usually through the use of antimicrobials or actions of other infectious organisms. *Lactobacillus* species, which normally predominate in the vaginal microbiome, do not synthesize IDO. They also produce a highly acidic H2O2-rich environment that, by its nature, inhibits chlamydial growth and development. (The use of yoghurt, as a douche and taken internally, can help restore or increase *Lactobacillus* populations in the vagina. A mixture of local wildflower honey mixed with yoghurt will produce even more effective outcomes.)

Unfortunately, IFN-y is also implicated in many of the negative effects from long-term chronic infection. The low-level inflammation that occurs over decades, often from continual IFN-y presence, is one of the factors in chlamydial scarring and physiological damage. A simple stimulation of IFN-y *in an attempt to kill the bacteria* can lead to more damage, not less. To make things more complicated, the activation of IFN-y and the subsequent depletion of tryptophan and iron are some of the factors that will cause the bacteria to take on the aberrant AB in which they will remain until the IFN-y, low iron, and low tryptophan conditions stop. (They then take on the infectious EB forms again.) The best intervention along these lines is the use of herbs that *modulate* IFN-y production, either direct IFN-y modulators or herbal adaptogens. Some of the best ones are *Withania, Rhodiola,* licorice (*Glycyrrhiza*), and *Scutellaria baicalensis*.

Chlamydiae inhibition of IFN-y-induced MHC-II expression is another strategy the bacteria use. This creates problems in immune recognition of the bacteria and the intracellularly infected cells. MHC-II is synthesized in the endoplasmic reticulum and then transported to the Golgi for use. The MHC-II system then takes parts of bacterial cells (antigens) and expresses them on antigen-presenting cells such as dendritic cells, mononuclear phagocytes, B cells, and some endothelial and epithelial cells. This programs those immune cells to look for and kill the bacteria. By inhibiting MHC-II expression, the antigen recognition process is, sometimes significantly, curtailed, allowing extended infection. This primarily affects CD4+ T helper T cells.

MHC-I, which is also inhibited, is present on nearly every nucleated cell. They take fragments of killed microbes and present those antigens on the surface of the infected cell. This brings CD8+ T cells primed for antigen recognition to that site where they engulf the infected cell. By inhibiting both MHC-I and -II, the *Chlamydiae* circumvent a primary mechanism the immune system uses to kill them. Besides inhibiting IFN-y, the bacteria also inhibit MHC production through the secretion of *Chlamydia* protease-like activity factor (CPAF). This compound degrades host transcription factors RFX5 and USF-1, both of which are required for MHC activation. Chlamydial inhibition of RFX5 is, in fact, essential to bacterial infection. Upregulation of RFX5, a DNA-binding protein, stimulates MHC-II expression and can help reduce infection. Two herbs that will inhibit this bacterial process are *Scutellaria baicalensis* and *Cordyceps* spp. Other herbs that will upregulate MHC-II are *Achyranthes bidentata, Astragalus mongholicus, A. membranaceus, Mori fructus* (mulberry), *Panax ginseng, Phellinus linteus,* and *Plantago asiatica*.

CD8+T cells, are produced in the spleen and are activated by MHC-I expression. They are specific for killing *Chlamydia*-infected fibroblasts. Supporting the spleen's production of T and B cells is crucial. The two best herbs for this are *Salvia miltiorrhiza* and *Ceanothus* (red root).

During active infections mild to moderate epithelial hyperplasia is common with a mixed inflammatory infiltrate of (mostly) macrophages with some T cells and polymorphonuclear leucocytes. Dendritic cells are often located deeper in the epithelium and underlying stroma. There is an increased expression of reactive oxygen species (ROS) in infected cells through upregulation of NADPH oxidase (NOX-1 and-4) and downregulation of superoxide dismutase-1 (SOD-1) and thioredoxin-1 (TRX-1). The production of ROS is used by host cells to restrict bacterial replication, but during chronic infection by persistent forms, vascular inflammation is exacerbated, leading to endothelial cell necrosis (over time). Curcumin and resveratrol (*Polygomun cuspidatum*) will help correct this.

A look at the cytokine cascade

Chlamydiae bacteria inhibit the production of some immune responses (e.g., IFN-y) and stimulate the production of others. They, like most intracellular bacteria, are extremely sophisticated at modulating the host immune system.

In cervical and colonic epithelial cells, the bacteria upregulate expression of IL-1a, IL-6, IL-8, GROu, and GM-CSF. IL-8 production is increased significantly (1.5- to 3.4-fold) and reaches a maximum 72 hours postinfection. IL-6, GROa, and GM-CSF also substantially increase within the same time period. As Rasmussen et al. (1997) comment . . .

> *Several of these cytokines are potent chemoattractants and activa-*
> *tors for neutrophils, monocytes, and T lymphocytes, while others*
> *have pleiotropic effects on cell functions associated with acute*
> *inflammation, including the induction of adhesion molecules on*
> *endothelial cells, the secretion of additional proinflammatory*
> *cytokines by macrophages and other cells, and the induction of*
> *acute phase proteins in epithelial cells and macrophages.*

During infection IL-1*a* levels increase three- to fourfold. This is a crucial cytokine; it initiates IL-8 production and amplifies the inflammatory response and initiates additional cytokine production by neighboring cells. Inhibition of IL-1*a* significantly reduces (up to 85 percent) the production of IL-8 and (up to 95 percent) the production of IL-6, GRO*a*, and GM-CSF. IL-1*a* inhibitors include *Polygonum cuspidatum, Zingiber officinalis, Pueria lobata, Salvia miltiorrhiza, Carthamus tinctorius,* and genistein.

During *C. pneumoniae* infection in the lungs, nearly the same cytokine cascade ensues; additional cytokines found include monocyte chemoat-tractant protein-1 (MCP-1), macrophage inflammatory protein 1*a* (MCP-1*a*), IL-12, tumor growth factor (TGF)-*B*, TNF-*a*, and a number of matrix metalloproteinases (MMPs) especially MMP-9. MMP-9 is strongly associ-ated with the increased scarring that can occur during infection. (MMP-9 inhibitors include *Cordyceps, Olea europaea, Polygonum cuspidatum, Punica granatum, Salvia miltiorrhiza, Scutellaria baicalensis,* and the supplements EGCG and NAC.)

C. pneumoniae infection of endothelial cells produces a very similar cascade: IL-1*a* followed by IL-8 and MCP-1 with parallel expression of endo-thelial-leukocyte adhesion molecule-1 (ELAM-1), intercellular adhesion molecule-1 (ICAM-1), and vascular adhesion molecule-1 (VCAM-1). Endo-thelial iNOS and subsequent NO production are high in chronic states – but low during acute infection.

Infection in the Fallopian tubes induces IL-1*b*. Inhibition of IL-1*b* can prevent pathology in human Fallopian tubes. (IL-1*b* inhibitors include *Cordyceps spp, Eupatorium perfoliatum, Polygala tenuifolia* (Chinese senega) root, *Polygonum cuspidatum, Pueraria lobata, Salvia miltiorrhiza, Scutellaria baicalensis,* and melatonin.) TNF-*a* and IL-10 are also present at high levels in the Fallopian tubes. While NO production is strongly antibacterial and is a primary immune response to infection, long-term overproduction in the Fallopian tubes can lead to scarring and persistent damage. Chronic, intense inflammation contributes to the tissue remodeling and scarring. Levels of iNOS, which stimulates NO production, also tend to be high during chronic infection – but low in acute, replicative infection. In most instances of chronic infection, NO levels tend to fluctuate. This tends to induce cytotoxicity and transcriptional disturbances in the tissues. The bacteria have mechanisms in place to reduce arginine levels (needed for NO production) during acute infections, which reduces NO levels, protecting the bacteria from NO damage. NO also directly inhibits IDO expression; it's part of how tryptophan levels in cellular tissue are reduced.

One of the primary, general, inflammatory pathways the bacteria intentionally activate is the MAP kinase/ERK 1/2/ cPLA2 pathway. Inhibition of this pathway has been shown to suppress chlamydial growth, inhibit acquisition of phospholipids, reduce host cPLA2 activity, and suppress bacterial-induced cytokine production. Some of the herbs useful for inhibiting this pathway are *Andrographis paniculata*, *Bidens pilosa*, *Cordyceps*, *Houttuynia*, *Salvia miltiorrhiza*, *Scutellaria baicalensis*, and *Silybum marianum*.

Activation of this pathway contributes to chronic inflammation through a couple of mechanisms. First, cPLA2 activation greatly increases arachidonic acid (AA) production in infected cells. AA is converted into prostaglandins, including prostaglandin E2 (PGE2). COX2 is also upregulated. AA and COX2 are inflammatory compounds (over-the-counter anti-inflammatories often act to reduce their levels). PGE2 can amplify this inflammation by inducing the production of other, different inflammatory cytokines and by suppressing IFN-y production. Some herbal PGE2 inhibitors are any of the various *Bidens* species (strongest), *Houttuynia*, *Polygala tenuifolia*, *Pueraria lobata* (kudzu), *Salvia miltiorrhiza*, and *Scutellaria baicalensis*.

The MAPK/ERK 1/2 pathway also upregulates interleukin-8 (IL-8), a rather potent inflammatory cytokine. IL-8 is an integral, early element of the cytokine cascade and is strongly correlated with the *Chlamydiae*-induced upregulation of intracellular IL-1 (both IL-1a and IL-1b). IL-1 is a rather potent immunostimulatory cytokine in its own right; it induces maturation, stimulation, and proliferation of B cells, release of IL-2, IL-3, numerous interferons, triggers fever, and affects chemotaxis of neurophils, lymphocytes, and monocytes. Most importantly for chlamydial infections, it promotes the formation of scar tissue and fibrosis. IL-1*a*, present in most infected parts of the body, significantly intensifies the cytokine-initiated inflammation.

Inhibiting IL-8 can significantly reduce this cytokine cascade, including IL-1 production. Inhibiting IL-8, as Darville and Hiltke (2010) note, "completely eliminates tissue destruction induced by the infection." IL-8 inhibitors include *Cordyceps* spp., *Isatis* spp, and *Polygonum cuspidatum*.

The bacteria also stimulate the production of IL-6, TNF-*a*, and caspase-1. Normally, NF-*k*B is dominant in generating IL-1, IL-6, IL-8, and TNF-*a*, but during chlamydial infection, NF-*k*B is unusually modulated. In some instances NF-*k*B is upregulated, in others inhibited and an alternate inflammatory pathyway is used; the bacteria utilize a MAP kinase pathway instead. Suppressing IL-6, and TNF-*a* can help limit inflammation in the affected cells and organs. Some IL-6 inhibitors are *Andrographis paniculata*, *Isatis* spp., *Pueraria lobata*, *Salvia miltiorrhiza*, and *Scutellaria baicalensis*. TNF-*a* inhibitors include *Andrographis paniculata*, *Cannabis* spp., *Cordyceps* spp., *Eupatorium perfoliatum* (boneset), *Glycyrrhiza* spp. (licorice), *Houttuynia spp*, *Panax ginseng*, *Polygala tenuifolia* (Chinese senega root), *Pueraria lobata* (kudzu), *Sambucus* spp. (elder), *Scutellaria baicalensis*, *Tanacetum parthenium* (feverfew), *Salvia miltiorrhiza*, and *Zingiber officinalis* (ginger).

Inhibition of caspase-1 produces significantly less severe pathology during chlamydial infection. *Scutellaria baicalensis* is particularly good for this.

Chlamydiae also inhibit apoptosis, thus keeping cells alive so that they remain infected. As Zhong (2009) comments . . .

> *These obligate intracellular parasites maintain a delicate balance between exploiting and protecting their host: they occupy intracellular space and acquire nutrients from the infected cells, but at the same time they have to maintain the integrity of the host cells for the completion of their intracellular growth. For this purpose, chlamydiae hijack certain signaling pathways that prevent the host cells from undergoing apoptosis induced by intracellular stress, and protect the infected cells from recognition and attack by host defenses.*

They do this through a variety of mechanisms, including inhibiting capase 3 activation, blocking mitochondrial cytochrome c release, modulating NF-kB behavior, disturbing Bax/Bcl balance, and inhibiting Bax/Bak activation. Intracellular BH3-only proteins are stress molecules (e.g., Puma and Bim), which migrate to the mitochondria when the cell is stressed. They activate pro-apoptic Bax and Bak, which negate the anti-apoptic actions of Bcl-2. The bacteria decrease Bax and Bak and increase BLC-2. Reversing this through the use of herbs strongly alters the infectious process and reduces infection. In fact, stimulating normal apoptosis can completely inhibit chlamydial development. Bax/bcl apoptosis pathway remodulators (which specifically increase Bax and reduce BCL-2) include *Artemisia* spp., *Glycyrrhiza* spp., *Goniothalamus cheliensis, Gynostemma pentaphyllum, Houttuynia,* spp., *Leonurus cardiaca* (motherwort), *Rhodiola* spp., *Scutellaria baicalensis,* and the isolated constituents arctigenin, beta-sitosterol, and curcumin. *Salvia miltiorrhiza* is particularly good for this. It is an apoptosis *modulator.* It modulates the actions of Bax/Bcl, decreasing or increasing the ratio as needed during inflammatory episodes; e.g, it increases apoptosis of cancer cells but decreases apoptosis of hypoxia damaged cells.

CHAPTER ELEVEN

NATURAL HEALING
OF CHLAMYDIA

*A class of herbal medicines, known as immunomodulators, alters
the activity of immune function through the dynamic regulation
of information molecules such as cytokines.*
Spelman et al., 2006

*The effects of plant based remedies may be due to one active
compound with a single mechanism of action, to compounds
that possess multiple modes of action, to the combined activity of
more than one active ingredient in a single species, or the syner-
gic interactions of different active ingredients from several plant
species as a medicinal formula.*
Elaine Elisabetsky, 2007

Despite the sophisticated modulation of the immune system that these
bacteria are capable of, it is quite possible to reverse it. Plant medicines
are very good at subtle remodulations of immune function, in fact much
better than pharmaceuticals. They are excellent for reducing the levels of
cytokines that cause inflammatory damage in the body while simultaneously upregulating immune-supporting cytokines that the bacteria have
inhibited. Plant medicines are also very effective at protecting the various
organ and cellular systems that have been adversely affected, helping them
heal any damage that has occurred and stimulating the organs to work
more efficiently. And finally, they are excellent for reducing or eliminating
many of the symptoms that infection causes.

> ### TREATING CHLAMYDIAE
>
> Please read the initial pages of Chapter Seven regarding natural treatment protocols. (It's important.) You can find the most crucial elements on pages 190–195

Natural healing of chlamydial infections

Each of the various human-infectious *Chlamydia* spp. are treated identically: (1) the use of antibacterial herbs specific for the bacteria; (2) herbs that modulate cytokine production to correct the cytokine cascade the bacteria generate; (3) herbs that protect the organs or cells targeted by the bacteria; (4) immune-enhancing herbs to support healthy immune function; and (5) herbs for specific symptoms.

Note: If your immune system is easily able to produce IFN-gamma, infection by chlamydial bacteria is significantly inhibited. The best herb for this is *Astragalus*, 1,000 mg daily, permanently. (This is also good for helping prevent Lyme infections.)

Antibacterial herbs for *Chlamydiae*

There are a number of herbs and herb combinations that are specific as antibacterials for all species of *Chlamydiae* (see the sidebar for a complete list). The two most important are: (1) any of the various berberine-containing plants and (2) *Scutellaria baicalensis* (Chinese skullcap root).

Of note: Retinoic acid, a metabolite of vitamin A (retinol) is also antibacterial in that it inhibits the ability of *Chlamydiae* to infect endothelial and epithelial cells. The compound also inhibits the development of atheromas in aorta. Our bodies naturally create that metabolite whenever we take vitamin A, so it should be used to supplement any protocols.

Berberine-containing plants

Both berberine and berberine-containing plants have been found active against chlamydial organisms in vitro and in vivo as well as effective in human trial. This includes such plants as goldenseal, phellodendron, and *Coptis chinensis*. Berberine plants have a number of other important uses in chalmydial infections: they protect Golgi structures from fragmentation (something

Chlamydiae regularly cause) through inhibition of Rho kinase (ROCK); inhibit inflammatory responses in macrophages induced by the bacteria; and inhibit MAPK activation. They also inhibit iNOS, COX-2, IL-1beta, IL-6, and TNF; and modulate apoptosis in affected cells. The berberines promote infected macrophage apoptosis (which is inhibited by many intracellular bacteria) through caspase activation, while at the same time reducing cellular apoptosis that intracellular bacteria also sometimes cause.

Because berberine is experienced by the body as a toxin, it is not very systemic; it does not easily pass the GI tract barrier. In consequence, only a tiny bit circulates systemically . . . if the herb is used over time. Nevertheless, this is not a huge impediment to the use of this group of herbs in treating chlamydial infections. The tiny amounts that do circulate systemically have tonic effects on the spleen, liver, lungs, and heart, helping them resist bacterial impacts.

Generally, however, to be effective, the berberine needs to touch the affected tissues; this is how it generates its most potent antibacterial effects. This makes it perfect for chlamydial infections because . . .

Firstly, the bacteria sequester themselves in the GI tract, usually in the cecum, specifically in its upper layer of epithelial cells. The GI tract *Chlamydia* do not normally pass beyond this location deeper into the body (they systemically infect other parts of the body through other mechanisms).

Berberine, when used internally, affects just this cell population, normalizing its functioning while at the same time providing antibacterial actions. Because the berberine-plant tinctures are so strongly antibacterial against the bacteria, they reduce the chances of reinfection from the bacteria in this sequestered location.

Berberine, as well, has a tendency to normalize the intestinal microflora, restoring healthy microbiome function.

Secondly, berberine-containing plants offer the same protections and actions when used vaginally in suppository form for treating *Chlamydia*-initiated STDs. Because the bacteria locate themselves in the surface of vaginal cells, the berberine will act as a direct antibacterial. It's very effective at eliminating the bacteria from the vaginal passage.

Thirdly, these plants perform similarly when used as aqueous decoctions or infusions as eyedrops in the treatment of *Chlamydia*-caused trachoma. As one example: a clinical study with fifty-one people suffering *C. trachomatis*-

initiated trachoma of the eye, compared the use of aqueous berberine eyedrops with sulfacetamide. Conjunctival scrapings from the sulfacetamide-treated group found they remained positive for chlamydial infection. However, the berberine group were clear and remained so one year later. There were no relapses. (*Note:* This study, oddly, insisted that the berberine was *not* antibacterial for *C. trachomatis.* Nevertheless, numerous studies in China and elsewhere, and my own experience, strongly contradict that finding.)

And finally, the systemic effects of berberine help restore tone and function in mucus membranes such as the lungs and genitourinary tract.

Note: Due to the many compounds in the plant and their complex nature, the berberine-containing plants *do not* tend to stimulate an alteration of the bacteria into AB forms. The use of the plant both in vivo and human use shows that in most cases, it clears the organisms rather than causing form alteration.

Scutellaria baicalensis

Chinese skullcap root is an extremely useful herb for the entire Lyme-group of stealth pathogens. It is strongly antiviral and moderately antibacterial, is a synergist, and powerfully modulates the cytokine disturbances caused by intracellular infections. It is a widely systemic herb, reaching tissues throughout the body. Importantly, the herb inhibits Golgi fragmentation (through ROCK inhibition), which itself strongly inhibits bacterial replication of *Chlamydiae.* It specifically inhibits the cytokine-initiated inflammation that *Chlamydiae* cause, as well as chlamydial cellular infection processes. It does this through blocking *Chlamydia* protease-like activity factor (CPAF) and upregulating RFX5, a compound degraded by CPAF. The chlamydial inhibition of RFX5 is essential to the bacterial infection process. Upregulation of RFX5, a DNA-binding protein, is essential to MHC-II expression during the immune response and thus helps eliminate the bacteria from the body.

Skullcap root also inhibits the TLR2 signaling pathway, as well as inhibiting iNOS and COX2, while modulating NF-kB expression. Use of the herb, in vivo, stops chlamydial genital tract infections in mice. Chinese skullcap root is also highly protective of endothelial and epithelial cell damage caused by intracellular cytokines, specifically TNF-a, normalizing their function.

Scutellaria baicalensis is not, in a sense, a *true* antibacterial because it does not, by direct action, kill the bacteria. It is rather what should be considered an indirect antibacterial. It interferes with the mechanisms the bacteria use to infect, fragment, and scavenge nutrients from host cells. The bacteria die because they cannot get the nutrients they need to survive. (Stealth antibacterial?)

Cytokine modulating herbs

Herbs that remodulate the body's production of cytokines, in and of themselves, can reduce severity of infection, protect cellular and organ health, and inhibit the growth of the bacteria by interfering with their ability to scavenge nutrients. Chinese skullcap root is the strongest of these, so strong in fact that its actions rise to antibacterial levels. There are some other good ones; the most broadly active is danshen, *Salvia miltiorrhiza*. Here is a list of those active for the most common cytokines the bacteria stimulate.

> ***TNF-a inhibitors:*** *Andrographis paniculata, Cannabis* spp., *Cordyceps* spp., *Eupatorium perfoliatum* (boneset), *Glycyrrhiza spp* (licorice), *Houttuynia* spp., *Panax ginseng, Polygala tenuifolia* (Chinese senega) root, *Pueraria lobata* (kudzu), *Sambucus* spp., (elder), *Scutellaria baicalensis, Tanacetum parthenium* (feverfew), *Salvia miltiorrhiza,* and *Zingiber officinalis* (ginger).
>
> ***MMP-9 inhibitors:*** *Polygonum cuspidatum* (Japanese knotweed) and *Salvia miltiorrhiza.*
>
> ***IL-1a inhibitors:*** *Carthamus tinctorius, Polygonum cuspidatum, Pueria lobata, Salvia miltiorrhiza, Zingiber officinalis,* and genistein.
>
> ***IL-1b inhibitors:*** *Cordyceps* spp., *Eupatorium perfoliatum, Polygala tenuifolia* (Chinese senega) root, *Polygonum cuspidatum, Pueraria lobata, Salvia miltiorrhiza,* and *Scutellaria baicalensis.*
>
> ***IL-6 inhibitors:*** *Andrographis paniculata, Isatis* spp., *Pueraria lobata, Salvia miltiorrhiza,* and *Scutellaria baicalensis.*
>
> ***IL-8 inhibitors:*** *Cordyceps* spp., *Isatis* spp., and *Polygonum cuspidatum.*

My approach for finding the strongest plants for treating these conditions is to note those that appear most often in the most categories in which the bacteria are active. From this, as you can see, *Andrographis, Cordyceps, Glycyr-*

Other herbs and herb combinations (Chinese and Indian) active against *Chlamydiae* bacteria: *Artemissia capillaris* (yin chin), *Arum maculatum* (root), chaga (primarily the constituent betulin), *Dianthus superbus* (qu mai), *Gardenia jasminoides* seeds (zhi-zi), *Glanthus nivalis* (snowdrop), *Houttuynia cordata, Kochia scoparia* fruit (di fu-zi), *Medicago truncatula, Melia azedarach* (Chinaberry), *Mentha arvensis* (wild or corn mint), *Mentha suaveolens* (applemint, essential oil), *Paeonia suffruticosa* (root cortex, mu-dan-pi), *Plantago asiatica* seeds (che-qian-zi), *Polyporus umbellatus* (zhu ling), *Poria cocos* (fu ling), *Rheum palmatum* root (da-huang), *Sophorae favescentis*, Praneem/Basant vaginal suppository (composed of *Emblica officinalis*, curcumin, aloe vera, and rose water extract), chuan-xin-lian (*Andrographis, Taraxacum officinale* (root), *Isatis*) and niao-lu-qing liquid (which is also strongly active against mycoplamal bacteria and a number of resistant microorganisms). Niao-lu-qing contains *Andrographis, Houttynia, Ileteropogon contortus, Pyrrosia sheareri, Zea mays, Poria cocos, Atractylodes macrocephalae,* and *Glycyrrhiza* spp. All are worth exploring.

Some of the ones that show up rather insistently as having strong activity, specific to *Chlamydiae,* are *Andrographis, Glycyrrhiza,* and *Houttuynia.*

rhiza spp., *Houttuynia* spp., *Polygala tenuifolia* (Chinese senega) root, *Pueraria lobata* (kudzu), *Scutellaria baicalensis, Salvia miltiorrhiza,* and *Zingiber officinalis* appear most often. Hence, the focus on those plants in these protocols.

Salvia miltiorrhiza

Salvia miltiorrhiza (danshen or red sage) is a rather remarkable Chinese herb that has been used for millennia. The herb tends to act as a cytokine normalizer (cytokine adaptogen is probably a better term), that is, it modulates cytokine expression during abnormal states. If cytokine activity is inappropriately high, it lowers it; if inappropriately low, it raises it. Thus, studies show that in some circumstances the herb lowers nitric oxide production; in others it raises it. In some circumstances it inhibits caspase activity; in others it raises it. In some instances, it stimulates apoptosis; in others it inhibits it.

Salvia miltiorrhiza appears then to be an immune-response adaptogen, specifically for use during altered, and unhealthy, cytokine responses to infection. Comparison of the herb's pharmacokinetic actions in both disease and nondisease states finds that during disease conditions, the herb's constituents localize to the sites of damage where they initiate modulation of the specific types of inflammation that is occurring there. Whereas in nondisease states, they don't seem to produce any cytokine modulating action at all.

For example, depth studies in mice found that the cytokine profile was unaltered in healthy mice when the herb was added (in various amounts) to their diets. However, when the mice were intentionally infected with *Listeria* bacteria, the herb modulated the exact cytokine alterations the organisms caused. Thus, again, the herb appears to work as a cytokine-specific adaptogen, that is, it normalizes cytokine responses to adverse events, such as microbial infection. A few of the other important actions of the plant are . . .

Danshen is also a strong modulator of unhealthy NF-*k*B behavior, which is one of the primary strategies of these bacteria. The herb modulates NF-*k*B expression and NF-*k*B binding activity by, when necessary, inhibiting NF-*k*B-inducing kinase, inhibiting the phosphorylation of I*k*Ba (i.e., nuclear factor of kappa light polypeptide gene enhancer in B-cells inhibitor-alpha) and mitogen-activated protein kinases (MAPKs) in a dose-dependent manner (i.e., you need to use high enough of a dose for long enough). *Note:* IkBa is functions as an inhibitor of NF-*k*B by masking signals that upregulate its expression, keeping nuclear localization signals of NF-*k*B proteins sequestered in cell cytoplasm. If IkBa is upregulated over long time lines, NF-*k*B becomes chronically active. This is what leads to the generation of lymphomas from low-level chronic infection with chlamydial bacteria over decades.

Organ and cellular protective herbs

The various organs affected by the bacteria can often be helped/protected by the use of a number of different herbs. The most specific are *Salvia miltiorrhiza* (danshen) and *Cordyceps*. And a note regarding hawthorn berries: Because of the bacterial impact on vascular function hawthorn can help, but the primary underlying dynamics are, I think, better addressed by danshen.

Salvia miltiorrhiza for organ protection

The herb is strongly protective (more so than skullcap root) of the Golgi structures of the cell, preventing fragmentation. (This alone will significantly reduce bacterial load.) The herb upregulates transforming growth factor-beta-1 (TGF-b1), which is a multifunctional cytokine, present in Golgi structures, and acts to protect them from fragmentation. Chlamydial bacteria inhibit this cytokine, more easily allowing them to fragement the Golgi. The herb also protects GM130, an important matrix protein that exists on the Golgi surface, stabilizing its structure and thus inhibiting Golgi fragmentation. It is involved in cellular processing and modification, vesicle transportation, cell migration, material exchange, mitosis, microtubule generation, and maintaining structural integrity of smooth surface mesh. During fragementation, from whatever cause, GM130 expression disappears. The herb is specific for, as researchers have noted, in maintaining the stability of Golgi morphology and structure.

The effects of the herb on neural cell Golgi structures is also profound, which makes the herb specific for neurological problems from the Lyme-group of coinfections. During neurological diseases such as ALS, Alzheimer's, and Parkinson's, the Golgi structures are damaged. Golgi damage during neurological Lyme, chlamydial, and RMSF (and other coinfectious bacteria) infections contributes to the generation of ALS/Alzheimer's-like diseases. The herb also inhibits Rho kinase (ROCK), also helping protecting Golgi structures. This has been found to protect heart and arterial tissues similarly to neural and general cell structure, again making the herb specific for chlamydial infections.

Note: the herb's action peaks and holds steady after seven days of use. It should be used long term during chlamydial infections to make sure it reaches peak and remains active throughout multiple reproductive cycles of the bacteria.

Salvia miltiorrhiza (danshen or red sage) is also specific for spleen protection, reducing inflammation while it also enhances spleen immune activity.

The herb restores mucosal integrity in mucosa-infected cells (in which these bacteria specialize), increases the population of healthy bacteria in the bowel (and the health of their biofilms – and no, it doesn't potentiate borrelial-biofilms), improves intestinal microcirculation, restores the ecology of the bowel, reduces unhealthy bowel bacteria overgrowth, and increases the levels of healthy bacteria throughout the bowel.

This particular salvia is highly protective of the reproductive tract. The use of the herb during *C. trachomatis* infections has been found to significantly inhibit fibrosis development in the genitourinary system during bacterial infection. It specifically reduces salpingitis, decreases tubal occlusion, and reduces hydrosalpinx formation. (*Note:* This herb is crucial to use during chlamydial infection of the reproductive tract.)

Salpingitis is an infection, and inflammation, in the Fallopian tubes, something this bacteria often causes. Hydrosalpinx is a Fallopian tube blocked with serous or clear fluid. The tube often becomes distended and bulges, somewhat like a sausage. This is one of the main causes of infertility during *C. trachomatis* infections. This same dynamic occurs in arteries surrounding the heart during chlamydial infections. Danshen is specific for preventing it, no matter the location. A study of endometriosis (with rats) found that the herb reduced the cytokine markers associated with that disease, relieving symptoms.

Several hundred human trials (at least) with the herb (or its constituents) have occurred in treating a variety of conditions. From this short review you can see how it would be useful for many of the problems that occur during a chlamydial infection. Specifically: pancreatitis, oral submucous fibrosis, fatty liver, polycystic ovary syndrome, hyper-androgenism, myocardial damage in people with severe burns, treatment of chronic artery disease among diabetics, coronary artery bypass, hypertension, platelet thrombin levels in chronic haemodialysis, chronic heart disease, hypercholesteremia, hyperlipidemia, vascular endothelial dysfunction, chronic hepatitis B, liver cirrhosis, Henoch-Schonlein purpura nephritis, primary nephrotic syndrome, portal hypertension, midsevere infantile hypoxic-ischemic encephalopathy, hypertensive cerebral hemorrhage, chronic asthma, cervical erosion, chronic hepatitis, whooping cough, schistosomal hepatomegaly, shock, scleroderma, allergic rhinitis, glaucoma, enlarged spleen, insomnia, and angina pectoris.

Cordyceps

Cordyceps is highly protective of sphingomyelin, the mitochondria, the lungs, the brain, and the kidneys.

The herb possesses a potent sphingomyelinase inhibitor that inhibits the breakdown of sphingomyelin in the body, making it specific for this infection. It strongly inhibits hydrogen peroxide oxidation and activity against cells, actively protects the mitochrondria (reducing oxidative stress and mitochondrial depolarization). It acts as an intracellular antioxidant, and is a strong hydroxyl radical scavenger. All these actions are dose dependent.

Cordyceps stimulates ATP generation by mitochondria, antioxidant activity, and modulates immune responses intracellularly. It protects mitochondria from ROS and enhances the mitochondrial antioxidant defenses.

Cordycepin strongly inhibits LPS-activated inflammation in microglia cells. It significantly inhibits the production of NO, PGE2, and proinflammatory cytokines in the microglia. It suppresses NF-kB translocation by blocking IkBa degradation and inhibits phosphorylation of Akt, ERK-1 and -2, JNK, and p38 kinase.

A blend of Cordyceps, Coptidis rhizoma (a berberine plant), and Scutellaria baicalensis (unsurprisingly) has been found in clinical trials to have powerful neuroprotective effects on bacterially activated microglial cells, inhibiting NO, iNOS, COX-2, PGE2, gp91(phox), iROS, TNF-a, IL-1b, and IkBa degradation. It upregulates HO-1 and increases cell viability and mitochondrial membrane potential. This three-herb combination was found to strongly protect neural cells from toxicity.

As well, Cordyceps has many protective effects on the lungs. It acts to normalize cellular function in airway epithelia via normalizing ion transport. It inhibits airway inflammation by blocking cytokine production in airway epithelia cells. It significantly reduces epidermal growth factor-stimulated mucous hypersecretion in lung mucoepidemoid cells by down regulating COX-2, MMP-9, and MUC5AC gene expression through blocking the relevant pathways. The herb strongly regulates the inflammation that can occur in the bronchii during infection also regulating bronchoalveolar lavage fluids. It is strongly protective of the lung's cilia.

Cordyceps is also highly protective of renal tubular epithelial cells through similar cytokine-regulating effects. And it suppresses the expression of diabetes-regulating genes.

Bidens pilosa

While B. pilosa seems to be the strongest species, most species of Bidens are very good at protecting mucus membrane structures from the negative effects of microbial infection, especially chronic, long-standing ones. In addition, the herb does possess some very good cytokine-modulating effects, especially on PGE2.

Immune-enhancing herbs

The best immune-normalizing herbs for this bacteria are, I think, *Astragalus* spp., *Cordyceps* spp., *Glycyrrhiza* spp., *Houttuynia* spp., *Rhodiola*, *Salvia miltiorrhiza*, *Scutellaria baicalensis,* and *Withania somnifera*. Of these, *Withania somnifera* is core.

Withania somnifera

This herb (also known as ashwaghanda) does have a nice range of actions, especially for coinfections. It is an immune tonic and modulator (especially good for modulating IL-10 overproduction), is stress protective, alterative, and anxiolytic; it is a nerve sedative, neural protector, chondroprotector, collagenase inhibitor, and a reliable tonic sedative for insomniac conditions (especially if caused by stress or disease); it is antifatigue, amphoteric, antioxidant, anti-inflammatory, haematopoietic, antibacterial, diuretic, antipyretic, antitumor, and astringent.

The leaves and stems are a nerve sedative, antipyretic, febrifuge, bitter, diuretic, antibacterial, antimicrobial, astringent, and antitumor. The seeds are hypnotic, diuretic, and coagulant. The fruit an immune tonic, antibacterial, alterative, and astringent.

Ashwagandha has been a major medicinal plant in India for at least three thousand years. They consider it tonic, alterative, astringent, and aphrodisiac and a nervine sedative. It has been used for TB, emaciation of children, senile debility, rheumatism, general debility, nervous exhaustion, brain fog, loss of memory, loss of muscular energy, and spermatorrhoea. Its primary use is to restore vigor and energy in a body worn out by long-term constitutional disease or old age.

Note: This herb may cause drowsiness, so take it at night the first few times to see how you do.

The core protocol and expanded repertory

I consider the primary herbs of the core protocol for all chlamydial infections to be the berberine-containing plants, *Scutellaria baicalensis*, and *Salvia miltiorrhiza*. This is the core around which treatment is based.

Core protocol

Note: Take *all* suggested tinctures and tincture combinations unless listed as optional. *For this organism, this is not a pick-and-choose process*, at least if you want to eliminate the infection. This protocol is for *all* forms of chlamydial infection, irrespective of the area of the body affected. Normally, most chlamydial infections will be eliminated in thirty days. The protocol, however, may be repeated as necessary.

1) Berberine-containing plant tincture, e.g., goldenseal:
   ½ teaspoon tincture, 3–6x daily, depending on severity
   of infection.
2) Combination tincture of *Scutellaria baicaleneis* and *Salvia miltiorrhiza*: 1 teaspoon 3–6x daily, depending on severity
   of infection.
3) Combination tincture of *Cordyceps*, *Withania somnifera*, and *Glycyrrhiza*. *Note:* Combination ratio is 1 part of the first
   two, ½ part of the third, (e.g., 1 ounce cordyceps, 1 ounce
   withania, ½ ounce licorice). One teaspoon of the combination 3–6x per day depending on severity of infection.
   If necessary dosage may be increased short term, i.e., 2
   teaspoons 3–6x daily, for up to thirty days.
4) *Bidens pilosa* or other *Bidens* species: ½ teaspoon 3–6x daily.
5) Vitamin A, 2,000 IU to 9,000 IU daily, depending on severity of infection. Best absorbed if taken with vitamin E and
   zinc. *Note:* May be toxic as it can bioaccumulate, especially
   if your food is well endowed with it. Limit use as supplement to the duration of the treatment for the infection.
6) This one is optional: Combination tincture of *Andrographis* and *Houttuynia*: ½ teaspoon 3–6x daily. Dosage can be
   increased to 1 teaspoon if desired. *Note:* Please see materia
   medica chapter for side effects of *Andrographis*.

Extended protocol, depending on type of infection

The following are *additions* to the core protocol and should also be taken if you are experiencing infection in the indicated parts of the body. All these protocols can be repeated if necessary.

Female Genital Tract Chlamydial-infection

1. Core protocol plus . . .
2. Daily use of herbal vaginal suppository for fourteen days

The vaginal suppository should be made this way . . .

Take two ounces *each* of powdered *Hydrastis canadensis*, i.e., goldenseal (or equivalent), *Echinacea angustifolia* (*note:* do *not* use *E. purpurea*), and *Scutellaria baicalensis*. Mix with enough glycerine so that you can shape the mixture into fourteen vaginal suppositories. Please note that the mix will be really sticky. Add enough flour to the mix to counteract the sticky. Then . . . place on a tray and put that in the freezer.

The next day, in the evening, take one suppository, and when you are ready for bed, lie down and insert the suppository up against the cervix. (It will be cold, still . . . some people *like* this.) The next morning, have ready ½ ounce of goldenseal tincture (or equivalent) and ½ ounce of *Bidens* tincture. Add the two tinctures to sufficient water to douche. Douche. Repeat this for fourteen days. If necessary you can repeat the fourteen day protocol as long as needed to help a vaginal chlamydial infection.

Chlamydial-induced poor semen quality

1. Core protocol plus . . .
2. L-arginine, 400–6,000 mg daily, plus . . .
3. L-carnitine, 500–2,000 mg daily, plus . . .
4. Acetyl-L-carnitine, 600–2,500 mg daily, plus . . .
5. *Panax ginseng* tincture, ½ tsp 3x daily.

All for two months minimum.

Trachoma

1. Core protocol plus . . .
2. Berberine-plant eyedrops. Dose 1-3 drops, in the eye, *throughout* the day.

To make: Take one ounce, chopped fairly fine but you don't need to be OCD about it, of any berberine plant (e.g., goldenseal root), place in heat-tolerant glass container with lid, and add five ounces of hot water. Close up tight and leave overnight. Next morning, strain by placing in cloth and wringing out the liquid. Then . . . strain the liquid through a coffee filter (you don't really want any plant chunks in your eye). Pour one ounce of the liquid in a tincture bottle that has a dropper lid. Put the rest in a closed container and keep refrigerated. Use the drops throughout the day for fourteen days, may be repeated if necessary.

CHAPTER TWELVE

THE SPOTTED FEVER RICKETTSIAE

The emergence and flux of RMSF and other tick-borne diseases can most often be traced to specific human activities and behaviors that disrupt ecosystems and place greater numbers of susceptible hosts into the environment.
Parola et al., 2013

Rocky Mountain spotted fever is among the most severe of human infectious diseases, with a mortality rate of 20 to 25 percent unless treated with an appropriate antibiotic. . . . Although, in theory, the disease is always curable by early, appropriate treatment, the case fatality rate is still 4 percent.
D.H. Walker, 1996

Rickettsia are intracellular, and are symbionts in the broad sense, having an intimate (but not necessarily beneficial) relationship with their hosts. Rickettsia species are the causative agents of numerous diseases of humans, including epidemic typhus, which is thought to have caused up to three million deaths in Russia alone, from 1917 to 1923.
Perlman et al., 2006

The stealth bacteria of the *Ricksettsia* genus are among the oldest medically known vector-borne diseases. Some of its members were identified as specific disease pathogens as early as the late 1800s. Despite that, and oddly enough, this group of coinfections is probably less well studied than any in the Lyme-group; sophisticated research only began during the last twenty-five years. Egregiously, there is very little of that.

As the rickettsial specialist David Walker comments . . .

> *In the United States, few infectious diseases specialists have focused investigative attention on rickettsial diseases. Isolation of rickettsiae from patients and prospective clinical studies are rarely undertaken. Diseases caused by such pathogens as the highly prevalent R. felis, which was shown to cause illness in humans more than a decade ago, and R. parkeri, which was discovered >60 years ago, remain virtually uninvestigated.*

The best known members of the genus, all identified in the nineteenth century, are Rocky Mountain spotted fever (*Rickettsia rickettsii*) and the two typhus organisms, *R. typhi* and *R. prowazekii*. For nearly a century these were considered to be the primary infectious agents of human beings. But the last twenty-five years has revealed, as it has with all the Lyme-group, the genus to be much larger, and more widely spread, than anyone suspected. Furthermore, many of its members are now understood to be, by researchers if not physicians, common sources of human infections. As researchers Parola et al. (2013) comment . . .

> *Several species of tick-borne* Rickettsiae *that were considered nonpathogenic for decades are now associated with human infections, and novel* Rickettsia *species of undetermined pathogenicity continue to be detected in or isolated from ticks around the world. . . . Finally, many well-characterized SFG* Rickettsia *species and recently or incompletely described* Rickettsiae *that were previously considered to be restricted to a specific tick host or geographical location have recently been detected on different continents and in various tick hosts.*

The organisms, while often found in wild arthropods who feed on forest and grassland animals, have a special affinity for arthropods that infect our domestic animals: dogs, cats, and a wide range of farm animals. And, unfortunately, the ticks and fleas that infect our companion and farm animals do transmit rickettsial infections to us. Additionally, the movement of people into formerly wild habitat because of human population increases is bringing more people into contact with wildland arthropods infected with the bacteria.

Part of the difficulty for researchers studying the bacteria is that the organisms appear to go through stages of virulence – sometimes they cause mild or no infections, sometimes severe infections. The bacteria, after they pass through birds (which spread them around the world) or, more problematical, *after overwintering in their tick hosts*, become more virulent. Eremeeva et al. (2001) comment that . . .

> *the isolates of* R. rickettsia *which exhibit different virulence for guinea pigs differ primarily because they were isolated during different phases of a normal cycle of adaptation to their verte-brate and invertebrate hosts. That is characteristic of the species.* R. sibirica *also has a complex cycle of maintenance in nature and distinct biotypes that differ in virulence for guinea pigs.*

So, when researchers captured wild ticks and studied the *Rickettsiae* within them, they, for decades, missed the crucial understanding that the bacteria undergo cycles of virulence. What they have been studying, and writing about, is not what they thought it to be. This contributes mightily to many of the common misunderstandings about rickettsial infections.

The *Rickettsiae*

are Gram-negative bacteria. However, due to some unusual features, they were long thought to be viruses or perhaps even an intermediate life-form somewhere between viruses and bacteria (like many in the pathogenic Lyme-group).

They are close relatives of two other Lyme coinfections (*Ehrlichia* and *Anaplasma*) and are very similar to mycoplasmal organisms in that they are very, very tiny. Like most intracellular bacteria, as they learned to live within other cells, they reduced the size of their genome, keeping only the most essential gene sequences. They began to use host cell machinery to meet their needs (rather than their own) and, over time, abandoned the parts of their genome they no longer needed. Like the rest of the Lyme-group, they are considered to be obligate, intracellular bacterial parasites.

Obligate because they are obligated to live inside other organisms. Intracellular because they live inside those organisms' cells.

These bacteria are descendants of an incredibly old family of microbes. Nearly one-fourth of all bacteria found in seawater are ancient, free-living, bacterial ancestors of the *Rickettsiae*. (The *Rickettsiae* are also close relatives of the mitochondria that power our cells and who, in a shocking instance of familial betrayal, they also sometimes infect.) Between 1 billion and 800 million years ago, some of the rickettsial ancestors split off and learned to live inside other organisms. Later, between 425 and 525 million years ago, more radiational splitting occurred, and some of those bacteria began to specialize in infecting arthropods such as ticks and fleas.

The arthropod-infecting *Rickettsiae* and their ancestral groups have had a long time to work with their hosts. Like many of the Lyme-group, they are transmitted from female ticks into their eggs and their developing embryos, a process known as vertical transmission. Many of them, very differently from the rest of the Lyme-group, have subsequently developed a unique strategy: they severely reduce the male population of arthropods during infection, stimulate the conversion of males to females, thus significantly increasing the numbers of females, eggs, and offspring they can infect. (As seen on the TV show, *Feminists Gone Bad*.) Some arthropod species (e.g., the booklouse) cannot even produce offspring without the help of the bacteria. As researchers (Pornwiroon et al., 2007) comment . . .

> *Sex ratio distortion (SRD), favoring female progeny as a continual means for vertical transmission of microorganisms, occurs through a variety of mechanisms including male killing, feminization, and parthogenesis. Additionally, cytoplasmic incompatibility (CI) is an alternative method for reproductive manipulation favoring vertical transmission of microorganisms.*

Over long evolutionary time, as new forms of life emerged out of the ecological background of the planet, the bacteria continued to innovate, adapting to life inside those newly emerging species. All that long time line, of course, they were learning how to effectively deal with the immune systems those life-forms possessed. Perhaps 150 million years ago the group of bacteria we now call the *Rickettsia* split off from their most immediate ancestral group. (The oldest, foundational member of that group is probably *Rickettsia belli*, which has the largest genome of them all.) Some 50 million years ago or so, there occurred what researchers call a "rapid radiation." This involved the rapid emergence (in evolutionary terms) of a large number of new subgroups, including what we now call the spotted fever *Rickettsiaes*.

Those millions of years of learning produced infectious organisms whose ability to find, infect, and subvert the immune systems of their hosts is tremendously sophisticated. As Azad and Beard comment (1998): "Rickettsial associations with obligate blood- sucking arthropods represent the highly adapted end-product of eons of biologic evolution." We humans, only around a million or so years, are, as usual, late on the scene. When we deal with these bacteria, we are encountering organisms that are immeasurably older than ourselves *and* our century-old pharmaceutical approaches to healing.

The rickettsial groups

Research on *Rickettsiae*, limited as it has been, has traditionally focused solely on the few members thought to cause human disease. The pervasiveness of the bacteria in nature, until recently, has remained invisible to the scientific eye. Deeper research over the past few decades has found however, that the *Rickettsiae* infect a wide range of life-forms . . . plants, amoebas, flies, beetles, weevils, moths, springtails, lacewings, lice, chiggers, mites, and ticks (hard and soft), as well as a vast array of vertebrates. They are an equal-infectious organism.

Unsurprisingly, the little that researchers (and physicians) did "know," even about the human-infectious *Rickettsiae*, has turned out to be either incorrect or distressingly oversimplified.

The infectious *Rickettsiae* were once believed to roughly fall into three groups: (1) the spotted fever group, (2) the typhus group – which counterintuitively also causes spots, and (3) the scrub typhus group (which inexplicably only contains one organism). But with the emergence of *Homo taxonomisii* (my least favorite subgroup of *Homo sapien sapien*) in the mid- to late-twentieth century, the family tree of the *Rickettsiae*, along with the family trees of all other life-forms on the planet, has found itself in disarray. As Vitorino et al. note (2007), "a robust and accurate phylogeny of this genus has not yet been accomplished and ambiguities remain in the phylogenetic position of some species." No kidding.

The scrub typhus organism *Rickettsia tsutsugamushi*, primarily found in Asia and which is transmitted by mites, has now been reclassified as *Orientia tsutsugamushi*. (It is no longer a member of the *Rickettsiae*.) And, of course, the rest of the genus has found itself mucked about with as well.

As of 2013, there are now (for a limited time only) four groups within the genus: (1) the spotted fever group (SFG); (2) the typhus group (TG), (3) the *Rickettsia bellii* group; and (4) the *Rickettsia canadensis* group. Of these the largest is the SFG group. (And, of course, there are some members of *Homo taxonomisii* who want to create an additional group, the transitional group *Rickettsiae* – TSG – just to make things even more difficult. This group would consist of the *Rickettsiae* that contain "phenotypic oddities" – much as *Homo taxonomisii* themselves do.)

The typhus group is generally believed to contain only two species, *Rickettsia prowazekii* and *R. typhi*. (The word "typhus," by the way, comes from an ancient Greek root meaning smoky or hazy, referring, I think, to taxonomists and not necessarily to the state of mind that develops in those infected by these organisms.) Simply to create confusion, some people insist on including *R. felis* in the typhus group; others, equally well degreed, do not. (Name calling at 6:00 p.m., behind the diner.) To make matters worse, some of the spotted fever group have common names (e.g., Indian tick typhus) with the word "typhus" in it. And even more irritating, the typhus organisms often cause spots identical to the spotted fever group. (Why have separate group names anyway?) And of course, just to make me consider taxonomicide, some of the spotted fever group *never* cause spots. This has stimulated desire among the taxonomist subgroup *Homo taxonomisii* var. *pleasegoawayii* to expand the *Rickettsiae* groups again, creating the *spotless* fever group. (Taxonomists are the one group of people on the planet that cannot, under any circumstances, count to potato.) The eminent *Rickettsiae* researcher, David Walker, whose work is refreshingly intelligent, shows a rare gift for taxonomic truth telling when he, gratifyingly, comments (2007) that . . .

> [t]he motivation driving the "genomic splitters" appears to be based on the gratifying experience of baptizing more organisms

> with creative names rather than using taxonomic criteria consis-
> tent with other similar organisms toward the aim of scientific
> utility. Any criteria for determining prokaryotic species are
> arbitrary.

Nevertheless, to continue. . .

Rickettsia prowazekii lives in human body lice and tends to spread via louse poop among the overcrowded, i.e., too many people living in squalid conditions (the poor, the jailed, soldiers in war). It is the source of epidemic typhus.

R. typhi lives in fleas and is most commonly spread from rats and mice to fleas to people. (The fleas bite you, pooping all the while, you scratch the bite, and into you the bacteria go, a strategy adopted by their close relatives the *Bartonellae*.) This endemic form of typhus usually occurs among the poor in coldish, third world countries. (It is sometimes called jail fever, which tells you a great deal about the conditions under which it is spread.) However (there is always a however), there is a form of *R. typhi*, loosely referred to as murine (essentially meaning "mouse") typhus, which appears most often in the south to southwestern United States, generally in California and Texas. The infected are usually those who are exposed to rat or mouse feces (when sweeping or cleaning – which is why I never sweep or clean). Fleas infected with this organism are, distressingly for cat lovers, not limited to rats and mice; they are common on house cats as well.

The *Rickettsiae* that infect flea and lice feces produce encysted-type forms that can remain viable for years. It is not yet known whether the tick-borne species do so. (I would suspect that they do.)

The symptoms of typhus infections, irrespective of species, are similar: abdominal pain, backache, high fever (104 degrees or higher), hacking dry cough, headache, chills, confusion, delirium, low blood pressure, joint and muscle pain, nausea, vomiting, spotted rash, and photosensitivity.

Rickettsia bellii and *Rickettsia canadensis* are, for now, the only members of their groups. *R. bellii* is widely distributed in ticks throughout North, Central, and South America; it is not yet known if they cause human infection (but they probably do). *R. canadensis* are found primarily in *Haemaphysalis leporispalustris* ticks in North and Central America. They are suspected to cause infections in people, but this has not been confirmed.

The spotted fever group (SFG)

is large and getting larger even as I speak. (In 2009 alone, twenty new strains were discovered.) There are (currently) twenty-six formally accepted species, six subspecies, thirty or more strains, sixteen recently identified *Rickettsiae* that are candidates (*candidatus*) for inclusion in the genus, and another fourteen (found in ticks) that have not yet been named, merely identified from their genetic structures as belonging to the genus. Most of these have been found in just the last ten years.

It was once thought, and unfortunately still is by many physicians, that very few of the SFG infected people. ("No, you cannot be infected with spotted fever, it doesn't occur around here, and I am not going to test you for it.") Distressingly, however, these infectious agents really are rather more common in people than realized. This is why the CDC has, finally, altered their reporting criteria. As Parola et al. (2013) comment: "Because some cases reported as RMSF might actually be diseases caused by other SFG *Rickettsiae*, the surveillance case definition for RMSF in the United States was modified in 2010 to encompass the broader category of spotted fever rickettsiosis."

Until recently, few physicians realized the extensive numbers of pathogenic bacteria in this genus; most still don't. Many SFG infections are mild and have been assumed to be "just a bout of the flu." They aren't.

It is important to note here that until somewhere between 1991 and 2012 most of these *Rickettsiae* were believed to *never* cause human infection. They had only been found in the wild, in ticks, during field research. Like most of the Lyme-group, the genus and its many members are much more commonly infectious of people than believed. As well, many of these species were thought to be geographically limited. Further research has found that their range is very wide – for most of them, the entire planet (excepting Antarctica so far). Most, but not all, are spread by ticks. Essentially, every hard tick species has been found to be infected with at least one rickettsial species.

In North and Central America, the ticks that most commonly spread the most virulent SFG member, Rocky Mountain spotted fever (RMSF), include the Rocky Mountain wood tick (*Dermacentor andersoni*), the American dog tick (*Dermacentor variabilis*), the Cayenne tick (*Amblyomma cajennense*), the brown dog tick (*Rhipicephalus sanguineus*), the Lone Star tick

(*Amblyomma americanum*), and several others including *Amblyomma imitator* (Mexico), *Dermacentor nitens* (Panama), and *Haemaphysalis leporispalustris* (Costa Rica).

These ticks are very common on dogs and that is the main route of transmission to people. Infection is especially frequent where wild or abandoned dogs are common.

Fortunately for humans, Rocky Mountain spotted fever organisms occur in relatively few numbers in the ticks they infect. This is part of the reason why RMSF infections in people tend to remain low. However, other *Rickettsiae* commonly infect close to 100 percent of the ticks tested. Those with the higher infection percentages are more easily infectious, those with lower less so.

Hard ticks, by the way, bite and travel on an incredibly wide range of animals, including birds during their winter and summer migrations. Thus these bacteria, like most of the Lyme-group of stealth pathogens, are to be found *everywhere*.

I, suspect as research continues to deepen, some of the species presumed to be solely tick borne will be found in other types of arthropods as well. Nobody has spent much time looking. In the very few instances they have, the bacteria were found in a wide range of arthropods.

Here is a look at the twenty-eight species, subspecies, and candidates currently known to cause disease in humans.

- *Rickettsia aeschlimannii* is found in eighteen different tick species in six different genera (so far). It causes a form of spotted fever in Sub-Saharan Africa, North Africa, and Europe and has been found in ticks in Israel and parts of Asia. It's often spread by migrating birds.
- *Rickettsia africae* has been found in thirteen different tick species in three different genera. It causes African tick bite fever in Sub-Saharan Africa, Asia, North and Central America, the Caribbean, and the Pacific Islands. Pathogen levels are generally very high in the ticks.
- *Rickettsia akari* is transmitted by the bite of mites who primarily live on house mice. It causes rickettsialpox, so-called because it strongly resembles chicken pox.

- *Rickettsia australis* is an Australian form that causes Queensland tick typhus. It is found, so far, in three *Ixodes* tick species.
- *Rickettsia conorii caspia* is found in four *Rhipicephalus* tick species and causes Astrakhan fever in Europe and Sub-Saharan Africa.
- *Rickettsia conorii conorii* is found in eight tick species in two genera and causes Mediterranean spotted fever in Europe, North Africa, Sub-Saharan Africa, and Asia. The brown dog tick is the primary arthropod that spreads it, but dogs, especially wild or abandoned ones, are considered to be primary vectors of the disease. Up to 72 percent of tested dogs have been found to be infected.
- *Rickettsia conorii indica* has been found in one tick species (*Rhipicephalus sanguineus*) in Europe and Asia and causes Indian tick typhus.
- *Rickettsia conorii israelensis* is found in that same tick species. It causes Israeli tick typhus in Europe, Asia, and North Africa. Unfortunately, dogs are competent vectors for the transmission of this species (via ticks) to people.
- *Rickettsia felis* is spread primarily by flea feces, similarly to *Bartonella* organisms. It's been found in a variety of flea species, including some that tend to reside on dogs (the horror). Still, the cat-residing flea, *Ctenocephalides felis,* lending credence to the widespread Internet belief that cats are evil, seems, currently, to be its most common host . . . well, it lives on opossums, too. (Everybody already knows opossums are evil – just look at a picture of one.) Infection rates in fleas tends to run from 43 to 93 percent in the populations studied. Unfortunately, for humans, the organism has also been found in twenty-four different species of ticks, lice, and mites. It is beginning to appear that infection with the organism is much more widespread than thought.
- *Rickettsia heilongjiangensis* has been found in four tick species in two genera and causes Far Eastern spotted fever in Asia, primarily in Russia, China, South Korea, and Japan.

- *Rickettsia helvetica* is found in *Ixodes* ticks and causes spotted fever infections (with no specific name) in Asia (so far only in Laos and Thailand) and Europe. It has been found in ticks in North Africa, Japan, and Turkey.
- *Rickettsia honei* is found in both *Ixodes* and *Bothriocroton* ticks and causes Flinders Island spotted fever in Asia, Australia, and the Pacific Islands.
- *Ricksettia honei marmionii* is carried by *Haemaphysalis novagyineae* ticks and causes Australian spotted fever in, well, Australia.
- *Rickettsia japonica* is found in seven ticks in three genera so far. It causes Oriental or Japanese spotted fever in Asia, primarily Japan and South Korea.
- *Rickettsia kellyi (candidatus)* has been found as the cause of a single case of spotted fever in India.
- *Rickesstia massiliae* is a very common tick-borne *Rickettsiae*. It is found widely in the tick genus *Rhipicephalus* (brown dog ticks) in North, Central America, and South America; Europe; Sub-Saharan Africa; Asia; and North Africa. It causes an as yet unnamed rickettsiosis.
- *Rickettsia monacensis*has been found primarily in *Ixodes* ticks in Europe and North Africa.
- *Rickettsia montanensis* is common in two tick genera in the US and Canada.
- *Rickettsia parkeri* is found primarily in *Amblyomma* and *Dermacentor* ticks in North, Central, and South America. It is a growing source of the inventively named *R. parkeri* rickettsiosis, primarily in the southeastern US, Argentina, and Uruguay.
- *Rickettsia philipii* has been found in *Dermacentor occidentalis* ticks in North and Central America, primarily in California. It causes an as yet unnamed rickettsiosis.
- *Rickettsia raoultii* is an Asian species found in *Dermacentor* ticks in North Asia and *Haemaphysalis* and *Amblyomma* ticks in South Asia. These ticks are common on domestic farm animals (sheep, goats, cattle) and tend to bite people who work with them.

- *Rickettsii riskettsii* is the most widely known of the spotted fever bacteria and the cause of the misnamed and always potentially severe Rocky Mountain spotted fever. It is found in a wide variety of hard ticks in North, Central and South America, most commonly in Canada, US, Mexico, Costa Rica, Panama, Argentina, Brazil, and Columbia. Dogs, especially roaming, wild, and abandoned ones, are especially good vectors of this pathogen.
- *Rickettsia sibirica mongolotimonae* is primarily in *Hyalomma* ticks in Europe, Sub-Saharan Africa, Asia, and North Africa. It causes a lymphangitis-associated rickettsiosis. The organism was first found in 1991 in China; most human infections have been diagnosed since 2005, most of those in Europe (two in North Africa). The organism commonly infects camels (possibly evil).
- *Rickettsia sibirica sibirica* causes Siberian tick typhus in Asia, primarily Russia, China, and Mongolia. It is found in a variety of hard ticks.
- *Rickettsia slovaca* is primarily found in *Dermacentor* ticks in Europe, Asia, and North Africa. It causes a tick-borne lymphadenitis. These ticks are common on domestic farm animals (sheep, goats, cattle) and tend to bite people who work with them.
- *Rickettsia* **species, strain Atlantic rainforest/strain Bahia**, is normally a South American strain, which infects a variety of *Amylyomma* ticks.
- *Rickettsia tamurae* has been found in *Amblyomma testudinarium* ticks in Laos and Japan. Typical hosts are wild and domestic pigs, but the ticks have been found on deer, cattle, livestock, and, of course, people.
- *Rickettsia tarasevichiae (candidatus)*, discovered in 2012 as the causal factor in a number of infections in northeastern China. The transmission vectors were found to be *Ixodes persulcatus* ticks.

Species not yet known to infect people

Here is a sampling of some of the many *Rickettsiae* species found in ticks worldwide that are not yet known to cause human infections. It is important to note that the majority of the human-infectious organisms in the preceeding list were once in this category. Current speculation is that many cases of Rocky Mountain spotted fever and/or fevers of unknown origin have been caused by some of these organisms. This additional list gives some idea of the tremendous prevalence of this genus in tick species throughout the world. It's not exhaustive. There are scores more, many not yet given a specific name.

- *Rickettsia amblyommii* is widely distributed in *Amblyomma americanum* ticks (and a large number of other genera and species) in North, Central and South America, especially in the US, Costa Rica, Panama, Brazil, Argentina, and French Guyana.
- *Rickettsia andeanae (candidatus)* is found in *Amblyomma maculatum* ticks in North and Central America, primarily in the southeastern US It occurs in a wide variety of other ticks in South America, primarily Peru, Chile, and Argentina.
- *Rickettsia antechini* has been found in *Ixodes antechini* ticks in Australia.
- *Rickettsia argasii* is an Australian species found in *Argas antechini* ticks.
- *Rickettsia cooleyi (candidatus)* is common in *Ixodes scapularis* ticks throughout the eastern, upper midwestern, and southern US.
- *Rickettsia derrickii* is found in *Bothriocroton hydrosauri* ticks in Australia.
- *Rickettsia* **unnamed species, strains G021 and G022** are common in Northern California and Oregon. They are found in *Ixodes pacificus* ticks.
- *Rickettsia guntherii* has been found in *Haemaphysalis humerosa* ticks in Australia
- *Rickettsia hoogstraalii* is found in a variety of ticks in Japan, Asia, Europe, and Sub-Saharan Africa.
- *Rickettsia monteiroi* has been found in *Amblyomma incisum* in

Brazil and is thought to possibly be a member of the *R. bellii* or *R. canadensis* group.

- **Rickettsia rhipicephali**, in a variety of hard ticks, has been found in Taiwan, and North, Central, and South America.
- **Rickettsia sauri** has been found in *Amblyomma hydrosauri* ticks in Australia.
- **Rickettsia tasmanensis** in *Ixodes persulcatus* ticks, has been found in Australia.

Symptoms of infection

Symptoms of infection with SFG pathogens run from a minimal febrile (feverish) illness, similar to a mild case of the flu, to septic shock and death. Many, but not all, of the SFG pathogens cause what is called an eschar, an unhealing, scabby, or necrotic-type wound at the inoculation site of the tick bite. This is one of the primary symptoms that can suggest an SFG infection. Some of the infectious organisms in this group are so new and the number of identified infections so uncommon (as yet) that very little has been written about their symptom picture. Here is a look at the general symptoms of the *Rickettsiae* that infect people.

Please note: Despite the name spotted fever group, a spotted-rash does not always occur; *its absence is often associated with poorer outcomes.*

- **Rickettsia aeschlimannii**, *R. aeschlimannii* spotted fever. Only one case found so far, similar symptoms to infection by *Rickettsia conorii conorii*.
- **Rickettsia africae,** African tick bite fever. An eschar-associated febrile illness, first identified in 1998 in the West Indies. North American tourists, hunters, and members of the military, visiting the Caribbean often return home infected with the organism. The disease begins five to seven days after tick bite and presents with sudden onset of fever, fatigue, headache, and myalgia. Inoculation eschars are not always present, but when they are, multiple eschars are common. The lymph nodes nearest to the inoculation site are often severely swollen, and the usual SFG spotting – a generalized maculopapular or papulocesicular rash

(and occasionally aphthous stomatitis) occurs. The disease is generally benign and rarely fatal though more severe complications can occur. This is especially true for the elderly (and in any other group with lowered immune function) where symptoms such as subacute cranial or peripheral neuropathy, chronic fatigue, internuclear ophthalmoplegia, myocarditis, and cellulitis can occur.

The disease, since 2005, is now known to be endemic in Sub-Saharan Africa, especially in indigenous cultures that raise cattle (who spread the infected ticks). Some 50 percent of indigenous populations apparently have antibodies to the organism. The ticks that carry it are extremely aggressive, emerging from their grassland homes and running toward potential hosts when they are in proximity. (They don't just climb a grass stalk with legs outstretched and wait.) I don't really like the image this creates in my mind, but one Japanese woman was found to have over one hundred infected ticks on her trunk and extremities.

- *Rickettsia akari*, rickettsialpox. A generally mild, flu-like illness characterized by eschar, fever, and a chickenpox-like rash. It primarily occurs in urban areas with large mouse populations whose mites transmit the disease. This species, like its close relatives the *Ehrlichiae*, primarily infects macrophages/monocytes instead of endothelial cells.

- *Rickettsia australis,* Queensland tick typhus. The first cases were identified in 1946; the species is pretty much limited to Australia. Symptoms are headache, chills, malaise, fever, maculopapular rash, and eschar. The disease covers the spectrum from mild to life threatening. Fatalities are rare.

- *Rickettsia conorii caspia,* Astrakhan fever, so named because it is common in the Astrakhan region (and nearby areas) around the Caspian Sea. The symptoms are similar to MSF (see next listing) but inoculation eschar is only present in about a quarter of infections, maculopapular rash is very common (91 percent), and petechiae occurs 20 percent of cases. There is fever, which at peak is sometimes accompanied by nasal hemorrhages and bleeding during medical treatment. There is lowered platelet aggregation, and thrombocytopenia (usually at height of fever). I have seen some reports that indicate this pathogen can be spread by aerosol inhalation.

• **_Rickettsia conorii conorii,_** Mediterranean spotted fever (MSF). This is one of the oldest recognized vector-borne infections. It is endemic in southern Europe but it has been spreading to northern, central, and, especially, eastern regions. There is an incubation period of approximately six days followed by abrupt onset. The disease is characterized by fever, flu-like symptoms, prostration, inoculation eschar, rash including soles of feet and palms of hands, and the usual spotted fever rash, either maculopapular or petechial. Fever, rash, and eschar are the most common symptoms. _However,_ this species has multiple strains, and many of them, depending on the geographic region, do not produce the rash; it's lacking in up to 40 percent of infections.

Studies have found an increasing aggressiveness in the brown dog tick that carries the bacteria, thought to be due to increased warming in the region. In consequence more infections and multiple eschars are becoming the norm. At the same time, more serious, atypical, and life-threatening symptoms seem to be occurring with greater frequency. These include cardiomyopathies (ecstasia of the arteries, tachycardia, myocarditis, and atrial fibrillation), ocular problems (uveitis, retinopathy, and retinal vasculitis), neurological symptoms (cerebral infarct, meningoencephalitis, sensorineural healing loss, tremors, limb weakness, stupor, mental confusion, acute quadriplegia secondary to axonal polyneuropathy, and motor and sensory polyneuritis), pancreatic problems, splenic rupture, acute renal failure, and hemophagocytic syndrome.

Risk factors for severe infection are advanced age, immunocompromise, chronic alcoholism, glucose-6-phosphate dehydrogenase deficiency, diabetes, treatment with sulfonamides, use of inappropriate antibiotics, and delay in effective treatment. *Fluoroquinolone treatment is associated with more severe infection and longer hospitalization.* Mortality rate, even with treatment, has reached 13 percent in Portugal; fatal outcome is associated with symptoms of confusion, obtundation, hyperbilrubinemia, acute renal failure, and *absence* of rash.

- *Rickettsia conorii indica,* Indian tick typhus. This has been most prevalent in India, however an infection in Europe, in a nontraveler, was caused by this organism in 2012. The disease is very similar to MSF (see *Rickettsia conorii conorii*). Complications including acute hepatitis and gangrene have occurred. In contrast to MSF, the rash is commonly purpuric; there is rarely an inoculation eschar.

- *Rickettsia conorii israelensis,* Israeli tick typhus. The symptoms are similar to MSF, *Rickettsia conorii conorii*, however inoculation eschar is only present in about 38 percent of cases, gastrointestinal symptoms (nausea and vomiting) are common, and in Portugal, the mortality rate is 29 percent.

- *Rickettsia felis,* R. *felis* spotted fever, cat-flea typhus, flea-borne spotted fever. This organism was only identified two decades ago and has now been found to be endemic to all continents except Antarctica (Antarctica means "no bears," another semiuseless fact). Testing for the bacterium is currently rare. However, its widespread presence in cat fleas indicates that infection with the organism could be very common.

  Symptoms tend to be fairly mild (so far). They include fever, fatigue, headache, maculopapular rash, and eschar. Researchers believe that the disease is commonly misdiagnosed, either as another spotted fever or "the flu."

- *Rickettsia heilongjiangensis,* Far Eastern spotted fever. Only a few cases have been found so far, in Russia, China, Japan, and Thailand, primarily due to the newness (to science) of the organism. The disease usually affects those over fifty and primarily shows as a mild rash with fever and eschar. However, one case of septic shock from the organism has occurred in Thailand.

- *Rickettsia helvetica,* unnamed spotted fever. Generally a mild, self-limiting infection accompanied by headache, myalgia, and only occasionally by rash and eschar. This species has, however, been found (in a number of people) to be the cause of idiopathic chronic perimyocarditis leading to sudden cardiac death. Emerging studies show this may be relatively common. A 2005 study of 84 sclerotic heart valves (in people undergoing aortic valve replacement) found 17 of the valves to be infected by *R. helvetica,* 22 with *Chlamydia pneumoniae,* and 6 with both organisms.
- *Rickettsia honei,* Flinders Island spotted fever. This species was identified in ticks in 1998. The first human infection was diagnosed in Australia in 1991. Since then infections have been reported in Australia, Tasmania, Thailand, and Nepal. Symptom picture is usually mild with fever, myalgia, headache, cough, and rash. More severe symptoms can occur and include encephalitis, pneumonitis, tinnitis, and deafness.
- *Ricksettia honei marmionii,* Australian spotted fever. Symptom picture includes fever, headache, arthralgia, myalgia, cough, maculopalular/petechial rash, nausea, pharyngitis, lymphadenopathy, and eschar.
- *Rickettsia japonica*, Oriental or Japanese spotted fever (Japan and South Korea so far). Usually this presents with fever, headache, eschar, and rash. However, more serious complications can occur, including severe neurological damage, mental dysfunction, seizure, and multiple organ failure.
- *Rickettsia kellyi (candidatus),* unnamed spotted fever. One case so far in a one-year-old child in India.
- *Rickesstia massiliae,* R. massiliae spotted fever, the first case was found in Spain in 2006. Only a few cases have been verified in Europe, however, a recent Polish study found some 15 percent of forest workers had antibodies to the organism. The infection rate is rather larger in western Siberia, Russia, China, Mongolia, and Kazakhstan. A few cases have now been reported in South Korea.

The species normally causes a mild to moderate febrile illness, i.e., "the flu." Generally, onset takes about four days. It is sudden and acute, accompanied by high fever, rash on the upper and lower extremeties, an inoculation eschar, and, commonly, an extremely swollen and painful lymph node near the eschar. More serious complications have occurred; acute visual loss and bilateral chorioretinitis have been reported in one case.

- *Rickettsia monacensis*, unnamed rickettsiosis. Two identified cases so far. Fever, flu-like symptoms, generalized rash on body including palms and soles of feet.

- *Rickettsia montanensis*, unnamed rickettsiosis. A single case, so far, it causes a mild, spotted fever-like illness, i.e., "the flu."

- *Rickettsia parkeri,* R. *parkeri* rickettsiosis causes an eschar-associated, low-to-moderate, febrile illness some-times accompanied by rash and lymphadenopathy (abnor-mal, usually swollen, lymph nodes). The first known case occurred in 2004; it is relatively new to researchers.

- *Rickettsia philipii,* unnamed rickettsiosis. The first identified case occurred in 2008 in Northern California. A relatively mild, eschar-associated infection accompanied by fever, headache, myalgia, and fatigue. It is thought that many of the cases in this region, thought to be RMSF, are, in fact, infections with this species.

- *Rickettsia raoultii,* unnamed spotted fever infection, however the term SENLAT has been proposed for both this infection and that of *Rickettsia slovaca*. SENLAT is unfor-tunately an acronym (caused by the common American disease, acronymitis), derived from "syndrome accompanied by scalp eschars and neck lymphadenopathy." (This makes me MADD.) Of course, this is the third acronym for the condition, former ones include TIBOLA (tick-borne lymph-adenopathy) and DEBONEL (*Dermacentor*-borne necrotic erythema and lymphadenopathy). (WTF!)

The incubation period is five to ten days, onset of the disease is accompanied by asthenia, headache, painful adenopathies, swollen lymph nodes near point of inoculation, painful scalp eschar surrounded by a perilesional erythematous halo (aka red region), low fever (sometimes), rash (only in 5 percent of infections), and face edema. Alopecia (hair loss) around the eschar can last for months. Prolonged or chronic asthenia (weakness) after successful treatment is common. Multiple eschars have been reported in one case.

- *Rickettsii riskettsii*, Rocky Mountain spotted fever. This is the most severe rickettsiosis known. Discussed in more depth below.

- *Rickettsia sibirica mongolotimonae,* mild, lymphangitis-associated (that is, extremely swollen lymph nodes) rickettsiosis – aka LAR. To date only twenty-five cases have been reported, most since 2005. Infection is accompanied by fever, asthenia, headache, generalized myalgia, arthromyalgia, rash, painfully enlarged lymph nodes, and single or multiple eschars. Rash is reported to be somewhat uncommon.

- *Rickettsia sibirica sibirica*, Siberian tick typhus. Typical incubation period is four days; the clinical picture is high fever, inoculation eschar, extremely swollen and painful lymph node near point of inoculation, and maculopapular rash. The disease is generally mild, rarely showing severe complications.

- *Rickettsia slovaca,* unnamed, tick-borne lymphadenitis – again, extremely swollen lymph nodes. See *Rickettsia raoultii* for symptom picture.

- *Rickettsia tamurae,* unnamed rickettsial disease. The first human infection was found in Japan in 2011. No symptom picture has yet been reported.

- *Rickettsia tarasevichiae (candidatus)*, unnamed rickettsial disease. First found infecting people in 2012 in northeastern China. Closely related to *R. canadensis*. High fever, asthenia, anorexia, nausea, headache, eschar, and lymphadenopathy were the most common symptoms. One of the infected experienced severe complications: meningitis, vomiting, neck stiffness, renal dysfunction, coma, respiratory acidosis, and, ultimately, death.

- *Rickettsia* species, strain Atlantic rainforest/strain Bahia, unnamed rickettsiosis. A mild to moderate febrile illness of the spotted fever group. Only two cases identified so far.

Some general comments on rickettsial infection

The information that follows about RMSF can be viewed, to some extent, as a generic look at the spotted fever group. In other words, you can use the depth look that occurs (symptom picture, cytokine cascade, organs affected, pharmaceutical treatment, effective natural treatments, diagnosis, and so on) as applicable to the entire genus. You just need to adjust treatment for severity of the symptoms.

The rickettsial genus utilizes similar infection strategies once the bacteria gain access to the body. They all cause a similar spectrum of symptoms, and they all are treated similarly by the medical industry.

If you look at the *Rickettsiae* as a whole, their symptom picture, within and across both species and genus, runs from mild flu-like infections to severe damage to organ systems, septic shock, and death. Some of the *Rickettsiae*, such as RMSF, as a rule, tend to have more serious symptoms. Nevertheless, some of those infected with RMSF only experience a mild case of "the flu." Other species, commonly presenting with mild, flu-like symptoms, can progress to severe disease, septic shock, and death. The spotted fever group needs to be viewed along a spectrum of expression, not as a grouping of species, each presenting a specific symptom picture.

Rickettsii riskettsii

This species, the cause of Rocky Mountain spotted fever (RMSF), is widely distributed in various tick species throughout North, Central, and South America; however it tends to be present in infected ticks in relatively low numbers. *This is the only reason infections from RMSF remain so low.* The CDC gives an infection rate of only about two thousand people per year (probably too low). Still, these numbers have shown a steady increase since 2001, paralleling the kinds of increases seen in the other members of the Lyme-group.

Similarly to the other members of the Lyme-group, there are a number of genetic types of the organism; five distinct phylogenetic clades have been found, each tending to locate in different geographical regions. Some of them are so genetically different that researchers think they should be thought of as subspecies, or variants or even as separate species entirely.

The primary host animals for transmission of the ticks to people are dogs, especially free-running dogs, those wild or abandoned. Both the American dog tick (*Dermacentor variabilis*) and the brown dog tick (*Rhipicephalus sangineus*) are common carriers in the United States, the latter is a primary carrier in Mexico. The cayenne tick (*Amblyomma cajennense*) is a common carrier in Central and South America. Its range, however, includes Mexico and the US, especially Texas. These ticks, unsurprisingly, are commonly infected with multiple species of *Rickettsiae*; they don't just spread this species.

Importantly: Most of these ticks easily transfer from dogs to people. This means that, in many instances, the ticks have already begun to feed. Studies on *R. rickettsia* transmission have found that *unfed* ticks need ten hours or more to transmit the disease. However, partially *fed* ticks need only about ten minutes to do so.

Rickettsia rickettsii infections have occurred in most of the contiguous US states but five of those states (North Carolina, Oklahoma, Arkansas, Tennessee, and Missouri) account for over 60 percent of infections.

The first decade of the twenty-first century saw the emergence of a rash of infections in eastern Arizona with a much higher mortality rate – ten percent of those infected died. Other states that commonly report RMSF infections are Idaho, Montana, Wyoming, Nebraska, Iowa, Illinois, Indiana, Mississippi, Alabama, Georgia, South Carolina, Maryland, New Jersey, Rhode Island, New York, Maine, and Washington, DC. As Parola et al. (2013) comment further . . .

> *Hyperendemic foci have been described repeatedly in commu-*
> *nities in the American southwest and northern Mexico, linked*
> *directly to large numbers of* R. rickettsii-*infected* Rhipiceph-
> alus sanguineus *ticks that result from unchecked popula-*
> *tions of stray and free-ranging dogs. . . . the case fatality rate*
> *[is] approximately four-times higher among American Indians*
> *than among members of other racial groups, related at least*
> *in part to the ecological dynamics created by large numbers of*
> Rhipicephalus sanguineus *and free-roaming dogs in perido-*
> *mestic environments.*

The groups of people most likely to be infected in the US are men, American Indians, and people forty years or older who have contact with free-roaming dogs and who live near wooded or high-grass areas. Fatal outcomes are most common in children under ten years of age, American Indians, those with low or compromised immune function, and those who receive delayed treatment.

RMSF (called *Brazilian* spotted fever in Brazil) is the primary and most serious of the tick-borne infections in South America. The disease is commonly misdiagnosed in South America as other, unrelated hemorrhagic fevers since, at later stages, that is exactly what RMSF becomes: a hemorrhagic fever.

Symptoms

It is important to understand that RMSF is (as are some of the other rickettsial species), in its later stages, a *hemorrhagic* fever, very similar to Ebola. It is considered to be a biosafety level three organism (BSL-3) – Ebola being BSL-4, the next level up. Researchers who work with RMSF bacteria typically don bacteria-resistant, sealed suits and breathe through a separate oxygen system. Four of the *Rickettsiae*, including RMSF, can be spread via aerosol – thus, several governments have developed them as biological warfare weapons.

Between two and fourteen days after tick bite, the first symptoms begin. As is common with the Lyme-group, more than half of the infected do not remember being bitten. The primary initial symptom is sudden onset of fever accompanied by headache. Most people who seek medical help at this point are generally misdiagnosed *and*, consequently, ineffectively treated. This is usually what leads to the development of severe infections, including mortality.

Normally, it is *only* if the infection becomes severe or if the typical spotted rash appears that an accurate diagnosis is made. (This tends to be true of all the *Rickettsiae*.) With RMSF, physicians are lucky (as are the infected); the spotted rash is commonly present in some 90 percent of the infected. (Nevertheless, misdiagnosis regularly occurs.) The rash usually emerges two to five days after the onset of fever and headache. It is important to note that *the longer treatment is delayed after the rash appears, the poorer the outcome.* In the 10 percent in whom rash does not occur, diagnosis is often significantly delayed, which is why the outcomes in this group tend to be so poor. Most of them are given broad-spectrum antibiotics, which, in some instances, make the infection worse.

Problematically, not all the spotted fever *Rickettsiae* produce a rash. In some, the rash is so mild as to be invisible. And in those with darker skins, the rash is often hard to see. In the pale skinned, the rash during RMSF looks a bit like a cross between chicken pox and measles. *It is also commonly present on the soles of the feet and palms of the hands.* This is a prominent feature in those in whom the rash appears, making a differential diagnosis nearly certain.

Here is a look at the most common symptoms . . .

- Fever (in nearly all cases)
- Headache (in nearly all cases – children tend to get headache less often)
- Rash (appears in 90 percent of cases – children tend to get the rash earlier than adults)
- Nausea
- Vomiting
- Abdominal pain
- Generalized myalgia
- Lack of appetite
- Red eyes (conjuntivitis)
- *Note:* an eschar is *extremely* **uncommon** during RMSF infections
- *Note:* enlarged and painful lymph nodes are *rarely* reported for RMSF

Cough, sore throat, and diarrhea, especially in children, can occur, promoting a physician tendency to misdiagnose the infection as "the flu."

The rash in RMSF typically appears a few days (two to five) after infection, initially as small, flat, pinkish, nonitchy spots (maculae) on the wrists, forearms, and ankles. It then spreads to the trunk, and eventually the palms and soles. The rash becomes more red to purple (petechiae) after day six and is a sign of the disease increasing in its severity.

The rickettsial rash is caused by bacteria infecting the endothelial cells that line the blood vessels of the body, in this case near to the skin surface.

The cells, which are normally bonded tightly to each other, inflame, and lose their bonds and fluids – including blood, which begins to leach into the surrounding tissues. (Blood vessel, i.e., vascular tissue, inflammation is what is meant by the term "vasculitis.") As the disease progresses in severity, this same kind of inflammatory process occurs throughout the body, including the organs. This is what leads, if the process is not stopped, to organ failure, septic shock, and death.

The range of possible impacts is large. These include arthritis, Bell's palsy, severe vertigo, sudden hearing loss, pulmonary edema and hemorrhage, myocarditis, pericarditis, cardiac tamponade, adult respiratory distress syndrome, cerebral edema and resulting neuropathies, hypotension, renal failure, disseminated intravascular coagulopathies, gangrene, seizures, septic shock, multiple organ failure, coma, and death.

During brain infection by the bacteria, scans have found focal arterial infarctions in the basal ganglia and left frontal region, diffuse edema, diffuse meningeal enhancement, and prominent perivascular spaces in the region of the basal ganglia. There are perivascular accumulations of mononuclear cells, white matter microinfarcts, hemiplegia, and a mononuclear cell-rich leptomeningitis. Neuronal necrosis of the hippocampi can occur along with gliosis and demyelination. The spinal cord can also be affected. Abnormal CT findings include diffuse white matter changes, sulcal effacement, and infarctions throughout the tissues. (Not all that different than neuroborreliosis.)

Despite CDC statistics insisting on a less than 1 percent death rate, Parola et al. (2005), looking more closely at records, note that "despite the current availability of an effective treatment and advances in medical care, an estimated 5% to 10% of U.S. patients die when infected with *R. rickettsia.*" Case fatality rates in Central America are much higher, 38 percent in Mexico alone. In Panama, from 2004 to 2007, the fatality rate was nearly 100 percent.

A severe symptom picture in South America tends to be more frequently reported and includes jaundice, central nervous system damage and impairment, respiratory distress, and acute renal insufficiency. The fatality rate in South America generally runs from 20 to 40 percent – up to 80 percent in outlying areas.

Risk factors for severe infection are advanced age, immunocompromise, chronic alcoholism, glucose-6-phosphate dehydrogenase deficiency, diabetes, treatment with a sulfonamide, use of inappropriate antibiotics, and delay in proper diagnosis/treatment.

Rickettsial diagnosis

Although there are some new testing techniques that will hopefully make the following statement obsolete (and which I will discuss in a moment), diagnosis of RMSF, and some of the other more serious SFG pathogens, within the limited time frame necessary to avoid severe courses of infection, is very difficult. As the CDC notes (CDC website, RMSF, 2015) . . .

There are several aspects of RMSF that make it challenging for health care providers to diagnose and treat. The symptoms of RMSF vary from patient to patient and can easily resemble other, more common diseases. Treatment for this disease is most effective at preventing death if started in the first five days of symptoms. Diagnostic tests for this disease, especially tests based on the detection of antibodies, will frequently appear negative in the first 7-10 days of illness. Due to the complexities of this disease and the limitations of currently available diagnostic tests, there is no test available at this time that can provide a conclusive result in time to make important decisions about treatment.

As they then emphasize (in bold) on their website . . .

The diagnosis of RMSF must be made based on clinical signs and symptoms, and can later be confirmed using specialized confirmatory laboratory tests. Treatment should never be delayed pending the receipt of laboratory results, or be withheld on the basis of an initial negative finding for R. rickettsii.

Because the organisms specialize in infecting the endothelial lining of the blood vessels, they do not, except in very severe infections, circulate in the blood in large enough numbers to be easily found. Blood specimens are not generally useful for diagnosis when using PCR or culture diagnosis. Routine hospital blood cultures, as the CDC notes, "cannot detect *R. rickettsii.*" (*Note:*

In the case of R. *africae* infections, seroconversion only occurs twenty-five to twenty-eight days after symptoms appear making this species even more difficult to diagnose.)

The worst diagnostic problem occurs with the rickettsial infections in which the spotted rash does not appear. This, in combination with two other factors, is the reason for the more serious complications that can occur from these bacteria. The other two factors are: (1) lack of awareness of rickettsial infections among physicians, and (2) the short time frame (eight to fifteen minutes) that most physicians spend with their patients during appointments (generally insufficient for any kind of effective diagnosis). See "Diagnostic and Treatment Failures" below.

Indirect immunofluorescence assay (IFA)

is the test most often used for RMSF and other members of the SFG. However, there are a number of problems with the test. It is, in actuality, an incredibly poor choice for effective diagnosis of *any* rickettsial infection.

IFA is a test that detects antibodies to infection. Unfortunately, during rickettsial infections *these do not occur at detectable levels until seven to ten days after the onset of symptoms.* As the CDC guidelines note, correctly for once, optimum outcomes occur when treatment begins within five days of symptom appearance.

For 85 percent of the infected, antibodies are *not* detectable during the first five to seven days of illness, which is, of course, when the testing is most commonly used. To make matters worse, at minimum, two IFA tests are necessary. The first occurs at initial consult, usually in the first week of symptoms, the second *two to four weeks later.* This is far past the time when effective treatment should take place and makes the test fairly useless for a proper diagnosis within the necessary time frame.

Further complicating the IFA test: high antibody levels may remain in the *previously* infected for months or years after infection. Up to 10 percent of healthy people in endemic areas show antibodies to the organism. In other words, people who do not have a rickettsial infection, if tested with IFA, can be misdiagnosed as having RMSF when they do not.

Normally, during an active infection, antibody titer will rise fourfold between the first test and the second. This is the primary diagnostic criteria for a RMSF infection, which, again, is generally useless for timely treatment.

Skin biopsy

is a much better approach than IFA. As Paola et al. (2013), observe: "Skin biopsy specimens (from rash and/or eschar) cultivated in a reference center can be positive even when molecular tests are negative." As they continue, "skin biopsy specimens should be sampled *before* treatment and early in the course of the disease and should be inoculated as soon as possible." This is the best test to use for RMSF, especially if the biopsy is examined via PCR.

Unfortunately, biopsies often cannot be performed by general practitioners in a consulting room or the patient's home; they normally need a more industrial setting. They are very unlikely to occur in developing countries or in the bush. This is part of the reason for the high mortality rates in Central and South America. A much easier, cheaper, and more reliable test for rickettsial infections is qPCR. Unfortunately, it is only useable if an eschar is present, which in RMSF is rare.

Quantitative, real-time PCR, a.k.a qPCR

This approach has been found to be exceptionally good for a quick diagnosis of the various spotted fever pathogens. While skin biopsy can be used for qPCR, it has been found that cutaneous swabs *from an eschar* are just as effective and much less invasive and painful.

Normally, a swab is used to break through the eschar scab (by rotating vigorously) to its base. (Recent studies have found that the eschar crust itself can be removed and used for diagnosis.) Unfortunately, this approach can only be used if an eschar is present, which it often isn't during RMSF infections (as it is with many of the other *Rickettsiae*). If no eschar is present then skin biopsy and symptom analysis are, at present, the best approaches to diagnosis.

There is some hope that better diagnostic tests for noneschar rickettsioses will occur in the future. Unfortunately, at this date, they do not exist.

Diagnostic and treatment failures

Few physicians understand the complexity of the Lyme-group of pathogens. This state of affairs is even worse with the spotted fever rickettsioses. It's especially true if the presenting symptoms do not include the spotted rash. Nevertheless, even with rash, diagnosis is often missed.

Perhaps the best account of this is by the physician Mark DiNubile (1996) who failed to appropriately diagnose a case of RMSF, which resulted in a fatal outcome. In this particular instance a rash eventually did occur on the trunk and palms (but not the soles). The patient, who was HIV positive, initially presented only with a four-day history of fever and chills. (His primary reason for seeking treatment was the HIV; he thought that was the cause.) Laboratory tests, as is common for spotted fever infections, showed nothing untoward. While hospitalized, the rash and headache did emerge, but the only other symptom he reported was a "feeling of fullness" in the head. By day six of the hospitalization, the man was nearly comatose. The physicians finally administered doxycycline, but it was too late; he died shortly afterward.

The most striking thing about the case are the comments by the physician, Mark DiNubile. He took the time to deeply examine what had occurred, why they had missed so obvious a diagnosis. Notably: despite IFA staining, the postmortem skin biopsies remained negative. However, a distraught colleague kept testing, even after the patient died. Eventually they found RMSF *Rickettsiae*. Rather poignantly, DiNubile says, "Luckily most patients will recover with (or despite) mediocre care." As he continues . . .

> *Why did we miss a diagnosis of Rocky Mountain spotted fever in a patient with fever, headache, and a rash involving the palms? The question continues to haunt and torment us, as we struggle to separate the real answers from the excuses, rationalizations, and post hoc justifications. When I first noticed the patient's palmar rash, I explicitly considered the diagnosis of RMSF. However, the absence of a history of myalgias, a severe headache, and exposure to ticks essentially eliminated the diagnosis from my mind. . . . [And] while pursuing an increasingly untenable diagnosis [of syphilis] that conveyed little urgency in its management, I never systematically reevaluated the remainder of the differential possibilities.*

DiNubile's long and rather deep self-examination leads him to the realization that the problem was one of arrogance and tunnel vision on his, and his colleagues, part as well as the way medical practice is conducted in the United States.

In an effort to attend to a large number of patients, many of whom probably did not require the expertise of a subspecialist in infectious diseases, we failed to devote sufficient contemplative time to our difficult diagnostic and management problems. This sad consequence constitutes part of the price we pay for indiscriminate consultation, although in a fee-for-service environment quantity – not quality – generates income.

DiNubile reveals that he is sharing the treatment team's failures in full, as many physicians refuse to do, "in the hope that errors of arrogance and tunnel vision might be avoided: Blessed are the humble physicians, for they will better see the ultimate diagnosis."

This case study could stand in as a generic example of the many errors in the treatment and diagnosis of Lyme-group infections. Unfortunately, very few physicians are willing to self-examine as DiNubile did, even fewer to publish that self-examination in a medical journal.

Medical treatment

Again, treatment is most effective if it occurs within the first few days. The longer infection remains untreated, the poorer the outcome, and the more severe the disease progression.

Doxycycline is considered to be the most effective antibiotic for adults and children, especially if given within the first five days of infection. Failure to treat by day eight after symptoms show, if the infection is severe, can be fatal. More severe infections often require IV antibiotics, prolonged hospitalization, and intensive care.

The normal dosage for non-IV doxycycline is 100 mg every twelve hours in adults, and for children under 100 pounds (45 kg), 2.2 mg/kg of body weight two times daily. *Note: In dogs, relapse after treatment with doxycycline has occurred.*

Chloramphenicol is sometimes used as most spotted fever organisms are susceptible to it. However, there are some severe adverse side effects associated with its use. As well, it is not really as effective, especially for RMSF, as doxycycline. Nonresponse to the drug and relapse after treatment has been found. There is a greater risk of fatal outcomes with its use.

The use of fluoroquinolones has been suggested as an alternative to doxycycline, but recently it has been found that their use produces extremely poor outcomes in the treatment of R. *conorii* due to the bacteria's upregulation of some unique toxins.

Broad spectrum antibiotics are not effective for the *Rickettsiae*; sulfa drugs may worsen the infection.

Mediterranean spotted fever, seemingly alone of the SFG, responds well to the use of ciprofloxacin and similar antibiotics.

Steroidal drugs will do nothing to alleviate rickettsial vasculitis and should be avoided.

Mild residual neurologic defects (polyneuropathies) can remain even after successful treatment with antibiotics. This is more frequent in those with abnormal neuroimaging readings.

Persistent infections

There are some fairly good studies finding that persistent infections do occur, even after appropriate doxycycline therapy. One of the main journal articles that explores this is Radulovic et al. (2002). As the authors comment . . .

> The host's immune responses to the rickettsial infection lead either to clearance of the pathogen or to the persistence of a subclinical infection. As an example of the latter, Rickettsia prowlazekii, the causative agent of louse-borne typhus, can persist in humans years after primary infection and/or appropriate antibiotic treatment. Persistence of the rickettsiae in otherwise healthy persons with subsequent reappearance of clinical symptoms (Brill-Zinsser disease) is one mechanism by which rickettsiae perpetuate in the absence of an animal reservoir.

In that study, the researchers examined R. *akari* and R. *typhi* infection of macrophages. R. *akari* was chosen because it primarily infects macrophages/monocytes, and they wanted to study the direct immune responses to infection. R. *typhi* was used as a comparative because, like other members of the *Rickettsiae*, it can and does infect a small number of macrophages/monocytes during the disease progression.

They found that *unactivated* macrophages were a source of persistent infection by *Rickettsiae*. Very few of those macrophages died either from lysis or necrosis. Death rates for the unactivated macrophages never topped

9 percent of infected cells. If the macrophages were activated by the addition of E. coli LPS, apoptosis increased substantially. The authors make some crucial observations . . .

> The inhibition of apoptosis at two levels, both in primary infection and after induction of proapoptotic immunological processes of acquired immunity, could set the conditions for persistent riskettsial infection. Surviving rickettsiae could then replicate within the macrophages remaining at a site of rickettsia-infected endothelium.

As they go on to note . . .

> Low rickettsial cytotoxicity toward host cells observed in this study not only provides ample opportunity for rickettsial spread to neighboring cells, but may also result in rickettsial persistence. Indeed we have been successful in isolating R. typhi from spleen and kidneys of wild-caught rats exhibiting high antirickettsial antibodies, which further confirms rickettsial persistence.

As with most of the Lyme-group, much of what is thought to be true about Rickettsiae bacteria is incomplete, incorrect, or overly simplistic. Persistence, as with other Lyme-group organisms, may be common.

CHAPTER THIRTEEN

SPOTTED FEVER RICKETTSIAE: A DEEPER LOOK

The clinical gravity of Rocky Mountain spotted fever is due to severe damage to blood vessels by R. rickettsii. *This organism is unusual among rickettsiae in its ability to spread and invade vascular smooth muscle cells as well as endothelium.*

D. H. Walker, 1996

From an ecologic and epidemiologic perspective, populations of the vector mite and rodent host [of R. akari*] are documented throughout the United States and various studies suggest that substantial rates of infection occur among inhabitants of other urban areas.*

Paddock et al., 2006

Humans are also highly susceptible to aerosol transmission of R. rickettsii . . . *[the organism] is 1000-fold more infectious than the spores of* Bacillus anthracis. . . . *Both* R. prowazekii *and* R. typhi *have stable extracellular forms that are present in louse and flea feces, respectively. These rickettsiae appear to remain infectious for a very long time.*

D. H. Walker, 2009

Compared to most of the other Lyme-group organisms, there is very little research exploring the subtleties of *Rickettsiae* infections. As Sahni et al. (2013) comment: "Despite more than 100 years of study, the mechanisms by which *Rickettsia* escapes the phagosome and establishes a successful intracellular infection still remain to be fully understood." From the little research that has occurred, the picture that emerges reveals, I think, that this group of organisms is one of the most subtle and sophisticated of all the Lyme-group in how they modulate the immune response and cytokine dynamics.

The *Rickettsiae* bacteria are transmitted to people by the bites of ticks and mites and the feces of lice and fleas. Once in the body they spread via the draining lymph nodes and bloodstream, infecting the endothelial cells that line the body's blood vessels. RMSF can also infect vascular smooth muscle cells, and all the *Rickettsiae*, to a minimal extent, will sometimes infect macrophages/monocytes and bone marrow stem cells. *(R. akari*, uniquely, infects macrophages/monocytes as its primary host cells.) However, normally, the bacteria's primary target is the body's endothelial cells. Once those cells are located, the bacteria move inside the target cells, multiply by binary fission, then exit in order to infect other, nearby cells. Sometimes the symptoms this causes are minor, sometimes life threatening. In all instances though, the dynamics of what happens are similar. Importantly, the symptoms they produce exist on a *spectrum*. As David Walker (2007) notes . . .

> *The clinical manifestations of most rickettsioses constitute a continuous spectrum. Indeed, even when the proportion of patients with an eschar is considered to be a clinical characteristic, the incidence [of eschar] varies for patients infected with the same strain in different geographic areas (e.g.,* R. conorii *strain Israeli in Portugal, where eschars are detected frequently, and that in Israel, where eschars are rarely identified). The latter example suggests that neither geography nor inconsistent clinical manifestations define the taxonomy of the microbial agent. The* R. sibirica *mongolotimonae strain, which has been found on 3 continents, is another example. The name "lymphagitis-associated rickettsioses" has been proposed for the disease caused by this strain, despite the fact that lymphangitis is observed in only 40% of cases.*

Specifics of intracellular infection

As with all of the Lyme-group, these bacteria take advantage of compounds found in tick saliva (and flea and louse feces) to facilitate their spread. Those compounds shut down many of the body's normal defenses against infection. Specifically, for this organism, they dampen normal Th1 responses, reducing and modulating the body's natural production of interferon-gamma (IFN-y) and tumor necrosis factor-alpha (TNF-a), which would normally counteract the infection.

The primary target of the bacteria, once they are in the body, is (except for *R. akari*) the endothelial cells lining the small- and medium-sized blood vessels. However, for those species that cause eschar at the inoculation point (tick bite), mononuclear phagocytes are the major cell types that are initially infected. (Importantly, the bacteria may also infect small numbers of these cells during disseminated infection as well as infecting bone marrow–derived dendritic cells.) This allows the bacteria to begin moving through the lymph and blood system deeper into the body, seeking out vascular endothelial cells. These cells, as Sahni et al. (2013) note, have . . .

> [n]ow emerged as key immunoreactive cells involved in host defense and inflammation, in part owning to their ability to synthesize and secrete many growth factors, cytokines, chemokines, adhesion molecules and vasoactive substances capable of exerting significant autocrine and/or paracrine effects on the microvascular, as well as other target cell functions.

The *Rickettsiae*, as all the intracellular Lyme-group do, sophisticatedly modulate cellular actions, in essence, coopting them for their own purposes.

The bacteria use chemotactic compounds to find their target cells, then use adhesins to attach themselves to the surface of the cells. Internalization of the bacteria occurs within minutes after they find a preferred host cell. The *Rickettsiae* stimulate the formation of a phagosome (a compartment in which they are sequestered) and its subsequent internalization by the cell. They enter the cell's cytosol region where nutrients such as adenosine triphosphate (ADP), amino acids, and nucelotides are available for their use. Once inside the cell, they disrupt the normal processes the cell uses to digest bacterially infected phagosomes.

The bacteria secrete phospholipase D and homolysin C, which disrupts the phagosomal membrane, permitting the escape of the bacteria to the interior of the infected cell. There they begin harvesting the nutrients they need to survive and reproduce. Once they reproduce, they relocate against the underside of the cellular membrane of the host cell, force the membrane to deform outward, bulging into the adjacent cell. They then repeat the infectious process.

During infection, most of the rickettsial bacteria remain sequestered inside cells and are never exposed to the extracellular environment or the immune responses that occur there. A few of the bacteria do enter the bloodstream, using it to travel to new locations in the body. A few others infect unactivated macrophages to create a persistent infectious niche. And still others infect some of the bone marrow's stem cells. This process is similar for nearly all the SFG *Rickettsiae*. (Typhus *Rickettsiae* are a bit different; they generally reproduce until the cell bursts open. They then enter the blood, infecting new endothelial cells in other parts of the body.)

Pathogenicity

of the SFG organisms is primarily due to the increased vascular permeability that the bacteria cause. This is probably the most important thing to keep in mind when treating rickettsial infections – it's the source of nearly every symptom they cause. Merely protecting endothelial structures from bacterial damage will reduce or eliminate both symptoms *and* the infection itself. It prevents the bacteria from gaining the nutrients they need to reproduce and spread.

The bacteria, once they adhere to and enter the endothelial cells, either release or cause the body's immune systems to generate a variety of cytokines and chemokines which alter the cell's structures and relationships. The various compounds that are generated inflame the vascular tissues, causing rickettsial vasculitis. One of the more damaging effects is the destruction of the adherens junctions between the cells (similarly to borrelial bacterial strategies). These junctions normally form a tight barrier that prevents blood in the vessels from leaking into the body. The adherens junctions are damaged through a number of mechanisms, including the movement of immune molecules (such as monocytes and neutrophils) to the inflamed area. The junctions become more porous, and this allows the leakage of fluids through the vascular walls (edema), which is a hallmark of the rickettsial infectious process. This can occur in many locations, e.g., the brain (cerebral edema) or the lungs (pulmonary edema). As the endothelial junctions become more porous, blood begins to leak more deeply into the body. This begins some eight days after symptoms occur. As it progresses, the infection becomes serious. Ultimately, it becomes a type of hemorrhagic infection, similar to ebola, as blood begins leaking out of the orifices.

Wherever the endothelial junctions are damaged is where symptoms occur: in the brain, encephalopathy; in the heart, cardiomyopathy; in the lungs, breathing problems.

The most effective healing approach to rickettsial infections (besides the use of doxycycline) is composed of two simultaneous interventions: (1) utilize substances that protect endothelial integrity, and (2) remodulate the unique cytokine cascade the bacteria use to damage the endothelial cellular bonds.

The *Rickettsiae* cytokines and endothelial dysregulation

The bacterial infection of vascular endothelial cells initiates a very specific cytokine cascade. This is what causes the inflammation in the vascular system. There are two, tightly interwoven elements to this, (1) the actual cytokines that the bacteria release, and (2) the bacterial modulation of the immune system's cytokine response, which creates a bacteria-initiated autoimmune-like process.

What is important to understand up front is that this group of bacteria are extremely sophisticated in their modulation of the immune system. Many of the Lyme-group strongly upregulate certain cytokines and downregulate others. This makes intervention strategies somewhat simple: the use of substances that downregulate the upregulated cytokines and upregulate the downregulated ones. The *Rickettsiae* are more subtle. Although there are differences between the various species, in general they *modulate* the cytokine levels, keeping them carefully within a certain range.

The cascade initiators are NF-kB, TNF-a, and p38 MAP kinase. These are the upstream factors that the bacteria depend upon for the infectious-inflammatory process. These compounds have a number of effects: inhibiting apoptosis (to keep cells alive while their nutrients are being harvested), protecting mitochondrial integrity (the loss of which is a factor in apoptosis), and stimulating the production a number of other, downstream, proinflammatory cytokines, for example IL-6, IL-8, monocyte chemoattractant protein-1 (MCP-1, aka CCL2), and E-selectin. The most crucial outcome is the dysregulation of the tight junctions that normally exist between endothelial cells.

Though there are a number of dynamics involved in the dysregulation, the primary one is the phosphorylation of VE-cadherin. Phosphorylation refers to the process by which the activity of certain proteins are turned on or off. In this instance what the bacteria are doing is inhibiting the normal function of VE-cadherin by turning it off.

VE-cadherin is shorthand for "vascular endothelial" cadherin. The word "cadherins" is a sort of acronym, created from "calcium-dependent adhesion proteins." Cadherins have a number of functions, among them is the forming of adherens junctions between cells, causing them to strongly adhere together. (Distressingly for many conservatives, VE-cadherin causes cells to become *homophilic* – rather than homophobic.) VE-cadherin is used by vascular cells to regulate the permeability of blood vessel walls, keeping a restrictive endothelial barrier in place or opening it up if substances need to penetrate deeper into the body. VE-cadherin is involved as well in healthy vascular development, a process known as angiogenesis, aka the formation of new blood vessels. When VE-cadherin function is turned off, the tight bonds (adherens junctions) between endothelial cells weaken, and the vessels begin to leak. In extreme cases this causes hemorrhage.

The bacteria enhance the dysregulation impacts of VE-cadherin phosphorylation by stimulating the body to upregulate and release angiogenin (ANG), primarily in the liver. The bacteria reach the liver, the main source of ANG, via the blood, subsequently infecting the liver's endothelial cells. Once in place, they stimulate the liver's hepatocytes to begin producing angiogenin. (This is the cause of the hepatitis, aka liver inflammation, that rickettsial infection sometimes causes.) Hepatocytes make up most of the liver's cells, and they are actively involved in the synthesis of various proteins, among them ANG. The bacteria-stimulated ANG is then released into circulation in the body. (Silymarin compounds in milk thistle seed, *Silybum marianum*, can inhibit this process, prohibiting it from occurring.) The stimulation of ANG (in the liver and throughout the body) reaches peak around seventy-two hours postinfection (p.i.). As researchers put it, an "intense" ANG signal occurs in endothelial tissues, localized to the sites of infection in the brain, liver, and lungs.

The circulating ANG is drawn to the rickettsial-infected endothelial cells where it is then pulled inside (endocytosis) the infected cells.

ANG is also held inside the nucleus of many cells, so the bacteria, redundantly, initiate other processes to withdraw ANG from that location. This begins 24 hours p.i., by 48 hours p.i., the ANG has begun to move into the cytoplasm of the cell, and at 72 hours p.i., ANG predominates in the cytoplasm.

The bacteria utilize the ANG to synergistically enhance the dysregulation of VE-cadherin. As Gong et al. (2013) put it: "Rickettsial infection initiated compartmentalized translocation of exogenous ANG in confluent human primary endothelial cells. [The] infection triggered cytoplasmic translocation of ANG, enhanced phosphorylation of VE-cadherin, reduced VE-cadherin stability, and attenuated endothelial barrier function."

VE-cadherins normally exist on the surface of the endothelial cells. The VE-cadherin molecule on one cell tightly binds to an identical one on the adjacent cell and so on throughout the vascular endothelium. The VE-cadherins form a kind of zipper-like structure along the cellular border, keeping a tightly joined cellular bond in place. These bonds begin to break down along a similar time line as that of the ANG production and translocation. It slowly begins at 24 hours p.i., the reduction in bonding accelerates considerably by 48 hours p.i., and becomes "dramatic" at 72 hours postinfection.

ANG is also strongly involved in breaking down what is called the basement membrane in vascular cells by degrading its laminin and fibronectin layers. Normally, this allows the movement of endothelial cells deeper into the perivascular tissues so that new blood vessels can form. The generation, translocation, and activation of ANG by the bacteria exacerbates this process. (*Asparagus officinalis* root can help prevent the negative effects of ANG.)

As the VE-cadherins are dysregulated, their bonds with each other break apart. The endothelial cells begin to "unzip." As the VE-cadherins are broken free from the exterior of the cell's surface membrane, the bacteria stimulate their movement into the cell's interior where the proteins that make them up can be utilized. The exogenous ANG that has been translocated to the site of the bacterial infection strongly increases both the dysregulation (phosphorylization) of the VE-cadherins and their cellular internalization. Some useful inhibitors of this process are Japanese knotweed (*Polygonum cuspidatum*) root, EGCG, *Crataegus* (hawthorn), *Pueraria lobata* (kudzu), and *Salvia miltiorrhiza*.

COX-2 is also upregulated during rickettsial infection. COX-2 increases the production of vasoactive prostaglandins PG12 and prostacyclin PGE2. PGE2 contributes to enhanced vascular permeability during infection. Inhibition of PGE2 will help stabilize the endothelial cellular structure. (Some good PGE2 inhibitors are *Salvia miltiorrhiza, Bidens pilosa, Houttuynia cordata, Polygala tenuifolia, Pueraria lobata,* and *Scutellaria baicalensis*.)

Once the *Rickettsiae* have sequestered themselves in the cells, E-selectin is also upregulated. This stimulates the recruitment of neutrophils to the infected endothelial cells, which contributes to the pathological alterations seen during infection. Reducing E-selectin upregulation can reduce the cellular inflammation that occurs during infection. (Some good E-selectin inhibitors are *Polygonum cuspidatum* [Japanese knotweed] root, *Pueraria lobata, Andrographis paniculata, Withania somnifera, Olea europeae* leaf and oil, quercetin, and piperine.)

The cytokine path that produces the vascular porousness common in rickettsial infection is NF-kB, TNF-a, p38 MAP kinase, and VE-cadherin dysregulation. *Inhibition of p38 alone has been found to stop it.* (Some good p38 inhibitors are *Cordyceps, Olea europeae* leaf and oil, *Polygonum cuspidatum, Schisandra, Scutellaria baicalensis,* N-acetyl-cysteine, EGCG, luteolin, and olive oil and leaf.) For a variety of reasons, discussed momentarily, inhibiting NF-kB and TNF-a is **absolutely not recommended**.

The vascular dysregulation process continues to escalate over time, which is why treatment within five days after rickettsial symptoms begin to show is so important. *Note:* Each rickettsial species, subspecies, and strain produces a different degree of endothelial dysregulation, hence the differences in the various organisms' impacts.

Another factor affecting the severity of symptoms is the immune health of the person. This is why the very old tend to get sicker; their immune systems are not as vital. Remodulating and enhancing immune function to counteract the bacteria is strongly suggested.

The bacteria utilize a number of processes for stopping cellular death. ANG has antiapoptic functions but the bacterial modulation of NF-kB plays a major role here. Once NF-kB is upregulated, it inhibits the expression of the antiapoptotic proteins caspase-8 and caspase-9 as well as the executioner enzyme caspase-3. As Baltadzhiev and Delchev (2013) comment: "Inhibition of apoptosis through activation of NF-kB is required for the early phase of the disease when *Rickettsiae* begin to proliferate in the microvascular endothelial cells." However, as they continue: "Later, when adaptive immunity is fully employed apoptosis is enhanced in infected endothelial cells."

So, again, the bacteria carefully modulate the levels and actions of NF-*k*B and TNF-*a* during infection, increasing or decreasing them as needed. One of the major ways the bacteria *increase* apoptosis later in infection is the modulation of Bcl/Bax expression by mitochondria. Bcl-2 levels are increased early in infection and inhibit apoptosis. Bax is upregulated later and promotes it. Remodulation of the Bcl/Bax balance with appropriate herbs can stop this rickettsial-alteration and inhibit infection.

In essence, the Bcl-2 group is upregulated, and Bax is downregulated early in the infection. This delays apoptosis of the mitochondria and thus interferes with one of the main methods of host cell apoptosis. (Mitochondria in infected cells are strongly motivated to stimulate cellular death as a mechanism to stop pathogenic infections.) Remodulation of Bax/Bcl-2, i.e., upregulating Bax and downregulating Bcl-2, has been found to reverse this process and increase apoptosis in affected cells. (Herbs and supplements useful for this are: *Artemisia* spp., *Glycyrrhiza* spp., *Goniothalamus cheliensis, Gynostemma pentaphyllum, Houttuynia cordata, Leonurus cardiaca* [motherwort], *Rhodiola* spp., *Scutellaria* spp., and the isolated constituents arctigenin, beta-sitosterol, and curcumin.)

The exact impacts of the other downstream cytokines during rickettsial infections are not yet understood. All of them play some role in the inflammatory processes the bacteria initiate, but no one has yet studied their subtleties during these infections. A list of the other cytokines upregulated are: IFN-*y*, IL-1*B*, IL-2, IL-6, IL-8, IL-10, IL-12, MCP-1, MIP-1. VCAM-1, ICAM-1, CCL2, CCL3, CCL4, CCL12, CXCL9, and CXCL10. Elevated levels of CXCL9 and -10 are normally present in the brains of people with fatal RMSF infections; however, their inhibition doesn't seem to have any effect on survival or degree of tissue damage.

The spleen, liver, and kidneys – all the organs that process blood — are infected during rickettsial diseases. Splenic immune activity (natural killer cells) is significantly increased during infection, especially the first week or so. Because of the damage these bacteria can cause to them, it is important to protect these organs.

A few rickettsial cytokine subtleties

Rickettsial infection is significantly different than some of the other Lyme-group infections in that the bacteria carefully initiate and maintain a low level of NF-kB, TNF-a, and IFN-y. They do so because these compounds are particularly antirickettsial. When these compounds are generated by macrophages NK cells and T lymphocytes, they stimulate the production of nitric oxide by endothelial cells to which the bacteria are very susceptible. Thus the behavior of the TNF-a, upregulated by the bacteria early in the infection, is carefully modulated.

TNF-a is a crucial cytokine for *stopping* the infection – mice deficient in TNF-a and IFN-y, for example, experience an unrestrained bacterial spread and a fatal, overwhelming infection. In people, *the use of a TNF-a inhibitor (sometimes used in treating rheumatoid arthritis) has been found to allow a low-level, undiagnosed, RMSF infection to become acute.*

Too much TNF-a will kill the bacteria; too little will kill the host. So the bacteria carefully keep the levels low enough to survive but high enough to keep the host alive (usually). They also use the cytokine to enhance the bacterial-induced vascular permeability. As Woods and Olano (2008) observe, "the addition of TNF-a, but not IL-1b or IFN-y, alone is sufficient to enhance *Rickettsiae*-induced microvascular permeability in a dose dependent manner."

The best approach to working with these cytokines is the use of cytokine-adaptogens, that is, herbs that will remodulate their behavior during infection. The best herbs for this are *Salvia miltiorrhiza*, *Scutellaria baicalensis*, *Rhodiola*, *Eleutherococcus senticosus*, and *Cordyceps*. *Salvia miltiorrhiza* is, very specifically, a cytokine adaptogen; its use is essential during rickettsial infections.

Studies have found that when human endothelial cells are activated by IFN-y, TNF-a, IL-1b, and RANTES, the intracellular *Rickettsiae* are killed through two mechanisms: the production of both nitric oxide (NO) and hydrogen peroxide (H_2O_2). The bacteria are exceptionally sensitive to both. To circumvent this the *Rickettsiae* utilize several strategies. Importantly, they don't inhibit but rather *dampen* the presence of those cytokines.

First, the bacteria convert the L-arginine the body uses to create NO to other compounds. Rather cleverly, they use the L-arginine to create polyamines that they then utilize for reproduction and infection.

Secondly, the *Rickettsiae*, to differing degrees, depending on the organism involved, cause a significant reduction of some key enzymes in the endothelial cells. Specifically, they reduce glucose-6- phosphate dehydrogenase (G6PD), catalase, and glutathione. As with NF-*k*B, TNF-*a*, and IFN-*y* the bacteria do not completely eliminate these compounds; they reduce the levels to within a specific range, one they can tolerate. This increases the numbers of reactive oxygen species (ROS), including nitric oxide (NO) and hydrogen peroxide (H2O2), circulating in the body. The bacteria hijack the process for their own ends, using this increase in ROS as an adjunct process in their dysregulation of adherins junctions.

G6PD is an enzyme that is used to maintain the levels of nicotinamide adenine dinucleotide phosphate (NADPH) in the body. NADPH, in turn, maintains the body's levels of glutathione, which is one of the major protectors of the body's cells, especially the red blood cells, from oxidative damage.

About five hundred million people around the world (one in fourteen), mostly those of Mediterranean or African descent, have a genetic deficiency of G6PD, primarily as an adaptation for countering malarial infections. The stronger the deficiency, the more resistant to malaria a person is. A side effect of the deficiency is that it predisposes its carriers to hemolysis, the spontaneous destruction of red blood cells. Unfortunately, people with this genetic deficiency are at tremendous risk during spotted fever (SFG) infections.

SFG infection normally lowers the levels of G6PD to within a certain range, but in those with G6PD deficiency the impact is extreme, how much so is directly proportional to the deficiency class they are in. There are five classes of deficiency (I–V), from very severe to very mild. The closer to severe deficiency a person is, the more serious the SFG infection is. Infection with SFG bacteria in those with a severe deficiency can cause jaundice, hemolytic crises, diabetic ketoacidosis, acute renal failure, organ failure, coma, and death in a very short period of time. During severe episodes, the damaged red blood cells are expressed out of the body by the kidneys, which is what leads to acute renal failure. This deficiency is nearly always carried by males.

Glutathione, whose levels are reduced during SFG infections, is an important antioxidant in the body. It is synthesized in the body from amino acids L-cysteine, L-glutamic acid, and glycine. As G6PD levels in the body drop, less glutathione is generated.

Glutathione has a number of functions. It is the primary antioxidant produced by the body's cells, neutralizing free radicals and ROS and maintaining the active forms of vitamins E and C. It is intimately involved in regulating the body's NO cycle and levels. It's essential to metabolic and biochemical reactions, such as protein synthesis, DNA synthesis and repair, prostaglandin synthesis, amino acid transport, and enzyme activation. Glutathione is also intimately involved in protecting tissues that are actively engaged in the biosynthesis of fatty acids, such as the liver, mammary glands, adrenals, and adipose (fat) tissues. Loss of healthy glutathione levels can have severe effects on the immune system, the neurological system, the GI tract, and the lungs.

Glutathione can be thought of as one of the body's primary detoxifiers. Besides reducing compounds that can cause oxidative damage, it removes toxins from tissues throughout the body, especially the liver. Many of the damaging impacts of SFG infections come from the reduction of G6PD, catalase, and glutathione in the body. Increasing the levels of glutathione in the body is essential during SFG infections.

Significant immune markers

Two of the immune molecules the body produces and which the *Rickettsiae* modulate are significant. They are IFN-beta (IFN-*b*) and interleukin-17 (IL-17). The first is downregulated during infection; the second is upregulated.

The rickettsial dampening of IFN-*b* upregulation during infection is one of the major strategies the bacteria utilize to spread and reproduce. IFN-*b*, when levels are sufficiently high, inhibits rickettsial replication in infected cells, reducing levels of infectious organisms. One of the more important supportive interventions is to increase the body's levels of IFN-beta during infection. (Herbs specific for this include *Polygonum cuspidatum, Astragalus,* and *Sambucus.*)

Researchers studying the cytokine dynamics in people (as opposed to in vitro or mouse studies) have found what they consider to be a cytokine core *and* a cytokine periphery that occur during infection. The cytokine *periphery* is the organism upregulation and subsequent modulation of NF-*k*B and TNF-*a*. The cytokine *core* is interleukin-17 (IL-17), which is strongly upregulated by the bacteria. This cytokine, similarly to IFN-*y*, is a potent mediator and acts to increase cytokine presence and action in tissues. It's a proinflammatory cytokine, highly synergistic with other cytokines such as TNF-*a* and IL-1. IL-17 induces the production of many other cytokines including macrophage inflammatory protein-1*B* (MIP-1*B*, aka CCL4), platelet derived growth factor (PDGF), granulocyte colony stimulating factor (G-CSF), and granulocyte macrophage stimulating factor (GM-CSF). These additional cytokines are also part of the *core* cytokine group.

IL-17 also induces the production of many other cytokines such as IL-6, IL-8, and TNF-*a* and the prostaglandin PGE2. The inhibition of IL-17 can significantly reduce symptoms of infection by the *Rickettsiae*. (Some good inhibitors are *Angelica sinensis, Hyssopus officinalis, Paeonia lactifolia, Salvia miltiorrhiza, Scutellaria baicalensis, Sophora flavescens*, and curcumin.)

Intravascular coagulation (not)

It has been claimed by a number of sources for a very long time that rickettsial infection causes disseminated intravascular coagulation in a majority of those infected. A deeper examination of the research reveals that this is rarely true. As Sahni et al. (2013) comment, the complications of ricksettial infection

> *lead to compromised vascular integrity and loss of barrier function, manifesting as noncardiogenic pulmonary edema, acute respiratory distress, complications of the CNS and failure of multiple organ systems, yet abnormalities, such as disseminated intravascular coagulation, are very rarely seen in severe, complicated cases of infection.*

David Walker (2007) notes that "careful analysis of such data reveals that disseminated intravascular coagulation occurs only rarely in persons with rickettsial infections." This is an important understanding as it affects treatment approaches. In general, it is not necessary to focus on coagulation as a problem during most rickettsial infections.

Septic shock

Unrestrained rickettsial infection, especially with RMSF, can lead to organ failure and death. Late infection can see a rebound in inflammatory cytokines, to extreme levels. The inflammation is so severe that the body's organs are severely damaged, septic shock, coma, and death often occur. As Clark et al. (2004) comment . . .

> *A point is reached at which the severity of the disease increases. . . . Unfortunately, this critical point does not immediately appear to lend itself to definition in the individual patient. . . . These changes [in the cytokine profile] have the characteristics of a self-perpetuating and amplifying system of functional derangement.*

I cover septic shock in depth in Chapter Eight of *Natural Treatments for Lyme Coinfections: Anaplasma, Babesia, and Ehrlichia* (Inner traditions, 2015), so I won't go into depth on it here. Treatment for it is included in the next chapter.

CHAPTER FOURTEEN

NATURAL HEALING OF RICKETTSIOSES INFECTIONS

Traditional medicines, such as Chinese medicine (CM), have long been used as multiple combinations of compounds in the form of processed natural products. Medicinal herbs relieve the symptoms of many different human diseases, including infectious diseases and have been used for thousands of years.
Kaio Kitazato et al., 2007

Doxycycline, so far, is extremely good at treating this group of bacteria. However, I have occasionally heard from people over the years who did not fully respond to antibiotic interventions and who still struggle with a low-level, recurring infection. As well, there is some indication in the literature that there may be more doxycycline failures than are recognized. And finally, for those in whom septic shock occurs there is a necessity for a wider range of options for effective intervention.

Besides doxycycline, the foundational approach for treating this group of organisms consists of: (1) protecting the endothelial cells and their adherens junctions; (2) remodulating the cytokine profile through the use of immune system or cytokine adaptogens; (3) inhibiting the production of p38 MAP kinase and IL-17; (4) upregulating IFN-beta; and (5) increasing glutathione levels in the body.

Other interventions that can help are inhibiting E-selectin, modulating apoptosis dysregulation, and inhibiting PGE2.

The more an herb has effects across multiple parameters of an infection, the better it is for that particular disease complex.

- The primary herbs for protecting the endothelial cells are: *Polygonum cuspidatum, Crataegus, Salvia miltiorrhiza, Puer-*

aria lobata, and the green tea constituent EGCG. All these herbs strongly suppress the phosphorylation of VE-cadherin, which the bacteria initiate.

- The primary herbs for remodulating the immune system and/or the cytokine profile are: *Cordyceps, Scutellaria baicalensis, Salvia miltiorrhiza, Rhodiola, Eleutherococcus senticosus,* and *Withania somnifera*. Of these *Salvia miltiorrhiza* is most specific; it's a cytokine adaptogen; *Scutellaria baicalensis* is nearly as good and is, as well, a very good synergist, enhancing the action of other herbs and supplements.

- The primary herbs and supplements for inhibiting the production of p38 MAP kinase are: *Cordyceps, Scutellaria baicalensis, Polygonum cuspidatum, Schisandra, Olea europae* leaf and oil, N-acetyl cysteine (NAC), luteolin, and EGCG.

- The primary herbs for downregulating IL-17 are *Scutellaria baicalensis, Paeonia lactiflora, Hyssopus officinalis, Salvia miltiorrhiza, Angelica sinensis, Echinacea angustifolia, Astragalus, Sambucus,* and the constituent curcumin.

- The primary herbs for upregulating IFN-beta are *Polygonum cuspidatum, Astragalus,* and *Sambucus*.

- The best herbs and supplements for increasing glutathione levels in the body are: *Silybum marianum,* N-acetyl-cysteine, vitamin D-3, vitamins B-6 and B-12, and selenium. Some people like to add vitamins C and E.

- The best herbs and supplements for modulating apoptosis dysfunction by regulating Bcl/Bax are: *Artemisia* spp., *Glycyrrhiza* spp., *Goniothalamus cheliensis, Gynostemma pentaphyllum, Houttuynia cordata, Leonurus cardiaca* (motherwort), *Rhodiola* spp., *Scutellaria* spp., and the isolated constituents arctigenin, beta-sitosterol, and curcumin.

- Some good PGE2 inhibitors are: *Salvia miltiorrhiza, Bidens pilosa, Houttuynia cordata, Polygala tenuifolia, Pueraria lobata,* and *Scutellaria baicalensis*.

- Some good E-selectin inhibitors are: *Polygonum cuspidatum, Pueraria lobata,* and *Andrographis paniculata, Withania somnifera, Olea europeae* leaf and oil, quercetin, and piperine.

Natural protocol for treating spotted fever rickettsioses

What follows is a good generic protocol for RMSF and most of the other rickettsioses organisms. *Note:* If you are treating *Rickettsia akari*, you should utilize the protocol for ehrlichiosis in *Natural Treatments for Lyme Coinfections: Anaplasma, Babesia, and Ehrlichia* (Healing Arts Press, 2015).

Please see side effects and contraindications for these herbs and supplements in the next chapter.

- *Polygonum cuspidatum (Japanese knotweed) root*
  Dosage: 1 tablespoon of the root powder 3x daily (my perference), or 2,000 mg resveratrol 3x daily (from *Polygonum cuspidatum* **NOT** grape seed), or 1 tablespoon of the tincture 3x daily.
- *Salvia miltiorrhiza (red sage, danshen) root*
  Dosage: 1 teaspoon of the tincture 3x daily.
- *Scutellaria baicalensis (Chinese skullcap) root*
  Dosage: 1 teaspoon of the tincture, 3x daily.
- *Cordyceps* spp.
  Dosage: 1 tsp 3x daily
- *Silybum marianum (milk thistle) seed, standardized*
  Dosage: 1,200 mg upon rising and again just before bed.
- *N-acetyl-cysteine (NAC)*
  Dosage: 650–800 mg 3x daily.
- *Vitamin D3*
  Dosage: 8,000 IU daily.
- *Vitamin B6*
  Dosage: 25–50 mg daily.
- *Vitamin B12*
  Dosage: 1,000 mcg daily, that is *micro*grams.
- *Selenium*
  Dosage: 60 mcg, 2x daily, that is *micro*grams.

Expanded repertory

Add the following to the core protocol, if the following conditions occur:

1.1 Chronic fatigue

    A. ¼ cup (in juice or water) of a blend of the chronic fatigue

herbal formula, outlined in the recipe section of Chapter
Eight.

1.2 Endothelial damage, severe

  A. EGCG (green tea catechins) Dosage: Try to get a supplement
   with at least 80 percent polyphenols and 50 percent or so of
   EGCG. A supplement with the natural green tea flavonoids
   would be even better. Dosage range is 400–800 mg daily.
   For greater effectiveness in treating *Rickettsiae*-generated
   endothelial cell damage, take it with 1,200 mg quercetin
   daily – both at the same time, in the morning. *Note:* there is
   about 100 mg EGCG in a cup of green tea. I would imagine
   that drinking green tea itself throughout the day would be a
   good approach, and it produces better bioavailability.

1.3 Fever

  A. *Corallorhiza maculata* (or similar species, aka coral root), 30
   drops each hour, or . . .
  B. *Eupatorium perfoliatum* (boneset), strong infusion, 1 cup
   every hour or two, or . . .
  C. *Mentha piperata* (peppermint) tea, 1 cup every hour or to, as
   needed.

1.4 Neurological impairment

  A. Both the *Salvia* and the skullcap root can be increased to
   1 tsp 6x daily. This will help lower inflammation in the
   neural system and reduce the impairment. You can also
   add, if needed . . .
  B. *Pueraria lobata* (kudzu) root tincture, 1 tsp 3x daily, and/
   or . . .
  C. *Hericium erinaceus* (lion's mane) tincture, ¼–½ tsp 3–6x
   daily, and/or . . .
  D. *Polygala tenuifolia* (Chinese senega root) tincture, 30 drops
   3x daily for thirty days.

1.5 Spleen impairment (especially with risk of rupture)

  A. Increase dose of *Salvia* to 1 tablespoon of the tincture 3–6x
   daily.
  B. *Ceanothus* (red root) tincture is also very good for this, ½
   tsp 3–6 times daily.

1.6 Sweats, fever/chills, malaria-like

A. *Eupatorium perfoliatum* (boneset) tea, 3–6x daily. Preparation: 3 tablespoons dried herb infused in cup of hot water
for 15 minutes, covered. *Note:* This will also stimulate
helpful immune responses to the infection.

1.6 Sepis/septic shock

You can read an indepth look at the dynamics of sepsis and septic shock
in *Natural Treatments for Lyme Coinfections: Anaplasma, Babesia, and Ehrlichia*
(Healing Arts Press, 2015). The protocol for sepsis is assertive; large doses
are necessary to turn the condition around. The protocol should be followed
until the cytokine storm stabilizes. The core protocol *except for the Japanese
knotweed root* should be *discontinued* and this intervention used in its stead.

1) Tincture combination of *Angelica sinensis* and *Astragalus*
   spp., equal parts, 1 tablespoon each hour.

2) Tincture of *Salvia miltiorrhiza*, one tablespoon each hour.

3) Tincture of *Pueraria lobata* and *Cordyceps* spp., equal parts,
   one tablespoon each hour.

4) Tincture of *Glycyrrhiza* spp. and *Scutellaria baicalensis*, equal
   parts, 1 tablespoon each hour.

5) Spleen protection is provided by the *Salvia miltiorrhiza*.
   This will also protect the liver to some extent, so will
   the licorice. The use of high dose standardized silymarin
   compounds is highly suggested to protect the liver's
   Kupffer cells from apoptosis. (Dosage: milk thistle, standardized tincture, 1 tablespoon, 6x daily.)

The tinctures may be mixed together in any liquid (pomegranate
suggested) and should be taken until sepsis ameliorates. *Note:* Such high
doses of licorice (*Glycyrrhiza* spp.) are strongly contraindicated for long term
use. This is a short term, acute condition intervention only.

CHAPTER FIFTEEN

THE MATERIA MEDICA

The continued discovery and development of new formula-tions of herbal medicines, containing a combination of multiple ingredients that synergistically act to potently and selectively inhibit [microbial] replication at different stages and strengthen impaired immune system, should be a potential therapeutic option in the future.
Kaio Kitazato et al., 2007

Patients with immunocompromised systems are at greater risk for a more prolonged and severe course of illness, especially with multiple infectious etiologies, illustrated here with Lyme disease and babesia. In these patients, reasoning to the single most likely cause of illness may not be the best approach to diagnosis and empiric treatment. Familiarity with tick-borne diseases is important and may become more so as the habitats of humans and ticks increasingly intersect.
Ya'aqov Abrams, 2008

I have done extensive monographs, in other works, on many of the herbs suggested in this book. Time and space limitations prohibit repeating them here. Herein, I will only include depth monographs on *Polygonum cuspidatum* (Japanese knotweed), *Uncaria tomentosa / Uncaria rhynchon-phylla* (cat's claw), and *Andrograhis paniculata*. While *Stephania* is still useful in some conditions, due to space limitations, I am not including the depth monograph, as I did in the first edition of this book, though there is a modified, semilong monograph on both it and motherwort (*Leonurus cardiaca*). Following those there is a quick look at the side effects, contraindications, and dosages of the other herbs that have been discussed.

Depth monographs of the herbs truly important in the treatment of these three conditions can be found in: *Herbal Antibiotics*, second edition (Storey Publishing, 2012), which contains *Bidens pilosa*, the berberines, *Cryptolepis sanguinolenta*, *Eleutherococcus senticosus*, *Eupatorium perfoliatum* (boneset), *Ganoderma lucidum* (reishi), *Glycyrrhiza* spp. (licorice), *Rhodiola* spp., *Sida acuta* (and related species), *Astragalus*, *Withania somnifera*, and *Ceanothus* spp. *Herbal Antivirals* (Storey Publishing, 2013) contains monographs on *Houttuynia* spp and *Scutellaria baicalensis* (Chinese skullcap) root. *Olea europa* (olive leaf and oil), including the constituents oleic and oleanolic acid are covered in depth in *Healing Lyme Disease Coinfections, Complementary and Holistic Treatments for Bartonella and Mycoplasma* (Healing Arts Press, 2013). *Salvia miltiorrhiza* is covered in depth in *Natural Treatments for Lyme Coinfections: Anaplasma, Babesia, and Ehrlichia* (Healing Arts Press, 2015).

Making your own medicines

I strongly suggest that, if you have any inclination at all to do so, you make your own herbal medicines. There are a number of reasons for this; the most obvious is cost: making you own will lower your cost significantly.

Although herbal medicines are extremely inexpensive compared to pharmaceuticals (and often more effective), treating a long-term, chronic condition can be expensive, especially if you buy them already prepared. This has become especially true as the FDA has begun to exert more control over herbal medicines via the good manufacturing practices act, aka the GMP (not necessarily a good thing). Making it worse, the larger herbal companies are beginning to consolidate their control over the marketplace (very much not a good thing). Those shifts are causing price increases in nearly every area. A small rant . . .

Small rant

The common and oft-repeated rationale for the GMP is that it will make the products safer for the public. This is not actually accurate. The main safety problems that occur with herbal products comes, and always has come, from two sources: (1) manufacturing errors by a large company (usually product contamination of one sort or another, always inadvertent) and (2) unscrupulous product creation (specifically: herbal energy pills, weight loss products, and muscle development formulations) by corporations of one sort or another. The small, herbalist-owned companies have never had these kinds of problems; their products are almost always better than those produced by the large companies, they often have a wider range of products, they are less expensive, and, based on the public record, much safer.

The GMP was developed, and supported, by the big herbal companies (as well as a number of large pharmaceutical companies and, interestingly companies such as Coca-Cola) in order to control the marketplace . . . and as a response to the FDA looking askance at those two problem areas within the natural products world. It wasn't really necessary to put the same restrictions on manufacturing on both the large and small companies – these are two different kinds of companies, with entirely different functions and behaviors – yet, they did. Unfortunately, over time, this will lead to the majority of the smaller companies going out of business; the FDA is already putting pressure on some of them. When that occurs, fewer herbal formulations will be available and those at a much higher price. Nevertheless, there are still many good small companies in business (the consolidation will take a few years); I recommend my favorites in Appendix Two.

Fortunately, neither the GMP or anything else prevents you, nor will prevent you, from making your own medicines. Not only will it be much cheaper for you, there is something exceptionally wonderful that happens when you work directly with a plant for your healing, when you find it in a field, or grow it in your yard (it may already be there, if you just look around), or even if you buy the plant from a grower (several really good ones in the supply section). *When your life is saved by a plant, nothing is ever the same again.* This is most especially true if you have developed a personal relationship with the plant while making it into medicine for yourself.

There are a number of good books on making plant medicines. I generally suggest my own depth look at it (inevitably), which is included in the second edition of *Herbal Antibiotics* (it contains, as well, an extensive formulary of over two hundred herbs), or Richo Cech's *Making Plant Medicines* (Horizon Herbs, third edition), or James Green's *Herbal Medicine Maker's Handbook* (Crossing Press). All are very good.

If you obtain a resale license from your state (easy and inexpensive) and give yourself a business name (e.g., The Get Rich Very Slowly Herb Company or The Make Tens of Dollars in Your Spare Time Herb Company), you will be able to buy herbs wholesale from nearly all wholesalers. This will lower your cost of the herbs by anywhere from one-half to nine-tenths of their retail price.

The materia medica

The materia medica begins with three depth monographs – in what I consider order of importance. These are followed by smaller monographs on stephania and motherwort. And finally: there is a quick look at the side effects, contraindications, substance interactions, and dosages for many of the other herbs and supplements discussed in the book.

Polygonum cuspidatum (Japanese knotweed)

FAMILY: Polygonacae

COMMON NAMES: The most common English terms for the plant are Japanese (or bushy) knotweed and (sometimes) Mexican bamboo or Chinese knotweed. Others of note include *hu zhang* (Chinese, meaning "tiger stick," no one knows why), *kojo* and *itadori* (Japanese), *hojang* (Korean), and Hancock's curse – no doubt for the man who originally planted it in the UK.

SPECIES USED: There are somewhere between 65 and 300 species in the genus. As usual, taxonomists are making life hard for, well, all living things. Emotive name calling has ensued about the members of the genus (the taxonomists – aka *Taxonomissii irritatious* – not the plants). In essence, the search for personal taxonomist immortality (and PhD degrees) has led to a frantic renaming of all Earth's organisms. ("Hey, over here, this one looks different!") Some members of *Taxonomissii irritatious*, tired of the same old names and the general lack of interest in their reordering of Earth's organisms, simply went ahead and created new genera: *Fagopyrum*, *Fallopia*, and *Persicaria* are some of them. Regrettably, my friend *Polygonum cuspidatum* is now sometimes known as *Fallopia japonica*. Some taxonomists insist that this really is the right scientific name for the plant and don't-use-the-other-one-anymore-we're-not-kidding.

Other (older) synonyms for the plant are *Polygonum japonicum*, *Polygonum reynoutria*, and *Reynoutria japonica*.

Scores of different *Polygonum* species have been used as medicinals, often for thousands of years. Because they are so closely related, many of them have similar medicinal actions. Still, I prefer *P. cuspidatum* for Lyme infections. It seems to be the most specific for the cytokine dynamics that these bacteria generate. After a decade of experience with it, it's pretty reliable in reversing symptoms for most of the people who use it.

Parts used

The root (rhizomes). The young shoots are edible, so if you are harvesting in the spring, don't just throw them away.

Preparation and dosage

There are three forms we have traditionally suggested for use during Lyme infections: standardized tablets, powder, and tincture. The standardized tablets were all that were available when the first edition of this book was released; they work fine. However, I prefer the bulk powder – primarily because the acids in the human GI tract are the best herbal extraction compounds that exist, much better than water and alcohol. In consequence, by taking the root in powdered form, you get the best range of constituents; the body pulls from the whole herb whatever it wants. Further, the bulk herb is much cheaper than tablets or tinctures.

Still . . . any form will work.

Root powder

The whole herb can be used directly, simply blended in juice or water. (Make sure you get it powdered, not cut and sifted. The chunks are unpleasant to swallow. If you can't get powder, you can make a very fine powder from using the combination of a Vitamix and a nut grinder, then sifting the result.)

My preferred dosage is 1 tablespoon of the powder in liquid of your choice 3x daily. You can also encapsulate it if you wish, but just taking the blended powder is faster and easier. *The dose can be increased or decreased* depending on personal response to the herb and the symptom picture. *Begin with one teaspoon 3x daily and work up to the larger dose over a few weeks.* For severe Lyme symptoms it usually takes 8–12 months to completely correct the condition. People often begin feeling better within a month, sometimes less, sometimes a bit longer.

The traditional Chinese medicine dosage is, as usual, much higher than the American: 9–30 grams (30 grams is a bit over an ounce) of the root daily, taken internally or as a decoction.

Note: The toxic dose – meaning the point where you begin to get a lot of GI tract disturbance – is pretty high, 75 grams (about 2.5 ounces), taken all at one time, by a 165-pound (75kg) person.

Standardized tablets

Standardized tablets are usually just called Resveratrol. Check the label to see that it is indeed formulated from knotweed root and not grapes. Grapes are sometimes used but knotweed root has the most resveratrol of any plant known. (The grape formulations, trust me on this, won't work for Lyme.) Resveratrol tablets from knotweed are simply a knotweed root formulation standardized for resveratrol content. They contain *all* of the plant's root constituents. Suggested dosage is 1–4 tablets 3–4x daily depending on severity of symptoms.

Begin at the lowest dose and increase incrementally every seven days, that is, begin with one tablet 3x daily, then after seven days, 2 tablets 3x daily, then 3 tablets 3x daily, then 4 tablets, 3x daily, then 4 tablets 4x daily.

> *Please note:* This is just a suggestion, some people need the high dose, some people never need more than one tablet 3x daily. If, on the increased dose, you start to feel worse, or your body just doesn't feel right, just go back down to where it seems to work best.

As symptoms decrease in severity, the dosage can be incrementally lowered to a maintanence dose. (If you begin to feel worse as you lower the dose, increase it again.) Maintain use of the herb for 8–12 months or until symptoms or infection is resolved.

Regarding sources: In the first edition of this book, the only reliable source I could find for a standardized knotweed tablet was Source Naturals brand. Those tablets contain 500 mg per tablet. However, a point of confusion arose (hundreds of emails); it came from the directions on the bottle. They list a serving *size* of *two* tablets, thus the *one gram* (1,000 mg) on the label. (They get that from multiplying 500 times two.) Each *serving* contains 8 percent total resveratrols (there is more than one kind), giving 80 mg total resveratrols with 20 mg of resveratrol itself. There is, as well, 5 mg of red wine extract (don't worry about this). This dosage works pretty well. If you get a different brand, it just needs to be somewhere in that range.

The Source Naturals brand worked just fine for most people, however . . .

Some people found that the Source Naturals resveratrol produced a number of unpleasant side effects for them. After switching to another brand (e.g., Paradise Herbs), the side effects disappeared.

Some people have reported that the use of knotweed root produced prob lems (massive herxing), which the resveratrol tablets did not, presumably this comes from the difference between a wild plant and a domesticated supplement.

Just be aware of how your body responds and adjust accordingly.

Tincture
Dosage: ½–1 teaspoon, 3–6x daily (1:5, 60 percent alcohol). Dose may be decreased or increased as needed for personal response and symptom picture.

Decoction
A number of people have been using a tea, and it seems to be working well for them. To make: four ounces herb (7 grams) in 32 ounces (1 liter) water, simmer for 20 minutes, strain, cool, and drink in four equal doses during the day.

Side effects and contraindications
Japanese knotweed is a very safe herb; however . . .
- The primary, bothersome side effect that seems to occur in about 1 percent of the people using the herb is loss of taste. (This can also occasionally occur when eating the fresh plant as food.) This will resolve once the herb is discontinued, though it may take up to a week or so to do so.
- Other occasional (and rare) side effects are primarily gastro-intestinal in nature: dry mouth, bitter taste in mouth, nausea, vomiting, abdominal pain, and diarrhea.
- This herb is contraindicated in pregnancy.

PROPERTIES OF JAPANESE KNOTWEED

Actions

Antibacterial, Antiviral, Antischistosomal, Antispirochetal, Antifungal, Immunostimulant, Immunomodulant, Anti-inflammatory, Angiogenesis modulator, Calcium channel adaptogen (modulates calcium channel signaling, raising it if it is depressed, decreasing it if it is too high), Central nervous system relaxant, Central nervous system (brain and spinal cord) protectant and antiinflammatory, Antioxidant, Antiathersclerotic, Antihyperlipidemic, Antimutagenic, Anticarcinogenic, Antineoplastic, Vasodilator, Inhibits platelet aggregation, Inhibits eicosanoid synthesis, Antithrombotic, Tyrosine kinase inhibitor, Oncogene inhibitor, Antipyretic, Cardioproctective, Analgesic, Antiulcer (slightly reduces stomach acid and protects against stress ulcers), Hemostatic, and Astringent.

Active Against

Polygonum cuspidatum is (mildly) active against *Leptospira* and *Treponema denticola* spirochetes, more strongly so against *Staphylococcus aureus, S. albus, Neisseria cattarrhalis, N. gonorrhoeae, N. meningitidis,* A and B Streptococci (twenty different strains, e.g., of *Streptococcus mutans* and *S. sobrinus.* The herb is directly antibacterial for this genus; it also inhibits bacterial glycolytic acid production and glucosyltransferase activity by the bacteria), *E. coli, Propionbacterium acnes, Proteus vulgaris, Pseudomonas aeruginosa, Salmonella typhi,* and *Shigella flexneri.* Part of its general antibacterial action is due to inhibiting bacterial DNA primase.

The ethanol extract of the herb (i.e., tincture), as researchers Zhang et al. (2013) note, has "significant protective effects against *Vibrio vulnificus* cytotoxicity and infection." *V. vulnificus*, a relative of the cholera organism, is one of the "flesh-eating' bacteria that is in the news every so often. It lives in seawater, as cholera does, and people are often infected when swimming. (It often causes loss of limbs. Yuck.) Researchers found that the extract inhibited the growth and survival of the organisms in seawater; pretreatment of mice protected six-week-old mice from infection by the bacteria. The root (as well as its constituent, emodin) is considered to be a significant antibacterial for this organism.

The herb is also (supposedly) broadly antifungal (part of resveratrol's function in the plant itself). It strongly inhibits the growth of *Candida albicans*, for example, but I haven't been able to find specifics on other fungal organisms it is active against.

In vitro studies have found a broad antiviral activity against a number of viruses including respiratory syncytial virus (RSV), various influenza viruses, e.g., H1N1 (inhibits replication via inhibiting hemagglutinin and neuraminidase and upregulating IFN-beta, which acts synergistically with the plant's compounds), enterovirus 71, Epstein-Barr virus, vaccinia virus, vesicular stomatitis virus, herpes simplex, and ECHO 11 (enteric cytopathic human orphan) viruses, the latter is inhibited by a 10 percent water decoction of the whole herb.

ECHO viruses, previously thought to be benign, are now known to cause a number of diseases, including: rashes, diarrhea, respiratory infections (colds, sore throat, bronchitis, bronchiolitis), muscle inflammation, meningitis, encephalitis, and pericarditis (inflammation of the membrane around the heart).

In other studies, a 2 percent water decoction of the plant strongly inhibited adenovirus type III, poliomyelitis virus type II, coxsackie A and B viruses, encephalitis B, HIV (strongly so), and the ECHO11 group viruses. Numerous tests have found the herb to be a specific antiviral agent for hepatitis B viruses (in a dose-dependent manner).

Biofilms: A number of Chinese studies have found the herb useful for *gently* breaking up biofilms in a slow, methodical, and irresistible manner – similar to the way its roots break through concrete foundations. The herb, when used over time, reduces the numbers of bacteria in biofilms *and* inhibits biofilm formation (both in a dose-dependent manner). The herb is both bacteriostatic and bactericidal. It helps prevent the formation of dental biofilms (plaque), which is why it has been used, traditionally, in Korea for millennia to improve oral health. If combined with other substances that also break up biofilms (e.g., fluoride), the actions are synergistic. Simply holding a decoction of the plant in the mouth, on the gums/teeth, for ten minutes every morning will break up plaque – and tone the gums as well. In tests, in the biofilms, biomass accumulation, water-insoluble polysaccharides, and intracellular iodophilic polysaccharides levels were all reduced.

Functions in Lyme Disease

A broadly systemic plant, Japanese knotweed modulates and enhances immune function, is active against a number of Gram-negative and Gram-positive bacteria, is potently anti-inflammatory, strongly protective of the body's endothelial cells – especially in the brain, is a very good cytokine modulator – reducing many of the most damaging cytokines the spirochetes initiate; it shuts down the exact pathways the bacteria utilize to generate the most damaging cytokines, helps protects the body against endotoxin damage, helps reduce Herxheimer reactions, and is a moderately good cardioprotector.

The pharmacokinetics of the plant are very good, that is, when taken orally the plant spreads easily and well throughout the body. (It shows two peaks in blood plasma, the first at one hour, the second at five.) Plant constituents pass the GI tract membrane quite well. (The use of piperine enhances this, increasing the medicinal effects of the plant, for example, in alleviating depression.) The herb's constituents flow throughout the body and tend to concentrate in the blood, stomach, duodenum, liver, kidney, brain, lungs, and heart. If the herb is used along with other herbs or pharmaceuticals, it "significantly" enhances the movement of those compounds throughout the body.

Polygonum cuspidatum's constituents cross the blood-brain barrier where they exert actions on the central nervous system: anti-microbial, anti-inflammatory, as protectants against oxidative and microbial damage, and as calming agents. The herb specifically protects the brain from inflammatory damage, microbial endotoxins, and bacterial infections.

Knotweed enhances blood flow especially to the eye, heart, skin, and joints. This makes it especially useful in Lyme as it facilitates blood flow to the areas that are difficult to reach to kill the spirochetes. It is a drug and herb synergist, facilitating the movement of other herbs and drugs into these hard-to-reach places when taken with them.

Thus, the herb has a number of specific actions in the treatment of Lyme disease: (1) stimulating microcirculation, especially to the eye, knees, heart, brain, and skin, which helps carry active constituents to those locations to affect spirochete presence; (2) reducing inflammation in tissues, thus lessening both skin and arthritic impacts from the spirochetes; (3) protecting and correcting heart function and reducing inflammation in heart tissue, especially helping with symptoms associated with Lyme carditis: lightheadedness, shortness of breath, palpitations, and chest pain; (4) reducing autoimmune reactions to Lyme; (5) promoting wide-spectrum antibiotic/antiviral action, including (mildly) against spirochetes; (6) enhancing healthy immune function; (7) acting as a synergist with other herbs or drugs in the treatment of Lyme; (8) protecting endothelial integrity from Lyme spirochetes and Lyme coinfectious agents such as *Bartonella*; (9) acting as a fairly gentle anti-biofilm agent; and, (10) most importantly, reducing inflammation in the brain and central nervous system, helping restore function during neuroborreliosis.

Other Uses

The plant is a good source of vitamin C (thus an antiscorbutic); in spring, the young shoots and leaves are eaten (by people and perhaps by pandas).

Many rural Japanese harvest the plants in the spring, gathering the newly emerging shoots (which look a bit like asparagus). The shoots are usually soaked in water for half a day or parboiled, then the tough outer skin peeled away. The inner shaft of the shoot is then cooked and eaten. The cooked shoots are reportedly sour (I haven't yet eaten them), some say extremely so. Japanese wild harvesters often pickle them as well. Some Southeast Asians smoke the leaves like tobacco.

The plant contains oxalic acid, hence its sour taste. Most sources suggest limiting the amount of oxalic-acid-containing plants that are eaten in the diet. Too much may aggravate conditions such as arthritis, gout, and kidney stones.

While not usually used, the stems and leaves of the plant contain many of the same constituents as the roots (though not as much) and are themselves usable as medicinals with the same range of actions as the root. Research has found that the antioxidant actions, as well as the plant's flavonoid content, of the stems and leaves are "significantly" higher than onion, broccoli, orange, carrot, and ginger.

Polygonum cuspidatum forms dense thickets and is especially good for erosion control in damaged landscapes. It is also a very good plant for phytoremediating industrial-damaged ecosystems as it tolerates and removes heavy metals such as arsenic and copper from contaminated soils. The metals are concentrated in the roots – *so don't harvest from such sites*.

Herb/drug interactions

   • Should not be used with blood-thinning agents. Discontinue
     use of the herb ten days prior to any surgery.

Habitat and appearance

The plant is very leafy and possesses a jointed stalk similarly to bamboo; it
does look a little like bamboo, hence some of its common names. It grows
quite insistently, often reaching a height of nine to twelve feet (three to four
meters).

   Native to Japan, North China, Taiwan, and Korea, the plant is an "invasive" botanical that is, to many people's dismay, exceptionally hard to eradicate. (It grows again from even the tiniest pieces of root; much like the Lyme
spirochetes themselves.) Introduced as an ornamental in 1825 in Britain and
the late 1800s in the US, it is now naturalized throughout much of mainland
Europe, the British Isles, at least thirty-nine states in the United States, as
well as Canada, New Zealand (where it's classified as an "unwanted" organism), the Russian federation, and Australia. It is considered, by phytoaryans,
to be one of the world's most invasive species.

   And to be fair, the plant root is an irresistible force that has not yet met an
immovable object. It can apparently work its way through any human-created,
land-altering object: concrete foundations, sidewalks, buildings, roads, paving,
retaining walls, and water-controlling fortifications. (The Gaian dynamics of
this apparently escapes the anti-invasive purists.) It loves riparian ecosystems
and certain side effects of human technology such as roadsides and waste
places.

   It can live pretty much in any type of soil, is resilient to cutting, will
vigorously resprout from even the tiniest piece of root left in the ground.
The plant likes to live along the edges of streams so that pieces of the root
can be carried off during floods – they then spread with gleeful abandon.

   In the UK, it is illegal to grow the plant *or* to allow it to remain on one's
property. Failure to remove it can get you an *ASBO*, that is, an "anti-so-
cial behavior order" from the authorities. Three of those, and you can
be forced to move out of the neighborhood. (And yes, chalk drawing on
the sidewalk by children, or children playing and laughing too loudly,
can get them, too. And don't even think of engaging in loud sex.) Mort-

gage companies regularly refuse to lend on properties that have the plant growing there. In Scotland, it is illegal to intentionally or *unintentionally* spread the plant. ("The seed was on my shoe, I didn't mean it." Sound of cell door closing.)

Apparently all the plants in Europe are clones of a single female plant, making the plant, as the Japanese Knotweed Alliance comments, "one of the biggest females in the world in biomass terms." A new concept of female measurement. (Speculation: Is the fanatical attempt to eradicate the plant by anti-invasive groups an unconscious misogynistic impulse?)

Cultivation and collection

Easily cultivated, primarily from pieces (often miniscule) of the rhizomes/roots. Seed cultivation is (reputedly) more difficult as male plants with fertile pollen are rare outside the Far East. But be cautious . . .

Considered an invasive species, the plant, and those who grow it, are diligently attacked with evangelical fervor by Native Purists who will often stop by your home, uninvited, to share their insights on eradication. (Hell hath no fury like an evangelical invasive activist scorned.) Cultivates internal strength in any who grow it intentionally. A powerful addition to the Western botanical pharmacopoeia.

The roots (rhizomes) are collected in the spring or fall. (Just make sure you don't gather them from heavy-metal-contaminated sites.) The root mass can be substantial; you won't need to harvest much unless you are making a lot of medicine. Roughly cut the roots into smaller sections and dry them out of the sun in a coolish location. (*Note:* the constituents in the root are highly susceptible to degradation by heat and sunlight.) Store in plastic bags in a plastic tub in a cool location. The stored root will last for years.

Plant chemistry

As of 2013, some sixty-seven compounds have been identified in Japanese knotweed, these include: 1-(3-O-B-D-glucopyranosyl-4,5-dihydroxyphenyl)-ethanone, 2,6-dihydroxybenzoic acid, 2-methoxy-6-acetyl-7-methyljuglone, aloe-emodin, astringin, catechin, catechin-5-O-B-D-glucopyranoside, chrysophanol, citreorosein, dimethylhydroxychromone, emodin, emodin

A COMMENT ON INVASIVES

In the Western world – most strongly among the adolescent offspring of the British empire – anti-invasive sentiments run extremely high. The UK, Canada, the United States, New Zealand, and Australia are particularly adamant advocates of the eradication of alien species (a perfect example of irony). While not as evangelical about it, the EU has feelings, too.

Humorously, I often remark that while conservatives in those regions are most outraged by illegal human immigrants, what outrages my liberal tribe are the illegal plant immigrants. Both want the aliens to go away (thus protecting our way of life) and will often go to extreme lengths to try and make them do so. Regrettably, this often extends to scientists who should know better. The problem, of course, is limited viewpoint, essentially a human-centric one.

Plants, as a general group, predate us by well over one hundred million years. They must have been doing something all that time besides waiting for us to emerge from the ecological background of the planet and suddenly notice they don't care about our rules of behavior. And, of course, they have been. They perform many crucially important ecological functions. In fact, they are the second-most important group of organisms (the first being bacteria) on the planet. Both actively maintain the human-livable state of the planet.

Few people know, or want to know, that evolution has not stopped or that we are fairly small players in the scheme of things. The planet exists as a self-organized, discrete ecosystem, in a remarkable state of balance. That balance point (aka homeodynamis) is maintained by *all* the organisms on the planet working in concert. But most important are the plants and the bacteria. Human disturbance of ecosystem homeodynamis is causing tremendous alterations in the functioning of the planet and its regional ecosystems. The mass movement of "alien" plant species, which most people consider an invasive process, is a response to that disturbance.

To make just one tiny point about it, the chemicals that plants generate in their millions are released into the ecosystems in which they live in order to modulate system responses to any disturbances of homeodynamis that occur. This keeps those ecosystems healthy and functioning as they are meant to do.

Despite the fact that landscapes (in places such as Vermont) appear to be healthy to the eye, they are not. Human population expansion, housing development, massive forest cutting in the nineteenth and early twentieth centuries, farming, industrialization, and a great many other factors have caused the loss of a tremendous number of plant species – long before people began to worry about Japanese knotweed. Those lost plant species performed essential functions in keeping those ecosystems healthy, including, as only one example, soil health. The many ecosystems damaged by human factors are no longer performing optimally; the planet is beginning to experience ever-wilder climate gyrations in response (global warming is the least part of it). The plants that are moving into these regions are doing so in order to restore ecosystem homeodynamis.

These "invasive" plants perform a wide variety of functions, here are five (just to give a sense of it): (1) They restore soil structure and health, damaged due to the loss of complex plant populations; (2) they remediate soils by removing industrial waste products; (3) they, very specifically, act to destabilize and degrade human-created structures, including industrial production plants, in order to reduce their impacts on ecosystems (and they act over long time lines, the Chinese got nothing on these guys); (4) they are potent medicinals for emerging disease complexes (they act on micro- as well as macroecological systems); and finally (5) most of them are extremely good (free) food plants, and believe me, we are all going to be getting a bit hungry by and by.

Some of the most important plants for emerging disease complexes are invasives: Russian elm, isatis, houttuynia, phellodendron (a berberine-containing tree now invasive in the regions where goldenseal was formerly dominant), Japanese knotweed, kudzu, and so on and on and on. (The most important thing to ask ourselves before we decide we know enough to eradicate a plant is "what is it *doing* here?")

Japanese knotweed has a number of specific actions in damaged landscapes. It bioconcentrates heavy metals such as arsenic and copper. It can grow in salt-heavy soils, part of the reason it is common along roadsides – that is where salt from winter road treatment concentrates. Salt concentrates in damaged soils; this is one of the major plants (tamarisk is another) that can reclaim them.

Crucially, the plant epigenetically alters itself to meet the needs of the diverse habitats which it "invades." This means that while the genome remains relatively stable, the environment in which the plant grows, in a complex and sophisticated conversation with it, turns certain genes on and others off – it affects how the cells read the genes. These epigenetic alterations are heritable, that is they are passed down to succeeding generations of plants. The plants are, in essence, altering themselves in order to more exactly interact with the specific ecosystem dysfunction present in each location in which it grows. (Soil makeup, the longer the plant grows there, alters itself considerably.) It is no surprise then that the chemical makeup of the roots (and rest of the plant) alters from one geographic location to the next. (This is in part why harvesting plants from the ecoregion in which you live makes sense; the plant contains the optimum constituent content for the organisms in its ecorange.) The chemical content of wild populations, while different, also tends to be higher than those grown domestically. Some researchers (e.g., Kirino et al., 2012) report that the resveratrol in knotweed roots differed in its biological functions "depending on its varieties and the countries in which the plant grew." (A fascinating insight, which, if true, has tremendous implications for reductionism; a chemical is not a chemical is not a chemical.) And a final note: P. cuspidatum is interbreeding with native Polygonums as it moves into new ecoregions, creating unique hybrids that themselves possess unique ecological functions. Oh, and knotweed . . . it tends to move into new regions about six months before Lyme disease becomes endemic there. These plants respond not only to the macroecology of a region but the micro-ecology of the organisms that live there. (Jacob Malcomb [2010?], while at the Cary Institute, did some interesting, and related, work on the "invasive" plant, garlic mustard, aka Alliaria petiolata. He comments, "Overall tick mortality suggests that garlic mustard exudates may have a direct role in reducing tick molting success from the nymphal to adult stage. . . . [The research indicates that] garlic mustard may be reducing populations of Ixodes scapularis.")

While I best understand plant invasives and their function, these kinds of effects are not limited to plants. Zebra mussels are another example of the complex ecological functions of "invasives."

Zebra mussels, originally from lakes in southern Russia, are now a potent "invasive" species in North America, the UK, and parts of Europe. They range in size from about that of a fingernail to some two inches across. And there are millions of them. What is nearly always missing when they are discussed is a non-human-centric ecological frame of reference.

The first thing to understand is that they are particularly invasive in polluted lakes (e.g., the Great Lakes in the US). Like most shellfish, zebra mussels are filter feeders. They remove particulate matter from water. Human behavior, the past three centuries, has increasingly degraded the ecology of most of the Great Lakes (and great rivers such as the Mississippi). The Great Lakes have been very polluted for a long time.

Yet, once zebra mussels moved into the lakes, the water began to clear. Zebra mussels filter about one quart (liter) of water per day per mussel (depending on their size). They use some of the particulate matter they filter as food; the rest is combined with mucus and feces and deposited on the lake floor, removing it from the water permanently. The food supplies on the lake floor thus increase substantially, stimulating a rise in fish populations. Since the introduction of zebra mussels, the water clarity in Lake Erie, one of the most polluted of the lakes, has increased from six inches to three feet . . . and it's still increasing.

The mussels also have a habit of clogging the intake and outflow pipes of the industrial factories that line the lakes; they also adhere to the bottom of ships, docks, and any other human-made structure they encounter. Over time, their numbers increase so much they begin to shut down the parts of human technology that are damaging waterways. (They are also very good eating.) As Henry David Thoreau once put it, "You must understand that nothing is what you have taken it to be."

monomethyl ether, emodin 8-O-B-D-glucopyranoside, emodin-1-O-gluco-
side, emodin-8-O-glucoside, fallacinol, gallic acid, glucofragulin, methyl-
courmarin, napthoquinone, polygonin, physcion, physcion-8-O-glucoside,
physcion-8-O-(6'-acetyl)glucoside, piceatannol glucoside, piceid, polydatin,
polyflavanostilbene A, polygonins A and B, protocatechuic acid, quercetin,
questin, questinol, resveratrol, resveratroloside, rheic acid, rhein, tachi-
oside, torachryson-8-O-glucoside, torachryson-8-O-(6'-acetyl)glucoside,
trans-resveratrol, trytophan, and numerous flavonoids, polysaccharides,
dicaffeoyl quinic acids (DCQAs), and condensed tannins.

Traditional uses of Japanese knotweed

The plant has been used in Asia for over 2000 years (especially in China,
Japan, and Korea) both as medicine and food. The root is traditionally used
in Korea for dental diseases, that use borne out by research finding that it
strongly inhibits biofilm (plaque) formation in the mouth. The leaves are
sometimes used as a smoking mix in India and Southeast Asia.

Nevertheless, there has been little use of the plant in the Western world
until recently – well, except for erosion control, as a garden ornamental,
and a focus of antialien sentiment. Research on and subsequent use of the
plant as a phytomedicinal have been primarily because of its high content of
resveratrol and, over the past decade, because of its effectiveness in treating
Lyme infections.

Resveratrol, as a concept, is relatively new. It came out of interest generated by the French "paradox." That is, while the French ate lots of cheese they
had very low cholesterol counts and comparatively few deaths from heart
disease, while we in the United States were dying like overweight flies in the
last days of autumn. Analysis tied the difference to the French propensity for
red wine consumption – red wine grapes contain quite a bit of resveratrol. (In
the US, when this is reported, the researchers make haste to say this does not
mean you should drink; in France they smile and continue to sip their wine.)

A number of compounds have been found to play a role in this "paradox," but resveratrol and trans-resveratrol seem to be the most important.
Red wine, particularly that made from pinot noir grapes, contain significant amounts of these resveratrols. The compounds easily move across the
gastrointestinal mucosa and circulate in the bloodstream. They also cross
the blood-brain barrier.

It should be stressed that while resveratrol does do amazing things, it is, by itself, not sufficient in effectively treating Lyme disease. *The whole herb is crucial.* Many other constituents in the plant (e.g., emodin, polydatin, and trans-resveratrol) all possess potent biological effects. As usual, depth research is showing that the plant's constituents' are highly synergistic and possess broad-spectrum actions that the single chemicals do not. As a whole herb, it is much more powerful than any constituent used alone.

Ayurveda

This particular species has not been used in traditional Ayurvedic practice though eleven other species of *Polygonum* are, many similarly to how *Polygonum cuspidatum* is used in TCM practice.

Traditional Chinese medicine

There are some 80 species of *Polygonum* used in traditional Chinese medicine (TCM). *Polygonum cuspidatum* is only one of them. Besides being used to treat specific conditions, the herb is considered a tonic and is used to increase general well-being and health.

The main traditional use for the herb is for invigorating and clearing the blood and reducing heat (i.e., inflammation). It is considered antipyretic, detoxicant, anti-inflammatory, antirheumatic, diuretic, expectorant, antitussive, and stasis eliminating and a channel deobstructant. It is primarily used in the treatment of jaundice, rheumatic pain, strangury with turbid urine, leukorrhea, dysmenorrhea, retained lochia, bleeding hemorrhoids, anal fissure, wounds, various injuries, scalds, and burns.

Other uses include: respiratory infections, damage to skin (burns, carbuncles, skin infections, snakebite – usually as a poultice), bacterial dysentery, acute infectious hepatitis with jaundice, hepatitis B surface antigen positive chronic active hepatitis, neonatal jaundice, cholelithiasis, cholecystitis (with damp heat or severe heat syndrome), trichomonas, bacterial vaginitis, hyperlipidemia, suppurative dermatitis, gonorrhea, athlete's foot, diarrhea, and psoriasis. (Basically, it is used to treat pathogenic heat in the blood, cough from lung heat, constipation from accumulated heat in GI tract, jaundice and liver inflammation due to damp heat, and accumulated heat in skin.)

Western botanic practice

This particular herb was unknown to Western botanic practice until recently (and is still unknown to most American and European botanic practitioners). The American Eclectics knew of and used (to some extent) nine different *Polygonum* species, primarily *Polygonum hydropiper* – water pepper. Many of them possess actions similar to that of Japanese knotweed, though they can't be used in a simple substitution for this particular species. Japanese knotweed is unique in a number of respects.

Scientific Research

Surprisingly, despite its recent introduction to the Western world, there are now (2015) some ten thousand studies on the plant and its constituents at Pubmed (and hundreds to thousands more on the Chinese database cnki). The studies in the West have primarily focused on the actions of resveratrol, followed by (in descending order) the whole plant, and the individual constituents: trans-resveratrol, emodin, and polydatin. Clinical and laboratory studies in China have mostly occurred with the whole plant and the single constituent polydatin. While the plant has a multitude of important actions (endothelial protecting, calcium channel modulation, and so forth), I think its most important functions for Lyme infections to be its cytokine modulation and its neuroprotective and regenerative actions.

First, a sample of findings that have occurred since the 2005 edition of this book.

Neurological effects

The root has been found to be a very specific inhibitor of CD40 expression on endothelial cells, primarily by inhibiting TNF-alpha activation of its expression. This protects endothelial junctions from degradation, significantly enhancing TEER strength.

The herb also inhibits senescence in endothelial progenitor cells (EPCs), essentially through increasing telomerase activity. EPCs are crucial for endothelial

health in that they are integral to endothelial repair after injury. In vivo studies have found that in the brain, resveratrol (and the herb) have a stabilizing and regeneration effect on endothelial cells, protecting the brain from recurrent strokes. The strength of the blood-brain barrier (BBB) is significantly enhanced when the herb is used.

In other in vivo studies (in mice), polydatin, a constituent, protected against motor degeneration in multiple rodent models of Parkinson's disease. Essentially, it attenuated dopaminergic neurodegeneration in a section of the brain known as substantia nigral and stimulated regeneration of the neurons. Other in vivo studies found that another constituent, emodin, had a potent neuroprotective effect against beta-amyloid toxicity in cortical neurons. The stillbenes and anthraquinones in the roots have a strong neuroprotective effect on transient middle cerebral artery occlusion in rats.

An extract of the root protects mitochondria from oxidative damage and improves locomotor function in a *Drosophila* Parkinson's disease model. Another constituent: emodin-8-O-beta-D-glucoside exerts neuroprotective effects on focal cerebral injury (from ischemia) in rats. Numerous studies have found that polydatin possesses the same actions, improving neurological deficits and reducing the volume of brain infarction. Other studies with that constituent found that the compound upregulated brain-derived neurotrophic factor and alleviated learning and memory impairments in neonatal rats with hypoxic-ischemic brain injury. If used prior to injury, it inhibited the damage.

Other constituents (e.g., naphthalene and flavan derivatives) also show neuroprotective effects. Resveratrol (and the herb) prevents impaired cognition induced by chronic, unpredictable stress in rats. Trans-resveratrol also reduces the impacts of stress in the nervous system. Analysis of brain function shows it increases the levels of serotonin, and function, in three distinct brain regions: the frontal cortex, hippocampus, and hypothalmus (three of the regions most impacted by neuroborreliosis). Noradrenaline and dopamine levels increased in the frontal cortex and the striatum. MOA-A was inhibited in the four brain regions, particularly the frontal cortex and hippocampus. The herb and this compound show a definite antidepressive effect. (This is increased by the use of piperine.)

Resveratrol also attenuates oxidative damage, ameliorating cognitive impairment in the brain of senescence-accelerated mice. Learning and memory are "significantly" improved, as are neuromuscular coordination and sensorimotor capacity. Polydatin protects learning and memory impairment in a rat model of vascular dementia. It alleviates the injury to neurons, decreases production of malondialdehyde, and increases SOD and catalase. Polydatin, in rats, improves neurological deficits and reduces the volume of brain infarction in rats. Levels of ICAM-1, VCAM-1, E-selectin, L-selectin, and integrins all decreased.

Numerous in vivo studies have found that the herb (and resveratrol and polydatin) substantially increase the stability of the BBD, restoring it whenever it is disrupted. Degenerative neurons "substantially" *decrease* if the plant is used during infections or insult; neuronal viability is enhanced.

Resveratrol completely protects endothelial junctions, TEER strength, F-actin, and microtubule cytoskeletons, as well as occludin and zona occludens-1 tight junctions in the brain. Decreases in mitochondrial membrane potential and intracellular ATP levels (important for energy) are normalized by the compound. Alterations in the Bcl-2/Bax balance were completely normalized in a number of studies.

A few human trials

There have only been a few human trials with the herb but 150 or so with the constituents, primarily resveratrol (though in China, studies on the effects of the herb in clinical use are very common – they just aren't very accessible).

A study of twenty male, healthy professional basketball players found that a standardized (20 percent trans-resveratrol) formulation of the root significantly reduced plasma levels of TNF-a and IL-6 in those who took it. A similar outcome was found in Brazilian firefighters. Another study with a standardized root formulation (40 mg resveratrol) in weight-normal healthy people found that its use for six weeks "significantly reduced" the generation of reactive oxygen species, the expression of p47 (phox), intranuclear factor kappa B binding, expression of jun-N-terminal kinase-1, inhibitor of kappaB-kinase-beta, phosphotyrosine phosphatase-1B, and suppressor of cytokine signaling-3 in mononuclear cells. TNF-a, IL-6, and C-reactive protein levels also decreased.

Another study, combining knotweed root and hawthorn berry for the treatment of heart disease, found that after six months carotid intima-media thickness and arterial plaque "decreased significantly." MMP levels also decreased.

There have been a number of resveratrol studies on cognition in people. The supplement increases cerebral blood flow and oxygen content of the blood in the brain. Another study with trans-resver-atrol found that the addition of piperine enhanced these effects. Another study with forty-six people found that resveratrol "significantly" enhanced word retention in healthy older adults. Neuroimaging found "significant increases" in hippocampal functional connectivity (FC). FC was also increased between the left posterior hippo-campus and the medial prefrontal cortex . . . this was directly related to increases in word retention scores.

"Robust improvement" of retinal struc-ture and function has occurred with the use of resveratrol in the treatment of macu-lar degeneration.

Resveratrol in healthy people enhanced endothelial gene expression, stabilizing its structure. There was a "significantly lower" mRNA expression of VCAM, ICAM, and IL-8. Another study with resveratrol found that it improves endo-thelial function in adults with metabolic syndrome (a disorder diagnosed by the presence of abdominal obesity, elevated blood pressure, elevated fasting glucose, high serum triglycerides, and low high-density lipoprotein).

There have been numerous studies on the effects of resveratrol on type 2 diabe-tes, all finding that it improves diabetic parameters. Insulin resistance "signifi-cantly" decreases, thus improving glucose sensitivity; glycemic control is improved. There is a "significant" increase in SIRT1 expression and p-AMPK to AMPK expres-sion ratio. Resting metabolic rate increases. A meta-analysis of 11 studies (Liu et al., 2014) with a total of 388 people found that "resveratrol significantly improves glucose control and insulin sensitivity in persons with diabetes."

There have been a number of human trials of the constituent in the treatment of cancer. The constituents seem to be drawn to the sites of cancer cells where they begin stimulating apoptosis (cell death). In one study, the supplement reduced colorectal tumor proliferation by 5 percent. Resvera-trol does seem to help, though the studies vary in their outcomes.

Another area of human trial has been with the constituent's cardiac effects. One study found that left ventricular diastolic function improved "significantly," as did endothelial function. Platelet aggregation decreased, LDL-cholesterol lowered, and unfavorable hemorheological changes were reduced. Another study found that taking resveratrol for a year improved the inflammatory and fibrinolytic status of the people taking it. C-reactive protein "significantly" decreased as did plasminogen activator inhibitor type 1, IL-6, and TNF-a. And yet another trial found that resveratrol (along with calcium fructoborate) alleviated angina pectoris. C-reactive protein levels decreased

There have also been a number of trials of the supplement in the treatment of obesity. Improvements in health status were common.

In vivo studies have found that the herb has significant analgesic and anti-inflam-matory effects in rats. Resveratrol has shown good effects in the treatment of nucleus pulposus-mediated pain. Transver-atrol helps prevent bone loss in ovariec-tomized rats (basically postmenopausal bone loss). Several studies have found that polydatin ameliorates diet-induced devel-opment of insulin resistance and hepatic steatosis in rats (fatty liver disease), primar-ily by inhibiting THF-a and SREBP-1c. The tincture of the plant root enhances innate immune responses in rats. Wound healing in rats is significantly enhanced when a salve of the root is applied topically. (Note: Over the past decade we have seen the rather remarkable healing capacity of the root salves. Anal fissures, which are tough to heal, do so incredibly quickly with the salve. So do all types of fissures and cuts in the fingers, feet, anyplace on the skin.)

The number of in vitro studies are legion, so, just a few. Resveratrol inhibits aggrecanase gene expression in chondrocytes (helping in the treatment of arthritic conditions). It is particularly good at inhibiting MMPs. The impacts of resveratrol on joint inflammation are profound. IL-1B and TNF-a stimulate matrix degrading enzymes such as MMPs and COX-2, through the activation of NF-kB, which is a main cause of cartilage matrix destruction, joint inflammation, RA, and OA. Resveratrol suppresses just those cytokines offering significant protection to chondrocytes. It blocks the activation of caspase-3, PARP cleavage, apoptosis, and accumulation of tumor suppressor gene protein p53 and induces its degradation. It suppresses NF-kB induction and IkB-a degradation. Accompanying in vivo trials found that resveratrol reduces cartilage tissue destruction, protecting against the development of OA. It can protect intervertebral discs from rupture, restoring them to healthy functioning after damage.

Resveratrol itself is a relatively slow-acting radical scavenger. Some of its other constituents (dacaffeoyl quinic acids, DCQAs) are twenty times faster in their actions. This points up, again, the synergistic nature of the whole root when used medicinally.

The herb is also a calcium channel adaptogen, that is, it modulates calcium channel signaling, raising it if it is depressed, decreasing it if it is too high. This is one of its major mechanisms for protecting endothelial cells from disruption. The modulation of calcium channel signaling increases TEER strength in the endothelial cellular bonds, making the junctions better able to withstand insult.

A few older studies, retrieved from the first edition

The herb has been used for a long time in China for the treatment of burns. It has been found in clinical trials to promote scabbing (eschar formation) and inhibit bacterial infections in the damaged skin. The herb reduces exudation, prevents water and electrolyte loss, and hastens wound healing. In one study, sixty people with second and third degree burns were treated with the herb. Ten to 71 percent of the body surface was burned, fifteen were suffering skin infections.

The 2nd degree burns healed in four to six days, third degree in twenty to forty to forty-two days. Other studies have shown similar outcomes. Reduced scarring and less tissue death is common with the use of the herb. This comes in large measure from its powerful angiogenesis modulating (blood-vessel-generating and -controlling) actions.

In burned skin, blood clots (thrombosis) within the capillaries lead to necrosis of the underlying tissues. Vasoconstriction, slow blood flow, and damage to underlying blood vessels are key conditions leading to thrombosis in burned skin. Clinical studies in China using special microscopes found that Japanese knotweed acted as a microcirculatory stimulant. It stimulated the blood flow into burned skin, expanded the blood vessels, stimulated the healing of old blood vessels, and initiated the development of new ones in burned skin.

Japanese knotweed is an angiogenesis *modulator*, that is, it stimulates the formation of new blood vessels and the healing of damaged ones but also stops the development of new vessels and blood flow in areas where they should not occur – specifically in malignant and benign tumor formation. It's a classic tonic herb in this respect, and the only one I am aware of for maintaining the blood vessels themselves. It has, as part of this mode of action, specific modulating and protectant actions on the endothelial cells that line blood vessels.

Polygonum acts as an angiogenesis stimulant in burns, chronic inflammations such as rheumatoid arthritis, debilitating ophthalmic disorders such as diabetic retinopathy and macular degeneration, in brain disorders such as stroke, and in various forms of heart disease such as coronary artery disease and angina. It acts powerfully as an angiogenesis inhibitor in both benign and malignant tumors. It may also come to soon play an important role in the treatment of a certain form of macular degeneration (MD), so-called wet MD, in which the growth of abnormal blood vessels occurs in the eye.

In studies of heart disease, researchers found that resveratrol, one of the primary components of *Polygonum*, protected the cardiovascular system against ischemic-reperfusion injury, promoted vasorelaxation, protected and maintained intact endothelium structures, was antiatherosclerotic, inhibited LDL levels, was an antioxidant, and suppressed platelet aggregation. Chinese researchers found that the constituent polydatin was also broadly active in the cardiovascular system. They noted that it strongly stimulated vasorelaxation throughout the body, including the bronchial capillaries.

Polydatin, they found, is especially effective in treating burn shock. It enhances cardiac and microcirculatory functions. It restores decreased cardiac functions: output, index, and stroke volume index. It restores pulse pressure to normal, decreases the number of adhesive white blood cells, and the amount of open capillaries returns to near normal. The degree of damage to scorched lung tissue was alleviated. It inhibits multiple organ failure from burn shock.

In vivo studies of polydatin and the whole herb on the cardiovascular system found that the herb markedly increases contraction amplitude levels even while lowering blood pressure. Coronary flow is increased while coronary resistance is significantly decreased. Both polydatin and the whole herb enhance cardiac and microcirculatory functions and restore decreased cardiac functions: output, index, and stroke volume index. Resveratrol has also been found to possess similar actions. It inhibits tissue factor expression in vascular cells in response to pathophysiological stimuli, including bacterial, thus reducing inflammation in the heart and vascular tissue. It normalizes vascular endothelium.

The whole herb and its constituent resveratrol are both strong antioxidants. Interestingly, resveratrol seems to be an antioxidant modulator in that it will increase antioxidant action when needed (most of the time) but will lower it in instances where necessary, e.g., in leukemia cells.

Resveratrol is a potent inhibitor of the dioxygenase activity of lopoxygenase. Lipoxygenase is involved in the synthesis of mediators in inflammatory, atherosclerotic, and carcinogenic processes. By its potent inhibition of the dioxygenase activity of lipoxygenase, the herb and its constituent resveratrol have pronounced effects on inflamatory processes such as arthritis, cholesterol levels in the blood, and cancer.

In part this is because resveratrol blocks eicosanoid production. Eicosanoids are powerful, very short-lived substances – quasi-hormones if you will – that are generated from three different fatty acids: dihomogammalinolenic acid, arachidonic acid, and eicosapentaenoic acid (EPA, common in fish and fish oils). Arachadonic acid is the predominate generator in mammals, being stored in cell membranes. Through cyclooxygenase (COX) enzymes, arachadonic acid is transformed into potent proinflammatory and platelet-aggregating thrombxanes and inflammatory prostaglandins. Through lipoxygenase (LOX) enzymes it becomes the potent inflammatory, and white-blood-cell-stimulating, leukotrienes, hepoxillins, and lipoxins. The herb inhibits both LOX and COX pathway inflammations.

Resveratrol specifically inhibits the generation of arachadonic acid metabolites. These metabolites are involved in a number of autoimmune and allergic reactions, in tumor development, and in psoriasis-like conditions of the skin. Not surprisingly, resveratrol causes a dose dependent inhibition of the biosynthesis of prostaglandin E immunoreactive material.

Recent research has found that the plant and its contituent resveratrol interfere with the actions of nuclear factor-kappaB (NF-kB). The herb apparently modulates the actions of NF-kB rather than acting simply as as suppressor. Resveratrol also modulates interferon-gamma-induced neopterin production and tryptophan degradation. It acts as an immunomodulator. It raises or reduces levels when necessary.

As an example of its stimulatory actions, knotweed has been found to raise white blood cell counts during radiation and chemotherapy. It was effective in treating leukopenia or low white blood cell counts (WBC) in sixty-seven people undergoing radiation and chemotherapy for tumors. Of the fifty-nine who had no break in radiation treatment 40 had an increase in WBC of 100/mm3. Of the eight who had a break in radiation treatment seven showed the same increase in WBC.

The herb also stimulates the formation of fibroblasts. These undifferentiated cells migrate to injury sites, especially (in this case) in the skin and collagenous tissues, and undergo alterations to form new cells necessary for healing. In arthritis and psoriasis, the herb reduces inflammation and stimulates the production of new fibroblasts and their translocation to the areas of damage.

Good therapeutic outcomes were found in China in a clinical trials of the herb for one hundred people with rheumatic arthritis, rheumatoid arthritis, lumbar hypertrophy, and osteoarthritis. The herb

has been found to be especially effective in acute inflammatory diseases such as appendicitis, appendiceal abscess, tonsillitis, and pneumonia. In forty-five people with pneumonia who were treated with the herb, body temperature dropped to normal in 1–1.5 days. In 26 cases of acute appendicitis, 14 cases of appendiceal abscess and 4 cases of perforated appendix complicated with peritonitis – all were cured by a decoction of the whole herb. Clinical studies have also found the herb to be effective in acute icteric viral hepatitis, inflammation of the bone and bone marrow, psoriasis, herpes, and cervix erosion.

In cancer studies, plant constituents from knotweed, primarily emodin and its derivatives: citreorosein, emodic acid, physcioin, fallacinol, chrysophanic acid, and rhein were found to be potent oncogene signal transduction inhibitors through inhibiting protein-tyrosine kinase and protein kinase C. Another constituent, resveratrol acts to inhibit tumor growth, metastasis of tumors, and angiogenesis in cancer. Resveratrol inhibits DNA synthesis in cancer cells (specifically Lewis lung carcinoma) and inhibits the binding of vascular endothelial growth factor to human umbilical vein endothelial cells. This constituent of the herb reduces the new blood vessels being created by cancerous clusters eventually cutting off their supply of blood. Resveratrol has been found to be a significant inhibitor of cancer formation in vitro and in vivo for both mouse mammary gland and skin cancers. Dose-dependently, resveratrol inhibited up to 98 percent of skin tumors in mice; the percentage of mice with tumors, at the highest dose range, was lowered by 88 percent.

Resveratrol affects cancer at three stages of its life cycle: initial, promotion, and progression. It inhibits metastasises, cuts off tumor blood supply, and helps normalize cell differentiation. It is strongly antimutagenic.

Uncaria tomentosa, U. Rhynchophylla (cat's claw)

FAMILY: Rubiaceae
COMMON NAMES: Cat's claw, uña de gato, Samento, saventaro.
SPECIES USED: There are 157 various *Uncaria* species around the world but most of these (maybe) are the same as other species just with a different name or else they might be subspecies or maybe they're variants or something, no one seems to know. It's pretty confusing. Taxonomists again.

> *Taxonomist: From two roots, the Ancient Greek taxis, meaning "arrangement" and an old German word for mist, meaning "a haze or film that obscures the vision or blurs perceptions." Thus: "People who create blurry or hazy arrangements that obscure our perceptions."*

Some say there are only 34, or perhaps 40, or maybe even 52 species in the genus. Another authoritative source (using a unique taxonomic addition technique) says there are 29, at minimum, in tropical Asia and Australia, 2 in Africa and Madagascar, 2 in South America, and 12 in China, giving a new total of 46.

All of the various species, however many there are, seem to be used medicinally in their respective regions, and for similar things. The Chinese seem to use all their species (they are often wild harvested by local herbalists who just use what grows near them), but the most focus in Chinese medicine, for millennia, has been on (in order of importance) *Uncaria rhynchophylla, U. macrophylla, U. hirsuta, U. sinensis,* and *U. sessilifructus. U. rhynchophylla* appears to have the longest history of use in the written texts, and it is that species upon which the most research has occurred.

Uncaria tomentosa and *U. guianensis* are (apparently) the only two Central/South American species. Both are used in traditional practice there. *U. tomentosa* has come to prominence from its use in the treatment of Lyme infections. (See the POA/TOA rant for more on this.)

We have focused on the use of (non-TOA-free) *U. tomentosa* over the past decade; it does help in Lyme infections. However . . . we currently consider *U. rhynchophylla* crucial in the treatment of neuroborreliosis. Both species should be used for Lyme infections. Thus . . .

PREFERRED SPECIES: *Uncaria tomentosa* **and** *Uncaria rhynchophylla*.

Parts used

The leaves are often used in China and other Asian countries for a variety
of things, but the predominant part of the plant used is (usually) the inner
bark of the vine. However, the Chinese have found that the *hooks* (aka, the
claw) of some species are exceptionally active medicinals; that is what you
will often get if you buy *Uncaria rhynchophylla*.

Preparation and dosage

The herb has been traditionally used (internally) throughout the world as
powders and infusions. Tinctures are now common as well but are mostly
found in the West.

Please note that the dosages below are only suggested dosages. Reduce
or increase them as needed, depending on personal response and severity
of infection. High dosages of *U. rhynchophylla* tincture (or infusion) may,
in some circumstances, be necessary if the neurological symptoms (e.g.,
seizures) are extreme. They can be lowered as the condition begins to
improve.

Again: some people have only needed to use 1–10 drops of the tinctures
during treatment. Please pay attention to how you respond and adjust
dosages accordingly.

Chinese dosages are predictably high, 10–15 grams at a time (approximately ⅓–½ half an ounce) up to 3x daily. They often (*very briefly*) decoct
the herb. That is, they bring it to a boil, then remove from heat, cover, and
allow to steep. *Boiling too long deactivates many of the constituents.*

Powder

Both species: 1 teaspoon 3–6x daily in juice or water. Start slow and work up,
see below. Dosage can be increased or decreased as necessary.

Capsules

Both species: One to four 500 mg (or close) capsules 3–4x daily for 8–12
months. Begin at lowest dose and increase incrementally every seven days,
i.e., after seven days take 2 capsules 3x daily, then 3 capsules 3x daily, then
4 capsules 3x daily, then 4 capsules 4x daily. Maintain this dosage range

for sixty days minimum. If desired, dosage can then be slowly decreased as Lyme symptoms subside. If symptoms worsen as dosage is lowered, increase dosage. This dosage modification minimizes chances of GI tract upset upon initially taking the herb – see "Side effects" below.

Note: Some people don't need more than 1 capsule 3x daily.

Tincture

(1:5, 60 percent alcohol)

U. tomentosa: ½–1 teaspoon 3–6x daily

U. rhynchophylla: ½ teaspoon–1 tablespoon 3–6x daily.

Note: The alkaloids in the plant are extracted much more easily if the water is on the acid side of the scale rather than the alkaline (alkaloid means alkaline-like). You can add 1 teaspoon of apple cider vinegar to the water, which will make sure it is acidified, when creating the alcohol/water ratio for extraction. Let it all macerate together for a few weeks before decanting.

Infusion (brief decoction)

Four ounces (7 grams) of the herb in 1 quart (1 liter) of water, bring to boil, immediately remove from heat, cover and let steep for one hour (or overnight). Strain, then drink in three divided doses over the day.

Again: this can be increased or decreased as necessary.

Side effects and contraindications

The *Uncaria*s are very safe herbs, however . . .

- Dosages of 3–4 grams of the herb at a time have sometimes caused intestinal upset such as loose stools, diarrhea, and/or abdominal pain. These effects tend to subside as the herb is used over time. Lower the dose of the herb if you experience these side effects. Discontinue use if diarrhea persists longer than three days.
- Because of the immune-stimulating actions, do not use if you have had an organ transplant or are using immunosuppressive drugs. Do not use if you are using blood-thinning medications or are scheduled for surgery. Cease use of the herb ten days prior to any surgery.

- Do not use if you are trying to become pregnant or are pregnant.
- A few sources are insisting that *Uncaria tomentosa* can cause kidney damage with resulting acute renal failure. This is based on a single report from South America (in a woman with systemic lupus); the cause was not definitively determined to be the herb (they guessed).

  Hundreds of thousands of people around the world have used the herb the past few decades and for millennia in South America. There are no reports of this kind of reaction from long-term use. In contrast to this report, Vattimo and da Silva (2011) note, "The results presented emphasize the protective effect of the plant *Uncaria tomentosa* in the renal function of rats submitted to the model of kidney ischemia . . . These data also reinforce that the phytotherapy may be considered a possibility . . . in situations of risk of imminent kidney injury as well." So . . . it is often used for kidney *healing*.
- Because *Uncaria rhynchophylla* is hypotensive, *caution* should be exercised if you have low blood pressure.

Herb/drug interactions

Not many, however . . . regarding *Uncaria tomentosa* . . .

- Do not use with immunosupprcsive herbs such as cyclosporin.
- The herb may potentiate the action of courmadin and other blood-thinning drugs.
- Some sources feel the *Uncaria* constituents are deactivated by stomach acid blockers or antiacids such as Pepto-Bismol. I indicated this in the first edition of the book; I no longer think the data on that is reliable. It may, or it may not, interact with acid blockers.
- Do not take *Uncaria rhynchophylla* if you are on blood-pressure-lowering medications; it may lower blood pressure too far when used in combination with pharmaceutical hypotensives.

PROPERTIES OF THE UNCARIAS

The chemical constituents in the various species differ, sometimes considerably. In consequence, the range of activity is different from species to species. The American species, geographically isolated from the Asian strains for millennia, do have a very different range of activity – they tend to be more immune potentiating than the Asian varieties.

Actions

(*Uncaria tomentosa*): Abortifacient, Analgesic, Anticoagulant, Antidepressant, Antidysenteric, Anti-inflammatory, Antileukemic, Antimutagenic, Antioxidant, Antitumor, Antiulcer, Antiviral, Diuretic, Hypocholesterolemic, Immune Stimulant, Vulnerary (wound healing).

Note: The primary actions of this species are as an anti-inflammatory in arthritic conditions, immune stimulation, and as an antineoplastic in the treatment of cancer.

(*Uncaria rhynchophylla*): Antibacterial, Anticonvulsant (anti-epileptic/antiseizure), Anti-inflammatory, Antiviral, Hypotensive, Neurological protectant, Sedative, Smooth muscle relaxant, Systemic tonic.

Note: The primary actions of this species is as a hypotensive (high blood pressure), anti-inflammatory (neurological), neurological protectant (antiepileptic/antiseizure).

Active Against

Uncaria species are not potent antimicrobial herbs. They have rarely been tested as such; still the various species are active against a few bacterial organisms. Those noted include: *Bacillus cereus, B.subtilis, Candida albicans, Enterococcus faecalis, Escherichia coli., Klebsiella pneumoniae, Staphylococcus aureus,* and *S. epidermina. Uncaria tomentosa* is active against dengue fever virus, vesicular stomatitis virus, and rhinoviruses. *U. rhynchophylla* is active against hepatitis B virus, HIV, and influenza A viruses. All the studies appear to be in vitro.

Use to Treat

Borrelial infections, arthritis, low immune function, neurological impairments, seizures, high blood pressure.

Habitat and appearance

Cat's claw likes the jungle. It is a woody vine (or liana), sometimes of massive size and length, that twists around trees, climbing up into the overstory in search of sunlight. It takes its name from the protruding, hook-like, usually paired, recurved thorns on the vines that it uses to climb the trees.

Of the two primary South American species, *U. guianensis* grows throughout Peru, Bolivia, Brazil, Guyana, Paraguay, Trinidad, and Venezuela. *U. tomentosa* has a much wider range: Colombia, Ecuador, Trinidad, Guyana, Venezuela, Panama, Suriname, Guatemala, and Costa Rica.

Cultivation and collection

In some regions of China, the plants are reportedly wild harvested *and* intentionally grown for medicinal use – though I have no information on how to cultivate them (no one seems to talk about that part of it much; most people just wild harvest the plants).

In South and Central America, the inner bark is normally used, collected when needed. The Chinese use the inner bark, the hooks themselves, and the leaves, all for various conditions in various formulations.

Plant chemistry

There is a great deal of overlap between the species' chemical constituents, especially in Asia. The Asian species have been in close contact for a long time; the South American species were isolated long ago. Nevertheless, the South American species do have some constituent overlap with the Asians. Still, the constituents and their synergistic dynamics appear to be very different in the two groups. Some constituents don't appear in the others at all. As is usual, the constituents among all the species worldwide vary depending on species, location, time of year.

Uncaria tomentosa: To date cat's claw has been found to possess seventeen different alkaloids, quinovic acid glycosides, flavonoids, sterol fractions, and numerous other compounds. These include: oxindole alkaloids (both pentacyclic and tetracyclic), beta-sitosterol, catechins, tannins, procyanidins, stigmasterol, campesterol, carboxy alkyl esters, ajmalicine, akuammigine, chlorogenic acid, cinchonain, coryantheine, corynoxeine, daucosterol, epicatichin, harman, hirsuteine, hirsutine, iso-pteropodine, pteropodine, loganic acid, lyaloside, mitraphylline, isomitraphylline, oleanolic acid, plamitoleic acid, pteropodine, rhynchophylline, iso-rhynchophylline (and their N-oxides), rutin, corynoxeine, iso-corynoxeine, rotundifoline, and iso-rotundifoline, speciophylline, strictosidines, uncarines A-F, and vaccenic acid.

Uncaria rhynchophylla: (From lowest to the highest concentration in the plant) 22-O-B-D-glucopyranosul isocorynoxeninic acid; its isomer; 18, 19-dehydrocorynoxinic acid; hyperoside; mitraphyllic acid 22-B-D-glycopyranosyl ester;   18,   19-dehydrocorynoxinic acid B; cadambine; 3a-dihydrocadambine; 3B-isodihydro-cadambine; 11-hydroxy-2-O-D-glucopyranosyl vincoside lactam; isocorynoxeine, strictosidine; isorhynchophylline; corynoxeine; corynoxine; corynoxeine-NO; cornoxine B; corynoxine

THE QUINOVIC ACID CONTROVERSEY

A rumor has spread that the quinovic acids in cat's claw are, at root, the same as quinolone antibiotics. The rumors say that this is why cat's claw is effective against Lyme spiro-chetes. Concern has been generated by this assertion because quinolone antibiotics, in some instances, can cause severe inflammation in tendons. So, the word is that cat's claw can cause tendonitis, resulting in tissue destruction over time. *This is all completely untrue.* The quinovic acids in cat's claw are structurally different than quinolone antibiotics. Molecularly, they are not the same at all; they do not do the same things.

B; isocorynoxine B; isocorynoxeine-NO; mitragynine; rhynchophylline; rhynchophylline-NO; isohyrhnchophylline-NO; isomer of rhynchophylline; dihydrocorynantheine; raubasine; strictosamide; yohimbine; geissoschizine methyl ether; hirsuteine; vincoside lactam; hirsutine.

Note: While *Uncaria tomentosa* does contain some of the same alkaloids as *U. rhynchophylla*, specifically hirsutine, rhynchophylline, and iso-rhynchophylline; the quantities vary considerably when compared to *U. rhynchophylla*. It is these compounds that exert the most potent neurological effects.

Traditional uses of *Uncaria*

Although related *Uncaria* species have been used in both India and China for millennia, the South American species, especially *Uncaria tomentosa*, appear to possess more specific and potent actions for the immune system, on inflammatory conditions, and in the treatment of cancer. It is these South American species that have been primarily used in treating Lyme infections.

Both South American *Uncaria* species have been known to indigenous peoples in the Amazon for millennia. The Aguaruna, Ashaninka, Casibo, Conibo, and Shipibo tribes of Peru have used it extensively for treating asthma, inflammations of the urinary tract, arthritis, rheumatism, bone pain, child birth recovery, curing deep wounds, general inflammation, gastric ulcers, treating tumors, diabetes, fevers, cirrhosis, dysentery, general disease prevention, prostatitis, shingles, skin disorders, and cancer, and as a kidney cleanser (again refuting it as damaging to kidneys), and, in a highly concentrated form, as a contraceptive.

Ayurveda

A related species, *Uncaria gambier*, is used in traditional Ayurvedic practice as a bitter astringent.

Traditional Chinese medicine

Five related species (most commonly *Uncaria rhynchophylla*) have been used in TCM for millennia. Other, similar species are used throughout China by traditional healers. (Ten of the Chinese species are commercially available in the country.) They are primarily used for healing damage to the central nervous system and correcting its symptoms (epilepsy, seizures, tremors, convulsions), for dizziness and vertigo, to lower blood pressure, for eclampsia, for fever and headache, and for liver disease.

Western botanic practice

The genus is of recent introduction to the Western medical world. The plant was unknown to the Eclectics, the great American botanical practitioners of the late nineteenth century. The first nonindigenous accounts of the plant and its medicinal actions seem to have begun in the 1930s with a young Bavarian immigrant to Peru, Arturo Brell. Brell treated hundreds of people for cancer with the herb and in the early 1960s, Brell shared much of his knowledge with an American professor, Eugene Whitworth. It was after Brell's death in 1974 that knowledge of the plant began to seriously engage with Western botanic practice, primarily from the work of the Austrian, Klaus Keplinger. Since the 1990s, it has found increasing use in the treatment of Lyme disease, cancer, AIDS, immune disorders, and arthritis.

Scientific research

Here is a brief look at some of the dynamics of both the *Uncaria* species recommended for use in Lyme infections:

Uncaria rhynchophylla: The herb has had extensive clinical use in China for millennia. There has been a great deal of in vitro and in vivo study on its actions; still, there have not been very many human clinical trials. I could find three in the cnki (Chinese) database. All were in the treatment of hypertension, either the herb, alone or in combination with others. Outcomes were very good.

There are a few papers that explore the use of the herb in traditional Japanese medicine for neurological problems (e.g., Tanaka and Sakiyama, 2013, and Matsumoto, et al, 2013). It is commonly used, with good results, in the treatment of dementia (Matsumoto); the Tanaka paper looked at three clinical cases of emotional and behavioral disorders in children (~11 years of age). The herb worked very well.

Again, my primary interest here is the herb's impacts on neurological impairments. Here is a brief review of some of the scores of relevant studies . . .

In vivo studies: The herb extract is strongly protective against excitotoxicity induced by N-Methyl-D-Aspartate in the rat hippocampus. The constituent rhynchophylline is highly neuroprotective against ischemic brain injury in rats. Treatment ameliorated neurological deficits, infarct volume, and brain edema. Both the herb and isorhynchophylline "significantly" improves the learning and memory impairments (including restoring spatial learning and memory) induced by D-galactose in mice. Levels of prostaglandin E2, nitric oxide, COX-2, and NF-*k*B all declined in the rat brains. The whole herb "significantly" increased the levels of acetylcholine and glutathione in the rat brains and was strongly protective of neurons against damage.

The herb reduces microglia activation, nNOS, iNOS, and apoptosis in neurons. Isorhynchophylline is also strongly protective of the heart against cardiac arrhythmias in rats and guinea pigs. Both isorhynchophylline and rhynchophylline reduce the inflammatory cytokines (such as TNF-a and IL-1beta) that are upregulated during brain inflammation and reduce the numbers of overactive microglia. It alters ERK and p38 MAPKs pathways and inhibits the degradation of I*k*B -alpha.

Both the whole herb and the constituent rhynchophylline improved kainic acid-induced epileptic seizures in rats by downregulating chemically increased levels of IL-1-beta and BDNF. The primary effects were found in the cerebral cortex and hippocampus. The herb attenuated glial cell proliferation, reduced neuronal death, and inhibited seizures.

The constituent geissoschizine methyl ester (GM) improves remyelination after chemically induced demyelination in the medial prefrontal cortex of adult mice. The compound "significantly" increased the numbers of mature oligodendrocytes (important in neuroborreliosis) and healthy microglia. It strongly reduced the myelin basic protein immunoreactivity in the brain (again, crucial during neuroborreliosis). GM was also found, by Japanese researchers, to ameliorate aggression and increase sociability in neurologically stress-damaged mice. (The actions appear to be on the amygdala – a part of the brain to which the plant constituents specifically adhere.) The compound is potently effective for activating serotonin (5-HT) receptors in the brain.

A number of other, recently discovered, compounds (not included in the list above, too many numbers to type) ameliorated scopolamine-induced memory impairment in vivo. The hook of the plant "significantly" reduced Parkinson-like effects in 6-OHDA-induced neurotoxicity in rats. Caspase-3 levels was reduced; neuronal loss was abated. The whole herb inhibits the development of atopic dermatitis-like skin lesions in mice.

In vitro studies have found that rhynchophylline is strongly protective of rat hippocampal neurons. The combination of the hook of the herb and licorice root protected neurons from the toxic effects of B-amyloid proteins.

Hirsutine, another constituent, inhibits inflammation-mediated neurotoxicity and microglial activation in the rat brain, strongly protecting hippocampal neurons from damage. Numerous inflammatory cytokines are downregulated. Hirsutine is also strongly protective of cardiomyocytes experiencing hypoxia.

Rhynchophylline protects cultured rat neurons against methamphetamine cytotoxicity. It also attenuates LPS-induced proinflammatory responses in primary microglia by downregulating MAPK/NF-kB signaling pathways.

In short, the herb and its compounds (which act synergistically) are strongly protective of neurons in the cortex and hippocampus (and act strongly in other parts of the brain as well, see below), downregulate inflammatory cytokines that could damage them, reduce microglial overactivation, inhibit inflammatory pathways, enhance remyelination of neurons, stimulate the regrowth of oligodendrocytes, and are strongly protective of the heart. (The herb is often combined with *Gastrodia elata* in the treatment of seizures and other neurological conditions; they work synergistically with each other. *Gastrodia* has a similar range of actions for such conditions; it's a good combination.)

The pharmacokinetics of the herb and its constituents are very good. Rhynchophylline can be detected in the brain and plasma from fifteen minutes to six hours after ingestion. It crosses the BBB just fine. Other studies have found that corynoxeine, isocornoxeine, isorhynchophylline, hirsutine, hirsuteine, and GM are all strongly present in both plasma and the brain as well. The constituents, e.g., GM, have specific binding sites in the frontal cortex, prefrontal cortical region (prelimbic cortex), hippocampus, caudate putamen, amygdala, central medial thalamic nucleus, dorsal raphe nucleus, and the cerebellum. They provide protection from inflammation in all these areas. You can't find a more specific herb for treating the neurological damage that occurs during neuroborreliosis.

Uncaria tomentosa: The main reason this species of cat's claw has come to be used in the treatment of Lyme infections is a single study with a number of people with Lyme patients that found the herb significantly alleviated symptoms of the disease; 85 percent of the patients, retested later, were found negative for Lyme infection. (The relevant study is Cowden et al. Pilot study of pentacyclic alkaloid-chemotype of *Uncaria tomentosa* for the treatment of

Lyme disease, December 28, 2002 - March 22, 2003. Presented at the International Symposium for Natural Treatment of Intracellular Micro Organisms, (March 29, 2003) Munich, Germany.)

This study is widely cited; however, despite our experience that this *Uncaria* does help in the treatment of Lyme infections, the study is seriously flawed.

Specifically: Twenty-eight patients with advanced chronic Lyme borreliosis (all of whom had previously used antibiotics) were enrolled in the study. All patients tested positive using western blot. Half were placed in a control group that used conventional antibiotic therapy during the course of the study. Three improved, three worsened, eight showed no change in their condition. The other fourteen patients received alternative treatments, one dropped out. Of the thirteen patients who used cat's claw, 85 percent tested negative for *Borrelia* after six months on the full alternative protocol, and three-quarters of all the patients reported improvements in nine parameters: fatigue, stomach pain, joint pain, memory problems, muscle pain, cisual disturbances, emotional irritability, peripheral neuropathy, and insomnia. This sounds great, but on examination a number of things are problematical with the study.

Of importance: The people in the alternative treatment group used a variety of treatment approaches, not just the (TOA-free) herb. Specifically: A blood-type diet, enzymes with meals, enzymes between meals, vitamin and mineral supplements, laser detoxification, light beam generator, skin brushing, bath detoxification, laughter, prayer, and emotional release.

The diets, enzymes, and vitamin and mineral supplements are not defined as to type or dosage. Laser and bath detoxification, and so on, are, as well, not defined either. The herb's dosage is not revealed. The study lasted six months; a preliminary report was given at the International conference in Germany after three months. In spite of diligent literature searches and emails to the study's initiator (in 2004), I never received a response, nor was able to find a full report of the study or an answer to a number of questions (e.g., dosage). A literature search in 2015 turns up a copy of the "study," the same one I found eleven years ago. However, it isn't really a study, not in any analytical or research sense of the term. It is really only a list of outcomes from three (perhaps four) of the people who used the herb, along with some testimonials. ("Studies" like this are what give herbal medicine a bad name.)

Other human studies with the herb: Half the male volunteers (numbers not stated) given a pneumonococcal vaccine also took a 350 mg capsule of C-MEd-100 2x daily for two months. C-Med-100 is a water-soluble extract of whole plant *Uncaria tomentosa* standardized to at least 8 percent carboxy alky esters. At five months the volunteers were retested. A statistically significant immune enhancement was found in those taking the herb: elevation in lymphocute/neutrophil ratios in peripheral blood and a reduced decay in the twelve serotype antibody titre responses to pheumonococcal vaccination.

Twelve human volunteers were separated into three groups, age and gender matched. One group took a 250 mg tablet daily of C-MEd-100, the second took a 350 mg tablet daily, the third group took nothing – for eight weeks. DNA repair after induction of DNA damage by a dose of hydrogen peroxide was tested. There was a statistically significant decrease of DNA damage and a concomitant increase in DNA repair in the supplement groups. There was also an increase in PHA-induced lymphocyte proliferation in the treated groups.

Thirteen people who were HIV positive and who refused to take conventional pharmaceuticals were dosed with 20 mg of cat's claw daily for five months. White blood cell counts were significantly increased.

And another study using cat's claw with AZT found that outcomes were better that with either alone, helping to reduce symptoms in AIDS patients.

Of forty-five people with osteoarthritis of the knee, thirty were treated with freeze-dried *Uncaria guianensis*, the remaining fifteen with a placebo over four weeks. Pain, medical, and subject assessment scores and adverse effects were collected at weeks one, two, and four. The antioxidant and ROS-scavenging action of the plant was checked as well as its inhibition of TNF-alpha and prostaglandin E2 production. No subjective or physiological side effects were found. Pain associated with activity, medical, and patient assessment scores were all significantly reduced. TN- alpha and PGE2 levels reduced, TNF-alpha the most.

A randomized, double-blind, placebo controlled fifty-two week, two phase trial of a POA chemotype *Uncaria* extract with forty people was conducted to assess its impacts in the treatment of rheumatoid arthritis. During the first phase, patients were treated with the extract or a placebo; the final twenty-eight weeks, all people received the plant extract. There was a significant reduction of pain compared to the placebo; the number of swollen and painful joints decreased.

Uncaria tomentosa extracts were used in the treatment of 273 people with different types of immune disturbances, including: secondary immune deficiency after low-dose radiation exposure (84), immune deficiency due to chronic bacterial or viral infection (92), allergic reactions (55), and acute lymphoid leukemia and lymphatic leukemia (10). In those with low-dose radiation exposure low CD4/CD8 ratios and suppresses NK cell activity improved as were CD3-CD16+ cell counts. TCR/CD3, HLA-DR, CD4 expression were all elevated after *Uncaria* use. Monocytes exhibited integrins ICAM-1 and LFA3 expression and CD4+ cells - LFA1.

The treatment of patients with immune deficiency due to chronic bacterial and viral infections found that the plant stimulated a normalization of immune response. There was a redistribution of the cells in the CD8+ subset, an increase of antigen-dependent cytotoxic effector cells, and an increase in CD56 and CD57 expression on natural killer cells. Humoral immunity showed a decrease of previously elevated B-cell (CD+19 sIgM+) counts. The quantity of differentiated cells expressing surface immunoglobulin G and IgG serum concentration increased. There was a decrease in IL-2 receptor, transferrin, and HLA-DR expression. Phagocytosis was enhanced.

In vivo studies: Water extracts of *Uncaria tomentosa* (C-Med-100) were used to treat rats with chemotherapy-induced leukenopenia. Neupogen-treated and untreated rats served as comparatives and controls respectively. Herb-treated rats received *Uncaria* for sixteen days; Neupogen (a pharmaceutical granulocyte colony stimulator) was given for 10 days. Both the C-MEd-100 and Neupogen groups recovered significantly sooner than the untreated group.

Calves treated with whole herb *Uncaria tomentosa* (4,200 mg per day for eight days) were examined (in relation to controls who received placebo) for changes in cellular immunity. The percentage of phagocytes in peripheral blood, their phagocytic index, and the values of random migration of meutrophils were significantly higher in treated calves than controls. There was a significant increase in the total number and percentage of CD2-T lymphocytes and CD4+T helper lymphocytes and a decrease in WC4+ B lymphocytes, PMNL, and MID cells.

Another study examined the effects of *U. tomentosa* on experimentally induced pneumonia in calves. Calves were separated into two groups. One received placebo, the other 3,600 mg per day for seventeen days of a whole herb extract. In the treated group, there was a significant increase in the total number and percentage of CD2+ and CD4+ cells. Temperature in the treated calves was lower. Researchers noted a "distinct inhibiting" of the synthesis and release of proinflammatory arachidonate (eicosanoids) and found it an effective modulator of the inflammatory process in the lungs of calves.

Both a freeze-dried water extract and a hydroalcoholic extract *of U. tomentosa* were tested for anti-inflammatory actions against induced inflammation in rats. The hydroalcoholic extract was found more potent; NF-kappa B was inhibited.

U. tomentosa has been found to significantly reduce edema in arthritic rats. Its anti-inflammatory effects are slightly better than the pharmaceutical drug indomethacine. The whole herb is significantly better as an anti-inflamatory than its isolated constituents. As usual, the whole plant's constituents posseses synergistic actions.

Studies with spontaneously hypertensive rats treated with *Uncaria* extracts found that the herb had a "protective effect for the endothelium against the influence of hypertension." Endothelium-dependent vasoconstriction decreased significantly in the treated group vs controls.

In vitro studies: A significant number of studies have found that *Uncaria* extracts inhibit human cancer cell proliferation and induce apoptosis. This has been borne out in decades of successful use of the herb in clinical practice for various forms of cancer.

The plant has been found to possess immunomodulatory activity. It modulates the immunochemical pathways induced by IFN-gamma, is a remarkably potent inhibitor of TNF-alpha production, is an effective antioxidant, stimulates interleukin-1 and -6 production in alveolar macrophages, and stimulates phagocytosis. The plant's quinovic alkaloids have shown antiviral activity, and broad antiinflammatory actions.

THE TOA/POA CONTROVERSY

If you begin looking into *Uncaria tomentosa* for the treatment of Lyme infections, you will soon come across "TOA-free Cat's Claw." There is, even after a decade, a fair amount of grandiosity about this product: "Only TOA-free cat's claw will work," "The TOAs will hurt you," "Don't use anything else." Unfortunately, this is just not accurate.

A review of the literature shows that a single series of *in vitro* studies – that is, in the laboratory only – found that the TOAs in a *very uniquely* prepared solution of isolated *Uncaria tomemtosa* constituents, in some circumstances, had negative impacts on POA activity.

Specifically what occurred was this: a blend of pentacyclic oxidole alkaloids (POAs – 28 percent pteropodine, 57 percent isopteropodine, 4 percent speciophyline, 6 percent uncarine F, 2 percent mitraphylline, and 3 percent isomitraphylline) was extracted from the herb and placed along with human endothelial cells in RPMI-1640 medium. This medium contained fetal calf serum, glutamine, penicillin, and streptomycin. This solution was allowed to stand for seven days to produce supernatants – a liquid layer floating above the solid matter – which was then filtered and stored for use in testing. This liquid was used to determine the activity of the POAs on a number of things, such as endothelial cells, and normal B and T lymphocytes. One of the tests run with this supernatant found that it caused "a yet to be identified factor" to be produced by endothelial cells which caused an increase in "normal resting or weakly activated human B and T lymphocytes. In contrast, the proliferation of B and T lymphocytes and Raji and Jurkat cell lines is significantly inhibited."

A supernatant of tetracyclic oxidole alkaloids (TOAs) was also prepared along the same lines as the POAs, containing 67 percent rhynchophylline and 33 percent isorhynchophylline (*very* high quantities btw). It was found that this supernatant "acted antagonistically" on the release of the "as yet to be identified factor" and, in a dose dependent manner, reduced the effect of the POA supernatant in Raji and Jurkat cells.

Raji cells are human B lymphocytes (Burkitt's lymphoma), Jurkat cells are leukaemic cells. To make an important point . . . it is the rhynchophylline and isorhynchophylline that are some of the strongest protectors of the brain and central nervous system in *Uncaria rhynchophylla*. Removing these from any *Uncaria* is simply idiotic. They make the TOA-free forms useless for treating neuroborreliosis.

There are only two papers that were published outlining this same series of tests; both are by very nearly the same authors. (See Wurm, Kacani, Laus, Keplinger, and Dierich, 1998, *and* Keplinger, Laus, Wurm, Dierich, and Teppner, 1999) The tests themselves were cited in three other publications (e.g., Reinhard, 1999). It is these five papers that are cited over and over as a justification for the statement that TOAs inactivate POAs.

No other researchers have found these kind of results; the tests themselves have never been duplicated by another laboratory. And they alone do not justify the statement that TOAs inactivate POAs. The TOA supernatant acted to inhibit the release of the unknown lymphocyte proliferation factor and reduced the POA supernatant inhibition of two *cancer* cell lines. That is all the studies (appear to) show in any event. This is a far cry from showing that TOAs inhibit the action of POAs in the human body.

As well, the TOAs used in the study are incomplete to the plant. Only two were used: rynchophylline and isorynchophylline. The plant also contains their N-oxides, corynoxeine, isocorynoxeine, rotundifoline, and isorotundifoline.) Scores of other studies in five countries, including the research for five patents, have shown that the whole herb (which naturally includes TOA alkaloids) stimulates the immune response. Other studies have found that the TOA alkaloid isorhynchophaylline, which naturally occurs in the plant and which was one of those whose supernatant was tested, stimulates immune function, specifically phagocytosis.

None of the many other researchers working with the plant for the past twenty-five years in scores of studies found that the naturally occurring TOA alkaloids inactivated the naturally occurring POAs. The majority of the studies on the plant have used the whole herb or other proprietary formulations that contain both TOAs and POAs.

For example, researchers using a water extract that does contain both TOA and POA alkaloids tested the growth inhibitory effects of the *Uncaria tomemtosa* preparation C-MED-100 on a human EBV-transformed B lymphoma cell line, i.e., Raji cells. This is the same cell line discussed earlier. These researchers (Sheng et al., 1998) found however that the "Raji cells were strongly suppressed in the presence of the C-Med-100."

Another study (Winkler et al., 2003) examined the effects of both TOA and POA and combined TOA/POA formulations as well as the whole herb. The authors note, "In our study, mixtures of POA and of TOA had similar influences on neopterin production and on tryptophan degradation. This finding contrasts earlier data showing a difference of POA and TOA [activity]." Specifically that the TOAs inhibited the function of POAs.

Of additional concern, for me, is that two of the authors of the TOA/POA studies (that led to the creation of TOA-free extracts) hold a patent on a process for removing TOAs from POAs and apparently have, as far as I can tell, an interest in the company that makes TOA-free cat's claw. (I did write and ask a number of years ago; I received no response.)

Without extensive in vivo studies and other laboratory replication of this original study *and the finding that it applies broadly in the body*, it is improper to determine that TOAs inactivate POAs in cat's claw. The evidence from other studies and millennia of use indicates that the assertion is incorrect.

The herb itself, without any fiddling around, will work exceptionally well, especially for Lyme disease. In part this is because the two different types of oxindole alkaloids offer a two-pronged impact on Lyme symptoms. The POAs enhance immune function, mainly the immunologic system cells, particularly those responsible for nonspecific and cellular immunity. The TOAs mainly affect the central and peripheral nervous system, helping with the neurological impacts of Lyme infection. *TOAs and POAs are both important in Lyme infection.* There is no need to seek out a TOA-free extract. You will, as well, save a great deal of money. The TOA-free extracts are, compared to the natural herb, exceptionally expensive.

Andrographis paniculata

FAMILY: The Acanthaceae, which comprises 240 genera and includes some 2,200 species spread throughout Asia, Indo-Malayasia, Africa, South and Central America.

COMMON NAMES: English: green chiretta (as opposed to sweet chiretta, which is another plant entirely), or andrographis (its usual English name in Western botanic practice). Also: chuan xin lian (TCM, China), senshinren (Japan), ch'onsimyon (Korea), kalmegh (ayurveda, Bengali), maha-tita (northeastern India), bhui-neem (India, because of its similar appearance, taste and uses to neem), karyat (Hindi), quasabhuva (Arabic), kariyatu (Gujarathi), nelaberu (Kannada), nelacepu or kiriyattu (Malayalam), oli-kiryata (Marathi), bhui-nimba (Oriya), naine-havandi (Persian), kalmegha or bhunimba (Sanskrit), nilavembu (Tamil and Telugu), and probably a whole lot more.

SPECIES USED: Well here we go again, there are 19 or maybe 44 species on the genus; no one seems to know though there is a lot of name calling going on. (We need a taxonomommy to sort out all this sibling conflict.) Nevertheless, for the heck of it, let's just use *Andrographis paniculata*.

Parts used

The aboveground, or aerial, parts of the plant (stems, leaves, flowers) are considered the most medicinally active, though the root is sometimes (rarely) used in traditional practice.

Preparation and dosage

This herb is known as "King of Bitters" or, sometimes, "Bile of the Earth." I would not recommend taking it as a tincture (unless you are really, really tough; I'm not, I cried). I would recommend capsules (rather than tablets, they taste just as vile). There is a decent brand, as an example, that offers 1,200 mgs (in a 2-capsule dose) of the herb. Most formulations are standardized for 10 percent andrographolides, I am not sure this is absolutely necessary, nevertheless, that's what's out there.

Please read carefully: There is one really nasty side effect to the herb; it can cause a massive course of hives (I will go into this in a bit). This only happens in about 1 percent of the people who use the herb but just to make sure . . .

Begin with a small dose and work up. I would recommend 600 mg (one capsule of the 1,200 mg formulation, for example) 3x daily to begin with, for one week. Then, if there are no side effects, increase the dose to 2 capsules 3x daily.

The herb should be taken for 8-12 months in the treatment of Lyme or until the disease is either under control or eradicated. You can reduce the dose, gradually, as you begin to feel better.

In traditional Chinese medicine 9–15 grams (⅓–½ an ounce) of the nonstandardized herb is used, usually in capsules. In India ½ to 1 fluid ounce of the infusion is used for those who can stand the taste. The concentrated juice of the fresh plant is also used in India (10–60 minims) as is the tincture (½–1 fluid drachm) – tough people. Traditional use in India emphasizes the expressed juice of the plant and water infusions – really tough people. The whole plant is often blended with other herbs (e.g., cardamom) for use in GI tract disturbances and, I suspect, to help them endure the taste.

Side effects and contraindications

- Allergic reactions. *Important:* When the first edition of this book was written, a depth look at both the historical record and every journal paper I could find revealed only two cases of allergic reactions in India, nothing serious. It was a shock then, when so many people began using the herb for Lyme infections to find that a number of people experienced rather severe hives from use of the herb. (They often went to the hospital where they were given calamine lotion and told that herbs are dangerous; neither the doctors' attitudes nor the calamine lotion helped much.)

  Finally, in 2014, a group of researchers in Thailand, where the herb is commonly used, took a serious look at allergic reactions to the herb. During the period from 2001 to 2012 they identified 243 allergic response categories in 106 people to oral intake of the herb. (To put this in perspective: that's about *ten* people per year, out of thousands, that had negative reactions to the herb.) Eighteen people were hospitalized; there were no fatalities. Reactions fell into the following categories:

1. 126 various types of skin and appendage disorders: urticaria (37), maculo-papular rash (31), rash (18), pruritis (16), erythematous rash (8), exfoliative dermatitis (1), skin exfoliation (2), Steven Johnson syndrome (1), excessive sweating (2), and one each of: acute generalized exanthematous pustulosis, bullous eruption, eosinophilia, fixed eruption, stomatitis ulcerative, allergic purpura, and generalized flushing.

2. 57 various types of a "general body" disorder: face edema (19), angioedema (4), anaphylactic shock (5), anaphylactic reaction (4), fatigue (6), mouth edema (5), fever (3), chest pain (3), oedema (2), periorbital oedema (1), back pain (1), peripheral oedema (3), and pain (1).

3. 22 various types of GI tract disorders: nausea (8), vomiting (4), abdominal pain (2), diarrhea (1), general GI tract disorder (1), dry lips or mouth (2), and melaena (1).

4. 15 various respiratory problems: Dyspnoea (6), coughing (6), bronchospasm (2), and increased sputum (1).

5. 15 types of central nervous system or behavioral effects: anorexia (4), somnolence (3), insomnia (1), headache (3) dysaethesia (2), and dizziness (2).

6. 8 varieties of various other reactions: muscle weakness (2), paralysis (1), vasculitis (1), hepatitis (1), urinary frequency (1), and local anaesthesia or anaesthesia of the mouth (2).

Our experience is that skin problems predominate among those who experience side effects. Please pay close attention to your responses to this herb. It is, in general, very safe. However, if you are one of the minority that has allergies to the herb, it can be unpleasant. Unfortunately, due to allergic reactions, the FDA in the US is considering banning the herb but has (thankfully) determined that more studies are necessary.

- *Abortifacient*: not to be used during pregnancy.
- *Contraceptive*: inhibits progesterone production, should not to be used by women when trying to conceive.
- The constituent, andrographolide, when injected as a pure compound (as it is sometimes in China) has induced acute kidney injury (which does not happen with the plant). So don't inject it.
- May cause mild constipation.
- Should not be used in active gall bladder disease.
- Very large doses may cause minor gastric upset.
- One in vivo study with rats found that the herb affected sperm production. Sperm production resumed upon discontinuance of the herb – further studies did not confirm this result but because it exists in the literature the herb is sometimes listed as antiandrogenic or spermatogenic. (It's not.)
- **If allergic responses occur, reduce dosage or discontinue the herb.**

Herb drug interactions
- *Andrographis* may have a synergistic effect with isoniazid, a pharmaceutical used for tuberculosis.
- It may increase clearance rate for theophylline.
- It does stimulate immune function, it may be contraindicated for use with immunodepressants (e.g., organ transplant drugs).

Habitat and appearance
Andrographis paniculata is native to Taiwan, China, India, various subtropical and tropical areas throughout Asia, Southeast Asia, a number of Caribbean islands, the West Indies, and a bit in the Americas. It is tremendously abundant in southern Asia and Southeast Asia, including India, Java, Sri Lanka, Pakistan, and Indonesia. It's heavily cultivated in India, China, Thailand, Brunei, Indonesia, Jamaica, Barbados, the Bahamas, Hong Kong, southern Nigeria, and a bit in the Americas.

A. *panniculata* is an annual, branching, erect herbaceous plant, growing up to three feet in height. The herb looks like your typical weedy-type bushy plant with spear-like (lanceolate) leaves. It prefers moist, warmish places, tropical habitats essentially, in which to grow. Still, it is a bit of an invasive once it gets going. It shows up, all on its own, in disturbed areas such as waste land, roadsides, and farms.

PROPERTIES OF *ANDROGRAPHIS PANICULATA*

Actions
Analgesic, Antibacterial, Antidiabetic, Antidiarrheal, Anti-inflammatory, Antifilarial, Antimalarial, Antispirochetal, Antithrombotic, Antitumor, Antiviral, Cardioprotective, Choleretic, Depurative, Expectorant, Hepatoprotective, Hypoglycemic, Immune stimulant, Sedative, Thrombolytic, Vermicidal.

Active Against
Bacillus lichenformis, Bacilus subtilis, Bordetella pertussis, Chlamydia trachomatis (strongly so, both intra- and extracellular forms), dengue fever virus serotype 1 (moderate), *E. coli* (including enterohemorrhagic), *Enterococcus faecalis,* Epstein-Barr virus, Herpes simplex type 1, HIV, human papillomavirus type 16, Influenza A, *Klebsiella pneumonia, Legionella pneumophila, Leishmania infantum, Leptospira* (moderate), *Mycobacerium smegmatis, Mycobacterium tuberculosis, Neisseria meningitis* (mildly so), *Plasmodium falciparum* (very good), *Plasmodium berghei, Proteus vulgaris, Pseudomonas aeruginosa* (mildly so), *Salmonella typhi, Salmonella typhimurium, Shigella boydii, Shigella sonnei, Staphylococcus aureus* (strongly so), *Streptococcus pyogenes, S. thermophilus, Trypanosoma brucei, Trypanosoma cruzi, Vibrio alginolyteus, Vibrio*

cholera, and various flaviviruses and pestiviruses. Studies for antimicrobial activity were in vitro and in vivo; clinically the herb has been used for millennia for treating malaria, leptospirosis, and other parasitic diseases.

Functions in Lyme Disease
Andrographis is the best antispirochetal for borrelial infections (at this point in time). It is moderately antispirochetal (people have reported Herxheimer reactions from use of the herb – most commonly during infection with *Borrelia miyamotoi*, which is very susceptible to this plant). The herb enhances immune function, protects heart muscle, is antiinflammatory (helping with arthritic symptoms), crosses the blood-brain barrier where it is active as both an antispirochetal and calming agent, enhances liver function, and protects the liver.

It is a widely systemic herb, making it good for these kinds of infections. It also has some decent effects (not as good as *Uncaria rhynchophylla*) in helping correct inflammation-mediated neurodegeneration in the brain. It does inhibit a number of the cytokines that become active during Lyme infections: E-selectin, TNF-a, IL-6, and IL-8.

Cultivation and collection

The plant is normally grown from seeds, apparently easily. It prefers moist and warmish climates (no snow and mild winters) with good sun access though it can grow pretty well in a bit of shade. *Andrographis* cultivates comfortably in all soils, including poor ones. Grows well in indoor pots in any climate. The germination rate is 70 to 80 percent though you have to be attentive. May to July is the normal sowing season.

The entire aerial (aboveground) plant is collected just before it blooms (in early fall) when the constituents are the strongest. In general, the plant contains the greatest amounts of andrographolide 110 days after cultivation. Cut the plant, dry in the shade, then bag in plastic, place in plastic tub, out of the sun in a coolish location. It will last just fine for several years.

Plant chemistry

Andrographis paniculata contains a number of unique chemicals, among which are andrographolide, dehydroandrographolide, neoandrographolide, deoxyandrographolide, andrographoside, hydroxytrimenthoxyflavone, andrographine, homoandrographolide, andrographosterol, andrographane, andrographone, paniculide A, B, and C, some novel flavonoids, a number of rare noriridoids, various quinic acids and xanthones, echiodinin, and apigenin.

Andrographolide is considered by most researchers to be the primary active constituent in the plant. It is highest in the leaves (about 2.5%), lowest in the seeds. Comprehensive studies, however, have shown significant synergistic activity between the plant's various constituents, and a number of studies have found that andrographolide alone is less active than the whole plant.

The usual reductive thinking that almost always occurs with plant medicines ("They're raw drugs!") has decided that the primary active constituents ("They're the most important!") are the "major" andrographolides ("These are the ones that are medicinal, the others do *nothing!*"), specifically: andrographolide, dehydroandrographolide, neoandrographolide, and deoxyandrographolide. These are what herbal companies generally standardize the plant for (10 percent). Again, I am not all that sure that this is necessary for this plant. After all, various Asian cultures have been using the plant for millennia, and it seems to have worked just fine for them before *Homo sapien var reductionistii* emerged in our midst.

Traditional uses of *Andrographis*

Andrographis has been used for hundreds to thousands of years in Ayurveda, TCM, and Unani medicine and in various traditional medicine systems in Japan, Malaysia, Bangladesh, and Thailand (among others). Many tribal peoples, wherever the herb grows, use it as well.

It's pretty much used in all places somewhat similarly: to reduce heat (inflammation) in the body, and for fevers, liver diseases, colds, diarrhea, dysentery, various GI tract problems, and infection by parasitic organisms (generally microbial). Western awareness of the herb is relatively new. By far the most extensive use has occurred in Ayurveda and TCM.

Ayurveda

In India, which has the longest tradition of use (it appears in texts 2000 years old), *Andrographis* has been extensively used in Ayurvedic, Siddha, and Unani systems of healing as well as by numerous tribes throughout the country. It's commonly used for malaria, syphilis, as an antiwormer (anthelmintic), for dysentery and bowel irregularity such as painful peristalsis and loose stools, nerve pain (neuralgia), liver disease, and sluggish liver.

It is considered potently effective for either acute or chronic infectious diseases (as an antiperiodic), especially for influenza and chronic relapsing infectious diseases such as malaria, related *Borrelia* infections such as East African relapsing fever, worm infestations, leptospirosis, syphilis, and chronic fatigue (i.e., general fatigue, debility, and weakness that will not resolve). *Andrographis* was the primary remedy used in India during the influenza pandemic of 1918 and is credited with reducing mortality rates from the disease.

Unani tradition uses it as an anthelmintic, anti-inflammatory, antipyretic, aperient, astringent, for boils, as a carminative, for chronic and seasonal fevers, for convalescence after fevers, as a diuretic, for dysentery, dyspepsia associated with gaseous distention, as an emmenagogue, emollient, a gastric and liver tonic, for general debility, for gonorrhea, irregular bowels, leprosy, loss of appetite, scabies, and skin eruptions.

Traditional Bangladeshi medicine (a blend of Ayurvedic and historical Islamic medicine) uses it for: acute diarrhea, anorexia, bloating with burning sensations in the chest (heartburn?), as a blood purifier, for colds and flu, constipation, cough, debility, diabetes, dysentery, edema, emesis, fever, headache, indigestion, intestinal worms, leucorrhea, liver disorders, loss of appetite, low sperm count (men are *not* mice . . . usually), urinary tract infections, lung infections, malaria, tonsillitis, skin disorders, spleen/liver inflammation, sinusitis, and vertigo.

Traditional Chinese medicine

Traditional Chinese medicine (TCM) uses the plant for lung infections and abscess, influenza-type illnesses, dysenteric disorders, painful urinary function, leptospirosis, general inflammation, fevers, burns, cervical erosion, chicken pox, colds and flu, cough with thick sputum, as a detoxicant, for diarrhea, dysentery, to dispel toxins from the body, eczema, epidemic encephalitis B, hepatitis, herpes, laryngitis, mumps, neuro-dermatitis, pelvic inflammation, pharyngitis, pneumonia, snake bites, sores, otitis media, tonsillitis, and vaginitis.

One of the specific indications for its use is "fire toxin manifestations on the skin," such as sores, ulcerations, or erythema migrans (EM), aka, the typical bull's-eye rash of Lyme disease. It's considered a primary herb to clear heat, relieve fire toxicity, and dry dampness, especially for such things as damp-heat dysenteric disorders.

Note: The plant is considered to be "cold" in this system and is contraindicated for those with a cold constitution.

Western botanic practice

While *Andrographis* was known to the nineteenth century Eclectic practitioners, it was rarely used or imported; they just didn't think it very sexy. The herb entered Western practice in the latter half of the twentieth century and is becoming increasingly popular in Europe, especially in Sweden and the Scandinavian countries for the treatment of colds and flu. In the United States the herb is now being used in combination with pharmaceuticals in the treatment of AIDS and alone in the treatment of colds, flu, and cancer.

Scientific Research

The literature is extensive; this is a brief overview.

Pharmacokinetics: Like many plants (not all) that have been traditionally used for malaria, *Andrographis paniculata* is a very good systemic. It spreads rather easily to all parts of the body, including the brain.

Radioactively labeled andrographolides have been used in clinical studies to track their movement in the human body. After forty-eight hours, the concentration of the compounds in various body tissues has been found to be: brain and spinal cord 20.9 percent, spleen 14.9 percent, heart 11.1 percent, lung 10.9 percent rectum 8.6 percent, kidney 7.9 percent, liver 5.6 percent, uterus 5.1 percent, ovary 5.1 percent, and intestine 3.2 percent.

Excretion of the herb is initially rapid but then slows. Half is excreted via the kidneys within two hours of ingestion, 80 percent within eight hours, 90 percent within forty-eight hours. Because of its rapid excretion the herb needs to be taken on a regular daily schedule, approximately every four hours.

Treatment of parasitic disease: The herb has shown reliable (and sometimes potent) actions in the treatment of parasitic diseases, especially microbial. *Andrographis* is active against *Leptospira* spirochetes in vitro and has been used successfully (clinically) in the treatment of leptospirosis. Prior to the introduction of antibiotics, it was used successfully (they say) in the treatment of syphilis (another spirochete) in traditional Indian practice. *Andrographis* gels have been found effective for the treatment of spirochetal periodontal disease organisms such as *Treponema denticola*.

Clinical trials and studies have found the herb to be active against a wide range of other parasitical organisms: *Plasmodium* species (malaria), *Leishmaniana* organisms (leishmaniasis), *Wuchereria bancrofti* and *Brugia malayi* (filariasis), *Ascaris lumbriocoides* (human roundworm), *Dipetalonema reconditum* (canine parasitic worm), and (again) *Leptospira* spirochetes (leptospirosis). Our experience the past ten years has shown that the herb is active against borrelial spirochetes, though it seems to work better against relapsing fever borrelias. Still, for about 60 percent of those with antibiotic refractory *Borrelia*, it seems to work well as an antiborrelial herb.

In clinical trials, 80 percent of leptospirosis patients treated with the whole plant or its isolated constituents were cured or experienced significant relief. The constituents used in clinical trials were: deoxyandrographolide, andrographolide, and neoandrographolide, all in tablet form. Andrographolide has been found to be specifically active against leishmanial parasites in both in vitro and in vivo studies, "producing a normal blood picture and splenic tissue architecture."

In vivo and in vitro studies have found *Andrographis* extracts to be effective against malarial parasites. The extract (composed of the four major andrographolides) was found to be more effective than chloroquine in its effects. The isolated constituents deoxyandrographolide and neoandrographolide were found to be the most powerful within the plant against malarial parasites. Pretreatment with neoandrographolide for two weeks prior to infection enhanced treatment outcomes. The whole plant extract was found to be as effective as the separated constituents in another study; two weeks of pretreatment with the herb suppressed later infection.

In one in vivo trial, dogs suffering from dipetalonemal infestation were injected with a water infusion of andrographis. Worm clearance from the blood was 85 percent within forty minutes.

A trial with 32 people suffering from stage 3 filariasis found that 25 people who used the protocol experienced reductions in swelling and symptomology (7 experienced a worsening of symptoms).

A clinical trail with 80 people suffering acute bacterial dysentery found andrographolide to be exceptionally effective. A dose of 165 mg of andrographolide was given 3x daily over six days accompanied by rehydration therapy. Of the 80 patients, 66 were cured (82.5%), 7 improved, and 7 did not respond. Another trial of andrographolide with 1,611 people suffering bacterial dysentery and 955 suffering diarrhea showed 91.3 percent effectiveness.

Andrographolide, in a number of studies, has been found to be especially effective for infectious *E. coli* bacteria. The whole herb is "exceptionally" active against *E. coli* enterotoxins, equivalent to standard pharmaceuticals. Andrographolide has been shown to be superior to the pharmaceutical loperamide for ST enterotoxin. As other researchers noted in other, similar studies, the herb "showed highly significant anti-secretory activity."

Chronic inflammation of the colon has responded well to enemas of the infused whole herb (combined with *Rhemannia glutinosa*) for a fourteen day period; 61 of 85 patients were cured, 22 had symptomatic relief.

In vivo studies have found that the plant has broad protective and healing actions for the heart and circulatory system. It inhibits arterial narrowing after angioplasty, decreases heart muscle damage after myocardial infarction, normalizes heart EEG readings, lowers blood pressure, inhibits noradrenaline induced hypertension, prevents clumping of platelets (and thus clots) in the blood vessels, and activates fibrinolysis, the process the body uses to dissolve clots.

Andrographis has been used in clinical trials to identify its effectiveness in both hepatitis A and B infections. A marked improvement in symptoms and liver function tests in the majority of patients was noted. In one trial in India 16 of 20 people with hepatitis A were cured by using a decoction of the whole herb daily for three weeks. In China 83 percent of 112 people with hepatitis were successfully treated with whole herb infusions. Other studies found that the whole herb combined with *Phyllanthus emblica* fruits (amalaki) taken 3x daily for thirty days was effective in the treatment of viral hepatitis. The plant is directly effective against the hepatitis B virus in vitro. In vivo studies have shown a broad liver protective action by *Andrographis paniculata* against a number of liver-damaging substances: carbon

tetrachloride, alcohol, galactosamine, and paracetamol. Researchers noted: "treatment of rats with 400 mg/kg, ip, 1, 4, and 7 h[ours] after paracetamol challenge leads to complete normalization of toxin-induced increase in the levels of all the five biochemical parameters." Other in vivo studies found that andrographis and its extracts are potent stimulators of gall bladder function, bile flow, bile acids, and bile salts.

In a clinical trial with 129 people with acute tonsillitis, 65 percent of those treated with andrographolide showed significant improvements. Of 49 pneumonia patients, 35 improved significantly and 9 completely recovered. Another trial with 111 pneumonia patients and 20 bronchitis patients showed an effectiveness of 91 percent with the use of the whole herb. The addition of andrographolide to rifampin in the treatment of tuberculosis reduced mortality rates 2.6 times.

Andrographis, in various studies, has been found as effective as nitrofurantoin in the treatment of pyelonephritis, inflammation of the kidney, though the herb had far fewer side effects.

In vivo studies have shown that the plant is strongly active against cobra venom, protecting mice from respiratory failure, increasing survival times considerably.

Andrographis has been found effective in clinical studies for infant cutaneous gangrene (study with 45 infants), leprosy (study with 112 people), herpes, chicken pox, mumps, neurodermatitis, burns, and vaginitis. An *Andrographis* gel has been developed for gum disease in Europe; trials have shown it as effective as metronidazole gel in the treatment of periodontal disease. The *Andrographis* gel has shown activity against a number of periodontal bacteria, including *Porphyromonas gingivalis* and *Treponema denticola* (a spirochetal organism).

The herb, in numerous studies, has shown general immune-enhancing activity, in essence, stimulating overall immunity and lessening autoimmune responses. Antibody production and phagocytosis increased.

The herb has repeatedly shown mast-cell stabilizing and anti-PCA activity. PCA (passive cutaneous anaphylaxis) refers to allergic reactions in cellular tissue. Researchers note that the herb stops "inappropriate recruitment of macrophages to sites of tissue injury." The herb, as researchers commented, "significantly decreased degranulation of mast cells." Of course, counterintuitively, the herb also *causes* this kind of reaction in a tiny number of its users.

Andrographolide has potent modulating effects on macrophage and neutrophil activity. The herb also extends this activity to the brain and central nervous system where it acts on the microglia. It's shown significant protective effects on inflammation-mediated neurodegeneration in the brain.

A number of double-blind trials have been conducted with the herb in the treatment of colds and flu. Consistent decrease in symptoms and improvement in recovery and recovery rates have been seen. The herb is often used in combination with *Eleutherococcus* for this in a particular mixture: *kan-yang*. Researchers in a randomized trial with 53 children in Sweden note that "in early acute noncomplicated respiratory disease Kay-Yang tablets relieves considerably the treatment course and promoted cure." Two other studies, randomized, double blind (this is where they put *both* the researchers' eyes out, but randomly), placebo controlled, with 46 and 179 people respectively, found similar outcomes. Headache, malaise, and nasal and throat symptoms responded significantly to the herb.

When taken to prevent the common cold, the herb showed significant activity in another randomized, placebo-controlled, double-blind study of 107 people. Dose was 200 mg taken five days per week for the three winter months. The *Andrographis* group had half as many colds.

The herb has been found to be active against the HIV virus in vitro and useful in human trials in reducing viral load and increasing the lowered CD4 cell counts that exist in AIDS patients. Use of *Andrographis* enhances AZT activity. Outcomes are better than with either alone.

It has also shown significant activity as an anticancer herb. The herb, in vitro and in vivo as well as in human clinical use, has shown a broad activity against different types of cancers: anal, stomach, melanoma, skin, breast, prostate, colon, and leukemia. In a 1977 trial of 60 skin cancer patients, 41 with metastases, 12 patients given *Andrographis* alone recovered. All other patients were given *Andrographis* along with standard drugs. There was no tumor regrowth in 47.

In vivo studies have found that andrographolide ameliorates diabetic retinopathy by inhibiting retinal angiogenesis and inflammation. It decreased the vascular endothelial growth factor (VEGF) in the blood, attenuated the breakdown of the blood-retinal barrier, reduced increased expression of retinal VEGF, reduced NF-kB levels, and inhibited IkB expression and IkB kinase. It decreased serum expression of TNF-a, IL-6, IL-8, and IL-1B.

Other in vivo studies found that andrographolide enhances proliferation of articular chondrocytes and prevents their de-differentiation, reducing edema and inflammation in arthritic conditions. It relieves destruction and degeneration of cartilage tissues during inflammatory processes. It promotes the expression of aggrecan, collagen II, and Sox9 genes.

Andrographolide reduces cognitive impairment in a mouse model of Alzheimer's disease. The constituent increases function in the hippocampus and inhibits the disease-caused depression of function. It reduces Abeta levels, altering the ontogeny of the amyloid plaques in the hippocampus and cortex, stimulated the recovery of spatial memory functions, and protected synaptic plasticity and synaptic proteins. It also protects astrocytes from IL-1B-stimulated upregulation of CCL5 and glial fibrillary acid protein. The herb has been found to have immunostimulant, cerebroprotective, and nootropic actions in normal and type-2 diabetic rats.

The whole herb (as well as andrographolide) is restorative, in rats, normalizing the physical alterations (including cytokine profiles) that occurs during chronic stress.

Andrographolide inhibits TNF-a-induced ICAM-1 expression in human endothelial cells, helping protect them from damage. It is also a pretty good MMP-9 inhibitor. Importantly, it also inhibits HMGB1-induced inflammation during a mouse model of polymicrobial sepsis.

The herb has a pronounced anti-quorum sensing effect on *Pseudomonas aeruginosa*, both inhibiting and breaking up biofilm formation.

The hydroalcoholic extract (tincture) protected rats from ischaemia-reperfusion induced myocardial injury. Andrographolide is strongly protective of LPS-induced acute lung injury, in vivo and in vitro.

Stephania root (*Stephania tetrandra, S. cepharantha*)

Stephania species may be able to play an effective role in Lyme borreliosis in that the plants are specific for nerve inflammations, acting as neuroprotectors in the brain from inflammatory conditions. They are also specific for arthritic inflammations that have an autoimmune dynamic such as rheumatoid arthritis. They have angiogenisis-modulating actions and exhibit a number of positive cardiovascular actions: helping with arrhythmia, infarction, coronary flow, and heart rate. These *Stephania* species, especially *S. tetrandra*, are specific for Lyme-initiated eye inflammations; in fact the whole range of ocular manifestations of Lyme can be successfully treated with the herb. The herbs also interfere with cellular adhesion and chemotaxis and protect endothelial cells. There is the potential that the herbs can interfere with the chemotactic and cellular adhesion dynamics of Lyme *Borrelia*. And finally the herbs have been found to potentiate the actions of antibiotics and other pharmaceuticals in the treatment of cancers and various diseases such as malaria. Drugs inactivated by the cancers or microbes through various resistance mechanisms are potently effective when readministered with either of these two species. Early findings also indicate that the herbs potentiate the actions of herbs as well.

The broad range of actions of these herbs, corresponding to many Lyme conditions, and the unusual nature of their underlying actions suggest that they are potentially significant herbs for use in the treatment of Lyme borreliosis. Regrettably, they are somewhat difficult to obtain, especially *S. cepha-rantha*. Bulk quantities of *S. tetrandra* can be ordered from a few Chinese medicine importers and generally must be prepared for use as capsules, tinctures, decoctions, or infusions. (See Resources, Appendix Two).

Dosage for Lyme infection

The herb powders easily and can be either encapsulated, made into tinctures, or cooked as an infusion or decoction for use. Tincture the herb (either herb individually, or a combination of the two, equal parts) in a 1:5, 65 percent alcohol/water solution. If encapsulating the herb, use 1–4 "00" capsules. For Bell's palsy, the most efficient form of the herb is the tincture or decoction.

Bell's palsy: 1 tsp 3x daily of the tincture

Neuroborreliosis: ½ tsp 3x daily of the tincture

Lyme arthritis: ½ tsp 3x daily of the tincture

Ocularborreliosis: ½ tsp 3x daily of the tincture, eye wash with the decoction daily.

Side effects

- Constipation. The herb is a strong calcium channel blocker. About half the people using pharmaceutical blockers experience the problem. If this occurs the herb should be taken with vitamin C or magnesium, dosed to bowel tolerance.

No other side effects have been reported; *however,* the plant has sometimes been confused with an Aristolochia species, *Aristolochia fangchi,* whose Chinese name is similar: *guang fang ji.* That *Aristolochia* species was sent, instead of stephania root, for instance, to a Belgian weight-loss clinic, which used it in treatment plans. A number of incidents of nephropathy with renal failure occurred among the patients at the clinic, and stephania root was blamed. Examination, however, showed that *Stephania* was not present, but rather *Aristolochia fangchi.* That particular plant contains aristolochic acid as a constituent, which can be a potent kidney toxin. Aristolochic acid–related nephropathy is a common side effect from improper use of aristolochic acid–containing plants. (The problem is exacerbated if the *Aristolochia* is tinctured, which it sometimes is in Western practice, and never is in China.)

Product safety: After those problems with adulterants, all *Stephania* herbal manufacturers and importers began testing the identity of the herb for accuracy prior to sale. Plum Brand, which is the primary source in the US is stringently tested prior to sale.

Contraindications

- Atrioventricular block. The constituents of these plants, especially tetrandrine, are potent calcium channel blockers, although their mechanism of action is decidedly unusual. They do not block through the same mechanisms of action as pharmaceuticals and are considered to be a new class of blocker. However, calcium channel blockers are contraindicated in atrioventricular block. There is no evidence that these plants would produce poor outcomes in AV block, but caution should be exercised in its use where AV block is present during Lyme infection.

Herb/drug interactions

- Not to be used with people taking pharmaceutical calcium channel blockers or beta-blocker drugs. Not for use with people taking digoxin. Not for use with people on antiarrhythmia medications. Not to be used if you are hypotensive.
- Drug/herb synergist. May potentiate the action of pharmaceuticals and other herbs. The plant and its constituents tetrandrine and cepharathine have generated interest because they have shown remarkable activity in potentiating the activity of pharmaceuticals.

Leonurus cardiaca (motherwort)

Motherwort is an important supportive herb in that it provides protection for mitochondrial integrity and function and is very good at reducing anxiety and sleeplessness. It also has some important protective actions in the brain.

Motherwort has been found to be strongly neuroprotective, especially in ischemia/reperfusion-induced mitochondrial dysfunctions in the brain, including the cerebral cortex. It significantly improves neurological outcomes and reduces ischemia/reperfusion damage in the brain. It decreases reactive oxygen species (ROS) levels in the brain mitochondria and, importantly, reduces mitochondrial swelling and restores mitochondrial membrane potential. Motherwort decreases the expression of a protein, B–cell lymphoma 2 (Bcl-2), in the brain. Increased Bcl-2 levels in the body have been implicated in the generation of various cancers including the prostate, as well as various psychiatric disorders of the CNS, and autoimmunity problems, all part of the coinfection symptom range. Part of the function of the Bcl-2 protein is interfering with apoptosis, that is, cell death. Motherwort decreases its expression and increases the levels of Bax. Bax is a protein, closely related to Bcl-2 that acts to increase apoptosis in cells. Bcl-2 and Bax normally exist in a modulated balance, and their expression is controlled by a protein, p53. This protein is intimately involved in controlling the emergence of cancers in the body as well as protecting the genome from damage. It is sometimes referred to as "the guardian of the genome."

Many of the Lyme-group alter p53/Bax/Bcl-2 as part of their infection strategy. This, quite often, results in damaged mitochondrial function. A major side effect of this is loss of energy due to mitochondrial malfunction. More crucially, it leads to damage in the brain that contributes to the psychiatric problems associated with this group of infections.

Motherwort stops this process and protects the mitochondria in the brain and, presumably, other cells in that location as well, since it also decreases the production, and impact, of ROS in the brain. The herb exerts anti-inflammatory actions throughout the CNS and also exerts a moderate pain-relieving action. Motherwort contains a number of chemical compounds among which is ursolic acid, which has been found to be a potent inhibitor of intracellular ROS induced by bacteria. Some studies have found that motherwort is higher in its antioxidative actions than both hawthorn and ginkgo.

Water extracts of motherwort completely inhibit tick-borne encephalitis (TBE) and induce resistance to the TBE virus in mice infected with it.

Motherwort slows and strengthens the heartbeat and has traditionally been used as a heart medicine. It is also a reliable and strong relaxant for anxiety. During anxiety episodes, the heart rate increases; motherwort calms it down through a variety of mechanisms. In combination with this, it also significantly decreases anxiety by its actions in the CNS. Double-blind studies have found it to significantly help in the treatment of anxiety. It also has been found to significantly decrease sensitivity to light (photophobia), a problem that often occurs during Lyme, *Bartonalla*, and *Mycoplasmal* infections.

Its actions are dose dependent.

Preparation: 1:2, 95 percent alcohol of the freshly harvested, *not* dried, plant. (The dried plant is not nearly as effective; I would not use it.)

Tincture dosage: ¼–½ tsp to 6x daily. *Fresh plant tincture only.* In acute situations we have used up to ½ ounce of the herb at a time. It is a benevolent medicinal.

Side effects and contraindications

The herb is contraindicated in pregnancy. Stomach irritation has been so rarely reported as to make me question the source, and I don't know what to make of the one report of diarrhea. Tremendously high dosage levels have been reported to cause uterine bleeding, but I can only find one source for this and nothing in the journal papers that are so often hysterical about herbs. The herb has traditionally been used as an emmenagogue, that is, a substance to start a delayed menstrual cycle, so perhaps this why it is reported to cause uterine bleeding.

The plant does lower blood pressure, so if you already have low blood pressure, be careful with it. But just to make things more difficult, the herb is also reported to raise blood pressure. I haven't seen this in practice in twenty-five years of use so am not sure what to make of that.

Herb/drug and herb/herb interactions

Will produce additive effects if taken along with blood-pressure-lowering pharmaceuticals.

Actions on the thyroid

Unfortunately, some assertions have arisen that motherwort is hypothyroidic (Lott, 2014). This is completely untrue and regrettably comes from a failure to understand the actions of the plant or why a few sources in the literature indicate it suppresses thyroid function. The mistaken assumption was derived by poor scholarship and a lack of understanding of herbal combinations, specifically why the herb is sometimes used in the treatment of *hyper*thyroidism. (It is because of the actions of the plant on the heart.) In many hyperthyroidic situations, heart and pulse rates increase, sometimes substantially. This increases the stress on the thyroid and overall system.

Traditionally, in Eclectic and German practice, motherwort has been used in a supportive role in the treatment of hyperthroydism. By lowering overall stress levels and both heart and pulse rate, the herb reduces the pressure on the system. It is merely a supportive adjunct for alleviating elevated thyroid function. *The herb does not, by itself, lower thyroid function.*

Because the herb is often used as a supportive adjunct during treatment for hyperthyroidism, some people have, unfortunately, assumed that the herb is hypothyroidic. Any intelligent examination of the data on the plant shows it is very much *not* a hypothyroidic medicinal. It use is *not* contraindicated during Lyme disease; it will not directly affect thyroid function.

Side effects/contraindications/dosages of some of the other herbs and supplements suggested in the book

Achillea millefolium (yarrow)
The only contraindication is allergy to yarrow or similar plants. No substance interactions noted.
DOSAGE: Tincture: 10–30 drops as often as needed.

Ailanthus altissima
Rarely: nausea, dizziness, vomiting, limb tingling, all from *very large* doses. No substance interactions noted.
DOSAGE: Depends on what you are using it for, tincture dose: 5 drops–1 tsp 6x daily. Higher doses are usually for GI parasites such as giardia.

Alpha lipoic acid (ALA)
Diabetics should use only after review with their physician. ALA strongly affects blood sugar levels and will affect medical protocols. N-acetyl cysteine (NAC) is an effective substitute for ALA in those who are diabetic.
DOSAGE: 600 mg daily.

Amni visnaga (khella)

Khellin, one of the active constituents of the herb, can cause skin sensitivity to light, and caution should be exercised by fair-skinned people, especially if you spend any time in the sun. In rare instances, the herb may cause mild liver inflammation or jaundice (AST and ALT levels can rise a bit). These conditions clear when the herb is discontinued. A few people have reported dermatitis, nausea, and vomiting from using the herb.

SUBSTANCE INTERACTIONS: Should not use with digoxin (it counteracts the drug to some extent) or drugs that cause photosensitivity.

DOSAGE: Normally, the herb is found standardized for its khellin content, 12 percent; 250–300 mg daily.

Angelica

No real side effects to the herb; it's contraindicated in pregnancy, especially the first trimester as it can stimulate menstruation. The herb does soften the bowel contents, not a good idea to use it during bouts of diarrhea.

SUBSTANCE INTERACTIONS: Shouldn't really be used with anticoagulants.

DOSAGE: The Chinese often prepare the herb as a decoction, 5–15 grams in water, divided into several doses daily. The powdered root is useful, 1–2 grams 3x daily. Dosage of the tincture of the dried root (1:5, 70 percent alcohol) runs ½ tsp–1 tbl 3x daily, depending on severity of the condition.

Apium graveolens (celery seed)

Diuretic, caution required if you are on diuretic drugs. Rarely: allergic reactions (usually to the plant itself, not the seed). If you can eat celery without trouble, the seed tincture should be fine.

SUBSTANCE INTERACTIONS: None noted.

DOSAGE: Tincture: ¼–½ tsp to 3x daily.

Arctium lappa (burdock)

This is a food-grade herb; the root is commonly eaten in many countries. No side effects noted, nor any substance interactions:

DOSAGE: High, it is like eating a turnip or a potato. Tiny amounts (tablespoon at a time) do work to help as a general tonic, but more can be taken, as desired.

L-ARGININE

L-arginine should be avoided in cases of active shingles or herpes as it can exacerbate the outbreak. L-arginine will not usually initiate an outbreak, but once an outbreak occurs, existing viruses can use arginine to enhance their replication.

SUBSTANCE INTERACTIONS: L-arginine can affect blood sugar levels and should be used with caution if you are diabetic. It can also lower blood pressure so should be used with caution if you are taking blood pressure medications.

DOSAGE: 1–2, 500 mg capsules 3x daily.

Artemisinin (*Artemisia annua*)

It can cause gastrointestinal upset, loss of appetite, nausea, cramping, diarrhea, vomiting. About 4 percent of people who take it experience these symptoms, usually in a more severe form than experienced when ingesting the herbal infusion. Very high doses (5000 mg day of artemisinin for three days) have caused liver inflammation, which corrects upon stopping the supplement. Artemisinin has a slightly chronotropic effect on the heart. It causes mild hypotension. This has not been, apparently, a problem in any users.

It should be used with caution in pregnancy, especially in the first trimester. In vivo studies have found a number of adverse effects in rats and mice if the herb is used in the first trimester. However, one clinical trial with sixteen patients in the first trimester of pregnancy found the miscarriage rate to be the same as that for the general population.

Caution: I have heard from several people with Lyme disease that they have been taking the herb for one to two years at relatively high doses. This is highly contraindicated and should **not** be done under any circumstances. I repeat: This is a really bad idea. Artemisinin is extremely safe when used appropriately, that is in doses around 1,200 mg daily for seven days (and it's probably fine for a month or two if you really want to do it that long). If used long term in high doses, there is significant risk of neurotoxicity, that is, damage to the central nervous system and brain. *Sida, Alchornea, Cryptolepis,* and *Bidens* are all much safer alternatives for long-term use, especially if you are treating any of the Lyme-group of microbes.

SUBSTANCE INTERACTIONS: *Artemisia annua*, like many antimicrobial plants, contains synergists that makes its compounds more active against microbial organisms. In this instance, chrysospenol-D and chrysophlenetin, two flavonols in the plant have been found to potentiate the activity of berberine and norfloxacin against resistant staph. *Artemisia annua* is a synergist with norfloxacin, potentiating the action of that drug.

Artemisinin does induce certain liver enzymes and may interact with drugs such as omeprazole.

DOSAGE: The effective dosage for malaria is 500–1000 mg on the first day and 500 mg daily thereafter for two to four more days. This will completely clear the malarial parasite from the blood. However at 400 mg per day for five days, the recrudence rate is 39 percent. Dosage at 800 mg drops the rate nearer to 3 percent. Chinese dosage runs from 500–1,600 mg for three days repeated in two weeks (to treat newly hatching parasites). I do think there is some evidential support for 800–1,200 mg for five to seven days, repeated for another five to seven days in two weeks. The relapse rate is definitely smaller at the higher dose.

Note: Artemisinin begins to become less present in the blood the longer it is taken; by day seven the constituent is only present at 24 percent of its day one levels. *The isolated constituent is not very effective if taken longer than seven days at a time for parasitical infections.* If it doesn't work for babesia (or whatever) within a few weeks to a month, it is not going to. Pulsing will not help.

Astragalus

No toxicity has ever been reported from the regular, daily use of the herb nor with the use of large doses. The Chinese report consistent use for millennia in the treatment of colds and flu and suppressed immune function without side effects.

It is contraindicated, however, *for some people*, in certain kinds of late stage Lyme disease because it can exacerbate autoimmune responses in that particular disease. For others it can alter the Th1/Th2 balance and reduce the autoimmune dynamics. Whether or not it acts as a modulator seems to depend on individual reactions to the herb; I haven't been able to find a reason why for some people it exacerbates their condition and for others it does not.

SUBSTANCE INTERACTIONS: A few.

- Synergistic actions: use of the herb with interferon and acyclovir may increase their effects. The herb has been used

in clinical trials with interferon in the treatment of hepatitis
B; outcomes were better than with interferon alone. It has
also shown synergistic effects when used with interferon
in the treatment of cervical erosion; antiviral activity is
enhanced.

- Use of the herb with cyclophosphamide may decrease effectiveness of the drug. Not for use in people with transplanted
  organs.

- Synergistic with echinacea and licorice in the stimulation of
  immune function.

DOSAGES: Generally used as tincture, tea, or powder.

Tincture: As a tonic, 30–60 drops to 4x daily. In chronic illness conditions,
1 tsp 4x daily. As preventative (from viral infection), 1 tsp 4–6x daily.
In acute conditions, 1 tsp 4–6x daily, generally every three hours.

Tea: Put 2–3 ounces of herb in a quart of hot water, let steep for two to
three hours, strain, then drink throughout the day.

Powder: In chronic conditions 1 tbl 3x per day. Acute: 2 tbl 3x per day.
Your body's own bile and stomach acids will extract the constituents.
You can go higher on these doses if you wish. The Chinese use very
large doses of the powdered root, from 15–60 grams per day, essentially ½–2 ounces per day.

Bacopa monnieri

Rarely (usually at high doses), thirst, nausea, muscle fatigue. No substance
interactions noted.

DOSAGE: 500 mg 2–3x daily.

Bidens pilosa

No adverse reactions/side effects noted in the literature.

SUBSTANCE INTERACTIONS: None noted, however . . . one study does show it
potentiating tetracycline. Caution should be exercised in using the plant
if you are on diabetic medications as it will alter your blood glucose and
insulin levels.

DOSAGE: Fresh plant tincture: 45–90 drops in water to 4x day. In acute conditions (malaria, systemic staph), ¼–1 tsp and up to 1 tbl in water to 6x daily
for up to twenty-eight days depending on severity.

Boswellia serrata

Rarely, diarrhea, rash, nausea. No substance interactions noted.

DOSAGE: Tincture: ¼–½ tsp 2–3x daily; capsules: 500 mg 2–3x daily.

Camellia sinensis (EGCG)

No side effects noted in the literature (hint: It's green tea), however . . . *massive* amounts of green tea catechins either from green tea ingestion or EGCG has been reported to cause hyperplasia of the thyroid. Caution should be exercised in ingesting either green tea or EGCG if you have a malfunctioning thyroid.

SUBSTANCE INTERACTIONS: None noted.

DOSAGE: Try to get one with at least 80 percent polyphenols and 50 percent or so of EGCG. A supplement with the natural green tea flavonoids would be even better. Dosage range is 400–800 mg daily. For greater effectiveness in treating *Bartonella*-generated endothelial cell damage, for instance, take it with 1,200 mg quercetin daily – both at the same time, in the morning.

Note: There is about 100 mg EGCG in a cup of green tea. I would imagine that drinking green tea itself throughout the day would be a good approach, and it produces better bioavailability.

L-carnitine

Generally very safe. At doses of 3 grams a day (just stay below this), nausea, vomiting, abdominal cramps, diarrhea, and "fishy" body odor have been reported. Much rarer side effects include weakness in those who are uremic and an increase in seizures in those with seizure disorders. *Avoid if there is a history of seizures.*

SUBSTANCE INTERACTIONS: Carnitine levels may be reduced by pivampicillin, phenobarbital, valproic acid, phenytoin, and carbamazepine, but no negative consequences have been noted.

DOSAGE: 500 mg 3x daily.

Ceanothus (red root)

No side effects have been noted however it is contraindicated in pregnancy. It is a blood coagulant and should not be used if there is excessive chance of intravascular coagulation. *Salvia miltiorrhiza* should be used instead.

SUBSTANCE INTERACTIONS: Red root should not be used with pharmaceutical coagulants or anticoagulants.

DOSAGE: Dry root tincture, 30–90 drops to 4x daily. In acute conditions, 1 tsp to 6x daily.

Centella asiatica (gotu kola)

Rarely, skin allergy, headache, stomach upset, nausea, dizziness, and drowsiness (usually on very high doses). *Cautions:* Liver disease: to reduce impact on liver, limit use to six weeks at a time, then a two-week break.

SUBSTANCE INTERACTIONS: Do not use with acetaminophen (you really should not take acetaminophen anyway; it's a main cause of liver damage in many countries). May enhance the actions of diuretics. May be additive to the actions of substances with sedative actions.

DOSAGE: Capsules: 500 mg 2–3x daily; tincture: ¼–½ tsp 2–3x daily.

Chelidonium majus (greater celandine)

Chelidonium is used by millions of people worldwide every day. In general, it is *very* safe. However, in recent years concern has been raised because it *occasionally* causes severe impacts on the liver. There are some forty instances, in the literature of *Chelidonium* causing liver disease, specifically cholestatic hepatitis. This is jaundice with bile stasis due to severely inflamed intrahepatic bile ducts. More women than men are affected by it, usually older (fifty-six years average), and the herb was taken for about a month before the first symptoms appeared. All recovered upon discontinuance of the herb. Because of this, the herb needs to be used with awareness. In general what the herb does, in those it affects this way, is to inflame the bile duct openings, causing them to swell and close. This creates the condition. This action of the herb is, in essence, an overstimulation. Many people use the herb to increase bile flow; for some people it just stimulates things too much. There has been a lot of overreaction to this, especially by herb-hostile physicians. So . . .

To put this in context, many antibiotic drugs will cause this condition; it is not uncommon – though with antibiotic drugs, the condition is not always reversible. Liver damage, often severe, is common as well with acetaminophen (i.e., Tylenol). Death and liver transplants are sometimes necessary. In contrast, this herb is extremely safe. Still . . .

The symptoms of cholestatic hepatitis are jaundice, itching, abnormal stools, and, sometimes, pain in the region of the gallbladder. In general, again, you have to take the herb for at least a month to develop symptoms. If you stop the herb, the condition will improve almost immediately, with no long-term effects. So . . .

Pay attention to the impact the herb makes on you and take action accordingly. In spite of this problem, greater celandine is a very good herb for coinfections; its use is warranted.

Contraindications: Obstructed bile duct, pregnancy.

SUBSTANCE INTERACTIONS: I would not use it with anything that causes inflammation in the liver, especially acetaminophen.

TINCTURE DOSAGE: The plant should be tinctured fresh, 1:2, 95 percent alcohol. Typical American dosage is 10–30 drops 3x daily for thirty days. English dosage is higher, generally 40–80 drops 3x daily. Chinese dosages are usually higher than that. I would begin with the American dosage and see how you respond. Then consider the English dosage if all goes well. In general, use for thirty days, wait a week, reinitiate use as necessary depending on physiological response to the herb.

Chlorella

When first using, it may cause diarrhea, nausea, gas and bloating, and/or digestive cramping. No substance interactions noted.

DOSAGE: Once you get used to it, a lot; it is a food-grade herb. In general: 1 tbl 3x daily.

Codonopsis pilosula

No side effects or substance interactions noted.

DOSAGE: Tincture: ¼–1 tsp to 3x daily.

Corallorhiza maculata (or similar species, aka coral root)

No side effects or substance interactions that I know of, none in the literature.

DOSAGE: Tincture: 30 drops up to 6x day, more for helping reduce acute fevers.

Cordyceps

There are no side effects noted in the literature. Up to 5 grams per kilo-gram of body weight per day have been used in rats long term with no side effects. That would be 350 grams – i.e., about 12 ounces or ¾ of a pound – in a person weighing 150 pounds. Double that dose was used with rabbits for three months with no side effects.

The only reported side effects I can find are occasional reports of dry mouth, nausea, and diarrhea. One case of an allergic reaction (a general allergy to fungi) that subsided when the herb was discontinued.

SUBSTANCE INTERACTIONS: *Cordyceps sinensis* is synergistic with cyclosporin A, and the amount of the drug needed is lessened if cordyceps is taken. The hypoglycemic actions of the herb also reduce the dosage needs for those on antidiabetic medications. There is some concern as well that cordyceps might be synergistic or additive with anitretroviral drugs, thus affecting dosage requirements, but nothing has yet been reported in the literature.

DOSAGE: *Cordyceps* needs to be viewed as a medicinal *food*, not a raw drug to be taken in minute doses. Again, the Chinese tonic dosages are normally rather large, 3–9 grams per day, and during acute disease conditions, they can go as high as 50 grams, nearly 2 ounces, per day.

If you think of the herb as a food, then eating 2 ounces, say, as you do of asparagus or potatoes, doesn't seem all that much. In China, *Cordyceps* is often added to soups and stews (just as *Astragalus* is) as a food ingredient for chronic illness. Sometimes the Chinese decoct it in water and drink it as a tea; however, traditional healers for millennia in Tibet and India (and in parts of China) used the herb only after soaking it in an alcohol/water combination, usually the local alcoholic drink. And in fact a number of the constituents are only extractable in alcohol (and bile acids) and not water.

To be effective, *Cordyceps must* be dosed appropriately. That means a minimum dose of 3 grams daily, but the best results occur with 6 grams daily as the baseline, especially in acute conditions. The renal studies usually used from 3–4.5 grams. This dose range can also work for lung problems, except in truly acute conditions when it should be 6–9.

The best way to use the herb is either as a powder preparation, taken directly by mouth (allowing the stomach acids and bile, etc., to extract for you), or as a tincture.

Note: There is a ridiculous herban (or is it urban) legend that if a person has a candida infection (or any kind of yeast or fungal infection or overgrowth, e.g. thrush), they can't take any kind of mushroom (IT'S A FUNGUS!) as it will cause the yeast/fungal infection to grow out of control. This is totally and completely untrue. It is akin to saying that I have an allergy to eggplant, so I can't eat any other plants. Some people do have allergic reactions to fungi; if so, don't use this one. But it will NOT, absolutely NOT, cause candida or any other kind of intestinal or systemic yeast or fungal infection to "bloom."

Bulk powder: For coinfections I would recommend you buy the powder in bulk from someone such as 1st Chinese Herbs and then use 3–4 table-spoons of the powder blended in water or juice 3x daily. The tepid US dosages, 500–1,000 milligrams daily, are useless for any active disease condition. I repeat: *useless.*

Capsules: The Chinese brands, if you buy capsules, run around 900–1,000 mg per capsule and the suggested dose is 6,000 milligrams (6 grams) per day – just for a tonic dose. If you want to use the capsules for *Myco-plasma*, I would double that.

Tinctures: (1:5, 50 percent alcohol) Tonic: ¼–½ tsp 3x daily; active infec-tion: ½–1 tsp 3–6x daily.

Some sources recommend taking cordyceps with vitamin C to help assimilation. There isn't anything in the scientific literature on this, and the Asians used the herb (and noted its beneficial effects) for thousands of years before vitamin C was discovered, so . . . not sure where that herban legend came from.

Corydalis spp.

Generally considered safe. There have been a few reports (very few) of some toxicity from the herb that can cause hepatitis (meaning simply inflamma-tion of the liver). Hence, it is *contraindicated* in active liver disease. Rarely, fatigue, vertigo, and nausea have been reported.

SUBSTANCE INTERACTIONS: It may, repeat *may*, add to the effects of pain relievers, sedatives, hypnotics, and drugs taken for abnormal heart rhythms. May interact with herbs and supplements containing tyramine. (I cannot find any specific instances of any of these interactions actually happening in the literature.

DOSAGE: ⅛–¼ tsp 3–4 x daily.

Crataegus oxyacantha (hawthorn):

Hawthorn is a food-grade herb; it is tremendously safe. It is about as dangerous as its close relative apples. An incredibly tiny number of people have experienced headache, nausea, and palpitations on the herb.

SUBSTANCE INTERACTIONS: The main problem is that hawthorn can lower blood pressure, so if you are taking blood pressure medications, caution is indicated. It may enhance the actions of digoxin. The herb is additive in its effects with knotweed and motherwort. Just take care if you are mixing the herb. Don't stand up suddenly as you might experience light-headedness. Stand s l o w l y .

DOSAGE: 120–900 mg of the herb daily or ¼–½ tsp 3x daily of the tincture (1:5, 60 percent alcohol). The dosage range in most clinical studies has been from 120–900 mg daily. Most of these have used nonstandardized (i.e., raw herb) extracts, either in capsules or as an alcoholic tincture. Some practitioners are suggesting that the extracts be standardized for 1.8 percent vitexin-4'-rhamnoside or 10 percent procyanidin content. I think that is a bit of overkill; the herb seems fine all on its own.

Cryptolepis sanguinolenta

None noted. Considerable research has taken place to determine the potential adverse reactions from using the plant; none have been found, either in human clinical use, or with in vivo testing on mice, rats, and rabbits. The plant is taken, often for years, as a general tonic by many people in Africa with no sign of adverse effects. However . . .

- Researchers in some instances have noted that people taking *Cryptolepis* have elevated levels of ALP (alkaline phosphatase) and uric acid, which return to normal after the herb is discontinued. There have been no reported adverse effects from this.
- There is one report in the literature of adverse effects of *Cryptolepis* in mouse pregnancy. There is nothing in traditional use that I can find that substantiates an extrapolation to humans nor any studies in the literature that shows negative effects in pregnancy in people.
- Cryptolepine has been found to be cytotoxic, which raises concerns in some people. A few points: (1) cryptolepine is

an isolated constituent and like most isolated constituents
that are made into pharmaceuticals there are side effects
from them that don't appear in the whole herb. Cryptolepis
itself has not been found to be cytotoxic to people; (2) cytotoxic,
when used in reports, generally means it kills cancer cells
and indeed cryptolepine does; 3) cryptolepine is cytotoxic
because it intercalates DNA. DNA is a double helix, two
joined, twisted ladders. Cryptolepine inserts itself between
the two ladders– that is, intercalates–and as a result interferes with cellular division, which is why it is useful in
cancer treatment. Cryptolepine is a potent inhibitor of
topoisomerase II, which it inhibits once it intercalates. The
function of topoisomerase II is to allow DNA replication by
unwinding the DNA helix, using it as a template, and then
winding it again after replication. If topoisomerase is inhibited, DNA replication, and cellular division, can't occur.

SUBSTANCE INTERACTIONS: None noted. However . . .

- *Cryptolepis* has been used in traditional medicine to help
  rectify insomnia. One mouse study has supported that
  effect of the plant. There is some potential for the plant to
  synergize with hypnosedatives or CNS depressants. Caution
  should be exercised. However, there have been no reported
  adverse effects in these situations to date.

DOSAGE: Can be taken as powder, capsules, tea, or tincture.

As a powder: For bacterial infections of the skin, wound sepsis, liberally
sprinkle the powder on the site of infection as frequently as needed.

Tincture: 1:5, 60 percent alcohol, 20–40 drops up to 4x daily.

For resistant staph: In the treatment of severe systemic staph infection the
usual dose is from ½ tsp–1 tsp 3x daily. In very severe cases up to 1
tbl 3x daily can be used. *Note:* I prefer to not use dosages this high for
longer than 60 days. That is usually sufficient.

For malaria/babesiosis: 1 tsp–1 tbl 3x daily for five days, repeat in fourteen
days.

As tea: As a preventative for malarial/babesial infection: 1 teaspoon in
6 ounces water to make a strong infusion, take 1–2x daily. In acute
conditions, up to 6 cups a day. *Note:* While the herb will work if

infused in cold water, studies have found that hot water extraction is more effective. It is nearly as strong as the alcohol tincture. *Note:* The alkaloids in cryptolepis are water soluble, but if the pH of the water is alkaline the alkaloids will not dissolve well. The pH scale is 1–14 where 1 is the most acidic, 14 the most alkaline, 7 is neutral. The word "alkaloid" means "alkaline-like." If you have hard water, aka alkaline, the more alkaline it is, the less the alkaloids will dissolve in it. You have to have a pH of at least 6 for the alkaloids to dissolve in the water. (A water softener makes hard water soft, that is acidic rather than alkaline.) If you have hard water (you can call your city's water department; they will tell you the average pH) or if you don't know, add a tsp of vinegar or lemon juice to the boiling water you are using to make your *Cryptolepis* tea.

As capsules: As preventative: three 00 capsules 2x daily; in acute conditions up to 20 capsules a day.

Note: The herb is taken as a regular tonic for years at a time in some parts of Africa and India. One or two cups a day of the tea or 2–3 droppers of the tincture (60–90 drops) a day are fine for extended, long term use.

Curcumin-bromelain combination

Rarely, digestive upset. No substance interactions I am aware of.

DOSAGE: These are available in many dosages, both separately and together. They are, however, often available in combination. The Internet is a good place to look for them. Try to get 400–600 mg of curcumin daily and 250–750 mg of bromelain daily in whatever combination you come up with.

DHEA

The supplement has been taken in doses up to 1,600 mg daily for a month with no side effects. The side effects for doses under that are minimal, if any. There is a slight potential for women to experience androgenization from intake of high DHEA levels. Higher dosage levels are contraindicated for adolescent men.

SUBSTANCE INTERACTIONS: I would be careful mixing it with other hormonal drugs and herbs.

DOSAGE: Men 50–200 mg daily; women 15–25mg daily.

Dipsacus sylvestris (teasel) root

Possible Herxheimer reactions; otherwise none are noted. No substance interactions noted.

DOSAGE: Generally used as a tincture. Matthew Wood, and many who have Lyme disease, uses tiny dosages: 1–3 drops, 1–3x daily. Other practitioners sometimes use higher dose ranges: 10–30 drops to 3x daily. The Chinese generally use 6–12 grams of the dried root daily.

Echinacea angustifolium

Large doses of *Echinacea* are normally well tolerated. However, because of its actions on hyalurodinase, excessive *Echinacea* doses may in very rare instances cause swelling in joint tissue. This normally occurs in people with *no* joint problems; they are taking *Echinacea* for immune-stimulating purposes and notice their shoe size has increased. The large doses of *Echinacea* cause hyaluronic acid buildup in the joints by interfering with its breakdown. This condition subsides when the herb is discontinued. This action of the herb, however, makes it perfect for cartilage and bursae problems.

SUBSTANCE INTERACTIONS: May be contraindicated for those on immunosuppressive drugs.

DOSAGE: 1 tsp tincture 3x daily until pain and swelling are reduced.

Eleutherococcus senticosus (formerly Siberian ginseng)

Insomnia and hyperactivity can occur with use of the stronger Russian formulation, especially when taken in large doses. *Do not take after 4 p.m.*, just an FYI on that one.

Eleutherococcus is, in general, completely nontoxic, and the Russians have reported the use of exceptionally large doses for up to twenty years with no adverse reactions. It is especially indicated for people with pale unhealthy skin, lassitude, and depression.

For almost all people, no side effects have been noted. A very small number of people have experienced transient diarrhea. It may temporarily increase blood pressure in some people. This tends to drop to normal within a few weeks. Caution should be exercised for people with very high blood pressure (180/90), especially if combined with other hypertensives such as licorice.

With extreme overuse: tension and insomnia.

SUBSTANCE INTERACTIONS: Increases the effects of hexobarbital, monomycin, and kanamycin.

DOSAGE: There are, in general, three primary forms of the herb that are used: (1) The Russian high concentration formulations, generally 2:1, 1:1, or 1:2; (2) lower strength 1:5 tincture formulations; and, finally, (3) capsules, usually standardized in some way or other (though I prefer the powdered herb myself).

If you are growing the plant and making your own extracts, the eleutheroside B content in the bark of woody stems is about 4x that of the roots, so use those rather than kill the plant to get the roots.

Russian/high-strength formulations and dosages: Most of the Russian studies were conducted using a 1:1 tincture in 30–33 percent alcohol. The dosage ranged from 2–20 milliliters per day (the smaller dose is a smidgeon under ½ tsp of tincture). This means people were taking from ¹⁄₁₆–⅔ of an ounce (and in some instances up to 1½ ounces) of tincture per day. At an average cost of seven to twelve dollars per ounce of tincture (in the US) this can be prohibitively expensive at the upper dosage ranges.

The Russians generally dosed 2–16 ml, 1–3x daily for sixty days with a two to three week rest period in between. Russian researchers, at these kinds of dosages, saw responses within a few days or even hours of administration.

In this concentration, and at those doses, eleuthero is an immune *stimulant*, not a tonic. Using it at those doses in this concentrated a form is, in my opinion, specific for debilitating diseases accompanied by severe fatigue, brain fog, depression, muscle weakness, tendency to start getting better with inevitable relapse, and chronically depressed immune function.

You can, of course, take lower doses of the concentrated extracts, which would indeed make the tincture more tonic in nature.

For the first thirty to sixty days: 1 tsp 3x daily, the last dose occurring no later than 4pm. This dose can be increased if necessary. After sixty days, discontinue the herb for two weeks. Then repeat if necessary.

If symptoms decrease after using the Russian formulation for awhile and immune function seems better, you can change to either an encapsulated form or a 1:5 alcohol-water tincture. Both of these are weaker, but more tonic, in their actions.

If symptoms and overall health are better on the stronger extract, or if the presenting symptoms are severe, then the extract may be a better choice for continual use instead. Continue the dosage of the stronger extract: thirty to sixty days on, two to three weeks off, thirty to sixty days on, and so on.

Tonic formulations and dosages: I have generally used, and prefer in conditions other than persistent chronic disease (e.g., Lyme disease) or severe chronic fatigue, a weaker tincture, as do many American herbalists and herbal companies, 1:5, 60 percent alcohol, full dropper (⅓ tsp) of the tincture 1–3x daily for up to a year.

In my experience, this dosage and pattern of use is less stimulating to the system and the long-term effects are better. The body gradually uses the herb to build itself up over time, the herb acting more as a long-term tonic and rejuvinative than an active stimulant. With this type of tincture, it is not necessary to stop every one to two months, nor have I seen any of the side effects that can occur with the stronger Russian formula. The Chinese, much less given to tincturing anyway, use 4.5–27 grams, often as a decoction or powder.

This weaker, American tincture, in my clinical experience, takes six months to become really effective and should be used at least that long; a year is better. It is great for long-term, mild chronic conditions that won't resolve that present, in Caucasians, with a pallid face, poor elasticity in the skin, mild skin eruptions, weak energy, monotonic voice, and general passivity.

Encapsulated herb: As an encapsulated form, I suggest 1,200 mg minimum daily. In acute conditions, 3x that amount. Some manufacturers used to standardize the herb to 0.8 percent eleutherosides B&E, but that is becoming less common as the herb is understood better. I am not sure it's necessary.

Powdered herb: I like this form of the root and, in conditions such as severe, long-term chronic fatigue, blend it with some other powdered herbs that I buy by the pound (Pacific Botanicals is good for this); see the recipe section in the Lyme protocol chapter.

Eupatorium perfoliatum (boneset)

Boneset is an emetic when taken in large doses, so an early sign that you may be taking too much is *nausea*. Generally, the cooler the tea, the less nausea. The herb *may* be contraindicated in pregnancy, but no one really seems to know why. *Sometimes* some people have an allergic reaction to plants in this family – such as chamomile, feverfew, ragwort, tansy – so if you are allergic to those, careful with this one.

SUBSTANCE INTERACTIONS: None noted.

DOSAGES: The herb is bitter and about as much fun to drink as a tea made from earwax. Honey helps considerably . . . and if you have the kind of flu where you can't taste anything. Generally, the herb is taken as tea or tincture, but few take the tincture directly on the tongue. Too bitter.

As cold tea: 1 ounce of herb in 1 quart boiling water; let steep overnight, strain and drink throughout day. The cold infusion is better for the mucous membrane system and as a liver tonic. If you want to help fevers, you need to take the tea hot.

As hot tea: 1 tsp herb in 8 ounces hot water, steep fifteen minutes. Take 4–6 ounces up to 4x per day. Boneset is only diaphoretic when hot and should be consumed hot for active infections or for recurring chills and fevers.

Tincture: Fresh herb in flower 1:2, 95 percent alcohol, 20–40 drops to 3x daily in hot water. Dry herb: 1:5, 60 percent alcohol, 30–50 drops in hot water up to 3x daily. In acute viral or bacterial upper respiratory infections: 10 drops of tincture in hot water every half hour up to 6x day. In chronic conditions where the acute stage has passed but there is continued chronic fatigue and relapse, 10 drops of tincture in hot water 4x day.

Galium aparine (cleavers)

No side effects or contraindications or substance interactions that I know of.

DOSAGE: Up to 1 tbl of the tincture 3x daily.

Gastrodia elata

Incredibly rarely, mild allergic reactions. No substance interactions noted.

DOSAGE: Tincture: ¼–½ tsp 3–6x daily.

Ginkgo biloba

Very seldom, intestinal upset, headache, or allergic skin reactions. The Germans, pretty conservative when it comes to side effects, don't note anything else; however, a few sources in the US attribute excess bleeding to the herb. I suppose caution is warranted. Some sources suggest discontinuing the herb prior to surgery.

SUBSTANCE INTERACTIONS: The Germans don't note any in their official compendium; however, the herb may be contraindicated along with blood thinners.

DOSAGE: Tincture (standardized), 1 tsp 3–6x daily, or standardized capsules: 600 mg 3x day.

Glucosamine sulfate (GS)

Rarely, upset stomach, nausea, heatburn, diarrhea, constipation. In essence, various bowel upsets. Sometimes: drowsiness, headache.

SUBSTANCE INTERACTIONS: May substantially increase warfarin's anticlotting action; do not use together.

DOSAGE: 500 mg 3x day

Glycyrrhiza (licorice)

Generally, licorice is nontoxic, even in high doses. However, long term use (more than four to six weeks in large doses), especially if you use the herb as a single (rather than in combination), and most especially if you use large doses, can cause a number of rather serious side effects. Even the use of a tea over several years will do so, and every now and then, due to the rather good range of effects the herb has, someone does. (This makes antiherb proponents *very* excited.)

The side effects can be severe: edema, weak limbs (or loss of limb control entirely), spastic numbness, dizziness, headache, hypertension, hypokalemia (severe potassium depletion) – especially in the elderly. Additional problems are: decreases in plasma renin and aldosterone levels, and at very large doses, decreased body and thymus weight and blood cell counts. Essentially, this complex of symptoms is a condition called pseudoaldosteronism, which licorice can and indeed does cause if you take too much of it for too long.

However: If you take licorice along with some other supplements, it *can* reduce or even eliminate the tendency of the herb to produce pseudoaldosteronism. There is an intravenous form of glycyrrhizin commonly used in China that contains 40 mg aminoacetic acid (glycine), 2 mg L-cysteine, 1.6 mg sodium sulfite, and 4 mg monoammonium glycyrrhizinate (glycyrrhizin) per 2 milliliter vial. Normal dosing is 40–60 ml IV and up to 100 ml. The oral therapeutic dose is as high as 200 mg daily. This combination eliminates pseudoaldosteronism as a side effect. You can add both glycine and L-cysteine to your protocol to limit the potential for pseudoaldosteronism if you are taking large doses of licorice for extended periods. (Glycine, minimum 2,000 mg daily; L-cysteine, minimum 500 mg daily.) The addition of potassium (5,000 mg daily) will also help prevent the hypokalemia. *Again:* Licorice should be taken in combination with other herbs – this reduces the tendency for side effects by itself. And, if you do need to take largish doses of licorice, even with other herbs, for severe infections, please add these supplements to your regimen and carefully monitor for side effects.

Because of licorice's strong estrogenic activity, it will also cause breast growth in men, especially when combined with other estrogenic herbs. Luckily, all these conditions tend to abate within two to four weeks after licorice intake ceases. Caution should be used, however, in length and strength of dosages.

There have been a number of studies finding that large doses of licorice taken long term during pregnancy has detrimental effects on unborn children. Low doses are apparently safe. Again, this plant should not be used in large doses or for lengthy periods of time *especially if you are pregnant*.

The herb is contraindicated in hypertension, hypokalemia, pregnancy, hypernatremia, and low testosterone levels. However, for short-term use in those conditions (ten days or less), in low doses combined with other herbs, it is very safe.

SUBSTANCE INTERACTIONS: The plant is highly synergistic. It is also additive. It should not be used along with estrogenic pharmaceuticals, hypertensive drugs, cardiac glycosides, diuretics such as thiazides, loop diuretics, spironolactone, or amiloride, corticosteroids, hydrocortisone.

DOSAGE: Used as tincture, tea, in capsules. *Again:* This herb is best used with other herbs in a combination formula.

One of the primary things to keep in mind when using licorice is that the higher the glycyrrhizin content, the more antimicrobial the herb will be. If using the herb as an antimicrobial you **should not** use deglycyrrhized licorice.

Tincture: Dried root, 30–60 drops up to 3x daily. In acute conditions: ½ tsp (2.5 ml) 3–6x daily – blended with other herbs – generally for a maximum of six weeks at this dose and only if you take the additional supplements described under contraindications.

As tea (infusion): ½–1 tsp of powdered root in 8 ounces water, simmer fifteen minutes, strain. To three cups a day. In acute conditions, every two hours.

As decoction: Traditional preparation in Japan (standard now in the Japanese pharmacopeia) is as follows: 6 grams powdered root in 500 ml (about 16 ounces) water, bring to a boil, uncovered, and let boil moderately until the liquid is reduced to 250 ml. (This will be fairly mucilaginous.) Then add enough water to bring the volume up to 1,000 ml. Drink throughout the day. Tests in Japan found that this preparation will have about 50 mg/g of glycyrrhizin. (I assume here that the powdered root they used conformed to the Japanese standard of 2.5 percent glycyrrhizin.)

As capsules or powder: 4,000 mg (i.e., 4 grams) daily in three divided doses. *Note:* ¼ teaspoon of the powder is about 2,000 mg. *However . . .* Chinese doses run high, as they tend to do, up to 9 grams daily. Oddly, the WHO monograph lists the dosage range as 5–15 grams daily, somewhat higher. Assuming that you are getting a 4 percent glycyrrhizin content in the root, that will give you 200–600 mg of glycyrrhizin daily, which is the WHO suggested limit. The European Union standards suggest people not consume any more than 100 mg of glycyrrhizic acid per day. In Japan glycyrrhizin intake is suggested to be kept to 200 mg per day. So, as usual, you have a range to choose from. *If* you are struggling with a severe infection for which this herb is specific, especially if it is severe encephalitis, there is no reason, keeping the contraindications in mind, to not use the higher WHO dose during limited treatment of four to six weeks duration. Again, please keep in mind the side effects and contraindications.

Harpagophytum procumbens (devil's claw)

No side effects or substance interactions of note. Possibly not safe in pregnancy.

DOSAGE: 1,000–2,000mg 3x daily

Hericium erinaceus (lion's mane)

No side effects or substance interactions that I know of and none in the literature. I have found one report of a person "feeling funny in their brain" when on the herb, condition alleviated upon discontinuing the herb.

DOSAGE: Tincture: ¼–½ tsp 3–6x daily.

Houttuynia cordata

Fishy smelling breath (maybe). The taste can be terrible to the point of gagging (some say). Other than the nausea from the taste, there are no other reported side effects in the literature from oral ingestion of the plant.

It does have emmenagogue actions (though oddly enough the herb is not traditionally used for starting menstruation), so it should not be used in pregnancy. However, a few individual reports from China say it can, very rarely, cause congestion in the vagina (but I can't really tell what that means).

The Chinese sometimes use it as an injectible, and there have been some severe anaphylactic reactions to that. So . . . don't inject it.

SUBSTANCE INTERACTIONS: None have been noted in the literature or in any anecdotal reports that I can find.

DOSAGE: The tincture of the fresh leaves is the most potent form of the plant as medicine, ¼–½ tsp up to 6x daily for viral infections, ½ tsp 3x daily for *Mycoplasma,* the same for *Bartonella* and other coinfections. I would not use a dried plant tincture unless that is all you can find.

Traditionally, the herb (sometimes the root) is used, either dried or fresh to make a decoction. For dried, 15–30 grams (about ½ to 1 ounce) of the dried plant is decocted (that is, briefly boiled) allowed to cool then consumed. Fresh, 30–50 grams of the fresh herb is decocted similarly. Examination of the decocted herb has, however, revealed that it loses much of its antibacterial/antiviral actions upon boiling (which is why the Chinese tend to boil it really, really briefly). If decocted intensively, the plant works well to stop diarrhea but is relatively inactive antimicrobially. Apparently, the Chinese boil it at all simply to alter the taste; the fishy taste is significantly reduced if even boiled briefly.

The fresh plant is much more antibacterial/antiviral (as is the tincture) and is traditionally pounded to make juice for oral administration internally, on wounds, or as eyedrops. The remaining mashed plant can be used as a paste applied topically to wounds and bites; the decoction (allowed to cool) can be used for an external wash. The Japanese use a tea, taken regularly, as a tonic medicine.

There are a few companies selling the tincture for absurd prices, which, given that the plant is an invasive and very easy to grow, I find obscene. You can also find the powder, sometimes concentrated at 5:1, sometimes just the regular old powdered herb, from some Chinese herb companies. You can encapsulate the powder if you cannot take the taste of the tincture. I have been unable to locate any preencapsulated forms on the market. The herb really isn't that popular at this point.

If you do encapsulate it yourself, use 00 capsules. I would begin with 2 capsules 3x daily and see how it goes, adjusting the dose depending on how it works for you. I have never been sure of how to dose the 5:1 concentrated powders that the Chinese often make, presumably you would take ⅕ the dose of the nonconcentrated form.

Juglans nigra (black walnut)

Side effects are uncommon, usually nut allergies. Should not use when pregnant. Contraindicated in Hashimotos. No substance interactions I am aware of.

DOSAGE: I prefer lower dosages of this herb, in tincture form: 5 drops to 1 tsp 2–3x daily. Usually, the lower side of that.

Kratom (Mitragyna speciosa)

The dose is crucial to avoid side effects, keeping it at ½ tsp or under there are rarely any. However, at higher doses, the most common are edginess and nervousness accompanied by sweating. At 1 tsp severe nausea can occur, sometimes leading to vomiting, especially at doses higher than that. Itching, constipation, tremors, and mental upsets of various sorts.

SUBSTANCE INERACTIONS: Do not take with any other stimulants of any sort.

DOSAGE: ½ tsp powder to 1–3x daily. I would not exceed this. It is a great herb if taken appropriately.

Maca (Lepidium meyenii)

At low doses, there are rarely any side effects at all. However, this herb is high in iodine. Too much of it can contribute to goiter formation and thyroid dysfunction. Rarely, nausea, increased heart rate, heartburn, and insomnia if taken too late in the day.

SUBSTANCE INTERACTIONS: None known, but I would not take with stimulants and be cautious if you are on thyroid medications.

DOSAGE: POWDER: 1 tsp 2–3x daily.

Mucuna pruriens

Generally if you take under a gram there should be few if any side effects. That said, high doses can cause vomiting, headaches, sleeplessness, high blood pressure, very rarely hair loss, and hallucinations. Contraindicated in those with schizophrenia.

SUBSTANCE INTERACTIONS: None noted but I would not take it with stimulants.

DOSAGE: 500 mg 1x daily in morning.

Melatonin

Take melatonin at night just before bed as it can cause grogginess, which is good as it is specific for helping Lyme-specific sleep disruption. *Do not take* at the same time you take zinc it will bind it. Take the zinc in the morning.

DOSAGE: 0.6–3 mg daily. People report various effects from taking melatonin, from hyperstimulation to feeling groggy the next day with a 3 mg dose. Some people find the 0.6 mg dose effective; for others it does nothing and higher doses are necessary. It is best to begin with the smallest dose and increase it slowly after you experience your individual response to the supplement. The smallest dose I have seen for sale is 600 mcg (aka .6 mg), the largest appears to be 3 mg. Start with either 0.6 mg or 1 mg and see how you do for a week or so.

Melissa officinalis (lemon balm)

A very benevolent herb, no side effects or substance interactions that I know of.

DOSAGE: Tincture: ¼ –1 tsp up to 3x daily.

Mentha piperata (peppermint)

A few people have allergic reactions to this plant. Otherwise, a benevolent friend, included in toothpaste and candies everywhere. No substance interactions that I am aware of. The tea will make you pee a lot, and it will make you sweat.

DOSAGE: Usually taken as tea, tincture, or essential oil.

Tea: Endless amounts.

Tincture: Up to ½ tsp 3–6x daily.

Essential oil: 1 drop on the tongue for severe stomach upset. I would not go over this. (Thus speaks the voice of experience.)

Mimosa pudica

No side effects that I can find in the literature, no substance interactions I can find either.

DOSAGE: Tincture: 20–60 drops daily.

Monotropa uniflora (Indian pipe)

May cause vivid, hallucinatory dreams. Other than that, none that I know of, even at doses of 1 ounce at a time (for extreme pain). No substance interactions that I know of.

DOSAGE: Tincture: ¼–½ tsp to hourly. Large doses in extreme pain may be used.

Moringa oleifera

At higher doses, may cause nausea. It has a laxative effect; too much can cause diarrhea and an upset stomach. Heartburn sometimes occurs.

SUBSTANCE INTERACTIONS: I would not use it with anything that loosens the bowels (such as vitamin C in large doses).

DOSAGE: Powder: 1 tsp in water up to 3x daily.

N-acetyl cysteine (NAC)

High doses may cause GI tract problems such as vomiting.

SUBSTANCE INTERACTIONS: None noted.

DOSAGE: 650–800 mg 3x daily. This can be increased during coinfections where there is significant neural damage.

NAC is a very good systemic; it is widely dispersed in the body within one hour and reaches peak at four hours. Levels remain high for twelve hours. It is predominantly concentrated in the liver, kidney, skin, thymus, spleen, eye, brain, and serum. It has strong protective effects against neurotoxicity throughout the CNS and can correct neurotoxic effects in the brain, especially in the hippocampus. It protects brain mitochondria from oxidative effects, eliminating membrane depolarization, keeping the mitochondria from swelling, bursting, and releasing ATP. It inhibits brain edema and as well acts throughout the entire peripheral nervous system to inhibit inflammation.

Paeonia lactiflora

Rarely: nausea, hives, skin rash, shortness of breath, chest pain, and mild GI tract disturbances, including occasionally diarrhea. Not for use during pregnancy or while on blood-thinning medications or those with bleeding disorders.

SUBSTANCE INTERACTIONS: It can be synergistic with anticlotting agents, such as *Ginkgo biloba*, aspirin, anticoagulants (warfarin, heparin), and clopidogrel. May interact with tamoxifen. May delay absorption of the antiseizure drug phenytoin.

DOSAGE: Chinese doses are, as usual, high. From 5–10 grams for tonic doses, 15–30 for acute conditions, decocted in water. Tincture dosage (1:5, 60 percent alcohol) is ½ – 1 teaspoon up to 3x daily. It is usually best combined with other herbs (e.g., *Angelica* for anemia, licorice for dysmenorrhea).

Passiflora incarnata (passion flower)

No side effects or contraindications I am aware of.

DOSAGE: Powder: 4–8 grams daily; tincture: ½ tsp to 6x daily.

Pedicularis spp. (lousewort, elephant's head)

No side effects I know of except at high doses an occasional goofiness. A very good muscle relaxant. No substance interactions I know of.

DOSAGE: Fresh plant tincture: I have used up to a half ounce at a time without problems. Normally, ½ tsp 3–6x daily. *Note:* I prefer the lousewort species; the elephant's head tastes, to me, like spoiled cabbage.

Petasites hybridus (butterbur)

The raw herb contains pyrrolizidine alkaloids, which are suspected to cause liver disease. I am not convinced by the science on this; still the products that are sold in stores have had the PA s removed, so not to worry. Normally, the side effects are mild: burping, headache, itchy eyes, mild GI tract upset, mild asthma, and drowsiness.

SUBSTANCE INTERACTIONS: None noted.

DOSAGE: 50 mg 3x day.

Phellodendron (or similar berberine-containing plants)

Caution is advised in pregnancy.

There is a tendency, because of the berberine plants poor absorption across the intestinal mucosa, to increase the dose of the plants substantially to try and get more alkaloids into the bloodstream. *This is a very bad idea.* Abdominal cramping, nervous tremors, and, most importantly, excessive drying of the mucous membranes will occur at high doses. You should not attempt to use these herbs as systemics.

SUBSTANCE INTERACTIONS: There are a number of them.

- The berberines are synergistic (or additive) with a number of pharmaceuticals such as fluconazole, ampicillin, and oxacillin. Repeated use of berberine *may* reduce the GI tract absorption of P-gp substrates including chemotherapeutic agents such as daunomycin. Berberine intake will *increase* the absorption of cyclosporine A if it is taken after long-term berberine use. Three mg/kg of berberine in six human volunteers taken twice daily for ten days increased the bioavailability of cyclosporine A by 19 percent. A randomized, clinical trial of fifty-two renal transplant patients for three months found that constant berberine intake significantly increased the amount of cyclosporine A in blood plasma.

- Conversely, P-glycoprotein inhibitors, such as piperine, will substantially increase (6x) the uptake of berberine across the intestinal mucosa. Sodium caprate, for example, will do so as well.

- Glutin, a fraction isolated from gluten, *increases* the transport of berberine alkaloids across the mucosa. Eating gluten-rich foods *may* increase the amount of berberine-type alkaloids moving across the intestinal mucosa. Gum arabic inhibits the crossing of most alkaloids other than berberine. *Coptis* interferes with the movement of constituents from radix scutellariae across the intestinal membrane.

DOSAGE: The alkaloids in the berberine plants, including berberine, are not very water soluble. (So, if you see a study of an aqueous extract of a berberine plant that is not effective as an antimicrobial, you now know why.) Tinctures need to use a higher alcohol content (generally 1:5, 70 percent alcohol, 30 percent water) and the water needs to be acidic, with a pH of 1–6. The addition of 1 tbl of vinegar to the tincture mix is recommended if your water is alkaline (hard) or if you don't know.

The berberine plants may be used as a powder for topical application, as a douche, a wash, a tincture, in capsules, and as a snuff.

As a powder: Apply to cuts, scrapes, or infected wounds.

As a douche: Add ⅓ ounce of tincture in 1 pint of water and douche once or twice daily.

As a wash: Add 1 ounce of tincture to 2 pints of water and wash the affected area morning and evening – especially good for helping acne and infected wounds.

As a tincture: Dried bark of *Phellodendron*, 1:5, 70 percent alcohol, 20–50 drops up to 4x daily. In acute dysenteric/diarrheal conditions: 1 tsp–1 tbl morning and evening until symptoms subside. Should be no longer than two days before improvement is seen, usually there will be some within eight hours.

As capsules: 00 capsules, 1–2 capsules up to 4x daily. In acute dysenteric/diarrheal conditions: To 25 capsules a day up to ten days.

As a snuff: Place two thin lines of root powder on a table and snort them vigorously – each line into a different nostril like those cocaine addicts on television, up to 3x daily for up to seven days. (May be helpful for staph infections in the nose.)

Pinus (pine pollen):

Rarely, pollen allergies. Not to be used for testosterone enhancement by men younger than middle age without a medical reason for doing so.

SUBSTANCE INTERACTIONS: Caution should be used in taking it with pharmaceutical androgens.

DOSAGE: The tincture should rarely be dosed more than 1 tsp 3x daily. To be effective for increasing testosterone levels, the tincture needs to be held in the mouth for a minute before swallowing. Do not add to water.

Piscidia spp. (Jamaican dogwood)

High doses can cause numbness, tremors, salivation, and sweating. At low doses, no side effects are noted.

SUBSTANCE INTERACTIONS: None noted.

DOSAGE: For the combined tincture formulation in this book, the dosage is tiny, less than ¹⁄₁₆–¹⁄₈ tsp 3x daily.

Polygala tenuifolia (Chinese senega root)

High doses, over 1 gram, can be emetic and irritating to the GI tract. The herb is an emmenagogue and uterine stimulant and should be avoided in pregnancy. Avoid in peptic ulcer and inflammatory bowel disease.

SUBSTANCE INTERACTIONS: None noted.

DOSAGE: 30 drops of the tincture of the dried root up to 3x daily, 1–3 grams daily of the dried herb.

Pregnenolone

At higher doses pregnenolone can cause agitation and overstimulation.

SUBSTANCE INTERACTIONS: Possibly not to be taken with other hormonal substances.

DOSAGE: 50–500 mg daily

Pueraria lobata (kudzu)

Kudzu root is a food-grade herb, in use for thousands of years in China. While great effort is being put forth to find negative outcomes from its use, none have been found in the real world (that I can find anyway).

SUBSTANCE INTERACTIONS: One study with rats found that the use of the herb with methotrexate was definitely contraindicated.

DOSAGE: In traditional chinese medicine the usual dose is 6–12 grams per day of the powdered root. Normally dosing in the West is usually one gram per day. Tincture dosage is ½ tsp 3–4x daily.

Kudzu (and puerarin) have targeted and potent effects on cytokine activated microglial cells and will reduce damage by cytokines in the CNS. They are strongly protective of the brain and CNS, especially in ischemia/reperfusion injury. The herb and its primary constituent have a strong protective effect against B-amyloid-induced neurotoxicity in hippocampal neurons, protect mitochondria from ROS, and stimulate peripheral nerve regeneration. Neuron pain receptors P2X(3) and P2X(2/3), similar to P2X(7), in the brain are inhibited by puerarin, making this a very good companion herb to use with greater celandine. The root is, in fact, strongly anti-inflammatory in the brain and CNS. It significantly inhibits neutrophil respiratory bursts, reducing autoimmune dynamics in the brain. Similarly to motherwort, it modulates Bax/Bcl-2 actions in the mitochondria in the brain and inhibits capase-3 and iNOS expressions. It is strongly neuroprotective during inflammation disturbances in the brain and CNS.

Pulsatilla patens (pasque flower, or similar species)

May cause nausea at higher doses. No substance interactions I am aware of.
DOSAGE: Tincture: 10–15 drops to each hour.

Quercetin

This supplement is well tolerated; high dosage taken daily for months produced no adverse side effects. It should not be taken along with digoxin; there is a possibility of negative side effects (speculative).
DOSAGE: 1,000 milligrams 2x daily during treatment of coinfections.

Rhodiola

Some people experience jitteriness from the herb; you should not take it at night until you know if you are one of them.
SUBSTANCE INTERACTIONS: None that I can find.
DOSAGE: Tincture: Dried root, 1:5, 50 percent alcohol . . .
   As a tonic: 30–40 drops 3–4x daily, usually in water.
   In acute conditions: ½–1 tsp 3x daily for 20–30 days, then back to the tonic dose.

Rumex crispus (yellow dock)

It's a laxative so it will loosen stools, too much and you get the typical too much laxative effects: nausea, cramping, diarrhea.
SUBSTANCE INTERACTIONS: I would not use it with anything likely to loosen your bowels.
DOSAGE: Tincture: ½–1 tsp to 3x daily.

Salix alba (white willow)

No real side effects at moderate doses, but I hate the taste. Contains salicylates (the word comes from "salix"), so too much can cause stomach ulceration (I can't find any instance of it, but . . .). People with allergic reactions to aspirin should not take the herb.

SUBSTANCE INTERACTIONS: Don't take it with aspirin.
DOSAGE: Tincture: ½ tsp 3x daily.

Sambucus spp. (elder)

Sometimes . . . diarrhea, nausea, vomiting, depending on the dose, what part of the plant you are using, how it is prepared, and your individual biological response to the medicinal. There are few reports of side effects from these plants except for that.

From individual reports, *S. mexicana* berry appears to be a bit more nausea inducing than the other varieties of blue- and black-berry species. There is one report of a group of people drinking juice pressed from "the berries, leaves, and stems" (juice from the leaves and stems? Are these crack babies?) and eleven of them, within fifteen, minutes, experienced weakness, abdominal cramps, nausea, and vomiting. Eight of them were taken (by helicopter for god's sake!) to the hospital where the physicians remarked on the dangerousness of self-medicating and the natural world in general (especially the intersection of the two). "All recovered quickly." Well, I guess so. Look, it will just make you vomit and only then if: (1) you take too much, or (2) you have an individual reaction to the plant, or (3) you take too much of the fresh or raw leaves, stem, or root, or, sometimes, the uncooked berries. Once the stuff is out of your system, that's it. No more trouble.

Because the individual response to the herb varies so widely, you should start with low doses and work up. Some people can take large amounts – that is, handfuls of raw (or dry) berries all day long, and large doses of the leaf tincture; with others, ten ripe, raw or dried, berries will cause nearly immediate vomiting.

SUBSTANCE INTERACTIONS: None have been noted but speculation abounds that it may exert additive actions when combined with laxatives or diuretics or decongestants or various jams and jellies (producing sugar overload, just an FYI on that one). A couple of reports say that, in rats, the herb interferes with the impacts of phenobarbitol and morphine, reducing their effects

Parts used: Most people these days are working with the berries only (a very few American herbalists use the flowers medicinally but not normally as a primary treatment approach). Usually what is used, especially in Germany – and probably because of German approaches everyplace else – is a standardized liquid extract (or standardized lozenge) or some other variation of the berry juice: expressed juice, syrups, a tea, or a juice decoction. Dosage usually being a cup of the tea or a glass of the juice or a couple tablespoons of the syrup for influenzal infections for reducing fever. I don't agree with this limitation on the medicinal use of the plant, but then I tend to be grumpy.

Rant: It is common in articles about elder to continually be exposed to the phytohysterical pronouncement that the plant is poisonous because it contains hydrocyanic compounds (HCN). Well, it is not. The various parts of the plant are emetic (and purgative if you take enough) *if used fresh.* That simply means that you will feel nauseous and possibly vomit if you take too much. The flowers are the least likely to cause any nausea or vomiting and thus are considered safe by phytohysterians everywhere. The berries may cause some degree of vomiting and nausea if you take too much at once or if you are especially susceptible to the compounds in the plant. But they are fairly safe in that respect, so the hysteria alert level is only Orange with the berries. The rest of the plant, however, is in the phytohysterian Red alert level range, and from reading about it, I am pretty sure the plant could kill off most of the Western Hemisphere with just a few drops of the leaf tincture.

The literature is rife with hysterical pronouncements about the plant's safety. The hysteria about the red berry (as opposed to the blue) varieties are even more pronounced, because the HCN in them exists in higher quantities. Nevertheless, they can be used as well . . . if you treat them just as the blackberry varieties, discussed below, are. Essentially you *heat* them.

The cyanogenic compounds in elder, which are also strongly present in cherries and apples, for example, *can* poison you . . . if you take them as isolated compounds. But the "poisoning" that most sources are talking about here merely consists of nausea, weakness, dizziness, and vomiting – the usual things that happen when you eat something that disagrees with you. The plant is *not* a poisonous plant the way hemlock is (see Socrates for more on this); it's an emetic (vomit) and in large doses a purgative (poop) and the word "poisonous" really should not be used to describe it.

The plant uses these compounds to protect itself from predators, especially vegetarians. When plant-eating animals forage too much from elder, they get dizzy and weak, and if that does not stop them and they keep at it, they eventually wander away to vomit. At that point, they pretty much forget about eating altogether, which is the point. If the plant were poisonous, it would just kill the animals, but it doesn't. In fact, it likes to be foraged a bit; it helps the growth and health of the plant (and the health of the animal). However, the compounds in the plant that cause vomiting occur in just the right amounts to stop foraging when the limit of the plant's tolerance is reached. The cyanide compounds in plants such as elder are normally held as separate compounds in different parts of the plant. When the animal chews the leaves, the crushing of the leaves, bark, and so on, frees the compounds and combines them together making, in the case of cherry, cyanide gas. Both this and HCN slow (or even paralyze) respiration by inhibiting an enzyme in the mitochondria of cells, cytochrome c oxidase. This is what makes the eater dizzy and a bit breathless. It is also why cherry bark is such a good herb for coughs, why it has antitussive actions (this is basically what *antitussive* means). In essence, it paralyzes the lungs, which is how it stops hacking coughs. If understood properly, elder can also be used as a potent antitussive herb for unremittant coughs.

Raw kidney beans (and a few other beans) are also considered poisonous unless they are cooked sufficiently by briskly boiling for at least ten minutes – after having been soaked for five hours. (Slow cookers that never reach high temperatures can increase the toxicity fivefold.) But you never see the same kind of phytohysteria about kidney beans that you do elder. People are simply told to cook them sufficiently to avoid the problem. So, let's stop it all right here and begin talking about what is true for this plant.

Boiling the plant (that is, the leaves, berries, bark, or root), beginning with cold water and raising the heat, for thirty minutes will reduce the cyanide (or HCN) content to nearly nothing. (With cassava root, for instance, the fresh leaves contain 68.6 mg/kg of HCN. Boiling them, beginning with cold water, for thirty minutes reduces this to 1.2 mg/kg, making them safe for use. If you start with hot water, the reduction is only to 37 mg/kg.) The longer the boil, the lower the cyanide compound content.

This is why, in the Asian traditions, they use the stems, leaves, and roots (of the *red* species no less) with impunity. To treat broken bones ½ to 1 ounce of the leaves are boiled in 3 cups of water until reduced to 1 cup, then that is consumed. And this is continued for two weeks. The root is used similarly for arthritic conditions. The boil time on this is long, much longer than thirty minutes. They are producing what is called a concentrated decoction.

The many chemical compounds contained in the plant are much stronger in the leaves, stems, and roots, and by this I am not just talking about the HCN content, but the antiviral compounds, the antibacterial compounds, the anti-inflammatory compounds, and so on. The best medicines are going to come from a much more sophisticated preparation process of the plant than any I have so far read of. To elucidate . . .

The leaves, like peach leaves, are a very reliable nervine. That is, they relax the nervous system. That is why the herb was used for epileptic fits and various dementias and uncontrollable movements by both the European and American herbalists for centuries. Dosage of the fresh leaf tincture runs from 5–10 drops, no more than each hour (though some people can take much higher doses – in fact up to one teaspoonful every hour).

Because the fresh stem, leaf, or root can cause nausea, they also cause sweating. This helps lower fevers and is very useful during viral infections. A tincture of the stem can be used to initiate sweating if you take just enough to cause that and not enough to start vomiting. This varies for each person, but in general, the dosage range is similar to the fresh leaf tincture. (I haven't yet worked with the root and so can't comment on it. However, the Asians use it, as a concentrated decoction, for arthritic inflammation, and given its constituents, it would be very good for that.) Oddly enough, in cases of excessive sweating, such as sometimes occurs during Lyme infection, just a few drops of the leaf tincture can help stop that dynamic.

The flowers are best if they are prepared as a hot infusion, covered. That is, put 1 ounce of the flowers, dried or fresh, in 1 quart of hot water, cover, and let sit until cool. This retains the floral, essential oil compounds of the flowers in the liquid, and they have unique antiviral qualities themselves. You can drink as much as you wish of it.

DOSAGE: Tincture, fresh leaves: 1–5 drops to 3x daily.

Schisandra sinensis

Rarely, abdominal upset, nausea, heatburn, skin rash. Very, very rarely.

SUBSTANCE INTERACTIONS: The herb does have some potentiation effects on pharmaceuticals. *Schisandra* is an inhibitor of CYP3A and affects the disposition of drugs metabolized by that system in the liver. It will increase the oral bioavailability of midazolam; paclitaxel bioavailability is increased three-fold. Caution should be exercised if you are using pharmaceuticals as the biopresence of the drugs may increase if you take *Schisandra* as well.

DOSAGE: ¼–½ tsp 3x daily.

Scutellaria baicalensis (Chinese skullcap)

Side effects from *Scutellaria* are rare, mostly gastric discomfort and diarrhea. It should not be used during pregnancy. Caution should be exercised if you are taking pharmaceuticals as it can increase the bioavailability of the drugs, thus increasing their impacts. It may interact additively with blood-pressure-lowering drugs. Type 1 diabetics should exercise strong caution with the herb as it can affect insulin and blood sugar levels.

SUBSTANCE INTERACTIONS: Lots. Chinese skullcap is a synergist, perhaps as efficacious as licorice, ginger, and piperine, and should probably be added to that category of herbs. Among other things it inhibits the NorA efflux pump, which inactivates some forms of antibiotic resistance. Like the other synergists I know of, it is also a strong antiviral, which is beginning to stimulate speculation. Nevertheless, the herb strongly effects pharmaceuticals and herbs taken along with it. *Some pharmaceutical synergies:* Baicalein, one of the major compounds in *S. baicalensis*, is synergistic with ribavirin, albendazole, ciprofloxacin, and amphotericiin B.

   S. baicalensis is strongly inhibitive of CYP3A4, a member of the cytochrome oxidase system. It is a type of enzyme, strongly present in the liver and is responsible for catalyzing reactions involved in drug metabolism. Many of the pharmaceuticals that are ingested are metabolized by the CYP3A4 system, meaning that some portion of the drug is inactivated. In some instances it is the metabolites created by CYP3A4 that are active as medicinals. Since the herb inhibits the CYP3A4 system, dose dependently, it can enhance the presence of a number of drugs in the system, specifically acetaminophen, codeine, cyclosporin, diazepam, erythromycin, and so on. It does affect the degree of antibiotics that enter the system.

   One of the herb's constituents, Oroxylin A, is a strong P-glycoprotein inhibitor. P-glycoprotein is strongly present in the blood-brain barrier, the lining of the GI tract, in renal tubular cells, and capillary endothelial cells, and the blood-testes barrier. It stops substances from crossing over those barriers. Additionally, cancer cells use P-glycoprotein as a form of efflux-pump in order to eject drugs designed to kill them from the cancer cells.

P-glycoprotein inhibitors allow more of a substance to cross over barriers high in P-glycoprotein. That means that oral ingestion of a substance will produce more of it in the bloodstream if it is also taken with a P-glyco-protein inhibitor. This means that Chinese skullcap will act through two mechanisms to increase drug and herb uptake in the body.

It will also increase the effectiveness of anticancer drugs by inhibiting P-glycoprotein-mediated cellular efflux. Paxlitaxel uptake, for example, was increased over two-fold when administered with oroxylin A.

The herb ameliorates irinotecan-induced gastrointestinal toxicity in cancer patients.

The herb will also help uptake of herbal medicines similarly, again by inhibiting the CYP3A4 system and P-glycoprotein.

DOSAGE: *S. baicalensis* is the primary species used in China and the one meant when Chinese skullcap is talked about. It most definitely *does not* mean the American skullcap, *Scutellaria lateriflora* – or any of the other American species. It is the root that is used, the leaves of the American species are not usable for coinfections (the roots may be, though no one seems to use the American roots). The herb reaches peak in the plasma and body organs in about one hour and only lasts in the body for about four hours, so you really do need to dose about every three to four hours.

Tincture: 1:5, 50 percent alcohol, ¼–½ tsp 3x daily. In acute conditions, double that.

Dried herb: The Chinese dosages are large, as usual, generally 3–9 grams at a time. Most of the clinical studies and trials used similar dosing. If you are using capsules, this is the dosage range you should be exploring, divided into three equal doses every four hours or so.

Selenium

Toxicity can occur if too much is taken. *Caution:* 400 *micrograms* per day (note: *micrograms*) is the highest dose that should be used; side effects can begin to occur beyond this dose range; 200 mcg is the best average daily dose in Lyme disease. Side effects from too much selenium are, nevertheless, pretty mild: GI tract distress, hair loss, white spots on nails, fatigue, and irritability. Under 400 mcg per day, no substance interactions of note.

DOSAGE: 200 mcg daily. Through a number of actions, it may also deplete the body's levels of zinc and copper. Take with a zinc-copper supplement.

Sida acuta

The main side effect I have seen is that, for some people, *Sida* can increase fatigue and symptoms of coinfection. If this occurs, reduce the dose. That will generally end the problem. This kind of side effect is not noted anyplace in the literature. My speculation is that *Sida* breaks biofilms, and that in diseases such as bartonellosis, once that happens, instead of the bacteria being limited to one location, they are then spread more widely throughout the body, increasing their negative impacts. In the literature, there are no side effects noted, known, or reported, however . . .

- The herb is used traditionally to prevent pregnancy. It does interfere with egg implantation in mice. The herb should not be used if you are trying to get pregnant or if you are newly pregnant.
- Even though the herb is traditionally used in pregnancy, caution should be exercised if you are pregnant. I would be uncomfortable using it if I were pregnant, but then, I would be uncomfortable anyway if I were pregnant.
- The herb contains ephedrine, although not in large quantities. There has been a lot of inaccurate, hysterical reporting on ephedra, even among researchers who should know better. Wikipedia is now among the worst offenders of overly conservative fear mongering – a departure from their original mission.

  Although the main reason cited for banning ephedra in the US is adverse effects, including death, what *is* accurate is that;

  1. Weight loss and "natural energy" companies were the ones who marketed the supplements containing the herb (usually along with caffeine and other stimulants). Herbalists did not support this use of the herb.
  2. People wanting to lose weight or increase their energy took the supplements – often in huge doses, far beyond sanity.

  Basically the herb was a way to make money off an aspect of the US's cultural insanity about how one should look to be beautiful or how much one should work to be useful, with, of course, predictable results.

In spite of this, the primary reason the herb was banned was that meth labs were using the herb to make meth. The adverse reactions from improper use of the herb were just the excuse. Ephedra is very safe when used properly; it really didn't need to be banned. The companies using it improperly just needed to be prohibited from doing so.

Nevertheless, just be aware that the herb contains *minute* (I repeat: *incredibly tiny*) amounts of ephedrine and that a mild raciness or wakefulness may occur from using the herb – but it probably won't.

SUBSTANCE INTERACTIONS: None known or reported, however:
- Since the herb is hypoglycemic, it *may* affect medications for diabetes. Just watch your blood sugar levels if you are diabetic.
- Since the herb contains ephedrine, it probably should not be used with pharmaceuticals that possess similar effects.

DOSAGE: Tincture and the hot water extracts are the strongest medicinal forms of the herb for internal use.

As a tincture: Dried leaf, 1:5, 60 percent alcohol, 20–40 drops up to 4x daily. In the treatment of severe systemic staph infection the usual dose is from ½ tsp–1 tbl 3–6x daily. I prefer to not use this high a dosage longer than sixty days. That is usually sufficient.

As hot tea: As preventative, 1–2 tsp of the powdered leaves in 6 ounces water, let steep fifteen minutes, drink 1–2x daily. In acute conditions to 10 cups a day.

Silybum marianum (milk thistle seed)

Milk thistle is a food-grade herb. It is about as dangerous as potatoes. An incredibly tiny number of people have experienced GI tract upsets of various sorts from it.

SUBSTANCE INTERACTIONS: None that I know of.

DOSAGE: I strongly prefer the use of standardized milk thistle during any disease condition. I feel the seeds themselves are fine for general tonic use, not so much so if you already are ill.

Standardized tincture: Standardized to somewhere around 80 mg silybum flavinoids (40 drops 3x daily) or 140 mg *Silybum* flavinoids (25 drops 3x daily).

Standardized capsules: 1,200 mg daily just before bed.

Note: These dosages can go much higher during acute liver damage.

Spirulina

Generally none, some sources cite rare side effects such as slight dizziness, thirst, constipation, stomach upset, skin, itch or rash. In thirty years I have never seen an instance of them, still . . . maybe they are out there, somewhere. *However:* Spirulina *may* be contraindicated for people with hyperparathyroidism and those with high fever.

SUBSTANCE INTERACTIONS: None known.

DOSAGE: Lots, many traditional peoples used it as a food. Generally, I use 1 tbl or so to 3x daily.

Tryptophan

At higher doses (over 5 grams daily), tremor, nausea, and dizziness can occur.

SUBSTANCE INTERACTIONS: Should not be taken along with SSRIs. This may cause "serotonin syndrome," delirium, involuntary muscle contractions, fever, coma.

DOSAGE: To 5 grams daily.

Turmeric

No real side effects are known, and there are no substance interactions I know of. *However:* The herb is contraindicated in cases of obstructed bile duct or if you have gallstone problems.

DOSAGE: Powder: 1.5–3 grams daily.

Urtica dioca (nettle)

No side effects or substance interactions of note.

DOSAGE: 1,200 mg daily.

Valeriana officinalis (valerian)

I don't know of any, nor any interactions, nor any contraindications, and the Germans don't seem to either. However . . . the herb stinks to high heaven (I don't like it for that reason), *and* if you take too much you may feel groggy the next day.

SUBSTANCE INTERACTIONS: It is usually used for sleep, so you might refrain from combining it with other sleep aids.

DOSAGE: Tincture: ¼–1 tsp daily, often just before bed. Historically, up to an ounce has been used in the treatment of severe epilepsy, but I don't think anyone does that any longer.

Verbena officinalis (vervain)

I don't know of any, nor any substance interactions either.

DOSAGE: Tincture: ¼–1 tsp as needed.

Vitamin A

In moderate, normal doses, very safe. Very high doses can cause liver damage, severe nause and vomiting, confusion, headache, dizziness, coma, pressure in space between skull and brain, visual changes.

SUBSTANCE INTERACTIONS: Acretin, Isotretinoin, topical tretinoin.

DOSAGE: 5,000–10,000 IU daily

Vitamin B complex

Excess B will come out in the urine, making it a brighter yellow or even slightly greenish yellow. It's pretty. No substance interactions of note.

DOSAGE: 1–2 tablets daily.

Vitamin B-12

There is no real toxic dose known for this one, the most common side effects (still rare) are headache, itching, swelling, nervousness/anxiety. At very high doses (5–10 mg daily) causes (very rarely) low potassium, congestive heart failure, blood clots in extremities, and anaphylactic shock.

SUBSTANCE INTERACTIONS: Leukeran (chlorambucil), prilosec (omeprazole), colchicine medications.

DOSAGE: 500–1,000 mcg (that is *micro*grams) daily, sublingual.

Vitamin C

Vitamin C at larger doses will cause flatulence and loose stools, upset stomach, or diarrhea. If you experience these symptoms, reduce the dose and begin to work up to higher doses as your body adjusts. Vitamin C is sometimes prescribed t.b.t – to bowel tolerance, meaning you take it until side effects occur.

Note: Many of the herbs and medications used to treat Lyme infections can cause constipation. Vitamin C is the best supplement to use to normalize bowel flow if this occurs. It corrects the constipation while adding a substance exceptionally useful to the body during Lyme infection.

SUBSTANCE INTERACTIONS: I would not take it with other substances that loosen the bowels.

DOSAGE: 1,000–3,000 mg daily. *Note:* I prefer a powdered, effervescent form of vitamin C.

Vitamin E

Uncommon side effects include nausea and vomiting, diarrhea, headache, rash, fatigue, blurry vision and . . . bleeding. Vitamin E is an anticoagulant, a blood thinner. So . . . avoid if you have a blood clotting disorder.

SUBSTANCE INTERACTIONS: Avoid using with warfarin and other anticlotting agents (aspirin, etc.).

DOSAGE: 400–800 IU daily.

Withania somnifera

Avoid high doses in pregnancy, may be abortifacient in large doses. May cause drowsiness. Take the herb after dinner to find out just how sleepy it makes you before using it during the day. In rare instances: diarrhea, GI tract upset, vomiting at large doses.

SUBSTANCE INTERACTIONS: May potentiate barbiturates (anecdotal); don't use with sedatives and anxiolytics.

DOSAGE: Usually as powder or tincture.

> *Tincture:* Dried root, 1:5, 70 percent alcohol, 30–40 drops to 3x daily. Higher dosages can be used if desired.
>
> *Powder:* ½–1 tsp 2–3x daily.

Zinc

At high doses, zinc can cause upset stomach, nausea, vomiting, metallic taste in mouth, dizziness, headache, drowsiness, sweating, hallucinations, and anemia.

SUBSTANCE INTERACTIONS: Do not take with amiloride. The supplement may have interactions with ACE inhibitors, and quinolone and tetracycline antibiotics, lowering their levels in the body.

DOSAGE: 25–40 mg day.

Zingiber officinalis (ginger)

No side effects other than a very spicy taste (don't get the juice on your hands and rub your genitals, experience speaking, just an fyi). No substance interactions that I know of. *However:* May be contraindicated if you have gallstone troubles.

DOSAGE: Fresh juice: no limit I can find, either in the literature or from experience.

FUTURE DIRECTIONS

Man's main task in life is to give birth to himself.
Eric Fromm

I remain in awe of the people who, infected with stealth infections, have refused to give up. They have struggled, often with little help or support, to find their way to health through an illness that, culturally, few understand. I am in awe of their courage and the willingness of so many to go outside the culturally accepted parameters of healing. Some, more than most people know, have turned to plants in that process. And many of those, as their healing has progressed, have, themselves, become people of the plant.

It is often like this when we are called to a new life path. Like so many of those who suffer from stealth pathogens, I found the world of plants over thirty years ago when I became ill and physicians could neither seem to diagnose nor help me. Oddly enough, a local herbalist had just that week introduced me to a plant on the land where I lived, one that was exceptionally good, she said, for intestinal cramping.

What I was experiencing was tremendously debilitating. If the spasms hit away from a couch or bed, I spent a lot of time on the floor. So, in desperation, I dug the root of the plant, carrying it with me, eating pieces of it from time to time. And little by little, the terrible intestinal cramping slowed and finally stopped. I was experiencing an extremely painful form of irritable bowel syndrome, though it would be many years before I understood that. After that initial treatment, the condition remained stable for over twenty years; when it did return, plants once again became my allies in healing, this time alleviating the condition permanently. (The secret? The fresh juices from a large slice of green cabbage and a few fresh plantain leaves from the front yard.)

Illness has a great many functions. It teaches us to be aware, to know ourselves, to understand how the world around us affects us each minute of our lives. It teaches us how to alter the fabric of our lives in order to become whole again . . . and how to remain that way. Illness also teaches us about the darkness that each one of us must face sometime during our lives. In the process, we learn (though all of us would avoid it if we could) how to enter the darkness and endure its touch. We learn about the territory of illness, the depths of depression that often accompany it, and struggle to face our own mortality. We acquire, often slowly and with great resistance, the qualities of character necessary to survive the journey. Personally, I would rather chew tacks. Still . . . all of us must learn, sooner or later, to eat the meal set before us. We learn to eat darkness. . . and eventually, to be unafraid of it. (I don't remember getting information about all this in the owner's manual when I was born.)

There are few of us who spend much time in that kind of experience who do not end up, in one form or another, becoming healers sooner or later. I did. For over a decade I was a psychotherapist, then for thirty years an herbalist.

During that time, I have watched the herbal world grow; it's changed considerably in the process. In those early years, I could buy every herbal book published in any particular year – there weren't many – and New York publishers produced none of them.

> I remember how groundbreaking it was when Christopher Hobbs published his first works on medicinal mushrooms, when Susun Weed first wrote about the Wise Woman Path; I remember hearing David Hoffmann, and Michael Moore, speak for the first time. . . . and Matthew Wood falling asleep while he was teaching. I remember meeting Rosemary Gladstar and her magical Sage Mountain for the first time and Ryan Drum and his seaweed and Pam Montgomery and the Green Nations conferences. And William LaSassier and Keewaydinoquay, too, and so many others.

I knew nearly everyone in the field (one way or another). The good, the bad, and the facially challenged. Now, nearly everyone in the United States has used herbs one time or another; the books published each year are too many to count.

The older generations (nearly all coming of age in the 1960s), many of them my friends, are beginning to pass. New generations are beginning to take their place. Among them, in their thousands, are those from the Lyme world. They know better than most the complexities involved in healing these kinds of chronic infections.

One of the things that the Lyme-group of pathogens teaches those of us who are willing to listen is the sophistication necessary for healing to occur, how much one must listen to the body (our often denigrated and terribly treated best friend without whom we could not exist), how subtly plant medicines work in altering what is happening in our bodies as we struggle toward health. Those from the Lyme world who are becoming herbalists are going to be some of the best healers the herbal world has ever known. I think a lot of people are going to be needing their skills before too long.

As for me, unless something very odd happens, this is the last medical herbal I will write. Over the past four years, including this book, I have written five very demanding medical herbals, plus the very long, depth look at the intelligence in Gaian ecosystems (*Plant Intelligence and the Imaginal Realm*, Inner Traditions, 2013). That latter volume is the final text in a four-book series that includes *Sacred Plant Medicine* (originally, Roberts Rinehart 1996), *The Lost Language of Plants*, and *The Secret Teachings of Plants* (all Inner Traditions, various dates). With its publication, I have finished the work I set out for myself some forty-five years ago. And to be truthful, at age sixty-two I am a bit worn out from the intense work load of the past four years, of the past forty-five years.

One of the primary goals I had set for myself (in writing these medical herbals) was to help bring herbal medicine to the level of sophistication that it is truly capable of. (I think, many of us are going to be needing that sophistication before too long.)

I have worked all these years to find a way to create a synthesis between the fundamentally holistic world of plant medicines and that of the reductionistic, mechanicalistic science that has, for far too long, held sway over our conceptions of the world and our practice of medicine. That reductive orientation (as I explore in depth in *Plant Intelligence* as well as this series of medical herbals) has far outlived its usefulness, especially when it comes to our successful habitation of this planet.

I felt such a synthesis was important because too many people were becoming ill with conditions their physicians could not effectively treat (whether systemic MRSA or chronic diseases caused by stealth pathogens). Such a synthesis, I felt, could help alleviate the uncertainty the many people who needed plant medicines had about herbs, specifically: that they were a superstitious holdover from a more primitive past. I believed that, within such a synthesis, they would be able to feel truths they intuitively knew to be true *and*, at the same time, experience the kind of analytical approach that they had been told throughout their lives was integral to any legitimate understanding of the world. I have believed for a long time that our capacity to reason does not mean we have to abandon our ability to feel (despite the terror that reductionists have of it). Both are necessary to becoming a full human being, to the practice of medicine, of herbalism, of science.

Such a synthesis was also intended to help the physicians who were open-minded enough to begin to overcome the antiplant bias in which they had been trained in medical school. And finally, the things I began to discover as I immersed myself deeper in the work, and which I then wrote of, set a higher bar, for the sophistication that we as herbalists are capable of.

When compared to the many herbal books in print, this series of books *is* very sophisticated. Yet, future generations of plant people will take this sophistication a great deal further, in directions I can only dimly imagine. (It is crucial that they do so.) These books will become, as so many herbals have throughout the centuries, dated in the extreme.

Nevertheless, to be clear, I believe that the hundreds of thousands of *community* herbalists that now exist in the United States (ultimately emerging in their present form through the early efforts of Rosemary Gladstar, William LaSassier, and Michael Moore) to be essential. I don't think we will ever get to the place where we don't need them. Further, I believe that, as a group, there is no need for them to train in a medical model of disease or use a reductive approach to understanding the dynamics of plant medicines. They fulfill in the United States the same kind of function that barefoot physicians once did in China. They are necessary, in just the form they are currently in. (Attempts to regulate them should be vigorously resisted – those who would regulate them have no one's best interests at heart, no matter how they present their arguments.) But we do need a more sophisticated body of knowledge, and no, the naturopaths will never provide it. (So, don't go there.) They don't, at this time, understand plant medicines all that well. While there are some notable exceptions (a number of whom I know and deeply respect), for the most part, the majority of licensed naturopaths are merely semidoctors, using supplements instead of pharmaceuticals. (This is mostly due to the demands of the accreditation committees that control what naturopathic colleges can teach.) Naturopaths are rarely herbalists, and I doubt, given their desires for licensure (at least the way licensure currently is), they ever will be. Nevertheless, our field is ripe for increasing the sophistication of our knowledge base.

Much still needs to be done; there are so many holes in our herbal knowledge still to be filled. Just off the top of my head, some of them are:

- We need a full and sophisticated look at the dynamics of cancer, whose long-term cytokine dynamics and cellular modulation make many of the Lyme-group's seem simplistic in comparison. (Most of those currently in print are embarrassingly oversimplified.)
- We need a depth look at the precipitation rates for herbal tinctures; just how fast do the constituents precipitate out of them? If the precipitate is ingested, does it still work medicinally?
- We need a depth exploration of the complex alterations that occur in plant medicine constituents as the plants grow, and especially, as they are picked, dried, and made into medicines. (Begun in a rudimentary way in this series of books, especially, in the analysis of *Salvia miltiorrhiza*, in the appendix to *Natural Treatments for Lyme Coinfections* [Inner Traditions, 2015].)
- We need to further develop the concept of plant synergists.
- The complex impacts that occur during the fermentation of plant medicines on their action as medicinals needs more work. Though it is early days yet, thankfully, some people are starting to make these kinds of medicines. (China is far ahead of us here.)
- We need more work on androgenic plants, especially those that contain testosterone. (Pine pollen certainly isn't the only one.)
- We need to develop the broad category of organ adaptogens, finding adaptogenic herbs for *every* organ system. (I think the word "tonic" is not specific enough here.) We have a few: for the heart (hawthorn), for the liver (milk thistle seed), for the endothelial cells (Japanese knotweed), the immune

system (*Eleutherococcus* and several others), and one for
cytokines (*Salvia miltiorrhiza*). We still need some for the
kidneys, the lungs, the pancreas – all the organs, big and
small. There is at least one herb that is truly adaptogenic for
every organ system in the body exists; it is just that no one
has been looking all that deeply for them.

• We need an accurate list of the most effective tincture ratios.
The approach we have been using (1:5 for the most part)
is not, I think, specific enough for our purposes. Someone
needs to actually work with every different plant, harvesting
it fresh and then drying and weighing it and calculating the
appropriate ratios. How much alcohol is really needed, how
much water? And what about those that need fats to extract
the constituents? Milk or a similar substance is more effective for some of them. What do we do with that truth? (And,
no, we do not need to, nor should we, get rid of kitchen herbalism and force all people to make their herbal formulations
in a lab.)

• We need to reclaim the sophistication once common to
every pharmacist in the United States. In 1900 *every* pharmacist could prepare a *Colchicum* tincture and determine the
exact amount of colchicine in it. (The National Formular-
ies are filled with similar, very sophisticated techniques of
herbal preparation.) There are no longer any pharmacists in
the United States that know how do so. The skill base has
been lost, abandoned to "progress." (Most pharmacists are
now simply trained as pill dispensers.) It is a skill base that,
as herbalists, we need to reclaim.

• We especially need a comprehensive diagnostic system that
is uniquely our own, not a modification of a reductive medical approach or the Chinese or the Ayurvedic systems. Most
of us in the United States have no real idea of *what* or *who* we
really are. We don't spend enough time in other cultures.

Our American herbal tradition is primarily a blend of indigenous tribal
practices, Thomsonian and Eclectic practice, English traditional medical

herbalism, a little bit of European practice from here and there, a bit from the South American, African, and Asian traditions, significant and unique developments that have occurred since the 1960s, *and* modern medical approaches. *It's unique.* As a people, we just don't know it. Yet it is out of that syncretic mix that our own diagnostic system must come. As Judy Garland once put it, it's much better to be a first-rate version of yourself than a second-rate version of someone else. Certainly, the world does not need us to become second-rate medical model, Ayurvedic, or TCM wannabes.

This life I have had – of working with plants as my teachers, my guides, my healing medicines, as living beings whom I have entrusted with my life – has been a rich one. Like most of us, I wandered into it one day without realizing what was going to happen to me. I became part of the long line of human beings who stretch back through time to the first person to whom a plant spoke and insisted it be used for healing. The only profession that moves me more, and has meant more to me, is that of storyteller, the life of a writer. But it was the plants that allowed that part of me expression, that allowed that seed in me to sprout, a seed that has not yet finished its growing.

Those of us who take up the mantle of becoming a plant person only do so for a while. Sooner or later it becomes incumbent on us to pass on to new generations what was passed into us. And that is what I do here. I pass it into you.

For many people, I suspect these words will have little meaning. But perhaps you are one of the ones who will hear them differently. If so, do as all people of the plant have done since time began . . . follow the genius inside you, not the maps your culture has given you; listen to the world – it is always speaking to those who would listen – and learn to understand what it's telling you; remain childlike so you can still ask the simple questions (which are the hardest, but most important, of all to find); seek the answers that you are uniquely meant to find; and find the work that is in you to do.

It is in our individual genius, all of us in our millions, that the way through the difficulties of our time will be found; it will never come from the pronouncements of topdown experts (as the stealth pathogens have taught us). Believe me, the journey is worth it.

The Gila Wilderness, 2015.

Ancient Herbals

Today, I read the description
of a medicinal plant
in a seventeenth-century herbal.
The words,
in intimate detail,
described *Potentilla*
and how the author used it to heal
long, long ago.

After I closed the book
and shut out the strange, time-distorted vocabulary
I took my staff,
and walked the fields
surrounding my home.
I do not know why I paused
and looked down
to see the same *Potentilla*
three hundred years later.

The description from the book,
like an insubstantial shadow in my mind,
arranged itself
over the five jagged fingers of *Potentilla's* leaves,
his straggly stem,
swaying yellow flowers,
and clicked into place.

Wind,
blowing down
a million years of plant medicine
brushed against me.
I flickered and was gone,
insubstantial shadow in the mind of Earth.

And for a moment
I was an old herbalist in 1720,
brushing back my cloak with my hand
as I bent to look
at a plant
that Hippocrates had used
2000 years before me.

SOME COMMENTS ON THE DYNAMICS OF COINFECTIONS

Hosts that are coinfected by multiple parasite species seem to be the rule rather than the exception in natural systems.
Andrea Graham et al., 2007

These emerging pathogens may represent the tip of the iceberg of a large number of as yet unknown intracellular pathogenic agents.
Baud and Greub, 2011

Interactions between pathogens in multiply-infected hosts strongly influence pathogen virulence, transmission, and persistence.
Dunn et al., 2014.

Lyme and its coinfections, instead of being thought of as they commonly are, should more properly be understood to be a closely cooperating group of stealth pathogens, what some researchers are calling second-generation pathogens. That is because they are very different than the bacteria (first-generation pathogens) for which antibiotics were created in the latter half of the twentieth century. Because Lyme disease was the first of this group to be recognized, it still takes center stage; nevertheless infections from mycoplasmal and chlamydial bacteria far exceed the number of Lyme infections. And a closer look at *Bartonella* bacteria reveals that they, too, are much more widely spread than is commonly recognized. At present the major members of this group of infectious microorganisms are *Anaplasma*, *Babesia*, *Bartonella*, *Borrelia*, *Chlamydia*, *Ehrlichia*, and *Mycoplasma*. Rocky Mountain spotted fever and the other *Rickettsia* are a growing presence as are a number of *Wolbachia* organisms. At least twenty others, which are much less well known and generally, at this point, significantly less common, are beginning to be recognized as growing threats. Coinfection can occur with any of them.

We are at a time in the history of the human species (and technological medicine) when these diseases are beginning to take a more prominent role. They are harder to treat than older bacterial infections (such as staph), cause a wide variety of chronic diseases, the infections are often long term – people are sometimes infected for years or decades, and they are common factors in the development of major chronic diseases: heart, lung, reproductive, and neurological conditions such as multiple sclerosis, Alzheimer's disease, amyotrophic lateral sclerosis (ALS), and cancer. The primary factor underlying their emergence is human population growth – past the point of sustainability. I have written about this in a number of my books; the recognition is no longer confined to the edges of our culture; mainstream researchers can no longer ignore the implications.

Over the coming decades, we will be seeing the emergence of more of these kinds of stealth pathogens. It's time for our approaches, and understandings, to become more sophisticated.

One of the most important understandings now facing us is accepting the limits of pharmaceuticals in the treatment of many of these emerging diseases. While antibiotics do still have a role, sometimes a very important one, they can no longer be relied on to provide the *sole* response to these kinds of infections as they spread through the human population. We have to approach treatment with a more sophisticated eye.

There are two important aspects to this. The first is realizing that single treatment approaches, most of which were developed out of an inaccurate nineteenth- and early-twentieth-century bacterial paradigm and were based on identifying the bacterial pathogen involved and then using a drug to kill it (i.e., monotherapy), are going to have to be abandoned as the primary method of treating these kinds of diseases. (Something that newer generations of physicians, especially in countries other than the United States, are beginning to understand.)

The second is coming to understand just *what* the bacteria do in the body and then designing a treatment protocol that is *specific* in counteracting it. In essence, this means designing treatment protocols that address bacterial cytokine cascades, the particular health or nonhealth of the person's immune system, and the specific symptom picture that is reducing the quality of the person's life.

Combined with antibacterials, of whatever sort, this creates the most sophisticated basic approach to the treatment of bacterial diseases. (If you add to that sophisticated human-human interactions oriented around deep caring and personal presence, something most physicians do not understand, you have the core of the most elegant and potent paradigm of disease healing that can occur.)

Some additional sophistications can occur for those who wish to go even deeper. Among them are the *synergy* that occurs among the healing agents that are used *and* those that exist between the different bacteria. The use of healing agents (pharmaceuticals *or* herbs) always involves synergy between the agents used – though this is rarely addressed in a positive light. It's usually the side effects of drug combination or drug-herb combination that are highlighted. However, herbs *are* synergistic with each other and can be positively synergistic with pharmaceuticals as well. For example, Chinese skullcap root (*Scutellaria baicalensis*) and licorice (*Glycyrrhiza* spp.) are synergists; they enhance the action of other herbs with which they are combined. Many herbs, as these do also enhance the action of pharmaceuticals. For example, Japanese knotweed (*Polygonum cuspidatum*) root, when used along with formerly ineffective antibiotics, can enhance the drugs' actions sufficiently to make them effective.

As well, the microbial pathogens are often synergistic with each other. That is, when infected by two or more Lyme-group organisms, the impacts on the body are often more severe. And this increase in severity is not additive; it tends to be more than the sum of the parts, that is, synergistic. This means that a simple linear approach will not give you an understanding of what they are doing in the body. As Telfer et al. (2010) comment . . .

> *Most hosts, including humans, are simultaneously or sequentially infected with several parasites. . . . Indeed, effects are typically of greater magnitude, and explain more variation in infection risk, than the effects associated with host and environmental factors more commonly considered in disease studies. We highlight the danger of mistaken inference when considering parasite species in isolation rather than parasite communities. . . . Single parasite studies may yield incorrect or incomplete*

conclusions. Nonetheless, most epidemiological studies, in animals and humans, still focus on single species.

Coinfection dynamics

To generate sophisticated, reliable interventions with these second-generation bacteria, there are a number of important fundamentals to understand. The primary ones are understanding the specific cytokine cascades that occur, the immune health (and preexisting conditions) in the host, the synergy between the various microorganisms, and their synergy with the vector of transmission.

Cytokines

The past several decades have seen a shift in the way many researchers (but regrettably few physicians) are approaching disease, nowhere more so than with the stealth pathogens that, due to their nature, often cause a wide range of symptoms. Researchers Ian Clark et al. (2004) for example, have done some marvelous work on the dynamics of cytokines specific to various disease conditions, especially malaria and its close relative babesia. They note that . . .

> *It is our view that focusing on malaria [and babesia and Lyme] in isolation will never provide the insights required to understand the pathogenesis of this disease. How can the illnesses caused by a spirochete and a virus be so clinically identical: typhoid readily diagnosed as malaria and malaria in returning travelers so commonly dismissed as influenza? . . . Understanding why these clinical confusions occur entails appreciating the sequence of events that led up to the cytokine revolution that has transformed the field over the last 15 years.*

Again, cytokines are small cell-signaling molecules released by cells that are damaged, cells of the immune system, and the glial cells of the nervous system that are important in intercellular communications in the body. As it turns out, many disease organisms have learned to use these for their own purposes.

In practical terms: when a bacteria touches a cell, the cell gives off a signal, a cytokine, that tells the immune system what is happening and what that cell needs. This calls on the immune system to respond (initially, the innate immune system), which then sends specific immune cells to that location to deal with the problem. Stealth pathogens subvert this process, enabling their successful infection of the body. As well, many stealth pathogens release, all on their own, many different types of cytokines, simply to jump-start the process.

As the microorganism enters the body, an initial, and very powerful, cytokine is often released into the body (for example tumor necrosis factor, aka TNF). That initial cytokine stimulates the production of others, and those generate still others – all of which have potent impacts on the body. Thus a *cascade* of cytokines occurs. This cascade (and any subsequent immune response) is carefully modulated by the pathogen to produce the exact effects it needs to facilitate its spread in the body, its sequestration inside our body's cells (thus hiding it from the immune system), to break apart particular cells in order to get nutrients, and to shut down the parts of our immune response that can effectively deal with the infection. It is this cascade of carefully modulated cytokines that, in fact, creates most of the symptoms that people experience when they become ill.

The cytokine cascade dynamics and its impacts alter depending on the animal host and its immune health. Clark et al. (2004) found that parasite load, that is the numbers of organisms in the body, counterintuitively, did not correlate to severity of illness, something that plays havoc with older bacterial theories of disease. They comment that . . .

Since P. falciparum *and* Babesia microti, *another hemoprotozoan protozoan, infect both humans and another host (the owl monkey, Aotus sp., and the mouse, respectively), it was possible to establish that the relationship [between severity of illness and parasite density] depended on a characteristic of the host, not the parasite species. This provided, for the first time, a plausible explanation for the long-standing puzzle that, although very low parasite densities cause onset of illness in first infections of human malaria and babesiosis and bovine babesiosis, mice withstand high parasite densities of several species of either*

*causative genus before onset of illness. In other words, previously
unexposed humans become ill after exposure to very few hemoprotozoan parasites whereas mice do not become ill until exposed
to many organisms. Similarly inexplicable had been the observation that incredibly high malaria parasite densities (sometimes
reaching a peak of 35,000 parasites per 10,000 red blood cells) do
not cause illness in reptiles.*

And in fact, very low densities of babesial (and spotted fever and chlamydial) organisms in people can (and do) cause serious disease. (This is also
why diagnosis is sometimes so difficult; there are so few organisms they
just can't be found during blood analysis or biopsy.) In some people high
densities occur but they remain asymptomatic. In others low densities exist
alone and still produce multiorgan failure, coma, and death.

The belief that a high density of infectious organisms is correlated with
severity of disease turns out to be inaccurate. The thought that very few
organisms could cause death did not, in older models of disease (and for
many physicians still does not), compute. Instead of parasite density, something else is involved in the development and seriousness of the disease
and its symptoms. And that something is cytokines. Clark et al. (2004) note
that . . .

> *the long-postulated malaria toxin did not cause illness directly,
> as had been assumed since the late 19th century, but did so
> through inducing the host to release a shower of LPS-inducible
> cytokines that, at lower concentrations, are an essential part of
> the host immune response.*

They continue . . .

> *Serum TNF level in East African and West African children at
> time of admission correlated with the severity of disease and
> mortality, even though serum TNF levels varied greatly. . . .
> Patients with complicated malaria (combined organ dysfunc-
> tion, hypotension, thrombocytopenia, and the highest parasite
> densities) and the longest durations between onset of clinical*

symptoms and diagnosis had significantly higher TNF levels than those in whom malaria ran a more benign course.

Cytokine researchers have found that even tiny alterations in existing cytokine profiles can cause significant shifts in disease symptoms. Clark et al. (2004) comment that, "In one IL-2 [interleukin-2] study, 15 of 44 patients developed behavioral changes sufficiently severe to warrant acute intervention and 22 had severe cognitive defects."

Although the news has not yet reached most medical doctors, many researchers are insisting that the most important thing is not the microbial source of infection but rather the cytokine cascade that is generated. This is especially true during coinfections with multiple stealth pathogens. One of the better articles on this is Andrea Graham et al., "Transmission consequences of coinfection: cytokines writ large," which appeared in *Trends in Parasitology*, volume 23, number 6, in 2007. They comment that "[w]hen the taxonomic identities of parasites are replaced with their cytokine signatures, for example, it becomes possible to predict the within-host consequences of coinfection for microparasite replication," as well as symptom picture, treatment approaches, and treatment outcomes.

(This, by the way, is the approach I use when exploring how best to treat the complex of Lyme-group coinfections. After more than a decade of experience, it turns out that interrupting the cytokine cascade these organisms initiate does in fact reduce or even eliminate both symptoms and infection.)

Immune health and preexisting conditions

Lyme-group parasites, like many stealth pathogens, utilize the immune responses of whatever mammal they infect as part of their infection strategy. As Graham et al. (2007) note: "The influence of cytokines on effector responses is so powerful that many parasites manipulate host-cytokine pathways for their own benefit," as is indeed the case with Lyme, the *Chlamydiae,* and Rocky Mountain spotted fever. Crucially, they continue, "the magnitude and type of cytokine response influence host susceptibility and infectiousness. Susceptibility to a given parasite will be affected by cytokine responses that are ongoing at the time of exposure, including responses to pre-existing infections." In other words, the bacteria utilize inflammatory processes that are already occurring in the body (e.g., preexisting arthritis) to facilitate successful infection.

But equally important is the overall *immune health* of the infected person. Telfer et al. (2009) comment that . . .

> *there is mounting evidence from experimental studies that the outcome of interactions during co-infections (for either the host or the parasite) is context dependent, potentially varying with different host or parasite genotypes or environmental conditions. Perhaps most critically, outcome can depend on the timing and sequence of infections. . . . Susceptibility is a property of an individual host at a given time. . . . the ability of a parasite to establish an infection successfully will depend on the initial immune response of the exposed host. On entry into the host, a parasite will experience an "immunoenvironment" potentially determined by both previous and current infections, as well as intrinsic factors such as sex, age, nutritional status and genotype. The immediate immuno-effectors in a naive host will be dominated by cells and molecules that comprise the innate immune response, and thus the efficiency of this arm of host immunity at reducing and clearing an infection will be influential in determining susceptibility.*

Resto-Ruiz et al. (2003) emphasize this as well, as do so many other researchers, "The reduced ability of the host's immune response to control bacterial infection apparently results in a bacteremia of longer duration . . . people with intact immune function who become infected with *B. henselae* usually" do not experience severe symptoms. In other words, the immune status of someone with coinfections *must be* addressed as part of any treatment protocol. Due to the synergistic nature of coinfections an inescapable truth exists: the weaker or more compromised the immune system, the more likely someone is to become infected and the more likely they are to have a debilitating course of illness.

Improving the immune status of those with chronic coinfections allows the immune system, refined over very long evolutionary time, to do what it does best, which is to use very elegant mechanisms to control and clear infection. Eventually, the healthy immune system begins to identify the outer membrane proteins of the bacteria and create antibodies to them. Due to the sophistication of the bacteria's subversion of the host immune system during coinfections, this can take anywhere from four to eight months. In those whose immune systems are very compromised, it may take longer, how long is directly proportional to the health of the immune system. Once the immune system creates the proper antigens, the bacteria are then eliminated fairly rapidly from the body. Reinfection is difficult as the antibodies remain in the body for some time.

This is a crucial element in addressing the treatment of coinfections, and it is one that technological medicine is generally unable to address. It is most definitely *not* a subject in which most physicians are trained.

Parasite synergy

Symptoms, length of illness, and its severity are all generally worse if infection occurs by more than one organism. Graham et al.'s research (2007) confirmed that, as the researchers put it, "coinfection increases the reproductive number for the incoming parasite species and facilitates its transmission through the host population." In other words, while the immune system is often compromised by the cytokine dynamics initiated by one type of bacteria, multiple, simultaneously initiated cascades are more potent in their impacts; infection is much more easily accomplished. This is, as Graham et al. (2007) comment, more common than otherwise. "Hosts that are coinfected by multiple parasite species seem to be the rule rather than the exception in natural systems and some of the most devastating human diseases are associated with coinfections that challenge immune response efficacy."

Another very fine paper on this is by Telfer et al., "Parasite interactions in natural populations: insights from longitudinal data," in *Parasitology*, volume 135, number 7, 2008. They echo Graham et al., when they note, "in natural populations 'concomitant' or 'mixed' infections by more than one parasite species or genotype are common. Consequently, interactions between different parasite genotypes or species frequently occur. These interactions may be synergistic or antagonistic with potential fitness implications for both the host (morbidity and/or mortality) and parasite (transmission potential)."

In other words, if you want to successfully treat someone who is infected with a vector-borne infection, you need to realize up front that it is usually the case that coinfection has occurred and you have to look at the interactive picture, not merely single infectious agents – we can no longer assume that bacterial organisms exist in a vacuum. They can't be studied in isolation.

Scott Telfer and his associates (2010), in another paper, explored the interactions and infection risks between cowpox virus, *Babesia microti, Bartonella* spp., and *Anaplasma phagocytophilum*. They note . . .

> *We found that this community of parasites represents not four independent infections but an interconnected web of interactions: Effects of other infections on infection risk were strong and widespread, and connectance within the parasite community was exceptionally high, with evidence detected for all possible pair-wide interactions.*

They found, as they note, that "the sizes of the effects of other parasites on infection risk were also similar to, and frequently greater than, other factors." Specifically, here, seasonal effects. That is, infection with Lyme-group coinfections is generally higher in certain months; it's three times higher for anaplasmal infections and fifteen times higher for babesial. Another crucial factor is the synergistic effects of multiple coinfections on host susceptibility. As they comment, "the most likely explanation for these effects is that interactions between these microparasites with individual hosts have a large impact on host susceptibility." That is, if there is more than one infectious organism involved, the easier infection in a new host will be.

The synergistic effects also contribute to symptom picture. If *Bartonella* is a coinfection with Lyme, for example, what you then get is assault on and resultant degradation of the collagen systems of the body by the Lyme spirochetes while a simultaneous assault on red blood cells occurs with a concomitant subversion and abnormalization of endothelial cells and their functions. So, the infected person is not only battling Lyme arthritis or neurological Lyme (both caused by collagen degradation) but a red blood cell infection (with potential anemia and lowered oxygen availability in the blood) and abnormal endothelial cell growth in the blood vessels themselves.

But the *Bartonella* also use what the Lyme bacteria are doing for their own purposes. This, as Telfer et al., noted, also affects host susceptibility. Once Lyme spirochetes damage collagen tissues, for instance in the joints of the knee, the body sends CD34+ cells to that site to help repair the damage. This is a normal part of the healing process when collagen is damaged. But *Bartonella* typically invade CD34+ cells, so some of those CD 34+ cells will be infected, and the *Bartonella* will take advantage of the local inflammation to establish a colony of its own in that location. The existing inflammation actually facilitates their growth. Once established, they will begin their own cytokine cascade, which will itself contribute to even more collagen degradation at that location. This tendency of the Lyme-group of pathogens to take advantage of existing inflammation is common.

The more coinfections, the more stress on the immune system. As Telfer et al. (2008) comment, "Attempts by the immune system to simultaneously counter the multiple parasite species involved in a co-infection can lead to immunopathological disease and pathology that are more than the simple additive pathogenic effects of the different parasite species." This is a crucial point. *The impact of multiple coinfectious organisms is **not** additive.* They are synergistic. They create effects that are more than the sum of the parts.

For example, infection with both *Babesia* and *Bartonella* are synergistically impactful on red blood cells and can reduce red blood cell counts up to 25 percent, leading to anemia, fatigue, breathlessness, and general weakness. In the immune-competent, neither bacteria will normally create this severe an impact by themselves. (One positive note, because both bacteria are competing for red blood cells, longer studies have found that the *Babesia*, over time, tends to clear the *Bartonella* infection by outcompeting them. Also: if someone is already infected by *Bartonella*, they are less likely to be infected with *Babesia*, and vice versa. Nevertheless, during infection with both, in the initial stages, the impact on red blood cells is immense.)

Babesia sequester themselves in the capillary networks of the spleen and liver. *Bartonella* species sequester themselves in the endothelial cells of the capillary networks of the spleen and liver. Both then seed the bloodstream from those locations at regular intervals. The impacts of infection with both parasites on the spleen and liver are much greater than either alone, and this has to be taken into account in any treatment approach. In other words, you have to design spleen- and liver-supportive interventions that are tightly focused on normalizing functioning in those organs. This protects them from cytokine damage *and* begins to reduce habitat for the bacteria, thus reducing bacterial load and presence in the body.

Studies of coinfection with *Anaplasma* and *Borrelia* have found that the deleterious impacts on immune function from such a double infection enhances the pathogenicity of the Lyme spirochetes and longterm infection. Researchers (Moro et al., 2002) note that "these effects may have a significant impact on the persistence of *B burgdorferi* and the immunologic selective pressure it is subjected to." Coinfection with Lyme spirochetes and anaplasmal bacteria produces synergistic effects on cytokine expression: IL-12, IFN-gamma, and TNF-a are more inhibited during early infection than with either bacteria alone; IL-6 levels are higher. Coinfection with these two organisms also produces more significant impacts in the brain and on brain function. There is a synergistically increased production and release of matrix metalloproteinases (MMPs) in the brain, specifically MMP-1, -3, -7, -8, and-9. IL-10 levels (which reduce effective innate immune responses and which are induced by the bacteria during initial infection) are significantly higher, and IL-8 and MIP-1a levels increase. Along with the MMPs, this leads to increased vascular permeability in the brain and CNS. This produces more inflammation deeper in the brain, with increased brain dysfunction and more serious neurocognitive defects. There is an increased bacterial burden throughout the body; symptom picture is generally worse.

Coinfection with *Borrelia* spirochetes and *Babesia microti* shows similar impacts and results both in increased severity of Lyme arthritis and its duration.

Telfer et al. (2010) also found that infection with *Anaplasma* (for example) made subsequent infection by *Babesia* much easier; in fact, it made it twice as likely. Reversing the order of infection found the same rate of increase – each organism paves the road for the other. The researchers also found that animals infected with one *Bartonella* species who were also infected by other *Bartonella* species were much more likely to have long-term infections, that is, a chronic illness.

An *Ehrlichia* infection, when combined with *Bartonella* (or *Babesia* or a hemoplasma) is often much more severe in the disease impacts than would be expected by looking at either alone. In this situation, both white and red blood cells are infected. Specifically, *Ehrlichia* infect neutrophils, the most abundant form of white blood cell in the body and an essential element of the innate immune system. Thus the immune system is fighting not only bacteria in the red blood cells and vascular tissues but bacteria inside its own immune cells. To make it worse, the bacteria cross-talk and engage in mutual support of each other, actually enhancing each others' impacts on the host and their resistance to antibiotics.

During coinfection with both *Mycoplasma* and *Bartonella*, there are going to be severe effects on the endothelial cells, the red blood cells, and the brain and CNS that are out of proportion to infection by either organism alone. Thus the cytokine impacts on those areas of the body are going to be stronger, synergistic, and more debilitating. Thus treatment regimens must be designed to reverse much stronger effects than would occur by either alone. This often calls for larger doses (or sometimes, counterintuitively, incredibly *tiny* ones), longer treatment duration, and more sophisticated intervention for symptom management. As only one example, such a double infection *may* simultaneously cause a form of regular epileptic seizures *and* periodic bouts of homicidal rage. Herbs that reduce the cytokine cascades involved *and* that are specific for these types of seizures *and* that are particularly calming to the nervous system, thus reducing extreme rage events, need to be used, and the doses, nearly always, need to be largish, continual, and very focused. (*Scutellaria baicalensis* and *Uncaria rhynchophylla* are specific examples of herbs that can reduce these symptoms.)

Researchers have also found that members of this coinfectious group tend to be present as coinfectious agents in many neurological conditions. Eighty percent of Gulf War veterans suffering from ALS were found to be infected with various mycoplasmal species. Fifteen percent of those were also infected with *Chlamydia pneumoniae* and 25 percent with *Borrelia burgdorferi*. Ninety percent of multiple sclerosis (MS) sufferers show immunological and cytokine characteristics of an infection. One of the most common findings is a chlamydial infection of the brain. Studies have found that as many of 80 percent of MS sufferers have intracellular infections from *Mycoplasma* spp., *Chlamydia pneumoniae*, *Borrelia burgdorferi*, and HHV-6. Most of them are infected with more than one organism. Children with autism spectrum disorder (ASD) also show infections with this group of organisms, often together. *Mycoplasma* spp., *Chlamydia pneumoniae*, *Borrelia burgdorferi*, and HHV-6 are again the most common.

In one study, the blood of one hundred people with Lyme disease were extensively studied for the presence of other microorganisms. The blood samples were sent to various laboratories for testing. In addition to *Borrelia* spp., in order of commonality, *Mycoplasma* spp was found in 45–70 percent (depending on lab used), *Ehrlichia* spp in 10-35 percent, *Bartonella* spp in 25–40 percent, *Babesia* spp in 8–20 percent, and *Chlamydia pneumonia* in 10 percent. The surprising thing (to me) is that all the labs that were used were considered top of the line . . . and they still varied widely in their findings. Still, studies such as these show that coinfection is the rule, not the exception. Researcher Garth Nicolson (2007) comments that . . .

> *[w]e and others have examined patients with various neuro-degernative and behavioral neurological conditions such as ALS, MS, and ASD and found evidence for systemic intracellu-lar bacterial and viral infections in a majority of patients. For example, examination of blood leukocytes for evidence of* Myco-plasma spp, Chlamydia pneumoniae, Borrelia burgdorferi *and other infections by PCR revealed high incidences of systemic co-infections that were not found in control subjects. . . . The most common co-infection found was* Mycoplasma *species in all of the conditions examined. In contrast, in the few control subjects that tested positive, only single infections were found. The results suggest chronic intracellular bacterial infections are common features of neurodegenerative and behavioral disorders, and treatment regimens should address the multiple infections present in these conditions.*

As Nicolson observes, "Coinfections complicate the diagnosis and produce different signs/symptoms of LD [Lyme disease]. These infections can also occur in various combinations. . . . When multiple infections are present, the number of signs/symptoms, their severity and duration, can be greater than in early stages of the disease."

A few other coinfectious interactions

- Malarial and relapsing fever (RF) coinfection decreases malarial burden but substantially increases (by twenty-one-fold) the number of RF spirochetes.
- Coinfection with *Anaplasma* increases the severity and dissemination of *Borrelia* in tissues and vice versa. Coinfection, researchers found (Grab et al., 2007), "enhanced reductions in transendothelial electrical resistance [TEER] and enhanced or synergistically increased production of metalloproteinases, cytokines and chemokines, which are known to affect vascular permeability and inflammatory responses." Coinfection with the two organisms increases bacterial burden, arthritic symptoms, and pathogen transmission to the vector. The impacts of neurological infection by *Anaplasma* are increased by *Borrelia* bacteria, specifically, IL-8 and MIP-1A levels are significantly augmented.
- Simultaneous infection by *Borrelia burgdorferi* ss and *Borrelia garinii* causes a more severe borreliosis.
- Prior infection with *Borrelia burgdorferi* enhances the replication of rickettsial organisms.
- Chlamydial and borrelial bacteria are commonly (more than 50 percent of the time) present together in the synovial fluid of people with early undifferentiated oligoarthritis.
- Borrelial infection in wild mouse populations lowers the ecological threshold for babesial parasites to become established in new ecoregions, increasing its emergence and expansion. They synergistically support each other in becoming endemic in new regions. (This appears to also be true in the microecological habitat of the human body.)

Ultimately, we have to look very closely and sensitively at the interactions that are occurring during infection if we wish to alter the course of the disease and return the people we work with to health. We need to create even more subtle interventions to counteract the impacts of multiple infectious organisms.

Herbal interventions

The protocols that I have developed in the three books on Lyme and its coinfections, as well as those in *Herbal Antivirals* (which covers, among other things, tick-borne encephalitis, another coinfectious organism), offer a perspective on how sophisticated herbal protocols can become.

The important thing to remember, to gain a sense of (this is a feeling thing, not a thinking thing), is that the herbal protocol you develop is similar to a bouquet of flowers. When combined it becomes a unique entity possessing specific effects. Slight modulation of the herbs produces an entirely different entity, with, sometimes, substantially different effects. The only way to get there is to *feel* your way to it. You may begin with an analytical understanding of what is happening and what you are creating, but once the protocol is generated for a particular person, it is mostly feeling that gets you where you are going, not thinking. The same is true for the disease complex itself. Each person has a slightly different form of infection, comprised, usually, of multiple coinfectious agents. You begin, again, with an analytical understanding, but your access to the reality of the disease in that person is the feeling sense, not the thinking mind.

Once you have a sense of these, you can begin to subtly modulate the process. It is a *conversation* not a monologue you are engaged in. You use the herbs to respond to what you are being told, the body and the organisms respond, and you take in and interpret what they are saying and then generate a new response. In this it is crucial to see the person in front of you every time they enter the office. They are *not* the same person they were the last time you saw them. Nor is the disease complex.

This is why true healing will always be more of an art than a science and why a combination of mind (thinking) and feeling are essential. Both are crucial in the process. Stealth infections need focus of mind, the ability to think deeply, in order to understand and treat them. But they also necessitate a well-trained and focused feeling sense as well. One without the other simply is not enough.

RESOURCES

Ooooh, look! A flower.
Four-year-old on a walk

*The tree which moves some to tears of joy is in the eyes of others
only a green thing that stands in the way.*
William Blake

Many of the herbs I have talked about in this book – and, of course, a great many others – grow wild. Even if you live in a city, you can find many of them co-habitating with you or only a short drive from your home. Since many of these herbs are invasives, most people will be glad for you to take them away.

If you need to buy your herbs, the Internet is a good way to seek them. I suggest running a web search for the herbs you are looking for to find the cheapest prices; if you are persistent you can often save half off normal retail.

If you are going to be buying a lot of herbs and you live in the US it makes sense to buy a resale license from your state. The price is often minimal (five dollars or so), and it will allow you to buy wholesale; most wholesalers will want a resale certificate before they will sell to you.

And, of course, you can grow them yourself. Once established most of the herbs in this book will provide medicine for you and your family forever.

Here are some of the best sources I know of for the herbs in this book. All of them are in the US:

- Woodland Essence: Kate and Don make wonderful tinctures and medicines and can sell you many of the herbal tinctures that I discuss in this book; if they don't have them, they can probably point you in the right direction. Woodland

Essence, 392 Teacup Street, Cold Brook, NY 13324, (315)
845-1515, www.woodlandessence.com.

- Horizon Herbs: Richo Cech has spent much of his life learning how to grow common and rare medicinals. He has seeds
or young stock for most of the plants in this book as well as
great information on how to grow them. Horizon Herbs,
P.O.Box 69, Williams, OR 97544, (541) 846-6704, www
.Horizonherbs.com.

- Pacific Botanicals: This is perhaps the best wholesaler (they
also sell retail) in the US. Their herbs are magnificent.
Normally, all are sold by the pound. Pacific Botanicals, 4840
Fish Hatchery Road, Grants Pass, OR 97527, (541) 479-7777,
www.pacificbotanicals.com.

- Zack Woods Herb Farm: Melanie and Jeff are wonderful
people and grow tremendously beautiful medicinal plants.
Very, very high quality herbs. Usually sold by the pound.
Zack Woods Herb Farm, 278 Mead Road, Hyde Park, VT
05655, (802) 888-7278, www.zackwoodsherbs.com.

- Healing Spirits Herb Farm: Matthias and Andrea Reisen have
been growing wonderful medicinal plants for years. The
plants just jump out of the bags and laugh when you open
them up. Healing Spirits Herb Farm, 61247 Rt 415, Avoca, NY
14809, (607) 566-2701, [www]healingspiritsherbfarm.com.

- Elk Mountain Herbs: Wonderful tinctures from local wild-
crafted Western plants. Elk Mountain Herbs, 214 Ord Street,
Laramie, WY 82070, (307) 742-0404, www.elkmountain
herbs.com.

- Sage Woman Herbs: They have some herbs otherwise hard
to get, especially isatis tincture (just the root though). Sage
Woman Herbs, 108 East Cheyenne Road, Colorado Springs,
CO 80906, (888) 350-3911, (719) 473-8873, www.sagewoman
herbs.com.

- 1st Chinese Herbs: Wonderful people with a very large selection of Chinese herbs, including most of those discussed in
this book. Most herbs by the pound. 1st Chinese Herbs, 5018

View Ridge Drive, Olympia, WA 98501, (888) 842-2049, (360) 923-0486, www.1stchineseherbs.com.

- Montana Farmacy: Wonderful herbs, wonderful people. P.O. Box 444, Trego, MT 59934. 406-882-4545. www.montana farmacy.com. (She carries the herbal tick repellant discussed in the Lyme protocol chapter.)
- Desert Tortoise Botanicals: John Slattery and friends. Another wonderful company with wonderful herbs (mostly southwestern). 4802 E. Montecito Street, Tucson, AZ 85711. www.deserttortoisebotanicals.com.
- Mountian Rose Herbs: a nice selection, sustainably produced. Moutain Rose Herbs, P.O. Box 50220, Eugene, OR, 1-800-879-3337, (541) 741-7307, www.mountainroseherbs.com.

A few good practitioners

Sometime ago, a wonderful woman by the name of Julie Genser created a website about my work on Lyme disease and its coinfections. Julie herself has been struggling with a number of chronic conditions over the years, but she still found the time to create a site that has helped a great many people. I don't, other than answering queries from time to time, have anything to do with that site, but it is a good source of information about practitioners that are knowledgeable about the protocols I suggest in my books on the Lyme-group of infections. In addition to the practitioners on that site (Buhnerhealinglyme.com; there are also a few Facebook groups), I also highly recommend my partner Julie McIntyre (Silver City, NM, who also offers phone consultations), Tommy Priester (MA, Bear Medicine Herbs), Neil Nathan, MD (Gordon Medical Associates, Santa Rosa, CA), and Tim Scott, LAc (Brattleboro, VT). All of them are very good; all are wonderful people who genuinely care about healing and their patients. Because contact information changes from time to time, I suggest Googling them for current contact information.

BIBLIOGRAPHY

Please note: The majority of the many citations in the first edition of this book are not relisted here due to space limitations (though some of them are); they are still relevant and can be found in that volume.

TEXTS

Aggarwal, Bhrat, et al. *Molecular Targets and Therapeutic Uses of Spices*, Singapore: World Scientific, 2009.

Atta-ur-Rahman, FRS. Studies in Natural Products Chemistry, volume 43, NY: Elsevier, 2014, Chapter 13, "Biologically Active Compounds from the Genus *Uncaria*."

Bergner, Paul. *Medical Herbalism*, all issues.

Blumenthal, Mark, et al. *The Complete German Commission E Monographs*, Austin, TX: American Botanical Council, 1998.

Brinker, Francis. *Herb Contraindications and Drug Interactions*, Sandy, OR: Eclectic Publications, 1998.

Bryan, L.E. *Bacterial Resistance and Susceptibility to Chemotherapeutic Agents*, Cambridge:Cambridge University press, 1982.

Buhner, Stephen Harrod. *Healing Lyme: Natural Healing and Prevention of Lyme Borreliosis and its Coinfections*, first edition, Silver City, NM: Raven Press, 2005.

Buhner. *Healing Lyme Disease Coinfections: Complimentary and Holistic Treatments for Bartonella and Mycoplasma*, Rochester, VT: Inner Traditions, 2013.

Buhner. *Herbal Antibiotics*, second edition, North Adams, MA: Storey Publishing, 2012.

Buhner. *Herbal Antivirals*, North Adams, MA: Storey Publishing, 2013.

Buhner. *Natural Treatments for Lyme Coinfections: Anaplasma, Babesia, and Ehrlichia*, Rochester, VT: Inner Traditions, 2015.

Caeser, Andrea. A Twist of Lyme: Battling a Disease that "Doesn't Exist." NY: Archway Publishing, 2013.

Cech, Richo. *Making Plant Medicine*, Williams, OR: Horizon Herbs Publication, 2000.

Ellingwood, Finley. *American Materia Medica, Therapeutics, and Pharmacognosy*, Cincinnati: Electic Publications, 1919.

Felter, Harvey and John Uri Lloyd, *King's American Dispensatory*, Cincinnati: Eclectic Publications, 1895.

Green, James. *The Herbal Medicine-Makers Handbook*, Fourth Edition, Forestville, CA: Wildlife and Green, 1990.

Haber, Mindy. *Lyme Rage: A Mother's Struggle to Save Her Daughter from Lyme Disease*, Rhinebeck, NY: Epigraph Publishing, 2014.

Harborne, Jeffrey, et al. *Phytochemical Dictionary: A Handbook of Bioactive Compounds from Plants*, Second Edition, London: Taylor and Francis, 1999.

Hoffmann, David. *The Herbal Handbook: A User's Guide to Medical Herbalism*, Rochester, VT:Healing Arts Press, 1988.

Hoffmann. *Medical Herbalism*, Rochester, VT: Healing Arts Press, 2003.

Hoffmann. *The New Holstic Herbal*, Rockport, MA: Element, 1992.

Horowitz, Richard. *Why Can't I Get Better? Solving the Mystery of Lyme and Chronic Disease*, NY, St. Martins, 2013.

Hson-Mon Chang and Paul Pui-Hay But. *Pharmacology and Applications of Chinese Materia Medica*, 2 vols, Singapore: World Scientific, 2001.

Jing-Nuan Wu. *An Illustrated Chinese Materia Medica*, NY:Oxford University Press, 2005.

Khan, Ikhlas, and Ehab Abourashed. *Leung's Encyclopedia of Common Natural Ingredients Used in Food, Drugs, and Cosmetics*, Hoboken, NJ: Wiley, 2010.

Langenheim, Jean. *Plant Resins: Chemistry, Evolution, Ecology, Ethnobotany*, Portland, OR: Timber Press, 2003.

Lott, Joey. *Healing Chronic Lyme Disease Naturally*, NP: Archangel Ink, 2014.

Makris, Katina. *Out of the Woods: Healing From Lyme Disease for Body, Mind, and Spirit*, NY: Helios Press, 2015.

Manandhar, Narayan. *Plants and People of Nepal*, Portland, OR: Timber Press, 2002.

Mitsuhashi, S. *Drug Action and Drug Resistance in Bacteria*, Tokyo: University of Tokyo Press, 1971.

Moore, Michael. *Herbal Materia Medica*, Albuquerque, NM: SWSBM, 1990.

Moore. *Herbal Repertory in Clinical Practice*, Albuquerque, NM: SWSBM, 1990.

Moore. *Herbal Tinctures in Clinical Practice*, Albuquerque, NM: SWSBM, 1990.

Moore. *Medicinal Plants of the Desert and Canyon West*, Santa Fe, NM: Museum of New Mexico Press, 1989.

Moore. *Medicinal Plants of the Mountain West*, Santa Fe: Museum of New Mexico Press, 1976.

Moore. *Medicinal Plants of the Pacific Northwest*, Santa Fe, NM: Red Crane Books, 1993.

Nadkarni, A.K. *Indian Materia Medica*, 2 vols, Bombay: Popular Prakashan, 1927.

Nathan, Neil. *Healing is Possible: New Hope for Chronic Fatigue, Fibromyalgia, Persisting Pain, and Other Chronic Illnesses*, Laguna Beach, CA: Basic Health Publications, 2013.

Rosner, Bryan and Kim Junker. *Freedom from Lyme Disease*, South Lake Tahoe, CA: Biomed Publishing Group, 2014.

Scott, Timothy Lee. *Invasive Plant Medicine*, Rochester, VT: Healing Arts Press, 2010.

Shiu-Ying Hu. *An Enumeration of Chinese Materia Medica*, Hong Kong: Chinese University Press, 1980.

Singleton, Kenneth. *The Lyme Disease Solution*, Charleston, SC: Book Surge Publishing, 2008.

Storl, Wolf. *Healing Lyme Disease Naturally*, Berkeley, CA: North Atlantic Books, 2010.

Strasheim, Connie. *Insights into Lyme Disease Treatment: 13 Lyme-Literate Health Care Practitioners Share Their Healing Strategies*, South Lake Tahoe, CA: Biomed Publishing, 2009.

Strasheim and Lee Cowden. *Beyond Lyme Disease: Healing the Underlying Causes of Chronic Illness in People with Borreliosis and Coinfections*, South Lake Tahoe, CA: Biomed publishing, 2012.

Stuart, G.A. *Chinese Materia Medica, Vegetable Kingdom*, Shanghai: American Presbyterian Mission Press, 1911.

Van Wyck, Ben-Erik and Michael Wink. *Medicinal Plants of the World*, Portland, OR: Timber Press, 2004.

Weintraub, Pamela. *Cure Unknown: Inside the Lyme Epidemic*, NY:St. Martins, 2008.

Weiss, Rudolph. *Herbal Medicine*, Sweden: Beaconsfield, 1988.

White, Shelly. *Cannabis for Lyme Disease & Related Conditions: Scientific Basis and Anecdotal Evidence for Medicinal Use*, South Lake Tahoe, CA: Biomed Publishing, 2015.

Willcox, Merlin, et al, editors. *Traditional Medicinal Plants and Malaria*, Boca Raton, FL: CRC Press, 2004.

Williams, J. E. *Viral Immunity*, Charlottesville, VA: Hampton Roads, 2002.

Williams, Mara. *Nature's Dirty Needle: What You Need to Know About Chronic Lyme Disease and How to Get the Help You Need to Feel Better*, SF, CA: Bush Street Press, 2011.

Winston, David and Steven Maimes. *Adaptogens*, Rochester, VT: Healing Arts Press, 2007.

You-Ping Zhu. *Chinese Materia Medica: Chemistry, Pharmacology and Applications*, Amsterdam: Harwood Academic Publishers, 1998.

Zhang Enqin. *Rare Chinese Materia Medica*, Shanghai: Shanghai University of Traditional Chinese Medicine, 1989.

JOURNAL PAPERS

The journal papers that cover these conditions, especially borrelial bacteria, are massive. This is only a sampling of what is available online; it's still rather extensive.

Lyme and Relapsing Fever

Aalto A. et al. Brain magnetic resonance imaging does not contribute to the diagnosis of chronic neuroborreliosis. *Acta Radiol.* 2007;48(7):755-62.

Aberer E. et al. Course of Borrelia burgdorferi DNA shedding in urine after treatment. *Acta Derm Venereol.* 2007;87(1):39-42.

Abraham S. et al. Brief, recurrent, and spontaneous episodes of loss of consciousness in a healthy young male. *Int Med Case Rep J.* 2010;3:71-6.

Abul-Kasim K. Neuroborreliosis with enhancement of the third, fifth, sixth and twelfth cranial nerves. *Acta Neurol Belg.* 2010;110(2):215.

Adeolu M., Gupta RS. A phylogenomic and molecular marker based proposal for the division of the genus Borrelia into two genera: the emended genus Borrelia containing only the members of the relapsing fever Borrelia, and the genus Borreliella gen. nov. containing the members of the Lyme disease Borrelia (Borrelia burgdorferi sensu lato complex. *Antonie Van Leeuwenhoek.* 2014;105(6):1049-72.

Adusumilli S. et al. Passage through Ixodes scapularis ticks enhances the virulence of a weakly pathogenic isolate of Borrelia burgdorferi. *Infect Immun.* 2010;78(1):138-44.

Agterof MJ. and ter Borg EJ. Erythematous pigmentation of the arm for more than ten years. *J Med.* 2008;66(4):176-79.

Aguirre JD. et al. A manganese-rich environment supports superoxide dismutase activity in a Lyme disease pathogen, Borrelia burgdorferi. *J Biol Chem.* 2013;288(12):8468-78.

Aher AR. et al. A case report of relapsing fever. *Indian J Pathol Microbiol.* 2008;51(2):292-3.

Al-Robaiy S. et al. Metamorphosis of Borrelia burgdorferi organisms—RNA, lipid and protein composition in context with the spirochetes' shape. *J Basic Microbiol.* 2010; 50 Suppl 1:S5-17.

Albrecht P. et al. A case of relapsing-remitting neuroborreliosis? Challenges in the differential diagnosis of recurrent myelitis. *Case Rep Neurol.* 2012;4:47-53.

Ali A. et al. Experiences of patients identifying with chronic Lyme disease in the healthcare system: a qualitative study. *BMC Fam Pract.* 2014;13:79.

Aliota MT. et al. The prevalence of zoonotic tick-borne pathogens in Ixodes scapularis collected in the Hudson Valley, New York State. *Vector Borne Zoonotic Dis.* 2014;14(4):245-50.

Alitalo A. et al. Lysine-dependent multipoint binding of the Borrelia burgdorferi virulence factor outer surface protein E to the C terminus of factor H. *J immunol.* 2004;172(10):6195-01.

Almodovar JL. et al. Acute bilateral painless radiculitis with abnormal Borrelia burgdorferi immunoblot. *J Clin Neuromuscul Dis.* 2012;14(2):75-7.

Amedei A. et al. Cerebrospinal fluid T-regulatory cells recognize Borrelia burgdorferi NAPA in chronic Lyme borreliosis. *Int J Immunopathol Pharmacol.* 2013;26(4):907-15.

Amore G. et al. Borrelia lusitaniae in immature Ixodes ricinus (Acari: Ixodidae) feeding on common wall lizards in Tuscan, Central Italy. *J Med Entomol.* 2007;44(2):303-7.

Andersson M. et al. In situ immune response in brain and kidney during early relapsing fever borreliosis. *J Neuroimmunol.* 2007;183(1-2):26-32.

Andersson M., Scherman K., Raberg L. Multiple-strain infections of Borrelia afzelii: a role for within-host interactions in the maintenance of antigenic diversity? *Am Nat.* 2013;181(4):545-54.

Ang CW. et al. Large differences between test strategies for the detection of anti-Borrelia antibodies are reveled by comparing eight ELISAs and five immunoblots. *Eur J Clin Microbiol Infect Dis.* 2011;30:1027-32.

Angel TE. et al. Proteome analysis of Borrelia burgdorferi response to environmental change. *PLoS One.* 2010;5(11):13800.

Antonara S., Ristow L., Conburn J. Adhesion mechanisms of Borrelia burgdorferi. *Adv Exp Med Biol.* 2011;715:35-49.

Arnaboldi PM., Sambir M., Dattwyler RJ. II. Decorin binding proteins A and B in the serodiagnosis of Lyme disease in North America. *Clin Vaccine Immunol.* 2014;21(10):1426-36.

Arruti M et al. Abdominal pain and wall distension as the onset form of neuroborreliosis. *Med Clin (Barc).* 2012;138(13):591-2.

Assous MV. et al. Molecular characterization of Tickborne relapsing fever Borrelia, Israel. *Emerg Infect Dis.* 2006;12(11):1740.

Atkinson SF. et al. A determination of the spatial concordance between Lyme disease incidence and habitat probability of its primary vector Ixodes scapularis (black legged tick). *Geospat Health.* 2014;9(1):203-12.

Aucott JN., Seifter A., Rebman AW. Probable late Lyme disease: a variant manifestation of untreated Borrelia burgdorferi infection. *BMC Infect Dis.* 2012;12:173.

Auwaerter PG. Point: Antibiotic Therapy Is Not the answer for patients with Persisting Symptoms Attributable to Lyme Disease. *Clin Infec Dis.* 2007;45:143-8.

Auwaerter PG. Scientific evidence and best patient care practices should guide the ethics of Lyme disease activism. *J Med Ethics.* 2011;37(2):68-73.

Auwaerter PG., Melia MT. Bullying Borrelia: when the culture of science is under attack. *Transact American Clin Climatol Assoc.* 2012;123:79-87.

Auwaerter PG. et al. Antiscience and ethical concerns associated with advocacy of Lyme disease. *Lancet Infect Dis.* 2011;11(9):713-9.

Bababeygy SR., Quiros PA. Isolated trochlear palsy secondary to Lyme neuroborreliosis. *Int Ophthalmol.* 2011;31(6):493-5.

Babady NE. et al. Percent positive rate of Lyme real-time polymerase chain reaction in blood, cerebrospinal fluid, synovial fluid, and tissue. *Diagn Microbiol Infect Dis.* 2008; 62(4):464-6.

Bachmann M. et al. Early production of IL-22 but not IL-17 by peripheral blood mononuclear cells exposed to live Borrelia burgdorferi: the role of monocytes and Interleukin-1. *PLoS Pathog* 2010;6(10):e1001144.

Bacino L. et al. Complete atrioventricular block as the first clinical manifestation of a tick bite in Lyme Disease. *G Ital Cardiol (ROME).* 2011;12(3):214-6.

Back T. et al. Neuroborreliosis-associated cerebral vasculitis: long-term outcome and health-related quality of life. *J Neurol.* 2013;260(6):1569-75.

Backenson, P, et al. Borrelia burgdorferi shows specificity of binding to glycosphingolipids. *Infect Immun* 1995; 63(8): 2811-7.

Bacon RM. et al Surveillance for Lyme disease—United States, 1992-2006. *MMWR Surveill Summ.* 2008;57(10):1-9.

Badger MS. Tick talk: unusually severe case of tick-borne relapsing fever with acute respiratory distress syndrome—case report and review of the literature. *Wilderness Environ Med.* 2008;19(4):280-6.

Ball R. HLA type and immune response to Borrelia burgdorferi outer surface protein a in people in whom arthritis developed after Lyme disease vaccination. *Arthritis Rheum.* 2009;60(4):1179-86.

Banerjee R., Liu JJ., Minhas HM. Lyme neuroborreliosis presenting with alexithymia and suicide attempts. *J Clin Psychiatry.* 2013;74(10):981.

Baranova NS. et al. Lesions of nervous systems in remote stages of Lyme borreliosis. *Zh Nevrol Psikhiatr Im S S Korsakova.* 2010;110(2):90-6.

Baranova NS. et al. Lyme disease in patients with multiple sclerosis: clinical, diagnostic and therapeutic features. *Zh Nevrol Psikhiatr Im S S Korsakova.* 2012;112(2Pt2):64-8.

Baranton G. and De Martino SJ. Borrelia burgdorferi sensu lato diversity and its influence on pathogenicity in humans. *Curr Probl Dermatol.* 2009;37:1-17.

Barbarese E. et al. Expression and localization of myelin basic protein in oligodendrocytes and transfected fibroblasts. *J Neurochem* 1988; 51(6): 1737-45.

Barbour AG. Phylogeny of a relapsing fever Borrelia species transmitted by the hard tick Ixodes scapularis. *Infect Genet Evol.* 2014;27:551-8.

Barbour AG. et al. Niche partitioning of Borrelia burgdorferi and Borrelia miyamotoi in the same tick vector and mammalian reservoir species. *Am J Trop Med Hyg.* 2009;81(6):1120-31.

Barcena-Uribarri I. et al. P66 porins are present in both Lyme disease and relapsing fever spirochetes: a comparison of the biophysical properties of P66 porins from six Borrelia species. *Biochimica Biophysica Acta* 1798.2010:1197-03.

Barclay SS., Melia MT., Auwaerter PG. Misdiagnosis of late-onset Lyme arthritis by inappropriate use of Borrelia burgdorferi immunoblot testing with synovial fluid. *Clin Vaccine Immunol.* 2012;19(11):1806-9.

Barie PS. Warning! Danger Will Robinson! Lyme disease clinical practice guidelines of the Infectious Diseases Society of America, activist patients, antitrust law, and prosecutorial zeal. *Surg Infect (Larchmt).* 2007;8(2):147-50.

Barmaki A. et al. Study on presence of Borrelia persica in soft ticks in western Iran. *Iran J Arthropod Borne Dis.*2010;4(2):19-25.

Barthold SW. et al. Ineffectiveness of tigecycline against persistant Borrelia burgdorferi. *Antimicrob Agents Chemother.* 2010;54(2):643-51.

Baud and Greub. Intracellular bacteria and adverse pregnancy outcomes, *Clin Microbiol Infect* (2011); 17(9):1312-22.

Baum E. et al. Diversity of antibody responses to Borrelia burgdorferi in experimentally infected beagle dogs. *Clin Vaccine Immunol.* 2014;21(6):838-46.

Baumann M. et al. Uncommon manifestations of neuroborreliosis in children. *Eur J Paediatr Neurol.* 2010;14(3):274-7.

Bazovska S. et al. Lyme borreliosis and demyelinating disease of the central nervous system. *Epidemiol Mikrobiol Imunol.* 2011;60(1):45-7.

Bednarova J. Cerebrospinal-fluid profile in neuroborreliosis and its diagnostic significance. *Folia Microbiol (Praha).* 2006;51(6):599-03.

Begon E. Lyme arthritis, Lyme carditis and other presentations potentially associated to Lyme disease. *Med Mal Infect.* 2007;37(7-8):422-34.

Behera AK. et al. Borrelia burgdorferi BBB07 interaction with integrin alpha3beta1 stimulates production of pro-inflammatory mediators in primary human chondrocytes. *Cell Microbiol.* 2008;10(2):320-31.

Beikin IaB. et al. Specifics of cytokine regulation in tick-borne encephalitis and Lyme borreliosis. *Vestn Ross Akad Med Nauk.* 2007;(9):16-9.

Belloni B. et al. 5-yr-old with borrelial lymphocytoma. *MMW Fortschr Med.* 2011;153(10):40.

Belot V. et al. Eosinophilic fasciitis associated with Borrelia burgdorferi infection. *Ann Dermatol Venereol.* 2007;134(8-9):673-7.

Belperron AA. et al. Dual role for Fcy receptors in host defense and disease in Borrelia burgdorferi-infected mice. *Front Cell Infect Microbiol.* 2014;4(75):1-12.

Belperron AA. et al. Marginal zone B-cell depletion impairs murine host defense against Borrelia burgdorferi infection. *Infect Immun.* 2001;75(7):3354-60.

Belum GR. et al. The Jarisch-Herxheimer reaction: revisited. *Travel Med Infect Dis.*2013;11(4):231-7.

Benedix F. et al. Early disseminated borreliosis with multiple erythema migrans and elevated liver enzymes: case report and literature review. *Acta Derm Venereol.* 2007;87(5):418-21.

Bennet L., Halling A., Berlund J. Increased incidence of Lyme borreliosis in Southern Sweden following mild winters and during warm, humid summers. *Eur J Clin Microbiol Infect Dis.* 2006;25(7):426-32.

Bennet L., Stjernberg L., Berlund J. Effect of gender on clinical and epidemiologic features of Lyme borreliosis. *Vector Borne Zoonotic Dis.* 2007;7(1):34-41.

Benoit VM. et al. Allelic variation of the lyme disease spirochete adhesin dbpa influences spirochetal binding to decorin, dermatan sulfate, and mammalian cells. *Infect Immun.* 2001;79(9):3501-3509.

Benoit VM. et al. Genetic control of the innate immune response to Borrelia hermsii influences the course of relapsing fever in inbred strains of mice. *Infect Immun.* 2010;78(2):586-94.

Beremell D. et al. Cerebrospinal fluid CXCL13 in Lyme neuroborreliosis and asymptomatic HIV infection. *Bio Med.* 2013;13:2(1-8).

Berende A. et al. Activation of innate host defense mechanisms by Borrelia. *Eur Cytokine Netw.* 2010;21(1):7-18.

Berghoff W. Chronic Lyme disease and Co-infections: differential diagnosis. *Open Neurol J.* 2012;6 (Suppl 1-M10):158-78.

Bernardino ALF., Kaushal D. and Philipp MT. The antibiotics doxycycline and minocycline inhibit the inflammatory responses to the Lyme disease spirochete Borrelia burgdorferi. *J Infet Dis.* 2009;199(9):1379-88.

Bernardino ALF. et al. Toll-Like Receptors: Insights into Their Possible Role in the Pathogenesis of Lyme Neuroborreliosis. *Infect Immun.* 2008;76(10):43855-95.

Berndtson K. Review of evidence for immune evasion and persistent infection in Lyme disease. *Int J Gen Med.* 2013;6:291-06.

Bestor A. et al. Competitive advantage of Borrelia burgdorferi with outer surface protein BBA03 during tick-mediated infection of the mammalian host. *Infect Immun.* 2012;80(10):3501-11.

Bettina P., Alroy J. and Huber BT. CD28 deficiency exacerbates joint inflammation upon Borrelia burgdorferi infection, resulting in the development of chronic Lyme arthritis. *J Immunol.* 2007;179(12):8076-82.

Bhambhani N., Disla E. and Cuppari G. Lyme disease presenting with sequential episodes of ruptured Baker cysts. *J Clin Rheumatol.* 2006;12(3):160-2.

Bhattacharjee A. et al. Structural basis for complement evasion of Lyme disease pathogen Borrelia burgdorferi. *J Biol Chem.* 2013;288(26):18685-95.

Bhide MR. et al. Complement factor H binding by different Lyme disease and relapsing fever Borrelia in animals and human. *BMC Res Notes.* 2009;2:134.

Biesiada G. et al. Levels of sVCAM-1 and sICAM-1 in patients with Lyme disease. *Pol Arch Med Wewn.* 2009;119(4):200-4.

Biesiada G. et al. Lyme disease: review. *Arch Med Sci.* 2010;8(6):978-82.

Biesiada G. et al. Neopterin in serum and cerebrospinal fluid in Lyme disease. *Przegl Lek.* 2009;66(9):508-10.

Biesiada G. et al. Neurobrreliosis with extrapyramidal symptoms: a case report. *Pol Arch Med Wewn.* 2008;118(5):314-7.

Binalsheikh IM. et al. Lyme neuroborreliosis presenting as Alice in Wonderland syndrome. *Pediatr Neurol.* 2012;46(3):185-6.

Binder SC., Telschow A., Meyer-Hermann M. Population dynamics of Borrelia burgdorferi in Lyme disease. *Front Microbiol.* 2012;3:104.

Biswas D. and Stafford N. Borrelia tonsillitis: common symptoms but uncommon organism. *Eur Arch Otorhinolaryngol.* 201;267(6):989-90.

Blaho VA. et al. 5-Lipoxygenase-deficient mice infected with Borrelia burgdorferi develop persistent arthritis. *J Immunol.* 2011;186(5):3076-84.

Blaho VA. et al. Cyclooxygenase-1 orchestrates germinal center formation and antibody class-switch via regulation of IL-17. *J Immunol.* 2009;183(9):5644-53.

Blaho VA. et al. Lipidomic analysis of dynamic eicosanoid responses during the induction and resolution of Lyme arthritis. *J Biol Chem.* 2009;284(32):21599-612.

Blaho VA., Mitchel WJ. and Brown CR. Arthritis develops but fails to resolve during inhibition of cyclooxygenase. *Arthritis Rheum.* 2008;58(5):1485-95.

Blaise S. et al. Lyme disease acrodermitis chronica atrophicans: misleading vascular signs. *J Mal Vasc.* 2014;39(3):212-5.

Blanc F. et al. Lyme neuroborreliosis and dementia. *J Alzheimers Dis.* 2014;41(4):1087-93.

Blanc F. et al. Lyme optic neuritis. *J Neurol Sci.*2010;295(1-2):117-9.

Blazejewicz-Zawadziniska M. et al. A retrospective analysis of 973 patients with Lyme borreliosis in Kuyavian-Pomeranian voivodship in 2000-2005. *Przegl Epidemiol.* 2012;66(4):581-6.

Blewett MM. Hypothesized role of galactocerebroside and NKT cells in the etiology of multiple sclerosis. *Med Hypotheses.* 2008;70(4):826-30.

Blowey, R, et al. Borrelia burgdorferi infections in UK cattle: a possible association with digital dermatitis. *Vet Rec* 1994; 135(24): 577-8.

Bockenstedt LK. et al. Detection of attenuated, noninfectious spirochetes in Borrelia burgdorferi-infected mice after antibiotic treatment. *J Infect Dis.* 2002;186(10):1430-7.

Bockenstedt LK. et al. Spirochete antigens persist near cartilage after murine Lyme borreliosis therapy. *J Clin Invest.* 2012;122(7):2652-60.

Boer A. et al. Erythema migrans: a reassessment of diagnostic criteria for early cutaneous manifestations of borreliosis with particular emphasis on clonality investigations. I *Br J Dermatol.* 2007;156(6):1263-71.

Bolin, C and Koellner, P. Human-to human transmission of Leptospira interrogans by milk. *Journal of Infections Disease* 1988; 158(1): 246-7.

Borchers AT. et al. Lyme disease: a rigorous review of diagnostic criteria and treatment. *J Autoimmun.* 2014;pii:S0896-8411(14)00133-4.

Borde JP. et al. CXXCL13 may improve diagnosis in early neuroborreliosis with atypical laboratory findings. *BMC Infect Dis.* 2012;12:344.

Borgermans L. et al. Relevance of chronic Lyme disease to family medicine as a complex multidimensional chronic disease construct: A systematic review. *Internat J Family Med.* 2014;138016:1-10.

Bouchard C. et al. Does high biodiversity reduce the risk of Lyme disease invasion? *Parasit Vectors.* 2013;6:195.

Boye T. What kind of clinical, epidemiological, and biological data is essential for the diagnosis of Lyme borreliosis? Dermatological and ophthalmological courses of Lyme borreliosis. *Med Mal Infect.* 2007;37 Suppl 3:S175-88.

Boylan JA, et al. Borrelia burgdorferi membranes are the primary targets of reactive oxygen species. *Mol microbiol.* 2008;68(3):786-99.

Bradley, et al. The persistence of spirochetal nucleic acids in active Lyme arthritis, *Annals of Internal Medicine,* 1994;120(6):487-9.

Bramwell KK. et al. Lysosomal b-glucuronidase regulates Lyme and rheumatoid arthritis severity. *J Clin Invest.* 2104;124(1):311-20.

Brangulis K. et al. Structure of an outer surface lipoprotein BBA64 from the Lyme disease agent Borrelia burgdorferi which is critical to ensure infection after a tick bite. *Acta Crystallogr D Biol Crystallogr.* 2013;69(Pt6):1099-107.

Bransfield RC. et al. The association between tick-borne infections, Lyme borreliosis and autism spectrum disorders. *Med Hypotheses.* 2008;70(5):967-74.

Bransfield and Kuhn. Autism and Lyme disease. *JAMA* 2013; 310(8): 856-7.

Bransfield RC. The psychoimmunology of Lyme / tick-borne diseases and its association with neuropsychiatric symptoms. *Open Neurol J.* 2012;6(Suppl 1-M3):88-93.

Bremell D. and Hagberg L. Clinical characteristics and cerebrospinal fluid parameters in patients with peripheral facial palsy caused by Lyme neuroborreliosis compared with facial palsy of unknown origin (Bell's palsy) *BMC Infec Dis.* 2011;11:215-21.

Brescia AC., Rose CD. and Fawcett PT. Prolonged synovitis in pediatric Lyme arthritis cannot be predicted by clinical or laboratory parameters. *Clin Rheumatol.* 2009;28(5):591-3.

Brinkerhoff RJ., Gilliam WF., Gaines D. Lyme disease, Virginia, USA. 2000-2011. *Emerg Infect Dis.* 2014;20(10):1661-68.

Brissette CA. et al. The Borrelia burgdorferi outer-surface protein ErpX binds mammalian laminin. *Microbiolgy.* 2009;155(Pt3):863-72.

Brissette CA. et al. Borrelia burgdorferi infection-associated surface proteins ErpP, ErpA, and ErpC bind human plasminogen. *Infect Immun.*2009;77(1):330-6.

Brissette CA. et al. Borrelia burgdorferi RevA antigen binds host fibronectin. *Infect Immun.* 2009;77(7):2802-12.

Brissette CA. et al. Lyme borreliosis spirochete Erp proteins, their known host ligands, and potential roles in mammalian infection. *Int J Med Mirobiol.* 2008;298 Suppl 1:257-67.

Brissette CA. et al. The multifaceted responses of primary human astrocytes and brain microvascular endothelial cells to the Lyme disease spirochete, Borrelia burgdorferi. *ASN Neuro.* 2013;5(3):221-27.

Brissette CA., et al. That's my story, and I'm sticking to it-an update on B. burgdorferi adhesins. *Front Cell Infect Microbiol.* 2014;4(41).

Brisson D. et al. Biodiversity of Borrelia burgdorferi Strains in Tissues of Lyme Disease Patients. *PLoS ONE* 2011;6(8):e22926.

Brisson D. et al. Genetics of Borrelia burgdorferi. *Annu Rev Genet.* 2012;46:1-13.

Broekhijsen-van Henten DM., Braun KP. and Wolfs TF. Clinical presentation of childhood neuroborreliosis; neurological examination may be normal. *Arch Dis Child.* 2010;95(11):910-4.

Broker M. Following a tick bite: double infections by tick-borne encephalitis virus and the spirochete Borrelia and other potential multiple infections. *Zoonoses Public Health.* 2012;59(3):176-80.

Bronson E. et al. Serosurvey for selected pathogens is free-ranging American black bears (Ursus ameicanus) in Maryland, USA. *J Wildl Dis.* 2014;50(4):829-36.

Brorson O. and Brorson SH. Grapefruit seed extract is a powerful in vitro agent against motile and cystic forms of Borrelia burgdorferi sensu lato. *Infection.* 2007;35(3):206-8.

Brorson O. et al. Destruction of spirochete Borrelia burgdorferi round-body propagules (Rbs) by the antibiotic Tigecycline. *PNAS* 2009;106(44):18656-61.

Brown CR. et al. Adenoviral delivery of interleukin-10 fails to attenuate experimental Lyme disease. *Infect Immun.* 2008;76(12):5500-7.

Brown RN. et al. Sylvatic maintenance of Borrelia burgdorferi (Spirochaetales) in Northern California: untangling the web of transmission. *J Med. Entomol.* 2006;43(4):743-51.

Brtkova J. et al. Borrelia arthritis and chronic myositis accompanied by typical chronic dermatitis. *JBR-BTR.* 2008;91(3):88-9.

Buchwald F. et al. Fatal course of cerbral vasculitis induced by neuroborreliosis. *Neurol India.* 2010;58:139-41.

Buczek A. et al. Threat of attacks of Ixodes ricinus ticks (Ixodida:Ixodidae) and Lyme borreliosis within urban heat islands in South-Western Poland. *Parasites Vectors.* 2014;7:562.

Buffen K. et al. Autophagy modulates Borrelia burgdorferi-induced production of Interleukin-1b (IL-1b). *J Biol Chem.* 2013;288(12):8658-66.

Bunikis I. et al. An RND-type efflux system in borrelia burgdorferi is involved in virulence and resistance to antimicrobial compounds. *PLoS Pathog.* 2008;4(2):e1000009.

Burbelo PD. et al Lack of serum antibodies against Borrelia burgdorferi in children with autism. *Clin Vaccine Immunol.* 2013;20(7):1092-3.

Bykowski T. et al. Coordinated expression of Borrelia burgdorferi complement regulator-acquiring surface proteins during the Lyme disease spirochete's mammal-tick infection cycle. *Infect Immun.* 2007;75(9):4227-36.

Cabello FC., Godfrey HP. and Newman SA. Hidden in plain sight: Borrelia burgdorferi and the extracellular matrix. *Trends Microbiol.* 2007;15(8):350-4.

Cadavid D. The mammalian host response to Borrelia infection. *Wien Klin Wochenschr.* 2006;118(21-22):653-8.

Cairns V. and Godwin J. Post-Lyme borreliosis syndrome: a meta-analysis of reported symptoms. *Int J Epidemiol.* 2005;34(6):1340-5.

Cameron D. Severity of Lyme disease with persistent symptoms. Insights from a double-blind placebo-controlled clinical trial. *Minerva Med.* 2008;99(5):489-96.

Campfield BT. et al. Follistantin-like protein 1 is a critical mediator of experimental Lyme arthritis and the humoral response to Borrelia burgdorferi infections. *Microb Pathog.* 2014;73:70-9.

Casjens, SR. Borrellia genomes in the year 2000. J. *Mol. Microbiol. Biotechnol.* 2000; 2(4): 401-10.

Casjens SR. Evolution of the linear DNA replicons of the Borrelia spirochetes. *Curr Opin Microbiol* 1999; 2(5): 529-34.

Casjens SR. et al. Whole genome sequence of an unusual Borrelia burgdorferi sensu lato isolate. *J Bacteriol.* 2011;193(6):1489-90.

Castaldo JE., Griffith E. and Monkowski DH. Pseudotumor cerebri: early manifestation of adult Lyme disease. *Am J Med.* 2008;121(7):e5-6.

Centers for Disease Control and Prevention (CDC). Acute respiratory distress syndrome in persons with tick borne relapsing fever—three states, 2004-2005. *MMWR Morb Mortal Wkly Rep.* 2007;56(41):1073-6.

Centers for Disease Control and Prevention (CDC). Press Release, August 19, 2013, "CDC provides estimate of Americans diagnosed with Lyme disease each year."

Centers for Disease Control and Prevention (CDC). Three sudden cardiac deaths associated with Lyme carditis – United States, November 2012-July 2013. *MMWR Morb Mortal Wkly Rep.* 2013;62(49):993-6.

Cepelova J. Lyme carditis—rare cause of dilated cardiomyopathy and rhythm disturbances. *Vnitr Lek.* 2008;54(4):430-3.

Cerar T. et al. Comparison of PCR methods and culture for the detection of Borrelia spp. in patients with erythema migrans. *Clin Microbiol Infect.* 2008'14(7):653-8.

Cerar T. et al. Diagnostic value of cytokines and chemokines in Lyme neuroborreliosis. *Clin Vaccine Immunol.* 2013;20(10):1578-84.

Cerar T. et al. Humoral immune responses in patients with Lyme Neuroborreliosis. *Clin Vaccine Immunol.* 2010;177(4):645-50.

Cerar T. et al. Validation of cultivation and PCR methods for diagnosis of Lyme neuroborreliosis. *J Clin Microbiol.* 2008;46(10):3375-9.

Cervantes JL. Phagosomal signaling by Borrelia burgdorferi in human monocytes involves oll-likreceptor (TLR) 2 and TLR8 cooperativity and TLR8-mediated induction of IFN-B. *Dept Pediatr Med Genetic and Deve Bio.* 2011;108(9):3683-3688.

Cervantes JL. et al. Human TLR8 is activated upon recognition of Borreia burgdorferi RNA in the phagosome of human monocytes. *J Leukoc Biol.* 2013;94(6):1231-41.

Cervantes JL. et al. Phagosomal TLR signaling upon Borrelia burgdorferi infection. *Front Cell Infect Microbiol.* 2014;4(55).

Chaconas G., Norris SJ. Peaceful coexistence amongst Borrelia plasmids: getting by with a little help from their friends? *Plasmid.* 2013;70(2):161-67.

Chan J., Ahmed A. and Stacey B. Acute abdominal pain: An unusual medical cause. *Acute Med.* 2009;8(1):26-8.

Chan K. et al. Comparative molecular analyses of Borrelia burgdorferi sensu stricto strains B31 and N40D10/E9 and determination of their pathogenicity. *BMC Microbiol.* 2012;12:157.

Chan K., Casjens S. and Parveen N. Detection of established virulence genes and plasmids to differentiate Borrelia burgdorferi strains. *Infect Immun.* 2012;80(4):1519-29.

Chan K., Marras SA. and Parveen N. Sensitive multiplex PCR assay to differentiate Lyme spirochetes and emerging pathogens Anaplasma phagocytophilum and Babesia microti. *BMC Microbiol.* 2013;13:295.

Chandra A. Anti-Borrelia burgdorferi antibody profile in post-Lyme disease syndrome. *Clin Vaccine Immunol.* 2011;18(5):767-71.

Chandra A. et al. Anti-Borrelia burgdorferi Antibody Profile in Post-Lyme Disease Syndrome. *Clin Vacc Immun.* 2011;18(5):767-71.

Chandra A. et al. Anti-neural antibody reactivity in patients with a history of Lyme borreliosis and persistent symptoms. *Brain Behav Immun.* 2010;24(6):1018-24.

Chandra A. et al. Epitope Mapping of Antibodies to VlsE protein of Borrelia burgdorferi in Post-Lyme Disease Syndrome. *Clin Immunol.* 2011;141(1):103-10.

Chanier S., Lauxerois M. and Rieu V. Back pain without radiculitis as an initial manifestation of Lyme disease: two cases. *Presse Med.* 2007;36(1 Pt 1):61-3.

Charles VS. et al. Poliomyelitis-like syndrome with matching magnetic resonance features in a case of Lyme neuroborreliosis. *BMJ Case Rep.* 2009; bcr 07 .2008.0527.0527.

Chauhan V. et al. A young healthy male with syncope and complete heart block. *Scott Med J.* 2013;58(2):e13-7.

Chauhan VS. et al. NOD2 plays and important role in the inflammatory responses of microglia and astrocytes to bacterial CNS pathogens. *Glia.* 2009;57(4):414-23.

Chauhan, VS. et al. Neurogenic Exacerbation of Microglial and Astrocyte Responses to Neisseria meningitidis and Borrelia burgdorferi. *J Immunol.* 2008;180(12):8241-49.

Chekili S. et al. Radiculalgia realing Lyme disease. *Tunis Med.* 2008;86(11):1023.

Chen I. et al. Increasing RpoS expression causes cell death in Borrelia burgdorferi. *PLoS One.* 2013;8(12):e83276.

Chmielewski T. and Tylewska-Wierzbanowska S. Interactions between Borrelia burgdorferi and Mouse Fibroblasts. *Pol J Microbio.* 201;59(3):157-60

Chmielewski T. et al. Bacterial tick-borne diseases caused by Bartonella spp., Borrelia burgdorferi sensu lato, Coxiella burnetii, and Rickettsia spp. among patients with cataract surgery. *Med Sci Monit.2* 2014;20:927-31.

Choa LL., Chen YJ. and Shih CM. First isolation and molecular identification of Borrelia burgdorferi sensu stricto and Borrelia afzelii from the skin biopsies of patients in Taiwan. *Intection.* 2011;39(1):35-40.

Chowdri HR. et al. Borrelia miyamotoi infection presenting as human granulocytic anaplasmosis: a case report. *Ann Intern Med.* 2013;159(1):21-7.

Chu CY. et al. Genetic diversity of Borrelia burgdorferi sensu lato isolates from Northeastern China. *Vector Borne Zoonotic Dis.* 2011;11(7)877-82.

Chu CY. et al. Novel genospecies of Borrelia burgdorferi sensu lato from rodents and ticks in southwestern China. *J Clin Microbiol.* 2008;46(9):3130-3.

Chung Y., Zhang N. and Wooten RM. Borrelia burgdorferi elicited-IL-10 suppresses the production of inflammatory mediators, phagocytosis, and expression of co-stimulatory receptors by murine macrophages and/or dendritic cells. *PLoS One.* 2013;8(12):e84980.

Ciuta C. et al. Lyme disease—unusual medical encounter for an urologist. *Rev Med Chir Soc Med Nat Iasi.* 2012;116(4):1101-5.

Clarissou J. et al. Efficacy of a long-term antibiotic treatment in patients with a chronic Tick Associated Poly-organic Syndrome (TAPOS). *Med Mal Infect.* 2009;39(2):108-15.

Clark KL., Leydet B. and Hartman S. Lyme borreliosis in human patients in Florida and Georgia, USA. *Int J Med Sci.* 2013;10(7):915-31.

Clark KL., Leydet BF. and Threlkeld C. Geographical and geospecies distribution of Borrelia burgdorferi sensu lato DNA detected in humans in USA. *J Med Microbiol.* 2014;63(pt.5):674-84.

Clegg S. et al. Isolation of digital dermatitis treponemes from hoof lesions in wild North American elk (Cervus elaphus) in Washington state, USA. *J Clin Microbiol* 2015; 53(1): 88-94.

Coburn J., Leong J. and Chaconas G. Illuminating the roles of the Borrelia burgdorferi adhesins. *Trends Microbiol.* 2013;21(8):372-79.

Codolo G. et al. Borrelia burgdorferi NapA-driven Th17 cell inflammation in Lyme arthritis. *Arthritis Rheum.* 2008;58(11):3609-17.

Codolo G. et al. Orchestration of inflammation and adaptive immunity in Borrelia burgdorferi-induced arthritis by neutrophil-activating protein A. *Arthritis Rheum.* 2013;65(5):1232-42.

Coipan EC. et al. Spatiotemporal dynamics of emerging pathogens in questing Ixodes ricinus. *Front Cell Infect Microbiol.* 2013;3:36.

Coleman JL. et al. Evidence that two ATP-dependent (Lon) proteases in Borrelia burgdorferi serve different functions. *PLoS Pathog.* 2009;5(11):e1000676.

Colin de Verdiere N. et al. Tick borne relapsing fever caused by Borrelia persica, Uzbekistan and Tajikistan. *Emerg Infect Dis.* 2011;17(7):1325-7.

Collighan, R, et al. A spirochete isolated from a severe virulent ovine foot disease is closely related to a Treponeme isolated from human periodontitis and bovine digital dermatitis. *Vet Microbiol* 2000; 74(3): 249-57.

Collins C. et al. Activation of yo Cells by Borrelia burgdorferi is indirect via a TLR-and Caspase-Dependent Pathway. *J Immunol.* 2008; 181(4):2392-2398.

Colombo MJ. and Alugupalli KR. Complement factor H-binding protein, a putative virulence determinant of Borrelia hermsii, is an antigenic target for protective B1b lymphocytes. *J Immunol.* 2008;180(7):4858-64.

Comstedt P. et al. Complex population structure of Lyme borreliosis group spirochete Borrelia garinii in subarctic Eurasia. *PLoS One.* 2009;4(6):e5841.

Comstedt P. et al. Design and development of a novel vaccine for protection against Lyme borreliosis. *PLoS One.* 2014;9(11):e113294.

Comstedt P. et al. Global ecology and epidemiology of Borrelia garinii spirochetes. *Infect Ecolog Epiderm.* 2011;1:9545.

Cook MJ. Lyme borreliosis: A review of data on transmission time after tick attachment. *Intern J Gen Med.* 2015;8:1-8.

Cotte V. et al. Differential expression of Ixodes ricinus salivary gland proteins in the presence of the Borrelia burgdorferi sensu lato complex. *J Proteomics.* 2014;96:26-43.

Cotte V. et al. Prevalence of five pathogenic agents in questing Ixodes ricinus ticks from Western France. *Vector Borne Zoonotic Dis.* 2010;10(8):723-30.

Coulon CL., Landin D. Lyme disease as an underlying cause of supraspinatus tendinopathy in an overhead athlete. *Phys Ther.* 2012;92(5):740-7.

Coumou J. et al. Tired of Lyme borreliosis. Lyme borreliosis in the Netherlands. *Neth J Med.* 2011;69(3):101-11.

Coutte L. et al. Detailed analysis of sequence changes occurring during vlsE antigenic variation in the mouse model of Borrelia burgdorferi infection. *PLoS Pathog.* 2009;5(2):e1000293.

Craig-Mylius KA. et al Arthritogenicity of Borrelia burgdorferi and Borrelia garinii: comparison of infection in mice. *Am J Trop Med Hyg.* 2009;80(2):252-8.

Crowder CD. et al. Prevalence of Borrelia miyamotoi in Ixodes ticks in Europe and the United States. *Emerg Infect Dis.* 2014; 1678-82.

Crowley JT. et al. Lipid exchange between Borrelia burgdorferi and Host Cells. *PLoS Path.*2013;9(1):e1003109.

Cruz AR. et al. Phagocytosis of Borrelia burgdorferi, Lyme disease spirochete, potentiates innate immune activation and induces apoptosis in human monocytes. *Infect Immun.* 2008;76(1):56-70.

Csallner G., Hofmann H., Hausteiner-Wiehle C. Patients with "organically unexplained symptoms" presenting to a borreliosis clinic: clinical and psychobehavioral characteristics and quality of life. *Psychosomatics.* 2013;54(4):359-66.

Cutler SJ. Myths, legends and realities of relapsing fever borreliosis. *Clin Microbiol Infect.* 2009;15(5):395-6.

Cutler SJ. Relapsing fever—a forgotten disease revealed. *J Appl Microbiol.* 2010;108(4):1115-22.

Czell D., Rodic B. and Imoberdorf R. Neuroborreliosis—a disease with many faces. *Praxi (Bern1994)*

Czupryna P. et al Ultrasonographic evaluation of knee joints in patients with Lyme disease. *Inf J Infect Dis.* 2012;16(4):e252-5.

Dame TM. et al. IFN-g alters the response of Borrelia burgdorferi-activated endothelium to favor chronic inflammation. *J Immunol.* 2007;10:1172-79.

Danielova V. et al. Integration of a tick-borne encephalitis virus and Borrelia burgdorferi sensu lato into mountain ecosystems, following a shift in the altitudinal limit of distribution of their vector, Ixodes ricinus (Krkonose mountains, Czech Republic. *Vector Borne Zoonotic Dis.* 2010;10(3):223-30.

Dattwyler RJ. A Commentary on the Treatment of Early Lyme Disease. *Clin Inf Dis.* 2010;50:521-2.

de Carvalho IL. et al. Molecular characterization of a new isolate of Borrelia lusitaniae derived from Apodemus sylvaticus in Portugal. *Vector Borne Zoonotic Dis.* 2010;10(5):531-4.

de Carvalho IL. et al. Vasculitis-like syndrome associated with Borrelia lusitaniae infection. *Clin Rheumatol.* 2008;27(12):1587-91.

de Heller-Milev M. et al. Borrelial erythema of the face. *Ann Dermatol Venereol.* 2008;135(12):852-4.

de Taeye SW. et al. Complement evasion by Borrelia burgdorferi: it takes three to tango. *Trends Parasitol.* 2013;29(3):119-28.

D'Elios MM. et al. Reply to letter by Nardelli and Schell commenting on the pathogenesis of Lyme disease. *Arthritis Rheum.* 2009;60(7):2205.

Delong AK. et al. Antibiotic retreatment of Lyme disease in patients with persistent symptoms: a biostatistical review of randomized, placebo-controlled, clinical trials. *Contemp Clin Trials.* 2012;33(6):1132-42.

Demirkan I. et al. Characterization of a spirochete isolated from a case of bovine digital dermatitis. *J Appl Microbiol* 2009; 101(4): 948-55.

Demirkan I. et al. The frequent detection of a treponeme in bovine digital dermatitis by immunocytochemistry and polymerase chain reaction. *Veterinary Microbiology* 1998; 60: 285-92.

Demirkan I. et al. Isolation and characterization of a novel spirochaete from severe virulent ovine foot rot. *J Med Microbiol* 2001; 50(12): 1061-8.

Demirkan I. et al. Serological evidence of spirochetal infections associated with digital dermatitis in dairy cattle. *Vet Journal* 1999; 157(1): 69-77.

Dennis VA. et al. Live Borrelia burgdorferi Spirochetes Elicit Inflammatory Mediators from Human Monocytes via the Toll-Like Receptors Signaling Pathway. *Infect Immun.* 2009;77(3):1238-45.

Dereler AM. et al. High prevalence of 'Borrelia-like' organisms in skin biopsies of sarcoidosis patients from Western Austria. *J Cutan Pathol.* 2009;36(12):1262-8.

Dersch R. et al. Efficacy and safety of pharmacological treatments for neuroborreliosis—protocol for a systemic review. *Bio Med.* 2014;3:117.

Deruaz M. et al. Ticks produce highly selective chemokine binding proteins with antiinflammatory activity. *J Exp Med.* 2008;205(9)2019-31.

DeSousa R. et al. Role of the lizard Teira dugesii as a potential host for Ixodes ricinus tick-borne pathogens. *Appl Environ Microbiol.* 2012; 78(10):3767-9.

Diaz JH. Endemic tickborne infectious diseases in Louisiana and the Gulf South. *J La State Med Soc.* 2009;161(6):325-6.

Dibernardo A. et al. The prevalence of Borrelia miyamotoi infection, and co-infections with other Borrelia spp. in Ixodes scapularis tics collected in Canada. *Parasit Vectors.* 2014;7:183.

Dickinson GS. et al. Efficient B cell responses to Borrelia hermsii infection depend on BAFF and BAFFR but not TACI. *Infect Immun.* 2014; 82(1):453-9.

Dickinson GS. et al. Toll-like receptor 2 deficiency results in impaired antibody responses and septic shock during Borrelia hermsii infection. *Infect Immun.* 2010;78(11):4579-88.

Dietrich T. et al. Borrelia-associated crystalline keratopathy with intracorneal detection of Borrelia garinii by electron microscopy an polymerase chain reaction. *Cornea.* 2008;27(4):498-500.

Divers TJ et al. Changes in Borrelia burgdorferi ELISA antibody over time in both antibiotic treated and untreated horses. *Acta Vet Hung.* 2012;60(4):421-9.

Djukic M. et al. The diagnostic spectrum in patients with suspected chronic Lyme neuroborreliosis— the experience from one year of a university hospital's Lyme neuroborreliosis outpatients clinic. *Eur J Neurol.* 2011;18(4):547-55.

Djunkie M. et al. Cerebrospinal fluid findings in adults with acute Lyme neuroborreliosis. *J Neurol.* 2012;259:630-36.

Dodson, B, et al. Wolbachia enhances west nile virus (WNV) infection in the mosquito Culex trasalis. *PLoS Neglected Tropical Diseases* 2014; 8(7): e2965.

Donta ST. Issues in the diagnosis and treatment of Lyme disease. *Open Neurol J.* 2012;6(Suppl 1-M8):140-45.

Donta ST. Lyme disease guidelines – It's time to move forward. *Clin Infect Dis.(LTTE).* 2007;44:1134-5.

Dopfer D, et al. Growth curves and morphology of three Treponema subtypes isolated from digital dermatitis in cattle. *Vet Journal* 2012; 193(3): 685-93.

Drecktrah D. et al. An inverted repeats in the ospC operator is required for induction in Borrelia burgdorferi. *PLoS One.* 2013;8(7):e68799.

Drouin EE. et al. Human homologues of a Borrelia T cell epitope associated with antibiotic-refractory Lyme arthritis. *Mol Immunol.* 20078;45(1):180-9.

Drouin EE. et al. Searching for borrelial T cell epitopes associated with antibiotic-refractory Lyme arthritis. *Mol Immunol.* 2008;45(8):2323-32.

Dubrey SW. et al. Lyme disease in the United Kingdom. *Postgrad Med J.* 2014;90(1059):33-42.

Dubska L. et al. Differential role of passerine birds in distribution of Borrelia spirochetes, based on data from ticks collected from birds during the postbreeding migration period in Central Europe. *Appl Environ Microbiol.* 2009;75(3):596-602.

Dumlao DS. et al. Dietary fish oil substitution alters the eicosanoid profile in ankle joints of mice during Lyme infection. *J Nutr.* 2012;142(8):1582-9.

Dunaj J. et al. The role of PCR in diagnostics of Lyme borreliosis. *Przegl Epidemiol.* 2013;67:35-39.

Dunn JM. et al. Borrelia burgdorferi promotes the establishment of Babesia microti in the Northeastern United States. *PLoS One.* 2014;9(12):e115494.

Dworkin MS. et al. Tick-borne Relapsing Fever. *Infect Dis Clin North Am.* 2008;22(3):449-viii.

Dykhuizen DE. et al. Short Report: The Propensity of Different Borrelia burgdorferi sensu stricto Genotypes to Cause Disseminated Infections in Humans. *Am J Trop Med Hyg.* 2008;78(5):806-10.

Earnhart CG. et al. Assessment of the potential contribution of the highly conserved C-terminal motif (C10) of Borrelia burgdorferi outer surface protein C in transmission and infectivity. *Pathog Dis.* 2014;70(2):176-84.

Ebnet, K, et al. Borrelia burgdorferi activates nuclear factor-kappa B and is a potent inducer of chemokine and adhesion molecule gene expression in endothelial cells and fibroblasts. *Journal of Immunology* 1997; 158(7): 3285-92.

Edwards AM. et al. Genetic relatedness and phenotypic characteristics of Treponema associated with human periodontal tissues and ruminant foot disease. *Microbiology* 2003; 149(pt 5): 1083-93.

Edwards AM. et al. From tooth to hoof: treponemes in tissue-destructive diseases. *J Appl Microbiol* 2003;94(5): 767-80.

Egberts F. et al. Multiple erythema migrans— manifestation of systemic cutaneous borreliosis. *J Dtsch Dermatol Ges.* 2008;6(5):350-3.

Eggers CH.et al. The coenzyme A disulphide reductase of Borrelia burgdorferi is important for rapid growth throughout the enzootic cycle and essential for infection of the mammalian host. *Mol Microbiol.* 2011;82(3):679-97.

Eisendle K., Grbner T. and Zelger B. Morphoea: a manifestation of infection with Borrelia species? *Br. J Dermatol.* 2007;157(6):1189-98.

Eisendle K. and Zelger B. The expanding spectrum of cutaneous borreliosis. *G Ital Dermatol Venereol.* 2009;144(2):157-71.

Eisendle K. et al. Detection of spirochaetal microorganisms by focus floating microscopy in necrobiosis lipoidica in patients from central Europe. *Histopathology.* 2008;52(7):877-84.

Eisendle K. et al. Possible role of Borrelia burgdorferi sensu lato infection in lichen sclerosus. *Arch Dermatol.* 2008;144(5):591-8.

Ekner A. et al. Anaplasmataceae and Borrelia burgdorferi sensu lato in the sand lizard Lacerta agilis and co-infection of these bacteria in hosted Ixodes ricinus ticks. *Parasit Vectors* 2011;4:182.

Elber H. et al. African relapsing fever borreliae genomospecies revealed by comparative genomics. *Front Pub Health.* 2014;2(43):1-8.

Elhelw RA., El-Enbaawy MI., Samir A. II. Lyme borreliosis: A neglected zoonosis in Egypt. *Acta Trop.* 2014;140:188-92.

Elsner RA., Hastey CJ., Baumgarth N.II. CD4+ T cells promote antibody production but not sustained affinity maturation during Borrelia burgdorferi infection. *Infect Immun.* 2015;83(1):48-56.

Embers ME., Narasimhan S. Vaccination against Lyme disease: past, present, and future. *Front Cell Infect Micbiol.* 2013;3(6):1-10.

Embers ME. et al. Persistence of Borrelia burgdorferi in rhesus macaques following antibiotic treatment of disseminated infection. *PLoS One.* 2012;7(1):e29914.

Endres S. and Quante M. Oedema of the metatarsal heads II-IV and forefoot pain as an unusual manifestation of Lyme disease: a case report. *J Med Case Rep.* 2007;1:44.

Eriksson P. et al. The many faces of solitary and multiple erythema migrans. *Acta Derm Venereol.* 2013;93(6):693-700.

Erol I., Saygi S., Alehan F. Acute cerebellar ataxia in a pediatric case of Lyme disease and a review of literature. *Pediatr Neurol.*2013;48(5):407-10.

Eshoo MW. et al. Direct molecular detection and genotyping of Borrelia burgdorferi from whole blood of patients with early Lyme disease. *PLoS One.* 2012;7(5):e36825.

Esposito S. et al. Borrelia burgdorferi infection and Lyme disease in children. *Internat J Infect Dis.* 2013;7:e153-58.

Evans NJ. et al. Differential inflammatory responses of bovine foot skin fibroblasts and keratinocytes to digital dermatitis treponemes. *Vet Immunol Immunopathol* 2014; 161(1-2): 12-20.

Evans NJ. et al. Three unique groups of spirochetes isolated from digital dermatitis lesions in UK cattle. *Vet Microbiol* 2008; 130(1-2):141-50.

Evans NJ, et al. Treponema pedis sp. nov., a spirochete isolated from bovine digital dermatitis lesions. *Int J Syst Evol Microbiol* 2009; 59(pt 5): 987-91.

Evans R. et al. More specific bands of the IgG western blot in sera from Scottish patients with suspected Lyme borreliosis. *J Clin Pathol.* 2010;63(8):719-21.

Fallon BA. et al. A comparison of Lyme disease serologic test results from 4 laboratories in patients with persistent symptoms after antibiotic treatment. *Clin Infect Dis.* 2014;59(12):1705-10.

Farshad-Amacker NA. et al. Brainstem abnormalities and vestibular nerve enhancement in acute Neuroborreliosis. *Bio Med.* 2013;6:551.

Feder HM, Jr. et al. A Critical Appraisal of "Chronic Lyme Disease". *New Engl J Med.* 2007;357:1422-30.

Fedorova N. et al. Remarkable diversity of tick or mammalian-associated Borreliae in the metropolitan San Francisco Bay area, California. *Ticks Tick Borne Dis.* 2014;5(6):951-61.

Feng, J, et al. Identification of novel activity against Borrelia burgdorferi persisters using an FDA approved drug library. *Emerging Microbes and Infections* 2014; 3: e49.

Feria-Arroyo TP. et al. Implications of climate change on the distribution of the tick vector Ixodes scapularis and risk for Lyme disease in the Texas-Mexico transboundary region. *Parasit Vector.* 2014;7:199.

Fernadez-Flores A. and Ruzic-Sabljic E. Granuloma annulare displaying pseudorosettes in Borrelia infection. *Acta Dermatovenerol Alp Pannonica Adriat.* 2008;17(4):171-6.

Fikrig E. et al. Toll-Like Receptors 1 and 2 Heterodimers Alter Borrelia burgdorferi Gene Expression in Mice and Ticks. *J Infect Dis.* 2009;200(8):1331-40.

Finsterer J. Myasthenia and neuroborreliosis and excessively high acetylcholine-receptor antibodies. *Scand J Infect Dis.* 2007;39(2):187-90.

Fischer RJ. et al. Identical strains of Borrelia hermsii in mammal and bird. *Emerg Infect Dis.* 2009;15(12):2064-6.

Fish D. Population ecology of Ixodes dammini. *Ecology and Environmental management of Lyme disease* 1993: 25-42.

Fisher JB. and Curtis CE. An unexpected case of Lyme disease in a soldier serving in northern Iraq. *Mil Med.* 2010;175(5):367-9.

Fisher JR., LeBlanc KT., and Leong JM. Fibronectin binding protein BBK32 of the Lyme disease spirochete promotes bacterial attachment to glycosaminoglycans. *Infect Immun.* 2006;74(1):435-41.

Floden AM. et al. Evaluation of RevA, a fibronectin-binding protein of Borrelia burgdorferi, as a potential vaccine candidate for Lyme disease. *Clin Vaccine Immunol.* 2013;20(6)L:892-9.

Foldvari G. et al. Detection of Borrelia burgdorferi sensu lato in lizards and their ticks from Hungary. *Vector Borne Zoonotic Dis.* 2009;9(3)331-6.

Foley J. et al. An Ixodes minor and Borrelia carolinensis enzootic cycle involving a critically endangered Mojave Desert rodent. *Ecol Evol.* 2014;4(5):576-81.

Fomenko NV., Borgoiakov Vlu. and Panov VV. Genetic features of Borrelia miyamotoi transmitted by Ixodes persulcatus. *Mol Gen Mikrobiol Virusol.* 2011;(2):12-7.

Fotso Fotso A. et al. Genome sequence of Borrelia crocidurae strain 03-02, a clinical isolate from Senegal. *Genome Announc.* 2014;2(6) pii:e01150-14.

Franke J., Hildebrandt A. and Dorn W. Exploring gaps in our knowledge on Lyme borreliosis spirochaetes—updates on complex heterogeneity, ecology, and pathogenicity. *Ticks Tick Borne Dis.* 2013;4(1-2):11-25.

Franke J. et al. Are birds reservoir hosts for Borrelia afzelii? *Ticks Tick Borne Dis.* 2010;1(2):109-12.

Fritz CL., Payne JR. and Schwan TG. Serologic evidence for Borrelia hermsii infection in rodents on federally owned recreational areas in California. *Vector Borne Zoonotic Dis.* 2013;13(6):376-81.

Gaito A. et al. Comparative analysis of the infectivity rate of both Borrelia burgdorferi in Anaplasma phagocytophilum in humans and dogs in a New Jersey Community. *Infec and Drug Resist.* 2014;7:199-01.

Gajovic O. et al. Lyme borreliosis—diagnostic difficulties in interpreting serological results. *Med Pregl.* 2010;63(11-12):839-43.

Gandhi, G et al. Interaction of variable bacterial outer membrane lipoproteins with brain endothelium, *PLOS One* 2010; 5(10): e13257.

Garcia-Monco JC., Benach JL. A disconnect between the neurospirochetoses in humans and rodent models of disease. *PLOS Path.* 2013;9(4):e1003288.

Garcia-Monco, JC, et al. Borrelia burgdorferi and other related spirochetes bind to galactocerebroside. *Neurology* 1992; 42(7): 1341-8.

Garcia-Soler P. et al. Severe Jarisch-Herxheimer reaction in tick-borne relapsing fever. *Enferm Infecc Microbiol Clin.* 2011;29(9):710-11.

Garment AR. and Demopoulos BP. False-positive seroreactivity to Borrelia burgdorferi in a patient with thyroiditis. *Int J Infect Dis.* 2009;145e373.

Gaubitz M. et al. Diagnosis and treatment of Lyme arthritis. Recommendations of the Pharmacotherapy Commission of the Deutsche Gesellschaft fur Rheumatologie (German Society for Rheumatology).

Gaultney RA. et al. BB0347, from the Lyme disease spirochete Borrelia burgdorferi, is surface exposed and interacts with the CS1 heparin-binding domain of human fibronectin. *PLoS One.* 2013;8(9):e75643.

Gautam A. et al. Different patterns of expression and of IL-10 modulation of inflammatory mediators from macrophages of Lyme disease-resistent and -susceptible mice. *PLoS One.* 2012;7(9):e43860.

Gautam A. et al. Interleukin-10 alters effector functions of multiple genes induced by Borrelia burgdorferi in macrophages to regulate lyme disease inflammation. *Infect Immun.* 2011;79(12):4876-92.

Geca A. et al. The role of complement factor H in the pathogenesis of Borrelia infection. *Postepy Hig Med Dosw (Online).* 2012;66:501-6.

Gelderblom H. et al. High production of CXCL13 in blood and brain during persistent infection with the relapsing fever spirochete Borrelia turicatae. *J Neuropathol Exp Neurol.* 2007;66(3):208-17.

Gelderblom H. et al. Role of Interleukin 10 during persistent infection with the relapsing fever spirochete Borrelia turicatae. *Am J Pathol.* 2007;170(1):251-62.

Ghandour M. and Skoff R. Expression of galactocerebroside in developing normal and jimpy ologodendrocytes in situ, *J Neurocytol* 1988; 17(4): 485-98.

Gidday J. et al. Leukocyte-derived matrix metalloproteinase-9 mediates blood-brain barrier breakdown and is proinflammatory after transient focal cerebral ischemia. *Am J Physiol Heart Circ Physiol* 2005; 289: H558-68.

Gilbert L., Aungier J.II. and Tomkins JL.III. Climate of origin affects tick (Ixodes ricinus) host-seeking behavior in response to temperature: implications for resilience to climate change? *Ecol Evol.* 2014;4(7):1186-98.

Gilmore RD. Jr. et al. Borrelia burgdorferi expression of the bba64, bba65, bba66, and bba73 genes in tissues during persistent infection in mice. *Microb Pathog.* 2009;45(5-6):355-60.

Girard YA., Fedorova N. and Lane RS. Genetic diversity of Borrelia burgdorferi and detection of B. bissettii-like DNA in serum of north-coastal California residents. *J Clin Microbiol.* 2011;49(3):945-54.

Girschick HJ., Morbach H. and Tappe D. Treatment of Lyme borreliosis. *Arthritis Research and Therapy* 2009;11(6):258.

Glatz M. et al. The clinical spectrum of skin manifestations of Lyme borreliosis in 204 children in Austria. *Acta Derm Venereol* 2014.

Goldberg S. and Katz BZ. Lyme disease presenting as ptosis, conjunctivitis, and photophobia. *Clin Pediatr (Phila)* 2011;51(2):186-7.

Golovchenko M. et al. Invasive potential of Borrelia burgdorferi sensu stricto ospC type L strains increases the possible disease risk to humans in the regions of the their distribution. *Bio Med.* 2014;7:538.

Gomez A. et al. An experimental infection model to induce digital dermatitis infection in cattle. *Journal of Dairy Science* 2012; 95(4): 1821-30.

Goodman JL. et al. Bloodstream invasion in early Lyme disease results from a prospective, controlled, blinded study using the polymerase chain reaction. *Am J Med.* 1995;99(1):6-12.

Gordillo-Perez G. et al. Borrelia burgdorferi infection and cutaneous Lyme disease, Mexico. *Emerg Infect Dis.* 2007;13(10):1556-8.

Gordon, LM. Leptospira interrogans serotype hardjo outbreak in a Victorian dairy herd and associated with infection in man. *Aust Vet J* 1977; 53(5): 227-9.

Grab DJ. et al. Anaplasma phagocytophilum-Borrelia burgdorferi coinfection enhances chemokine, cytokine, and matrix metalloprotease expression by human brain microvascular endothelial cells. *Clin Vac Immun.* 2007;14(11):1420-24.

Grab DJ. et al. Human brain microvascular endothelial cell traversal by Borrelia burgdorferi requires calcium signaling. *Clin Microbiol Infect.* 2009;15(5):411-6.

Grabe HJ et al. No association of seropositivity for anti-Borrelia IgG antibody with mental and physical complaints. *Nord J Psychiatry.* 2008;62(5):386-91.

Greene NP. et al. Structure of an atypical periplamic adaptor from a multidrug efflux pump of the spirochete Borrelia burgdorferi. *FEBS lett.* 2013;587(18):2984-2988.

Grinager HS., Krason DA. and Olsen TW. Lyme disease: resolution of a serous retinal detachment and chorioretinal folds after antibiotic therapy. *Retin Cases Brief Rep.* 2012;6(3):232-4.

Groshong AM. et al. BB0238, a presumed tetratricopeptide repeat-containing protein, is required during Borrelia burgdorferi mammalian infection. *Infect Immun.* 2014;82(10):4292-306.

Grosskinsky S. et al. Borrelia recurrentis employs a novel multifunctional surface protein with anti-complement, anti-opsonic and invasive potential to escape innate immunity. *PLoS One.* 2009'4(3):e4858.

Grosskinsky S. et al. Human complement regulators C4b-binding protein and C1 esterase inhibitor interact with a novel outer surface protein of Borrelia recurrentis. *PLoS One.* 2010;4(6):e698.

Grusell M., Widhe M. and cytokines interleukin-12 and interleukin-18 in cerbrospinal fluid but not in sera from patients with Lyme neuroborreliosis. *J Neuroimmunol.* 2001;131(1-2):173-8.

Grygorczuk S. et al. Activity of the caspase-3 in the culture of peripheral blood mononuclear cells stimulated with Borrelia burgdorferi antigens. *Przegl Epidemiol.* 2008;62(1):85-91.

Grygorczuk S. et al. Failures of antibiotic treatment in Lyme arthritis. *Przegl Epidemiol.* 2008;62(3):581-8.

Grygorczuk S. et al. Increased expression of Fas receptor and Fas ligand in the culture of the peripheral blood mononuclear cells stimulated with Borrelia burgdorferi sensu lato. *Ticks Tick Borne Dis.* 2014;pii:S1877-959x(14)00222-2.

Gualco F. et al. Intersitial granuloma annulare and borreliosis: a new case. *J Eur Acad Dermatol Venereol.* 2007;21(8):1117-8.

Gubertini N., Bonin S. and Trevisan G. Lichen sclerosus et atrophicans, scleroderma en coup de sabre and Lyme borreliosis. *Dermatol Reports.* 2011;3(2):e27.

Guenther F., Bode C. and Faber T. Reversible complete heart block by re-infection with Borrelia burgdorferi with negative lgM-antibodies. *Dtsch Med Wochenschr.* 2009;134(1-2):23-6.

Gugliotta JL. et al. Meningoencephalitis from Borrelia miyamotoi in an immunocompromised patient. *N Engl J Med.* 2013;368(3):240-5.

Guo BP. et al. Relapsing fever Borrelia binds to neolacto glycans and mediates rosetting of human erythrocytes. *PNAS* 2009;106(46):19280-85.

Guo X. et al Inhibition of neutrophil function by two tick salivary proteins. *Infct Immun.* 2009;77(6);2320-9.

Gupta RS., Mahmood S. and Adeolu M. A phylogenomic and molecular signature based approach for characterization of the phylum Spirochaetes and its major clades: proposal for a taxonomic revision of the phylum. *Front Microbio.* 2013;4(217):1-18.

Gyllenborg J. and Milea D. Ocular flutter as the first manifestation of Lyme disease. *Neurology.* 2009;72(3):291.

Habek M., Mubrin Z., Brinar VV. Avellis syndrome due to borreliosis. *Eur J Neurol.* 2007;14(1):112-4.

Haenel, Dylan. Antimicrobial effects of lactoferrin and cannabidiol on *Borrelia burgdorferi*. Np, nd but probably 2012/2013, Department of Biology and Environmental Science/Biotechnology. University of New Haven.

Hallstrom T. et al. CspA from Borrelia burgdorferi inhibits the terminal complement pathway. *mBio.*2013;4(4):e00481-13.

Halperin JJ. Diagnosis and treatment of the neuromuscular manifestations of Lyme disease. *Curr Treat Options Neurol.* 2007;9(2):93-100.

Halperin JJ. Lyme disease: a multisystem infection that affects the nervous system. *Continuum (Minneap Minn).* 2012;18(6Infectious Diseases):1338-50.

Halperin JJ. Nervous system Lyme disease. *Handb Clin Neurol.* 2014;121:1473-83.

Halperin JJ. Nervous system Lyme disease: diagnosis and treatment. *Rev Neurol Dis.* 2009;6(1):4-12.

Halperin JJ. Nervous system Lyme disease: is there a controversy? *Semin Neurol.* 2011;31(3):317-24.

Halperin JJ. Neurologic manifestations of Lyme disease. *Curr Infect Dis Rep.* 2011;13(4):360-6.

Halperin JJ. et al. Practice parameter: treatment of nervous system Lyme disease (an evidence-based review): report of the Quality Standards Subcommittee of the American Academy of Neurology. *Neurology.* 2007;69(1):91-102

Halpern MD. et al. Simple objective detection of human Lyme disease infection using immuno-PCR and a single recombinant hybrid antigen. *Clin Vaccine Immunol.* 2014;21(8):1094-105.

Hammerschmidt C. et al. Versatile roles of CspA orthologs in complement inactivation of serum-resistant Lyme disease spirochetes. *Infect Immun.* 2014;82(1):380-92.

Hanincova K. et al. Borrelia burgdorferi sensu stricto is clonal in patients with early Lyme borreliosis. *Appl Environ Microbiol.* 2008;74(16):5008-14.

Hanincova K. et al. Multilocus sequence typing of Borrelia burgdorferi suggests existence of lineages with differential pathogenic properties in humans. *PLoS One.* 2013;8(9):e73066.

Hansen ES. et al. Interleukin-10 (IL-10) inhibits Borrelia burgdorferi-induced IL-17 production and attenuates IL-17-mediated Lyme arthritis. *Infect Immun.* 2013;81(12):4421-30.

Hansen K., Crone C., Krostoferitsch W. Lyme neuroborreliosis. *Handb Clin Neurol.* 2013;115:559-75.

Hansford KM. et al. Borrelia miyamotoi in host-seeking Ixodes ricinus ticks in England. *Epidemiol Infect.* 2014;14:1-9.

Hansmann Y. et al. Feedback on difficulties raised by the interpretation of serological tests for the diagnosis of Lyme disease. *Med Mal Infect.* 2014;44(5):199-05.

Harris G. et al. Borrelia burgdorferi protein BBK32 binds to soluble fibronectin via the N-terminal 70-kDa region, causing fibronectin to undergo conformational extension. *J Biol Chem.* 2014;289(32):22490-9.

Harrison BA. et al. Recent discovery of widespread Ixodes affinis (Acari: Ixodidae) distribution in North Carolina with implications for Lyme disease studies. *J Vector Ecol.* 2010;35(1):174-9.

Hartiala P. et al. Borrelia burgdorferi inhibits human neutrophil functions. *Microbes Infect.* 2008;10(1):60-8.

Hartiala P. et al. Tlr2 utilization of Borrelia does not induce p38- and IFN-b autocrine loop-dependent expression of cd38, resulting in poor migration and weak Il-12 secretion of dendritic cells. *J Immunol.*2010;184:5732-42.

Hartiala P. et al. Transcrptional response of human dendritic cells to Borrelia garinii-defective CD38 and CCR7 expression detected. *J Leukoc Biol.* 2997-82(1):33-43.

Hasle G. et al. Transport of Ixodes ricinus infected with Borrelia species to Norway by northward-migrating passerine birds. *Ticks Tick Borne Dis.* 2011;2(1):37-43.

Hassett AL. et al. Psychiatric comorbidity and other psychological factors in patients with "chronic Lyme disease." *Am J Med.* 2009;122(9):843-50.

Hassett AL. et al. Role of psychiatric comorbidity in chronic Lyme disease. *Arthritis Rheum.* 2008;59(12):1742-9.

Hastey CJ. et al. Delays and diversions mark the development of B cell responses to Borrelia burgdorferi infection. *J Immunol.* 2012;188(11):5612-22.

Hastey CJ. et al. MyD88- and TRIF-independent induction of Type I interferon drives naive B Cell accumulation but not loss of lymph node architecture in Lyme disease. *Infect Immun.* 2014;82(4):1548-58.

Haupl T. et al. Persistence of Borrelia burgdorferi in ligamentous tissue from a patient with chronic Lyme borreliosis. *Arthritis and Rheumatism* 1993; 36(11):1621-1626.

Haven J., Margori K. and Park AW. Ecological and in host factors promoting distinct parasite life-history strategies in Lyme borreliosis. *Epidemics.* 2012;4(3):152-7.

Haven J. et al. Pervasive recombination and sympatric genome diversification driven by frequency-dependent selection in Borrelia burgdorferi, the Lyme disease bacterium. *Genetics.*2011;189(3):951-66.

Hawley K. et al. Macrophage p38 mitrogen-activated protein kinase activity regulates invariant natural killer T-cell responses during Borrelia burgdorferi infection. *J Infect Dis.* 2012;206.

Hawley KL. et al. CD14 cooperates with complement receptor 3 to mediate MyD88-independent phagocytosis of Borrelia burgdorferi. *Proc Natl Acad Sci USA.* 2012;109(4):1228-32.

Hawley KL. et al. CD14 targets complement receptor 2 to lipid rafts during phagocytosis of Borrlia burgdorferi. *Int J Biol Sci.* 2013;9(8):803-10.

He M. et al. Regulation of expression of the fibronectin-binding protein BBK32 in Borrelia burgdorferi. *J Bacterio.* 2007;189(22):8377-80.

Heilpern AJ. et al. Matrix metalloproteinase 9 plays a key role in lyme arthritis but not in dissemination of Borrelia burgdorferi. *Infect Immun* 2009;77(7):2643-49.

Hellgren O., Andersson M. and Raberg L. The genetic structure of Borrelia afzelii varies with geographic but not ecological sampling scale. *J Evol Biol.* 2011;24(1):159-67.

Henningson AJ. et al. Indications of Th1 and Th17 responses in cerebrospinal fluid from patients with Lyme neuroborreliosis: a large retrospective study. *J Neuroinflamm.* 2011;8(36).

Henningsson AJ. et al. Laboratory diagnosis of Lyme neuroborreliosis: a comparison of three CSF anti-Borrelia antibody assays. *Eur J Clin Microbiol Infect Dis.* 2014;33(5):797-03.

Henry B. et al. How big is the Lyme problem? Using novel methods to estimate the true number of Lyme disease cases in British Columbia residents from 1997-2008. *Vector Borne Zoonotic Dis.* 2011;11(7):863-8.

Hentzer M. and Givskov M. Pharmacological inhibition of quorum sensing for the treatment of chronic bacterial infections, The Journal of Clinical Investigation 2003; 112(9): 1300-1307.

Herrmann C. and Gern L. Search for blood or water Is influenced by Borrelia burgdorferi in Ixodes ricinus. *Institute Bio.* 2000.

Herrmann C., Voordouw MJ. and Gern L. Ixodes ricinus ticks infected with the causative agent of Lyme disease, Borrelia burgdorferi sensu

lato, have higher energy reserves. *Int J Parasitol.* 2013;43(6):477-83.

Hersh MH. et al. Co-infection of blacklegged ticks with Babesia microti and Borrelia burgdorferi is higher than expected and acquired from small mammal hosts. *PLoS One.* 2014;9(6):e99348.

Herzberger P. et al. Human pathogenic Borrelia spielmanii sp. nov. resists complement-mediated killing by direct binding of immune regulators factor H and factor H-like protein 1. *Infec Immun.*2 2007;75(10):4817-25.

Herzer P. et al. Lyme borreliosis. *Internist (Berl).* 2014;55(7):789-802.

Heylen D. et al. Songbirds as general transmitters but selective amplifiers of Borrelia burgdorferi sensu lato genotypes in Ixodes rinicus ticks. *Environ Microbiol.* 2014;16(9):2859-68.

Heymann WR., Ellis DL. Borrelia burgdorferi infections in the United States. *Clinical Aesthetic.* 2012;5(8):18-28.

Hikita, T, et al. Cationic glycosphingolipids in neuronal tissues and their possible biological significance. *Neurochem Res* 2002; 27(7-8): 575-81.

Hildenbrand P. et al. Lyme neuroborreliosis: manifestations of a rapidly emerging zoonosis. *Am J Neurodiol.* 2009;30:1079-87.

Hinterseher I. et al. Presence of Borrelia burgdorferi sensu lato antibodies in the serum of patients with abdominal aortic aneurysms. *Eur J Clin Microbiol Infect Dis.* 2012;31:(5):781-9.

Hjetland R. et al. Seroprevalence of antibodies to Borrelia burgdorferi sensu lato in healthy adults from western Norway: risk factors and methodological aspects. *APMIS.* 2014;122(11):1114-24.

Ho K., Melanson M. and Desai JA. Bell palsy in Lyme disease-endemic regions of Canada: a cautionary case of occult bilateral peripheral facial nerve palsy due to Lyme disease. *CJEM.* 2012;14(5):321-4.

Hoa Q. et al. Distribution of Borrelia burgdorferi sensu lato in China. *J Clin Microbiol.* 2011;49(2):647-50.

Hodzic E., Feng S. and Barthold SW. Assessment of transcriptional activity of Borrelia burgdorferi and host cytokine genes during early and late infection in a mouse model. *Vector Borne Zoonotic Dis.* 2013;13(10):694-711.

Hodzic E. et al. Persistence of Borrelia burgdorferi following antibiotic treatment in mice. *Antimicrob Agents Chemother.* 2008;52(5):1728-36.

Hodzic E. et al. Resurgence of persisting non-cultivable Borrelia burgdorferi following antibiotic treatment in mice. *PLoS One.* 2014;9(1):e86907.

Hoffmann AK. et al. Daam1 is a regulator of filopodia formation and phagocytic uptake of Borrelia burgdorferi by primary human macrophages. *FASEB J.* 2014;28(7):3075-89.

Hofmann H. The variable spectrum of cutaneous Lyme borreliosis. Diagnosis and therapy. *Hautarzt.* 2012;63(5):381-9.

Holl-Wieden A., Suerbaum S. and Girschick HJ. Seronegative Lyme arthritis. *Rheumatol Int.* 2007;27(11):1091-3.

Homouz D. et al. Crowded, cell-like environment induces shape chages in aspherical protein. *Proc Natl Acad Sci U S A.* 2008;105(33):11754-9.

Hoogers SE., Wirtz PW., Koppen H. Subacute anterior horn disease caused by neuroborreliosis. *Neurol Sci.* 2013;34(6):1019-20.

Hoon-Hanks LL. et al. Borrelia burgdorferi malQ mutants utilize disaccharides and traverse the enzootic cycle. *FEMS Immunol Med Microbiol.* 2012;66(2):157-65.

Horka H. et al. Tick saliva affects both proliferation and distribution of Borrelia burgdorferi spirochetes in mouse organs and increases transmission of spirochetes to ticks. *Int J Med Microbiol.* 2009;299(5):373-80.

Hornok S. et al. Occurrence of ticks and prevalence of Anaplasma phagocytophilum and Borrelia burgdorferi s.l. in three types of urban biotopes: forests, parks and cemeteries. *Ticks Tick Borne Dis.* 2014;5(6):785-9.

Hovius JW. et al. Coinfection with Borrelia burgdorferi sensu stricto and Borrelia garinii alters the course of murine Lyme borreliosis. *FEMS Immunol Med Microbiol.* 2007;49(2):224-34.

Hovius JW. et al. The urokinase receptor (uPAR) facilitates clearance of Borrelia burgdorferi. *PLoS Pathog.* 2009;5(5):e1000447.

Hsieh YF. et al. Serum reactivity against Borrelia burgdorferi OspA in patients with rheumatoid arthritis. *Clin Vaccine Immunol.* 2007;14:1437-41.

Huda S., Wieshmann UC. Protracted neuroborreliosis—an unusual cause of encephalomyelitis. *BMJ Case Rep.* 2012;2012:pii bcr1120115206.

Hufschmidt A. et al. Prevalence of taste disorders in idiopathic and B. burgdorferi-associated facial palsy. *J Neurol.* 2009;256(10):1750-2.

Huppertz HI. et al. Rational diagnostic strategies for Lyme borreliosis in children and adolescents: recommendations by the committee for infectious diseases and vaccinations of the German Acadamy for Pediatrics and Adolescent Health. *Eur J Pediatr.* 2012;171(11):1619-24.

Hutschenreuther A. et al. Growth inhibiting activity of volatile oil from Cistus creticus L. against Borrelia burgdorferi s.s. in vitro. *Pharmazie.* 2010;65(4):290-5.

Hvidsten D. et al. Ixodes ricinus and Borrelia prevalence at the Arctic Circle in Norway. *Ticks Tick Borne Dis.* 2014;5(2):107-12.

Hyde JA. et al. Bioluminescent imaging of Borrelia burgdorferi in vivo demonstrates that the fibronectin-binding protein BBK32 is required for optimal infectivity. *Mol Microbiol.* 2011:82(1):99-113.

Hyde JA. et al. The BosR regulatory protein of Borrelia burgdorferi interfaces with the RpoS regulatory pathway and modulates both the oxidative stress response and pathogenic properties of the Lyme disease spirochete. *Mol Microbiol.* 2009;74(6):1344-55.

Hynote ED., Mervine PC., and Stricker RB. Clinical evidence for rapid transmission of Lyme disease following a tickbite. *Diagnostic Microbiology and Infectious Disease.* 2012;72(2):188-92.

Hytonen J. et al. CXCL13 and neopterin concentrations in cerebrospinal fluid of patients with Lyme diseases that cause neuroinflammation. *J Neuroinflamm.* 2014;11:103.

Iliopoulou BP., Alroy J. and Huber BT. Persistent arthritis is Borrelia burgdorferi-infected HLA-DR4-positive CD28-negative mice post-antibiotic treatment. *Arthritis Rheum.* 2008;58(12):3892-901.

Iliopoulou BP., Guerau-de-Arellano M. and Huber BT. HLA-DR alleles determine responsiveness to Borrelia burgdorferi antigens in a mouse model of self-perpetuating arthritis. *Arthritis Rheum.* 2009;60(12):3831-40.

Illiopoulou BP. and Huber BT. Emergency of chronic Lyme arthritis: putting the breaks on CD28 constimulation. *Immunopharmacol Immunotoxicol.* 2009;31(2):180-5.

Imai DM., et al. Dynamics of connective-tissue localization during chronic Borrelia burgdorferi infection. *Lab Invest.* 2013;93(8):900-910.

Imai DM. et al. The early dissemination defect attributed to disruption of decorin-binding proteins is abolished in chronic murine Lyme borreliosis. *Infect Immun.* 2013;81(5):1663-73.

Ivanova LB. et al. Borrelia chilensis, a new member of the Borrelia burgdorferi sensu lato complex that extends the range of this genospecies in the South Hemisphere. *Environ Microbiol.* 2014;16(4):1069-80.

Iyer R. et al. Detection of Borrelia burgdorferi nucleic acids after antibiotic treatment does not confirm viability. *J Clin Microbiol.* 2013;51(3):857-62.

Iyer R. et al. Stage-specific global alterations in the transcriptomes of Lyme disease spirochetes during tick feeding and following mammalian host adaptation. *Mol Microbiol.*2014.

Izadi H. et al. c-Jun N-terminal kinase 1 is required for Toll-like receptor 1 gene expression in macrophages. *Infect Immun.* 2007;75(10)5027-34.

Jacek E. et al. Increased IFN-a activity and differential antibody response in patients with a history of Lyme disease and persistent cognitive deficits. *J Neuroimmunol.* 2013;255(1-2):85-91.

Jackman, N, et al. Myelin biogenesis and oligodendrocyte development: Parsing out the roles of blycosphingolipids. *Physiology* 2009; 24: 290-7.

Jackson CR. et al. Evidence of a conjugal erythromycin resistance element in the Lyme disease spirochete Borrelia burgdorferi. *Int J Antimicrob Agents.* 2007;30(6):496-504.

Jacquot M. et al. Comparative population genomics of the Borrelia burgdorferi species complex reveals high degree of genetic isolation among species and underscores benefits and constraints to studying intra-specific epidemiological processes. *PLoS One.* 2014;9(4):e94384.

Jacquot M. et la. High-throughput sequence typing reveals genetic differentiation and host specialization among populations of differentiation and host specialization among populations of the Borrelia burgdorferi species complex that infect rodents. *PloS One.* 2014;9(2):e88581.

Jaenson TG. and Lindgren E. The range of Ixodes ricinus and the risk of contracting Lyme borreliosis will increase northwards when the vegetation period becomes longer. *Ticks Tick Borne Dis.* 2011;2(1):44-9.

Jain S. et al. Borrelia burgdorferi harbors a transport system essential for purine salvage and mammalian infection. *Infect Immun.* 2012;80(9):3086-93.

Jairath V. et al. Lyme disease in Haryana, India. *Indian J Dermatol Venereol Leprol.* 2014;80(4):3200-3.

James MC. et al. The heterogeneity, distribution, and environmental associations of Borrelia sensu lato, the agent of Lyme borreliosis, in Scotland. *Front Public health.* 2014;2:129.

Jarefors S. et al. Decreased up-regulation of the interleukin-12Rb2-chain and interferon-g secretion and increased number of forkhead box P3-expressing cells in patients with a history of chronic Lyme borreliosis compared with asymptomatic Borrelia-exposed individuals. *Clin Experiment Immun.* 2006;147l:18-27.

Jares TM., Mathiason MA., Kowalski TJ. Functional outcomes in patients with Borrelia burgdorferi reinfection. *Ticks Tick Borne Dis.* 2014;5(1):58-62.

Jiang Y. et al. Interpretation criteria for standardized Western blot for the predominant species of Borrelia burgdorferi sensu lato in China. *Biomed Enviorn Sci.* 201;23(5):341-9.

Johnson BJ., Pilgard MA., and Russell TM. Assessment of new culture method for detection of Borrelia species from serum of Lyme disease patients. *J Clin Microbiol.* 2014;52(3):721-4.

Johnson L. and Sticker RB. Attorney General forces Infectious Diseases Society of America to redo Lyme guidelines due to flawed development process. *J Med Ethics.*2009;35(5):283-8.

Johnson L. et al. Severity of chronic Lyme disease compared to other chronic conditions: a quality of life survey. *Peer J.* 2014;2:e322.

Jones KL. et al. Analysis of Borrelia burgdorferi genotypes in patients with Lyme arthritis: High frquency of ribosomal RNA intergenic spacer type 1 strains in antibiotic-refractory arthritis. *Arthritis Rheum.*2009;60(7):2174-82.

Jones KL. et al. Higher mRNA levels of chemokines and cytokines associated with macrophage activation in erythema migrans skin lesions in patients from the United States than in patients from Austria with Lyme borreliosis. *Clin Infect Dis.* 2008;46(1):85-92.

Jordan BE. et al. Detection of Borrelia burgdorferi and Borrelia lonestari in birds in Tennessee. *J Med Entomol.* 2009;46(1):131-8.

Jurtras BL. and Chenail AM., Stevenson B. Changes in bacterial growth rate govern expression of the Borrelia burgdorferi OspC and Erp Infection-associated surface proteins. *J Bacteriology.*2013;195(4):757-64.

Kadam P. et al. Delayed onset of the Jarisch_ Herxheimer reaction in doxycycline-treated disease: A case report and review of its histopathology and implications for pathogenesis. *Am J Dermatopathol.* 2014.

Kameda G. et al. Diastolic heart murmur, nocturnal back pain, and lumbar rigidity in a 7-year-old: an unusual manifestation of Lyme disease in childhood. *Case Rep Pediatr.* 2012;2012:976961.

Kaneda, K, et al. Glycosphingolipid-binding protein of Borrelia burgdorferi sensu lato. *Infect Immun* 1997; 65(8): 3180-5.

Kaneda, K, et al. Infectivity and arthritis induction on SCID mice and immune competent mice: possible role of galactocerebroside binding activity on initiation of infection. *Microbiol Immunol* 1998; 42(3): 171-5.

Kannian P. et al. Antibody responses to Borrelia burgdorferi in patients with antibiotic-refractory, antibiotic-responsive, or non-antibiotic-treated Lyme arthritis. *Arthritis Rheum.* 2007;56(12):4216-25.

Kannian P. et al. Decline in the frequencies of Borrelia burgdorferi OspA161 175-specific T cells after antibiotic therapy in HLA-DRB1*0401-positive patients with antibiotic-responsive or antibiotic-refractory Lyme arthritis. *J Immunol.* 2007;179(9):6336-42.

Kariu T. et al. BB0323 and Novel virulence deteminatnt BB0238: Borrelia burgdorferi proteins that interact with and stabilize each other and are critical for infectivity. *J Infect Dis.* 2015;211(3):462-71.

Karmacharya P., Aral MR. Heart stopping tick. *World J Cardiol.* 2013;5(5):148-50.

Karna SL. et al. Contributions of enviornmental signals and conserved residues to the functions of carbon storage regualtor A of Borrelia burgdorferi. *Infect Immun.*2013;81(8):2972-85.

Karosi T. et al. Recurrent laryngeal nerver paralysis due to subclinical Lyme borreliosis. *J Laryngoi Otol.* 2010;124(3):336-8.

Katchar K., Drouin EE., Steere AC. Natural killer cells and natural killer Tcells in Lyme arthritis. *Arthritis Res Ther.* 2014;15(6):R183.

Kawabata H. et al. Multilocus sequence typing and DNA similarity analysis implicates that a Borrelia valaisiana-related sp. isolated in Japan is distinguishable from European B. valaisiana. *J Vet Med Sci.* 2013;75(9):1201-7.

Kawano Y. et al. Case of Borrelia brainstem encenalitis presenting with severe dysphagia. *Rinsho Shinkeigaku.* 2010;50(4)·265-7.

Kelesidis T. et al. The cross-talk between spirochetal lipoproteins and immunity. *Front Immun.*2014;5(310):1-12.

Kemperman MM., Bakken JS. and Kravitz GR. Dispelling the chronic Lyme disease myth. *Minn Med.*2008;91(7):37-41.

Kempf W., Kazakov DV. and Kutzner H. Lobular panniculitis due to Borrelia burgdorferi infection mimicking subcutaneous panniculitis-like T-cell lymphoma. *Am J Dermatopathol.* 2013;35(2):e30-3.

Kempf W. et al. Cutaneous borreliosis with T-cell-Rich infiltrate and simultaneous involvement by B-Cell chronic lymphocytic leukemia with t(14;18) (q32;q21). *Am J Dermatopathol.* 2014.

Kenedy MR. and Akins DR. The OspE-related proteins inhibit complement deposition and enhance serum resistance of Borrelia burgdorferi, the Lyme disease spirochete. *Infect Immun.*2011;79(4):1451-7.

Kenedy MR., Lenhart TR. and Akins DR. The role of Borrelia burgdorferi outer surface protein. *FEMS Immunol Med Microbiol.* 2012;66(1):1-19.

Kenedy MR. et al. CspA-mediated binding of human factor H inhibits complement deposition and confers serum resistance in Borrelia burgdorferi. *Infect Immun.* 2009;77(7):2773-82.

Kern A. et al. Tick saliva represses innate immunity and cutaneous inflammation in a murine model of Lyme disease. *Vector Borne Zoonotic Dis.*2011;11(10):1343-50.

Khatchikian CE. et al. Evidence for strain-specific immunity in patient treated for early Lyme disease. *Infect Immun.* 2014;82(4):1408-13.

Kim MH., Kim WC., Park DS. Neurogenic bladder in Lyme disease. *Int Neurourol J.* 2012;16(4):201-4.

Kindler W. et al. Peripheral facial palsy as an initial symptom of Lyme neuroborreliosis in an Austrian endemic area. *Wien Klin Wochenschr.* 2015;10.

Kirmizis D., Chatzidimitriou D. Comment on 'Membranous glamerulonephritis secondary to Borelia burgdorferi infection presenting as nephrotic syndrome. *Nephrol Dial Transplant.* 2010, Letter to the Editor:1723-4.

Kisand KE. et al. Propensity to excessive proinflammatory response in chronic Lyme borreliosis. *APMIS.* 2007;115(2):134-41.

Kishimoto M. et al. Lyme disease presenting as ruptured synovial cysts. *J Clin Rheumatol.* 2007;13(6):365-6.

Kisova-Vargova L. et al. Host-dependent differential expression of factor H binding proteins, their affinity to factor H and complement evasion by Lyme and relapsing fever borreliae. *Vet Microbiol.* 2011;148(2-4):341-7.

Klemen S. et al. Borrelia burgdorferi RST1(OspC Type A) Genotype Is Associated with Greater Inflammation and More Severe Lyme Disease. *Americ J Pathology.* 2011;178(6):2726-39.

Klitgaard, K, et al. Discovery of bovine digital dermatitis-associated Treponema spp. In the dairy herd environment by a targeted deep-sequencing approach. *Appl Environ Microbiol* 2014; 80(14): 4427-32.

Klitgaard, K, et al. Evidence of multiple Treponema phylotypes involved in bovine digital dermatitis as shown by 16S rRNA gene analysis and fluorescence in situ hybridization. *Journal of Clinical Microbiology* 2008; September: 3012-20.

Klitgaard, et al, Targeting the treponemal microbiome of digital dermatitis infections by high-resolution phylogenetic analyses and comparison with fluorescent in situ hybridization. *Journal of Clinical Microbiology* 2013; 51(7): 2212-9.

Knauer J. et al. Borrelia burgdorferi potential activates bone marrow-derived conventional dendritic cells for production of IL-23 required for IL-17 release by T cells. *FEMS Immunol Med Microbiol.* 2007;49(3):353-63.

Knauer J. et al. Borrelia burgdorferi potently activates bone marrow-derived conventional dendritic cells for production of IL-23 required for IL-17 released by T cells. *FEMS Immunol Med Microbiol.* 2007;49(3):353-63.

Knauer J. et al. Evaluation of the preventive capacities of a topically applied azithromycin formulation against Lyme borreliosis in a murine model. *J Antimicrob Chemother.* 2011;66(12):2814-22.

Kochling J. et al. Lyme disease with lymphocytic meningitis, trigeminal palsy and silent thalamic lesion. *Eur J Paediatr Neurol.* 2008;12(6):501-4.

Koenigs A. et al. BBA70 of Borrelia burgdorferi is a novel plasminogen-binding protein. *J Biol Chem.* 2013;288(35):25229-43.

Koening CL. et al. Toll-like receptors mediate induction of hepcidin in mice infected with Borrelia burgdorferi. *Blood.* 2009;114(9):1913-8.

Konopka M. et al. Unclassified cardiomyopathy of Lyme carditis? A three year follow-up. *Kardiol Pol.* 2013;71(3):283-5.

Korotaevskiy AA., Hanin LG. and Khanin MA. Non-linear dynamics of the complement system activation. *Math Biosci.* 2009;222(2):127-43.

Kosik-Bogacka DI. et al. Ticks and mosquitoes as vectors of Borrelia burgdorferi s.l. in the forested areas of Szczecin. (3-4):143-6.

Kovalchuka L. et al. Associations of HLA DR and DQ molecules with Lyme borreliosis in Latvian patients. *BMC Res Notes.* 2012;5:438.

Kowacs PA. et al. Chronic unremitting headache associated with Lyme disease-like illness. *Arq Neurropsiquiatr.* 2013;71(7):470-3.

Kowalski TJ. et al. Antibiotic treatment duration and long-term outcomes of patients with early Lyme disease from a Lyme disease-hyperendemic area. *Clin Infect Dis.* 2010;50(4):512-20.

Krabbe NV., Ejlertsen T. and Nielsen H. Neuroborreliosis recurrence: reinfection or relapse? *Scand J Infect Dis.* 2008;40(11-12):985-7.

Kramer F. et al. Serological detection of Anaplasma phagocytophilum, Borelia burgdorferi sensu lato and Ehrilichia canis antibodies and Dirofilaria immitis antigen in a countrywide survey in dogs in Poland. *Parasitol Res.* 2014;113(9):3229-39.

Krause DL., Muller N. The relationship between Tourette's symdrome and infection. *Open Neurol J.* 2012;6:124-8.

Krause PJ. et al. Blood transfusion transmission of the tick-borne relapsing fever spirochete Borrelia miyamotoi in mice.*Transfusion.* 2014;10.

Krause PJ. et al. Borrelia miyamotoi infection in nature and humans. *Clin Microbiol Infect* 2015 (Feb 18): epub ahead of print.

Krause PJ. et al. Borrelia miyamotoi sensu lato seroreactivity and seroprevalence in the Northeastern United States. *Emerg Infect Dis.*2014;20(7):1183-90.

Krause PJ. et al. Human Borrelia miyamotoi infection in the United States. *N Engl J Med.* 2013;368(3):291-93.

Krim E. et al. Retrobulbar optic neuritis: a complication of Lyme Disease? *J Neurol Neurosurg Psychiatry.* 2007;78(12):1409-10.

Kritchevskaya GI. et al. The rate of detection and diagnostic significance of antibodies to Borrelia burgdorferi in patients with eyes diseases of inflammatory nature. *Klin Lab Diagn.* 2014;(2):53-6.

Krol CG. et al. Acrodermatitis chronica atrophicans: late manifestation of Lyme borreliosis. *Ned Tidschr Geneeskd.* 2010;154:A2012.

Krugman P. The Civility Whine, Krugman Blog, *NY Times*, October 18, 2014.

Krugman P. Reckonings: Bait and Switch, Krugman Blog, *NY Times*, November 1, 2000.

Krull A. et al. Deep sequencing analysis reveals temporal microbiota changes associated with development of bovine digital dermatitis. *Infection and Immunity* 2014; 82(8): 3359-73.

Krupka M. et al. Biological aspects of Lyme disease spirochetes: unique bacteria of the Borrelia burgdorferi species group. *Biomed Pap Med Fac Univ Olomouc Czech Repub.* 2007;151(2):175-86.

Krupna-Gaylord MA. et al. Induction of Type I and Type III Interferons b Borrelia burgdorferi correlates with pathogenesis and requires linear plasid 36. *PLoS One.* 2014;9(6):e100174.

Kubanek M. et al. Detection of Borrelia burgdorferi sensu lato in endomyocardial biopsy specimens in individuals with recent-onset dilated cardiomyopthy. *Eur J Heart Fail.* 2012; 14(6):588-96.

Kudryashev M. et al. Evidence fo direct cell-cell fusion in Borrelia by cryogenic electron tomography. *Cell Microbiol.* 2011;13(5):731-41.

Kuenzle S. et al. Pathogen specificity and autoimmunity are distinct features of antigen-driven immune responses in neuroborreliosis. *Infect Immun.* 2007;75(8):3841-7.

Kuhn M., Bransfield R. Divergent opinions of proper Lyme disease diagnosis and implications for children co-morbid with autism spectrum disorder. *Med Hypotheses.* 2014;83(3):321-5.

Kuhn M. et al. Long term antibiotic therapy may be an effective treatment for children co-morbid with Lyme disease and autism spectrum disorder. *Medical Hypothesis* 2012; 78(5): 606-15.

Kumi-Diaka J. and Harris O. Viability of Borrelia burgdorferi in stored semen. *British Veterinary Journal* 1995; 151(2): 221-4.

Kuo J. et al. Interleukin-35 enhances Lyme arthritis in Borrelia-vaccinated and -infected mice. *Clin Vaccine Immunol.* 2011;18(7);1125-32.

Kwiatkowska E. et al. Minimal-change disease secondary to Borrelia burgdorferi infection. *Case Rep Nephrol.* 2012;294532:1-2.

Kyckova K., Kopecky J. Effect of tick saliva on mechanisms of innate immune response against Borrelia afzelii. *J Med Entomol.* 2006;43(6):1208-14.

Labato E. et al. Seabirds and the circulation of Lyme borreliosis bacteria in the North Pacific. *Vector Borne Zoonotic Dis.* 2011;11(12):1521-7.

Lakos A., Igari Z. and Solymosi N. Recent lesson from a clinical and seroepidemiological survey: low positive value of Borrelia burgdorferi antibody testing in a high risk population. *Adv Med Sci.* 2012;57(2):356-63.

Lakos A. and Solymosi N. Maternal Lyme borreliosis and pregnancy outcome. *Int J Infect Dis.* 2010;14(6);e494-8.

Lalosevic D. et al. Borrelia-like organism in heart capillaries of patient with Lyme-disease seen by electron microscopy. *Int J Cardiol.* 2010;145(3):e96-8.

Lammano E. et al. Tick-borne pathogens in ticks collected from breeding and migratory birds in Switzerland. *Ticks Tick Borne Dis.* 2014;5(6):871-82.

Lane RS. Western gray squirrel (Rodentia: Sciuridea): a primary reservoir host of Borrelia burgdorferi in Californian oak woodlands? *J Med Entomol.* 2005;42(3):388-96.

Lantos PM. Chronic Lyme disease: the controversies and the science. *Expert Rev Anti Infect Ther.* 2011;9(7):787-97.

Lantos PM. Lyme disease vaccination: are we ready to try again? *Lancet Infect Dis.* 2013;13(8):643-4.

Lantos PM. and Auwaerter PG., Wormser GP. A systematic review of Borrelia burgdorferi morphologic variants does not support a role in chronic Lyme disease. *Clin Infect Dis.* 2014;58(5):663-71.

LaRocca TJ. et al. Cholesterol lipids of Borrelia burgdorferi form lipid rafts and are required for the bactericidal activity of a complement-independent antibody. *Cell Host Microbe.* 2010;8(4):331-42.

LaRocca TJ. et al. Proving Lipid Rafts Exist: Membrane Domains in the Prokaryote Borrelia burgdorferi have the Same Properties as Eukaryotic Lipid Rafts. *PLoS Path.* 2013;9(5):e1003353.

Larsson C. and Bergstrom S. A novel and simple method for laboratory diagnosis of relapsing fever borreliosis. *Open Microbiolo J.* 2008;2:10-12.

Larsson C., Lundqvist J. and Bergstrom S. Residual brain infection in murine relapsing fever borreliosis can be successfully treated with ceftriaxone. *Microb Pathog.* 2008;44(3):262-4.

Larsson C. et al. First record of Lyme disease Borrelia in the Arctic. *Vector Borne Zoonotic Dis.* 2007;7(3):453-6.

Lawaczeck EW. et al. Tickborne relapsing fever in a mother and newborn child—Colorado, 2011. *Cent Dis Control Prevent.* 2012;61(10):174-6.

Lawrence KA. et al. Borrelia burgdorferi bb0426 encodes a 2'deoxyribosyltransferase that plays a central role in purine salvage. *Molecul Microbiol.* 2009;72(6):1517-29.

Lazarus JJ. et al. IL-10 deficiency promotes increased Borrelia burgdorferi clearance predominantly through enhanced innate immune responses. *J Immunol.* 2006;177(10):7076-85.

Lazarus JJ. et al. Viable Borrelia burgdorferi enhances interleukin-10 production and suppresses activation of murine macrophages. *Infec Immun.* 2008;76(3):1153-62.

Lee DH and Vielemeyer O. Analysis of overall level of evidence behind Infectious Diseases Society of American practice guidelines, *Archives of Internal Medicine* (2011) 171(1): 18-22.

Lee JK. et al. Detection of a Borrelia species in questing Gulf Coast ticks, Amblyomma maculatum. *Ticks Tick Borne Dis.* 2014;5(4):449-52.

Lee K. et al. A relapsing fever group Borrelia sp. similar to Borrelia lonestari found among wild sika deer (Cervus nippon yesoensis) and Haemaphysalis spp. ticks in Hokkaido, Japan. *Ticks Tick Borne Dis.* 2014;5(6):841-7.

Lee SH. et al. Detection of borreliae in archived sera from patients with clinically suspect Lyme disease. *Int J Mol Sci.* 2014;15(3):4284-98.

Lee SH. et al. DNA sequencing diagnosis of off-season spirochetemia with low bacterial density in Borrelia burgdorferi and Borrelia miyamotoi infections. *Int J Mol Sci. et al.* 2014;15(7):11364-86.

Lee WY. et al. An intravascular immune response to Borrelia burgdorferi involves Kupffer cells and iNKT cells. *Nat Immunol.* 2010;11(4):295-302.

Lee Y. et al. A case of atrophoderma of pasini and pierini associated with Borrelia burgdorferi infection successfully treated with oral doxycycline. *Ann Dermatol.* 2011;23(3):352-6.

LeFrance ME. et al. The Borrelia burgdorferi intergrin ligand p66 affects gene expression by human cells in culture. *Infect Immunt.* 2011;79(8):3249-61.

Legatowicz-Koprowska M. et al. Borreliosis—simultaneous Lyme carditis and psychiatric disorders—case report. *Pol Merkur Lekarski.* 2008;24(143):433-5.

Legatowicz-Koprowska M. et al. Lyme carditis—a bitter lesson or a delayed diagnostic success—a case report. *Kardiol Pol.* 2007;655(10):1228-30.

Lelovas P. et al. Cardiac implications of Lyme disease, diagnosis and therapeutic approach. *Int J Cardiol.* 2008;129(1):15-21.

Lenormand C. et al. Species of Borrelia burgdorferi complex that cause borrelial lymphacytoma in France. *Br J Dermatol.* 2009;161(1):174-6.

Lescot M. et al. The genome of Borrelia recurrentis, the agent of deadly louse-borne relapsing fever, is a degraded subset of tick-borne Borrelia duttonii. *PLoS Genet.* 2008;4(9):e1000185.

Lesnicar G. and Zerdoner D. Temporomandibular joint involvement caused by Borrelia burgdorferi. *J Craniomaxillofac Surg.* 2007;35(8):397-400.

Leverkus M. et al. Metastatic squamous cell carcinoma of the ankle in long-standing untreated acrodermatitis chronica atrophicans. *Dermatology.* 2008;217(3):215-8.

Levy S. The Lyme disease debate. Host biodiversity and human disease risk. *Environ Health Perspect.* 2013;121(4):A120-A125.

Li X. et al. Burden and viability of Borrelia burgdorferi in skin and joints of patients with erythema migrans or Lyme arthritis. *Arthritis Rheum.* 2011;63(8):2238-47.

Liba Z., Kayserova J., Komarek V. Th1 and Th17 but no Th2-related cytokine spectrum in the cerebrospinal fluid of children with Borrelia-related facial nerve palsy. *BioMed.* 2013;10:30.

Liebold T., Straubinger RK. and Rauwald HW. Growth inhibiting activity of Lipophilic extracts from Dipsacus sylvesris Huds, roots against Borrelia burgdorferi s.s. in vitro. *Pharmazie* 2011;66(8):628-30.

Lieskovska J., Kopecky J. Effect of tick saliva on signaling pathways activated by TLR-2 ligand and Borrelia afzelii in dendritic cells. *Parasite Immunol.* 2012;34(8-9):421-9.

Lieskovska J. and Kopecky J. Tick saliva suppresses IFN signalling in dendritic cells upon Borrelia afzelii infection. *Parasite Immunol.* 2012;34(1):32-9.

Ligor M., Olszowy P. and Buszewski B. Application of medical and analytical methods in Lyme borreliosis monitoring. *Anal Bioanal Chem.* 2012;402(7):2233-48.

Lilenbaum, W, et al. Detection of Leptospira spp. in semen and vaginal fluids of goats and sheep by polymerase chain reaction. *Theriogenology* 2008; 69(7): 837-42.

Lin YP. et al. Glycosaminoglycan binding by Borrelia burgdorferi adhesion BBK32 specifically and uniquely joint colonization. *Cell Microbiol.* 2014.

Lin YP. et al. Strain-specific variation of the decorin-binding adhesin DbpA influences the tissue tropism of the Lyme disease spirochete. *PLoS One.* 2014;10(7):e1004238.

Literak I. et al. Larvae of chigger mites Neotrombicula spp. (Acari: Trombiculidae) exhibited Borrelia but no Anaplasma infections: a field study including birds from the Czech Carpathians as hosts of chiggers. *Exp Appl Acarol.* 2008;44(4):307-14.

Little SE. et al. Canine infection with Dirofilaria immitis, Borrelia burgdorferi, Anaplasma spp., and Ehrlichia spp. in the United States, 2010-2012. *Parasit Vectors.* 2014;7:257.

Littman MP. Lyme nephritis. *J Vet Emerg Crit Care (San Antonio).* 2013;23(2):163-73.

Liu H. et al. Induction of distinct neurologic disease manifestations during relapsing fever requires T lymphocytes. *J Immunol.* 20100;184(10):5859-64.

Livengood JA. et al. Global trascriptome analysis of Borrelia burgdorferi during association with human neuroglial cell. *Inf Immun.* 2008;76(1):298-07.

Liveris D. et al. Comparison of five diagnostic modalities for direct detection of Borrelia burgdorferi in patients with early Lyme disease. *Diagn Microbiol Infect Dis.* 2012;73(3):243-45.

Ljostad U., Mygland A. CSF B—lymphocyte chemocattractant (CXCL13) in the early diagnosis of acute Lyme neuroborreliosis. *J Neurol.* 2008;255(5):732-7.

Ljostad U., Mygland A. The phenomenon of 'chronic Lyme': an observational study. *Eur J Neurol.* 2012;19(8):1128-35.

Lledo L. et al. A seventeen-year epidemiological surveillance study of Borrelia burgdorferi infections in two provinces of northern Spain. *Int J Environ Res Public Health.* 2014;11(2):1661-72.

Lochhead RB. et al. Endothelial cells and fibroblasts amplify the arthritogenic Type I IFN response in murine Lyme disease and are major sources of chemokines in B. burgdorferi-infected joint tissue1. *J Immunol.* 2012;189(5):2488-501.

Lochhead RB. et al. MicroRNA-14-146a provides feedback regulation of Lyme arthritis but not carditis during infection with Borrelia burgdorferi. *PLoS Pathog.* 2014;10(6):e1004212.

Londonon D. et al. Il-10 helps control pathogen load during high-level bacteremia. *J Immunol.* 2008;181(3): 2076-2083.

Londono D. et al. IL-10 Prevents apoptosis of brain endothelium during bacteremia. *J Immunol.* 2011;186(12):7176-86.

Londono D. et al. Interleukin 10 protects the brain microcirculation from spirochetal injury. *J Neuropathol.* 2008;67(10):976-983.

Londono D. et al. Relapsing fever borreliosis in interleukin-10-deficient mice. *Infect Immun.* 2008;76(12):5508-13.

Lopez JE. et al. Acquisition and subsequent transmission of Borrelia hermsii by the soft tick Ornithodoros hermsi. *J Med Entomol.* 2011;48(4):891-5.

Lopez JE. et al. A novel surface antigen of relapsing fever spirochetes can discriminate between relapsing fever and Lyme borreliosis. *Clin Vaccine Immunol.*2010;17(4):564-71.

Lopez JE. et al. Real-time monitoring of disease progression in rhesus macaques infected with Borrelia turicatae by tick bite. *J Infect Dis.* 2014;210(10):1639-48.

Love AC. et al. Induction of indoleamine 2,3-dioxygenase by Borrelia burgdorferi in human immune cells correlates with pathogenic potential. *J Leukoc Biol.* 2014;pii:jib.4A0714-339R.

Love AC., Schwartz I., Petzke MM. Borrelia burgdorferi RNA induces Type I and III interferons via toll-like receptor 7 and contributes to production of NF-KB-Dependent Cytokines. *Infect Immun.* 2014;82(6):2405-16.

Lovett JK. et al. Neuroborreliosis in the South West of England. *Epidemiol Infect.* 2008;136(12):1707-11.

Luger, S. Lyme disease transmitted by a biting fly, *New England Journal of Medicine* 1990; 322(24):1752.

Luigetti M. et al. Lumbosacral multiradiculopathy responsive to antibiotic therapy: description of four patients with lumbar spondylosis and a superimposed Lyme disease. *Acta Neurol Belg.* 2014;114(4):297-01.

Lundquist J. et al. Concomitant infection decreases the malaria burden but escapes relapsing fever borreliosis. *Infect Immun.* 2010;78(5):1924-30.

Lusitana, D, et al. Borrelia burgdorferi are susceptible to killing by a variety of human polymorphonuclear leukocyte components, *The Journal of Infectious Diseases* 2002; 185: 797-804.

Ma Y. et al. Borrelia burgdorferi arthritis-associated Locus Bbaa1 regulates Lyme arthritis and K/B x N serum transfer arthritis through intrinsic control of type 1 IFN production. *J Immunol.* 2014;193(12):6050-60.

Macauda MM. et al. Long-term Lyme disease antibiotic therapy beliefs among New England residents. *Vector Borne Zoonotic Dis.* 2011;11(7)857-62.

Macdonald AB. Alzheimer's disease Braak Stage progressions: reexamined and redefined as Borrelia infection transmission through neural circuits. *Medical Hypothesis* 2007; 68(5): 1059-64.

Macdonald AB. Alzheimer's neuroborreliosis with trans0synaptic spread of infection and neurofibrillary tangles derived from intraneuronal spirochetes. *Medical Hypothesis* 2007; 68(4): 822-5.

MacDonald AB. Plaques of Alzheimer's diseases originate from cysts of Borrelia burgdorferi, the Lyme disease spirochete. *Medical Hypothesis* 2006 (article in press).

Macdonald A. and Miranda J. Concurrent neocortical borreliosis and Alzheimer's disease. *Human Pathology* 1987; 18(7): 759-61.

Mackensen F. et al. Difficulties of interpreting Borrelia serology in patients with uveitis. *Ocul Immunol Inflamm.* 2011;19(4):227-31.

MacQueen DD. et al. Genotypic diversity of an emergent population of Borrelia burgdorferi at a coastal Maine island recently colonized by Ixodes scapularis. *Vector Borne Zoonotic Dis.* 2012;12(6):456-61.

Maczka I. et al. Tick-borne infections as a cause of heart trasplantation. *Pol J Microbiol.*2011;60(4):341-3.

Magnarelli LA. and Anderson JF. Ticks and biting insects infected with the etiologic agent of Lyme disease, Borrelia burgdorferi. *Journal of Clinical Microbiology* 1988; 26(8): 1482-1486.

Magnarelli LA., Anderson JF., and Barbour AG. The etiologic agent of Lyme disease in deer flies, horse flies, and mosquitoes. *Journal of Infectious Disease* 1986; 154(2): 355-8.

Maheshwari P. and Eslick GD. Bacterial infection and Alzheimer's disease: a meta-analysis. *J Alheimers.* 2015;43(3):957-66.

Malawista SE. and de Boisfleury Chevance A. Clocking the Lyme spirochete. *PLoS One.* 2008;3(2):e.1633.

Malkiel S. et al. The Loss and Gain of Marginal Zone and Peritoneal B Cells Is Different in Response to Relapsing Fever and Lyme Disease Borrelia. *J Immunol* 2009;182:498-506.

Marchal C. et al. Antialarmin effect of tick saliva during the transmission of Lyme disease. *Infect Immun.*2011;79(2):774-85.

Marchal CM. et al. Defensin is suppressed by tick salivary gland extract during the in vitro interaction of resident skin cells with Borrelia burgdorferi. *J Investig Dermatol.* 2009;129:2515-17. Letter to the editor.

Margos G. et al. Borrelia bavariensis sp. nov. is widely distributed in Europe and Asia. *Int J Syst Evol Microbiol.* 2013;63(Pt11);4284-8.

Margos G. et al. Borrelia kurtenbachii sp. nov., a widely distributed member of the Borrelia burgdorferi sensu lato species complex in North America. *Int J Syst Evol Microbiol.* 64(Pt1):128-30.

Margos G. et al. Long-term in vitro cultivation of Borrelia miyamotoi. *Ticks Tick Borne Dis.* 2014;pii:S1877-959X(14)00219-2.

Margos G. et al. Multilocus sequence analysis of Borrelia bissettii strains from North America reveals a new Borrelia species, Borrelia kurtenbachii. *Ticks Tick Borne Dis.* 2010;1(4):151-8.

Margos G. et al. A new Borrelia species defined by multilocus sequence analysis of housekeeping genes. *Appl Environ. Microb.* 2009;75(16):5410-6.

Margos G. et al. Population genetics, taxonomy, phylogeny and evolution of Borrelia burgdorferi sensu lato. *Infect Genet Evol.* 2011;11(7):1545-63.

Margos G. et al. Two boundaries separate Borrelia burgdorferi populations in North America. *Appl Environ Micrbiol.* 2012;78(17):6059-67.

Margulis L. et al. Spirochete round bodies, syphilis, Lyme disease & AIDS: Resurgence of the great imitator. *Symbiosis* 2009; 47: 51-8.

Marinez-Balzano CD., Greenberg B. Bilateral vocal cord paralysis requiring tracheostomy due to neuroborreliosis. *Chest.*2014;146(5):e153-5.

Markeljevic J., Sarac H. and Rados M. Tremor, seizures and psychosis as presenting symptoms I a patient with chronic lyme neuroborreliosis (LMB). *Coll Antropol.* 2011;35(1):313-8.

Marks DH. Neurological complications of vaccination with outer surface protein A (OspA). *Int J Risk Saf Med.* 2011;23(2):89-96.

Marques A. Chronic Lyme Disease: An appraisal. *Infect Dis Clin North Am.* 2008;22(2):341-60.

Marques A. et al. Natural killer cell counts are not different between patients with post-Lyme disease syndrome and controls. *Clinical and Vaccine Immunology* 2009; August: 1249-50.

Marques A. et al. Xenodiagnosis to detect Borrelia burgdorferi infection: a first-in-human study. *Clin Infect Dis.* 2014;58(7):937-45.

Marre ML. et al. Role of adrenomedullin in Lyme disease. *Infec Immun.* 2010;78(12):5307-13.

Martolff L. et al. Recurrent nerve palsy due to Lyme disease: report of two cases. *Rev Med Interne.* 2010;31(3):229-31.

Marvin S. et al. Interpretation criteria in Western blot diagnosis of Lyme borroliosis. *Br J Biomed Sci.* 2011;68(1):5-10.

Mason LM. et al. Menage a trois: Borrelia, dendritic cells, and tick saliva interactions. *Trends Parasitol.* 2014;30(2):95-03.

Matera G. et al. Chronic neuroborreliosis by B. garinii: an unusual case presenting with epilepsy and multifocal brain MRI lesions. *New Micrbiolog.* 2014;37:393-7.

Mathers A. et al. Strain diversity of Borrelia burgdorferi in ticks dispersed in North America by migratory birds. *J Vector Ecol.* 2011;36(1):24-9.

Mattsson N. et al. Neuroinflammation in Lyme neuroborreliosis affects amyloid metabolism. *BMC Neurology* 2010; 10: 51.

Mayne P. et al. Evidence for Ixodes holocyclus (acarina: Ixodidae) as a vector for human Lyme borreliosis infection in Australia. *J Insect Sci.* 2014;14:271.

Mayne PJ. Clinical determinants of Lyme borreliosis, babesiosis, bartonellosis, anaplasmosis, and ehrlichiosis in an Australian cohort. *Int J Gen Med.* 2014;8:15-26.

Mayne PJ. Investigation of Borrelia burgdorferi genotypes in Australia obtained from erythema migrans tissue. *Clin Cosmet Investig Dermatol.* 2012;5:69-78.

McAuliffe L. et al. Biofilm formation by mycoplasma species and its role in environmental persistence and survival. *Microbiology* 2006; 152: 913-22.

McCall JW. et al. The ability of a topical novel combination of fipronil, amitraz and (S)-methoprene to protect dogs from Borrelia

burgdorferi and Anaplasma phagocytophilum infections transmitted by Ixodes scapularis. *Vet Parasitol.* 2011;179(4):335-42.

McKay G., Gill I. and Chauhan S. Lyme disease: and an unusual case of peripheral nerve palsy. *J Bone Joint Surg Br.* 2010;92(5):713-5.

McVeigh K., Vakros G. Case report: papillitis as the sole ocular sign in Lyme disease. *Clin Ophthalmol.* 2012;6:1093-7.

Mearini M. et al. Spinal cord stimulation for the treatment of upper and lower extremity neuropathic pain due to Lyme disease. *Neuromodulation.* 2007;10(2):142-7.

Mechai S. et al. Phylogeographic analysis reveals a complex population structure of Borrelia burgdorferi in Southeastern and South Central Canada. *Appl Environ Microbiol.* 2014;pii:AEM.03730-14.

Mediannikov O. et al. Borrelia crocidurae infection in acutely febrile patients, Senegal. *Emerg Infect Dis.* 2014;20(8):1335-8.

Meer-Scherrer, L, et al. Lyme disease associated with Alzheimer's disease. *Curr Microbiol* 2006; 52(4): 330-2.

Meng Z. et al. Detection of co-infection with Lyme spirochetes and Spotted fever group rickettsiae in a group of Haemaphysalis longicornis. *Zhongha Liu Xing Bing Xue Za Zhi.* 2008;29(12):1217-20.

Menten-Dedoyart C. et al. Neutrophil extracellular traps entrap and kill Borrelia burgdorferi sensu stricto spirochetes and are not affected by Ixodes ricinus tick saliva. *J Immunol.* 2012; 189 (11):5393-401.

Mercer, G, et al. Detection of Borrelia burgdorferi DNA by polymerase chain reaction in urine specimens of patients with erythema migrans lesions. Mol Cell Probes 1997; 11(2): 89-94.

Merilainen L. et al. Morphological and biochemical features of Borrelia burgdorferi pleomorphic forms. *Microbio papers press.* 2015;14.

Michel ML. et al. Identification of an IL-17-producing NK1.1(neg) iNKT cell population involved in airway neutrophilia. *J Exp Med.* 2007;204(5):995-1001.

Middelveen MJ. and Stricker RB. Filament formation associated with spirochetal infection: a comparative approach to Morgellons disease. *Clin Cosmet Invest Dermat..* 2011;4:167-77.

Middelveen MJ. et al. Association of spirochetal infection with Morgellons disease. *F100Research.*2013;2(25):1-15.

Middelveen MJ. et al. Characterization and evolution of dermal filaments from patients with Morgellons disease. *Clin Cosm Investig Dermatol.* 2013;6:1-21.

Middelveen MJ. et al. Culture and identification of Borrelia spirochetes in human vaginal and seminal secretions. *F1000 Research 3* (2015).

Mikkila HO. et al. The expanding clinical spectrum of ocular Lyme borreliosis. *Ophthalmology.* 2000;107(3):581-7.

Miklossy J. Alzheimer's disease – a neurospirochetosis. Analysis of the evidence following Koch's and Hill's criteria. *Journal of Neuroinflammation.* 2007;8:90.

Miklossy J. Alzheimer's disease – a spirochetosis? *Neuroreport* 1993;4(7):841-8.

Miklossy J. Chronic inflammation and amyloidogenesis in Alzheimer's disease: The role of spirochetes. Ph.D thesis. 2005.

Miklossy J. Chronic inflammation and amyloidogenesis in Alzheimer's disease – role of spirochetes. *Journal of Alzheimer's Disease* 2008; 13(4): 381-91.

Miklossy J. Chronic or late Lyme neuroborreliosis: Analysis of evidence compared to chronic or late neurosyphilis. *Open Neurology J.* 2012;6(Suppl 1-M9):146-57.

Miklossy J. Emerging roles of pathogens in Alzheimer disease. *Expert Rev Mol Med.* 2011;13:e30.

Miklossy, J, et al. Borrelia burgdorferi persists in the brain in chronic lyme neuroborreliosis and may be associated with Alzheimer disease. *Journal of Alzheimer's Disease* 2004; 6: 639-49.

Miklossy J. et al. Persisting atypical and cystic forms of Borrelia burgdorferi and local inflammation in Lyme neuroborreliosis. *J Neuroinflam.* 2008;5:40.

Miller JC. et al. A critical role for type 1 IFN in arthritis development following Borrelia burgdorferi infection of Mice. *J Immunol.* 2008;181(12):8492-503.

Miller JC. et al. The Lyme disease spirochete Borrelia burgdorferi utilizes multiple ligands, including RNA, for interferon regulatory factor 3-dependent induction of type I intrferon-responsive genes. *Infect Immun.* 2010;78(7):3144-53.

Mlynarcik P. et al. Deciphering the interface between a CD 40 receptor and borrelial ligand OspA. *Microbiol Res.* 2015;170:51-60.

Modjtahedi SP. et al. Neuroretinitis associated with serologies positive for Bartonella henselae and Borrelia burgdorferi. *Retin Cases Brief Rep.* 2009;3(3):243-4.

Moiuszko A. et al. Co-infections with Borrelia species, Anaplasma phagocytophilum and Babesia spp. in patients with tick-borne encephalitis. *Eur J Clin Microbiol Infect Dis.* 2014;33:1835-41.

Molin S., Ruzicka T. and Prinz JC. Borreliosis mimicking lupus-like syndrome during infliximab treatment. *Clin Exp Dermatol.* 2010,35(6).631-3.

Monari P., Farisoglio C. and Calzavara Pinton PG. Borrelia burgdorferi-associated primary cutaneous marginal-one B0cell lymphoma: a case report. *Dematology.* 2007;215(3):229-32.

Mongodin EF. et al Inter- and intra-specific pan-genomes of Borrelia burgdorferi sensu lato: genome stability and adaptive radiation. *BMC Genomics.* 2013;14:693.

Moniuszko A. et al. Coinfection of tick cell lines has variable effects on replications of intracellular bacterial and viral pathogens. *Ticks Tick Borne Dis.* 2014;5(4):415-22.

Moniuszko A. et al. Evaluation of CXCL8, CXCL10, CXCL11, CXCL12 and CXCL13 in serum and cerebrospinal fluid of patients with neuroborreliosis. *Immunol Lett.* 2014;157(1-2):45-50.

Moniuszko A. et al. Post Lyme syndrome as a clinical problem. *Pol Merkur Lekarski.* 2009;26(153):227-30.

Moniuszko AM. et al. Concentration of soluble

forms of selectins in serum and in cerebrospinal fluid in group of patients with neuroborreliosis—a preliminary study. *Pol Merkur Lekarski.* 2007;23(135):174-8.

Montandon CE. et al. Evidence of Borrelia in wild and domestic mammals form the state of Minas Gerais, Brazil. *Rev Bras Parasitol Vet.* 2014; 23(2): 287-90.

Moore MW. et al. Phagocytosis of Borrelia burgdorferi and Treponema pallidum potentiates innate immune activation and induces gamma interferon production. *Infect Immun.* 2007;75(4):2046-62.

Morgan A., Wang. X. The novel heparin-binding motif in decorin-binding protein A from strain B31 of Borrelia burgdorferi explains the higher binding affinity. *Biochemistry* 2013;52(46):8237-45

Morgenstern K. et al. In vitro susceptibility of Borrelia spielmanii to antimicrobial agents commonly used for treatment of Lyme disease. *Antimicrob Agents Chemother.* 2009;53(3):1281-4.

Moriarty TJ. et al. Real-time high resolution 3d imaging of the Lyme disease spirochete adhering to and escaping from the vasculature of a living host. *PLoS Pathog.* 2008; 4(6): e1000090.

Mormont E. et al. Abdominal wall weakness and lumboabdominal pain revealing neuroborreliosis: a report of three cases. *Clin Rheumatol.* 2001;20(6):447-50.

Mukhacheva TA. et al. Borrelia spirochetes in Russia: genospecies differentiation by real-time PCR. *Ticks Tick Borne Dis.* 2014;5(6):722-6.

Muller KE. Damage of collagen and elastic fibers by Borrelia burgdorferi—known and new clinical and histopathological aspects. *Open Neurology J.* 2012;6(Suppl 1-M11):179-86.

Murillo G. et al. Oculopalpebral borreliosis as an unusual manifestation of Lyme disease. *Cornea.* 2013;32(1):87-90.

Myers TA., Kaushal D. and Phillipp MT. Microglia Are mediators of Borrelia burgdorferi-induced apoptosis in SH-SY5Y neuronal cells. *PLoS One* 2009;5(11):e1000659.

Mylonas I. Borreliosis during pregnancy: a risk for the unborn child? *Vector Borne Zoonotic Dis.* 2011;11(7):891 8.

Nadelman RB. et al. Differentiation of reinfection from relapse in recurrent Lyme disease. *N Engl J Med.* 2012;367(20):1883-90.

Naesens R. et al. False positive Lyme serology due to syphilis: report of 6 cases and review of the literature. *Acta Clin Belg.* 2011;66(1):58-9.

Nafeev AA. et al. Cutaneous manifestations of the late stage of Lyme disease. *Klin Med.* 2011:89(2)59-60.

Naj X. et al. The formins FMNL1 and mDia1 regulate coiling phagocytosis of Borrelia burgdorferi by primary human macrophages. *Infect Immun.* 2013;81(5):1683-95.

Narasimhan S. et al. Gut microbiota of the tick vector Ixodes scapularis modulate colonization of the Lyme disease spirochete. *Cell Host Microbe.* 2014;15(1):58-71.

Nardelli DT., Callister SM. and Schell RF. Lyme arthritis: current concepts and a change in paradigm. *Clin and Vac Immunol.* 2008; 15(1):21-34.

Nardelli DT. et al. Role of IL-17, transforming growth factor-beta, and IL-6 in the development of arthritis and production of anti-outer surface protein A borreliacidal antibodies in Borrelia-vaccinated and -challenged mice. *FEMS Immunol Med Microbiol.* 2008;53(2):265-74.

Nefedova VV., Korenberg El. and Gorelova NB. Genetic variants of Borrelia garinii, a widely spread Eurasian pathogen of Ixodic tick borreliosis. *Mol Gen Mikrobiol Virusol.* 2010;(3):7-12.

Nefedova V. et al. Studies on the transovarial transmission of Borrelia burgdorferi sensu lato in the taiga tick Ixodes persulcatus. *Folia Parasitol (Praha)* 2004; 51(1): 67-71.

Nejedla P. et al. What is the percentage of pathogenic borreliae in spirochaetal findings of mosquito larvae? *Ann Agric Environ Med.* 2009;16(2):273-6.

Nelson C. et al. Concerns regarding a new culture method for Borrelia burgdorferi not approved for the diagnosis of Lyme disease. *MMWR Morb Mortal Wkly Rep.* 2014;63(15):333.

Netusil J. et al. The occurrence of Borrelia burgdorferi sensu lato in certain ectoparasites (Mesostigmata, Siphonapter) of Apodemus flavicollis and Myodes glareols in chosen localities in the Czech Republic. *Acta Parasitol.* 2013;58(3):337-41.

Nguyen KT. et al. Zinc is the metal cofactor of Borrelia burgdorferi peptide deformylase. *Arch Biochem Biophys.* 2007;468(2):217-25.

Ni XB. et al. Lyme borreliosis caused by diverse genospecies of Borrelia burgdorferi sensu lato in Northeastern China. *Clin Microbiol Infect.* 2014;20(8):808-14.

Nicolson, Garth. Systemic intracellular bacterial infections (Mycoplasma, Chlamydia, Borrelia species) in neurodegenerative (MS, ALS) and behavorial disorders (ASD), *Infectious Disease Newsletter* (2007).

Nieto NC., and Teglas MD. Relapsing fever group Borreilia in Southern California rodents. *J Med Entomol.* 2014;51(5):1029-34.

Nieto NC. et al. Detection of relapsing fever spirochetes (Borrelia hermsii and Borrelia coriaceae) in free-ranging mule deer (Odocoileus hemionus) from Nevada, United States. *Vector Borne Zoonotic Dis.* 2012;12(2):99-05.

Nigrovic LE. et al. Clinical Predictors of Lyme disease among children with a peripheral facial palsy at an emergency department in a Lyme disease-endemic area. *Pediatrics.* 2008;122(5):e1080-5.

Nimmrich S., Becker I., Horneff G. Intraarticular corticosteroids in refractory childhood Lyme arthritis. *Rheumatol Int.*2014;34(7):987-94.

Niscigorska-Olsen J. et al. Genospecies of Borrelia burgdorferi sensu lato in patients with erythema mirans. *Ann Agric Environ Med.* 2008;15(1):167-70.

Nordberg M. et al. Cytotoxic mechanisms may play role in the local immune response in the central nervous system in neuroborreliosis. *J Neuroimmunol.* 2011; 232(1-2):186-93.

Norman MU. et al. Molecular mechanisms involved in vascular interactions of the Lyme disease pathogen in a living host. *PLoS Pathog.* 2008;4(10):e1000169.

Normark J. et al. Maladjusted host immune responses induce experimental cerebral malaria-like pathology in a murine Borrelia and Plasmodium co-infection model. *PLoS One.* 2014;9(7):e103295.

Norris SJ. How do Lyme Borrelia organisms cause disease? The quest for virulence determinants. *Open Neurol J.* 2012;6(Suppl 1-M8):119-23.

Norte AC. et al. The importance of lizards and small mammals as reservoirs of Borrelia lusitaniae in Portugal. *Environ Microbiol Rep.* 2014.

Novak EA. et al. The cyclin-di-GMP signaling pathway in the Lyme disease spirochete Borrelia burgdorferi. *J Biol Chem.* 2014;4(56).

Ogden NH. et al. Investigation of Genotypes of Borrelia burgdorferi in Ixodes scaplaris Ticks Collected during Surveillance in Canada. *Appl Enviro Microbio.* 2011;77(10):3244-54.

Ogden NH. et al. Projected effects of climate change on tick phenology and fitness of pathogens transmitted by the North American tick Ixodes scapularis. *J Theor Biol.* 2008;254(3):621-32.

Ogrinc K. et al. Suspected early Lyme neuroborreliosis in patients with erythema migrans. *Clin Infect Dis.* 2013;57(4):501-9.

Oksi J. et al. Borrelia burgdorferi detected by culture and PCR in clinical relapse of disseminated Lyme borreliosis. *Ann Med* 1999;31(3):225-32.

Oksi J. et al. Duration of antibiotic treatment in disseminated Lyme borreliosis: a double-blind, randomized, placebo-controlled, multicenter clinical study. *Eur J Clin Microbiol Infect Dis.* 2007;26(8):571-81.

Oldak E., Rozkiewicz D. and Sulik A. Clinical manifestation of Lyme borreliosis in children with positive and negative western blot results. *Przegl Epidemiol.* 2008;62 Suppl 1:77-82.

Oldak E. et al. Unusual clinical manifestation of Lyme disease—report of 2 cases. *Przegl Lek.* 2007;64(12):1031-2.

Oliveira AD. et al Growth, cysts and kintics of Borrelia garinii (Spirochaetales: Spirochaetacea) in different culture media. *Mem Ins Oswaldo Cruz, Rio de janeiro.* 2010;105(5):717-19.

Oliver JH., Gao L. and Lin T. Comparison of the spirochete Borrelia burgdoreri S.L. isolated from the tick Ixodes scapularis in southeastern and northeastern United States. *J Parasitol* 2008;94(6):1351-6.

Olson CM. et al. p38 mitogen-activated protein kinase controls NF-kappaB transcriptional activation and tumor necrosis factor alpha production through RelA phosphorylation mediated by mitogen-and stress-activated protein kinase 1 in response to Borrelia burgdorferi antigens. *Infect Immun* 2007; 75(1): 270-7.

Olson CM Jr. et al. Local production of IFN-gamma by invariant NKT cells modulates acute Lyme carditis. *J Immunol.* 2009;182(6):3728-34.

Onder O. et al. OspC is potent plasminogen receptor on surface of Borrelia burgdorferi. *J Biol Chem.* 2012;287(20):16860-8.

O'Rourke M. et al. Quantitative detection of Borrelia burgdorferi sensu lato in erythema migrans skin lesions using internally controlled duplex real time PCR. *PLoS One.* 2013;8(5):e63968.

Oosting M. et al. Borrelia species induce inflammasome activation and IL-17 production through a caspase-1-dependent mechanism. *Eur J Immunol.* 2011;41(1):172-81.

Oosting M. et al. Innate immunity networks during infection with Borrelia burgdorferi. *Crit Rev Microbiol.* 2014;25:1-12.

Oosting M. et al. Recognition of Borrelia burgdorferi by NOD2 is central for the induction of an inflammatory reaction. *J Infect Dis.* 2010;201(12):1849-58.

Oosting M. et al. Role of Interleukin-23 (IL-23) Receptor Signaling for IL-17 Responses in Human Lyme Disease. *Infect Immun.* 2011;79(11):4681-87.

Oscarsson J. et al. Proinflammatory effect in whole blood by free soluble bacterial components released from planktonic and biofilm cells. *BMC Microbiology* 2008; 8: 206.

Ostfeld RS. et al. Life history and demographic drivers of reservoir competence for three tick-borne zoonotic pathogens. *PLoS One.* 2014; 9(9):e107387.

Ott-Conn CN. et al. Pathogen infection and exposure, and ectoparasites of the federally endagered Amargosa vole (Microtus californicus scirpensis), California USA. *J Wildl Dis.* 2014;50(4):767-76.

Ouyang Z. et al. BosR (BB0647) governs virulence expression in Borrelia burgdorferi. *Mol Microbiol.* 2009;74(6):1331-43.

Ouyang Z. et al. A manganese transporter, BB0219 BmtA), is required for virulence by the Lyme disease spirochete, Borrelia burgdorferi. *Proc Natl Acad Sci U S A.* 2009;106(9):3449-54.

Padgett K. et al. Large scale spatial risk and comparative prevalence of Borrelia miyamotoi and Borrelia burgdorferi sensu lato in Ixodes pacificus. *PLoS One.* 2014;9(10):e110853.

Palecek T. et al. Presence of Borrelia burgdorferi in endomyocardial biopsies in patients with new-onset unexplained dilated cardiomyopathy. *Med Mcrobiol Immunol.* 2010;199(2):139-42.

Palma M. et al. Borrelia hispanica in Ornithodoros erraticus, Portugal. *Clin Micobiol Infect.* 2012;18(7):696-701.

Palmer GH., Bankhead T. and Lukehart SA. 'Nothing is permanent but change' – antigenic variation in persistent bacterial pathogens. *Cell Microbiol.* 2009;11(12):1697-705.

Pancewicz SA. et al. Concentrations of pro-inflammatory cytokines IFN-gamma, IL-6, IL-12 and IL-15 in serum and cerebrospinal fluid in patients with neuroborreliosis undergoing antibiotic treatment. *Pol Merkur Lekarski.* 2007;22(130):275-9.

Panelius J. et al. Expression and sequence diversity of the complement regulating outer surface protein E in Borrelia afzelii vs. Boreelia garinii in patients with erythema migrans or neuroborreliosis. *Microb Pathog.* 2011;49(6):363-8.

Panic G., Stanulovic V. and Popov T. Atrio-ventricular block as the first presentation of disseminated Lyme disease. *Int J Cardiol.* 2011;150(3):e104-6.

Parma, A, et al. Tears and aqueous humor from horses inoculated with Leptospira contain antibodies which bind to cornea. *Vet Immunol Immunopathol* 1987; 14(2): 181-5.

Parola P. et al. Relapsing fever Borrelia I Ornithodoros ticks from Bolivia. *Ann Trop Parasitol.* 2011;105(5):407-11.

Parthasarathy G., Fevrier HB. and Philipp MT. Non-viable Borrelia burgdorferi induce inflammatory mediators and apoptosis in human oligodendrocytes. *Neurosci Lett.* 2013;556:200-3.

Parthasarathy G. and Philipp MT. The MEK/ERK pathway is the primary conduit for Borrelia burgdorferi-induced inflammation and P53-mediated apoptosis in oligodendrocytes. *Apoptosis.* 2014;19(1):76-89.

Patrican, LA. Acquisition of Lyme disease spirochetes by cofeeding Ixodes scapularis ticks. *Am J Trop Med Hyg* 1997; 57(5): 589-93.

Patton TG., Brandt KS. and Gilmore RD Jr. Borrelia burgdorferi visualized in Ixodes scapularis tick excrement by immunoflorescence. *Vector Borne Zoonotic Dis.* 2012;12(11):1000-3.

Patton TG., Dietrich G. and Gilmore RD., Jr. Detection of Borrelia burgdorferi DNA in tick feces provides evidence for organism shedding during vector feeding. *Vector Borne Zoonotic Dis.* 2011;11(3):197-00.

Peeters N. and Colnot DR. In response to letter to the editor: Lyme disease associated with sudden sensorineural hearing loss: case report and literature review. *Otol Neurotol.* 2013;34(8):1544

Peeters N. et al. Lyme disease associated with sudden sensorineural hearing loss: case report and literature review. *Otol Neurotol.* 2013;34(5):832-7.

Perronne C. Lyme and associated tick-borne diseases: global challenges in the context of a public health threat. *Frontier Cell Infect Micro.* 2014;4(74).

Peterson SH. et al. Anti-p19 antibody treatment exacerbates Lyme arthritis and enhances borreliacidal activity. *Clin Vaccine Immunol.* 2007;14(5):510 7.

Petke MM. et al. Recognition of Borrelia burgdorferi, the Lyme disease spirochete, by TLR9 induces a type I IFN response by human immune cells. *J Immunol.* 2009;183:5279-92.

Petnicki-Ocwieja T. and Kern A. Mechanisms of Borrelia burgdorferi internalization and intracellular innate immune signaling. *Cell Infect Microbio.* 2014;4(175):1-7.

Petnicki-Ocwieja T. et al. Nod2 suppresses Borrelia burgdorferi mediated murine Lyme arthritis and carditis through the induction of tolerance. *PLoS One.* 2011;6(2):e17414.

Petnicki-Ocwieja T. et al. TRIF mediates toll-like receptor 2-dependent inflammatory responses to Borrelia burgdorferi. *Infect Immun.* 2013;81(2):402-10.

Pettersson J. et al. Purine salvage pathways among Borrelia species. *Infect Immun.* 2007;75(0):3877 84.

Pfister HW., Rupprecht TA. Clinical aspects of neuroborreliosis and post-:yme disease syndrome in adult patients. *Int J Med Microbiol.*2006;296Suppl40:11-6.

Phillips SE. et al. A proposal for the reliable culture of Borrelia burgdorferi from patients with chronic Lyme disease, even from those previously aggressively treated. *Infection* 1998;26(6):354-357.

Picha D. et al. DNA persistence after treatment of Lyme borreliosis. *Folia Microbiol (Praha).* 2014;59(2):115-25.

Picha D. et al. Examination of specific DNA by PCR in patients with different forms of Lyme borreliosis. *Int J Dermatol.* 2008;47(10):1004-10.

Piesman J. and Hojgaard A. Protective value of prophylactic antibiotic treatment of tick bite for Lyme disease prevention: an animal model. *Ticks Tick Borne Dis.*2012;3(3):193-6.

Piesman J. et al. Efficacy of an experimental azithromycin cream for prophylaxis of tick-transmitted Lyme disease spirochete infection in a murine model. *Antimicrob Agents Chemother.* 2014;58(1):348-51.

Pisanu B. et al. High prevalece of Borrelia burgdorferi s.l. in the European red squirrel Sciurus vuslgaris in France. *Ticks Tick Borne Dis.* 2014;5(1):1-6.

Platonov AE., Maleev VV. and Karan' LS. Relapsing borrelioses fevers: forgotten and new ones. *Ter Arkh.* 2010;82(11):74-80.

Policastro PF., Raffel SJ., Schwan TG. Contransmission of divergent relapsing fever spirochetes by artificially infected Ornithodoros hermsi. *Appl Environ Microbiol.* 2011;77(24):8494-9.

Pollock AA. Accuracy of recommendations in the Infectious Diseases Society of America clinical practice guidelines for Lyme disease. *Clin Infect Dis. (LTTE).* 2007;44:1135.

Pollock H. et al. Perivascular spaces in the basal ganglia of the human brain: their relationship to lacunes. *Journal of Anatomy* 1997; 191: 337-46.

Portmann A. et al. Isolated intracranial hypertension as the presenting sign of Lyme disease. *J Fr Ophtalmol.* 2012;35(9):720.

Postic D. et al. Expanded diversity among Californian Borrelia isolates and description of Borrelia bissettii sp. nov. (Formerly Borrelia group DN127). *Journal of Clinical Microbiology* 1998; December: 3497-3504.

Pratt CL. and Brown CR. The role of eicosanoids in experimental Lyme arthritis. *Front Cell Infect Microbiol.* 2014;4(69).

Prinz JC. et al. "Borrelia-associated early-onset morphea": a particular type of scleroderma in childhood and adolescence with high titer antinuclear antibodies? Results of a cohort analysis and presentation of three cases. *J Am Acad Dermatol.* 2009;248-55.

Pulzova L. and Bhide MR. Outer surface proteins of Borrelia: peerless immune evasion tools. *Curr Protein Pept Sci.* 2014;15(1):75-88.

Pulzova L., Bhide MR., and Andrej K. Pathogen translocation across the blood-brain barrier, *FEMS Immunol Med Microbiol* 2009: 57: 203-13.

Pulzova L. et al. OspA-CD40 dyad: ligand-receptor interaction in the translocation of neuroinvasive Borrelia across the blood-brain barrier. *Scientif Rep.* 2011;1(86).

Qui WG. and Martin CL. Evolutionary genomics of Borrelia burgdorferi sensu lato: findings, hypotheses, and the rise of hybrids. *Infect Genet Evol.* 2014;27:576-93.

Qui WG. et al. Wide distribution of a high-virulence Borrelia burgdorferi clone in Europe and North America. *Emerg Infect Dis.* 2008;14(7)1097-104.

Radolf JD. and Caimano MJ. The long strange trip of Borrelia burgdorferi outer-surface protein C. *Mol Microbiol.* 2008;69(1):1-4.

Radolf JD. et al. Of ticks, mice and men: understanding the dual-host lifestyle of Lyme disease spirochaetes. *Nat Rev Microbiol.* 2012;10(2):87-99.

Radzisauskiene D., Ambrozaitis A. and Marciuskiene E. Delayed diagnosis of Lyme neuroborreliosis presenting with abducens neuropathy without intrathecal synthesis of Borrelia antibodies. *Medicina (Kaunas)* 2013;49(2):89-94.

Raju BV. et al. Oligopeptide permease A5 modulates vertebrate host specific adaptation of Borrelia burgdorferi. *Infect Immun.* 2011;79(8):3407-20.

Ramesh G. et al. Interaction of the Lyme disease spirochete Borrelia burgdorferi with brain parenchyma elicits inflammatory mediators form glial cells as well as glial and neuronal apoptosis. *Amer J Pathol.* 2008;173(5):1415-27.

Ramesh G. et al. The Lyme disease spirochete Borrelia burgdorferi induces inflammation and apoptosis in cells from dorsal root ganglia. *J Neuroinflam.* 2013;10(88):1-14.

Ramesh G. et al. Possible role of glial cells in the onset and progression of Lyme neuroborreliosis. *j Neuroinflam.* 2009;6:23(1-16).

Ranka R. et al. Fibronectin-binding nanoparticles for intracellular targeting addressed by B. burgdorferi BBK32 protein fragments. *Nanomedicine.* 2013;9(1):65-73.

Rashmir-Raven A., et al. Papillomatous pastern dermatitis with spirochetes and Pelodera strongyloides in a Tennessee walking horse. *J Vet Diagn Invest* 2000; 12(3): 287-91.

Rebaudet S. and Parola P. Epidemiology of relapsing fever borreliosis in Europe, *FEMS Immjnol Med Microbiol* 2006; 48(1):11-15.

Redman AW. et al. Characteristics of seroconversion and implications for diagnosis of post-treatment Lyme disease syndrome: acute and convalescent serology among a prospective cohort of early Lyme disease syndrome: acute and convalescent serology among a prospective cohort of early Lyme disease patients. *Clin Rheumatol.* 2014;13.

Rey V. et al. Multiple ischemic strokes due to Borrelia garinii meningovasculitis. *Rev Neurol (Paris).* 2010;166(11):931-4.

Rhee H. and Cameron DJ. Lyme disease and pediatric autoimmune neuropsychiatric disorders associated with streptococcal infections (PANDAS): an overview. *Intern J Gen Med.* 2012;5:163-74.

Rhodes RG., Atoyan JA. and Nelson DR. The Chitobiose transporter, chbC, is required for chitin utilization in Borrelia burgdorferi. *BMC Microb.* 2010;10:21(1-14).

Ritzman AM. et al. The chemokine receptor CXCR2 ligand KC (CXCL1) mediates neutrophil recruitment and is critical for development of experimental Lyme arthritis and carditis. *Infect Immun.* 2010;78(11):4593-600.

Rizzoli A. et al. Lyme borreliosis in Europe. *Euro Surveill.* 2011;16(27):pil=19906.

Rocha R. et al.. Neuroborreliosis presenting as acute disseminated encephalomyelitis. *Pediatr Emerg Care.* 2012;28(12):1374-6.

Rodionova NN. et al. Effect of proteins from the spirochete Borrelia burgdorferi sensu lato on myelinated nerve excitability. *Bull Exp Biol Med.* 2007;143(1):36-9.

Rogers EA. et al. Rrp1, a cyclic-di-GMP-producing response regulator, is an important regulator of Borrelia burgdorferi core cellular functions. *Mol Microbiol.* 2009;71(6):1551-73.

Rogovskyy AS, and Bankhead T. Variable VlsE is critical for host reinfection by the Lyme disease spirochete. *PLoS One.* 2013;8(4):e61226.

Rogovskyy AS., Bankhead T. Bacterial heterogeneity is a requirement or host superinfection by the Lyme disease spirochete. *Infect Immun.* 2014;82(11):4542-52.

Rolla D. et al. Post-infectious glomerulonephritis presenting as acute renal failure in a patient with Lyme disease. *J Renal Inj Prev.* 2013;3(1):17-20.

Rollend L., Fish D., and Childs JE. Transovarial transmission of Borrelia spirochetes by Ixodes scapularis: a summary of the literature and recent observations. *Ticks Tick Borne Dis.* 2013;4(1-2):46-51.

Rosa Neto NS., Gauditano G., and Yoshinari NH. Chronic lymphomonoctytic meningoencephalitis, oligoarthritis and erythema nodosum: Report of Baggio-Yoshinari syndrome of long and relapsing evolution. *Rev Bras Reumatol.* 2014;54(2):148-51.

Roy-Dufresne E. et al. Poleward expansion of the white-footed mouse (Peromyscus leucopus) under climate change: implications for the spread of Lyme disease. *PLoS One.* 2013;8(11):e80724.

Rudenko N. et al. Borrelia carolinensis sp. nov., a new (14th) member of the Borrelia burgdorferi sensu lato complex from the southeastern region of the United States. *J Clin Microbiol.* 2009;47(1):134-41.

Rudenko N. et al. Borrelia carolinensis sp. nov., a novel species of the Borrelia burgdorferi sensu lato complex isolated from rodents and a tick from the South-Eastern USA. *Int J Syst Evol Microbiol.* 2011;61(Pt2):381-3.

Rudenko N. et al. Delineation of a new species of the Borrelia burgdorferi sensu lato complex, Borrelia americana sp. nov. *J Clin Microbiol.* 2009;47(12):3875-80.

Rudenko N. et al. Detection of Borrelia bissettii in cardiac valve tissue of a patient with endocarditis and aortic valve stenosis in the Czech Republic. *J Clin Microbiol.* 2008;46(10:3540-3.

Rudenko N. et al. Divergence of Borrelia burgdorferi sensu lato spirochetes could be driven by the host: diversity of Borrelia strains isolated from ticks feeding on a single bird. *Parasit Vectors.* 2014;7:4.

Rudenko N. et al. Molecular detection of Borrelia bissettii DNA in serum samples from patients in the Czech Republic with suspected borreliosis. *FEMS Microbiol Lett.* 2009;292(2):274-81.

Rudenko N. et al. The rare ospC allele L of Borrelia burgdorferi sensu stricto, commonly found among samples collected in a coastal plain area of the Southeastern United States, is associated with Ixodes affinis ticks and local rodent hosts Peromyscus gossypinus and Sigmodon hispidus. *Appl Environ Microbiol.* 2013;79(4):1403-6.

Rudenko N. et al. Updates on Borrelia burgdorferi sensu lato complex with respect to public health. *Ticks Tick Borne Dis.* 2011;2(3):123-28

Rudolf I. et al. Salivary gland extract from engorged Ixodes ricinus (Acari:Ixodidae) stimulates in vitro growth of Burgdorferi sensu lato. *J Basic Microbiol.* 2010;50(3):294-8.

Rupprecht TA. et al. Borrelia garinii induces CXCL13 production in human monocytes through Toll-like receptor 2. *Infect Immun.* 2007;75(9):4351-6.

Rupprecht TA. et al. CXCL13: a biomarker for acute Lyme neuroborreliosis: investigation of the predictive value in the clinical routine. *Nervenarzt.* 2014;84(4):459-64.

Rupprecht TA. et al. The pathogenesis of Lyme neuroborreliosis: from infection to inflammation. *Mol Med.* 2008;14(3-4):205-12.

Rupprecht TA., Birnbaum T. and Pfister HW. Pain and neuroborreliosis: significance, diagnosis and treatment. *Schmerz.* 2008;22(5):615-23.

Russell TM. and Johnson BJ. Lyme disease spirochaetes possess an aggrecan-binding protease with aggrecanase activity. *Mol Microbiol.* 2013;90(2)228-40.

Russell TM. et al. Borrelia burgdorferi BbHtrA degrades host ECM proteins and stimulates release of inflammatory cytokines in vitro. *Mol Microbiol.* 2013:90(2):241-51.

Sabino GJ. et al. Interferon-γ influences the composition of leukocytic infiltrates in murine Lyme carditis. *Am J Pathol.* 2011;179(4):1917-28.

Sadik CD. et al. Systematic analysis highlights the key role of TLR2/NF-kappaB/MAP kinase signaling for IL-8 induction by macrophage-like THP-1 cells under influence of Borrelia burgdorferi lysates. *Int J Biochem Cell Biol.* 2008;40(11):2508-21.

Sahay B. et al. CD134 signaling reciprocally controls collagen deposition and turnover to regulate the development of Lyme arthritis. *Am J Pathol.* 2011;178(2):724-34.

Sahay B. et al. CD14 signaling restrains chronic inflammation through induction of p38-mapk/socs-dependent tolerance. *PLoS pathog.* 2009;5(12):e1000687.

Saito K. et al. Case report: Borrelia valaisiana infection in a Japanese man associated with traveling to foreign countries. *Am J Trop Med Hyg.* 2007;77(6):1124-7.

Sajanti EM. et al. Lyme borreliosis and deficient mannose-binding lecting pathway of complement. *J Immunol.* 2014;pii:1402128.

Salazar JC. et al. Activation of Human Monocytes by Live Borrelia burgdorferi Generates TLR2-Dependent and -Independent Responses Which Include Induction of IFN-b. *PLoS Pathog.* 2009;5(5):e1000444.

Salkeld DJ. et al. Seasonal activity patterns for the Western black-legged tick, Ixodes pacificus, in relation to onset of human Lyme disease in Northwestrn California. *Ticks Tick Borne Dis.* 2014;5(6):790-6.

Salo J. Decorin binding by DbpA and B of Borrelia garinii, Borrelia afzelii, and Borrelia burgdorferi sensu stricto. *J Infect Dis.* 2011;201(1);65-73.

Samimi S., Salah S and Bonicel P. Acquired nystagmus in a 12-year-old boy as initial presentation of Lyme disease. *J Fr Ophtalmol.* 2011;34(5):325.e1-3.

Sandholm K. et al. Early cytokine release in response to live Borrelia burgdorferi sensu lato spirochetes Is largely complement independent. *PLoS One.* 2014;9(9):e108013.

Santiago-Moreno, J, et al. Potential impact of diseases transmissible by sperm on the establishment of the Iberian ibex (*Capra pyrenaica*) genome resource banks. *Eur J Wildl Res* 2011; 57: 211-16.

Santino I. et al. Detection of different Borrelia burgdorferi genospecies in serum of people with different occupational risks: short report. *Int J Immunopathol Pharmacol.* 2009;22(2):537-41.

Santos M. et al. Antibody reactivity to Borrelia burgdorferi sensu stricto antigens in patients from the Brazilian Amazon region with skin diseases not related to Lyme disease. *Int J Dermatol.* 2010;49(5):552-6.

Santos M. et al. Presence of Borrelia burgdorferi "sensu lato" in patients with morphea from the Amazonic region in Brazil. *Int J Dermatol.* 2011;50(11):1373-8.

Sapi E. et al. Characterization of biofilm formation by Borrelia burgdorferi in vitro. *PLOS One.* 2012;7(10):e48277.

Sapi E. et al. Evaluation of in-vitro antibiotic susceptibility of different morphological forms for Borrelia burgdorferi. *Infect Drug Resist.* 2011;4:97-113.

Sarkar A. et al. Borrelia burgdorferi resistance to a major skin antimicrobial peptide is independent of outer surface lipoprotein content. *Antimicrob Agents Chemother.* 2009;53(10):4490-4.

Sarksyan DS. et al. Clinical presentation of "new" tick-borne borreliosis caused by Borrelia miyamotoi. *Ter Arkh.* 2012;84(11):34-41.

Sato K. et al. Human infections with Borrelia miyamotoi, Japan. *Emerg Infect Dis.* 2014;20(8):1391-3.

Sauer A., Speeg-Schatz C. and Hansmann Y. Two cases of orbital myositis as a rare feature of Lyme borreliosis. *Case Rep Infect Dis.*2011;2011:372470.

Sauer A. et al. Five cases of paralytic strabismus as a rare feature of Lyme disease. *Clin Infect Dis.* 2009;48(6):756-9.

Sauer A. et al. Ocular Lyme disease occurring during childhood: five case reports. *J Fr Ophtaimol.* 2012;35(1):17-22.

Schafers M. et al. Diagnostic value of sural nerve biopsy in patients with suspected Borrelia neuropathy. *J Periper Nerv Syst.* 2008;13(1):81-91.

Scheckelhoff MR. et al. Borrelia burgdorferi intercepts host hormonal signals to regulate expression of outer surface protein A. *Proc Natl Acad Sci U S A.* 2007;104(17):7247-52.

Schmidt B. et al. Detection of Borrelia burgdorferi DNA by polymerase chain reaction in the urine and breast mild of patients with Lyme borreliosis. *Diagn Microbiol Infect Dis* 1995; 21(3): 121-8.

Schmidt B. et al. Detection of Borrelia burgdorferi-specific DNA in urine specimens from patients with erythema migrans before and after antibiotic therapy. *J Clin Microbiol* 1996; 34(6): 1359-63.

Schmidt C. et al. A prospective study on the role of CXCL13 in Lyme neuroborreliosis. *Neurolog.* 2011;76(12):1051-8.

Schmit VL., Patton TG and Gilmore RD Jr. Analysis of Borrelia burgdorferi Surface Proteins as Determinants in Establishing Host Cell Interactions. *Front Microbiol.* 2011; 2:141.

Schnar, S, et al. Chlamydia and Borrelia DNA in synovial fluid of patients with early undifferentiated oligoarthritis. *Arthritis and Rheumatism* 2001; 44(11): 2679-85.

Schneider SC. et al. Assessing the contribution of songbirds to the movement of ticks and Borrelia burgdorferi in the Midwestern United States during fall migration. *Ecohealth.* 2014.

Schollkopf C. et al. Borrelia infection and risk of non-Hodgkin lymphoma. *Blood.* 2008;111(12):5524-9.

Schott M. et al. Molecular characterization of the interaction of Borrelia parkeri and Borrelia turicatae with human complement regulators. *Infect Immun.*2010;78(5):2199-208.

Schramm F. et al. First detection of Borrelia burgdorferi sensu lato DNA in king penguins (Aptenodytes patagonicus halli). *Ticks Tick Borne Dis.* 2014;5(6):939-42.

Schramm F. et al. Microarray analyses of inflammation response of human dermal fibroblasts to different strains of Borrelia burgdorferi sensu stricto. *PLoS One.* 2012;7(6):e40046.

Schroder NW. et al. Immune responses induced by spirochetal outer membrane lipoproteins and glycolipids. *Immunobiology.* 2008;213(3-4):329-40.

Schuijt TJ. et al. A tick mannose-binding lectin inhibitor interferes with the vertebrate complement cascade to enhance transmission of the Lyme disease agent. *Cell Host Microbe.* 2011;10(2):136-46.

Schuijt TJ. et al. The tick salivary protein Salp15 inhibits the killing of serum-sensitive Borrelia burgdorferi sensu lato isolates. *Infect Immun.* 2008;76(8):2888-94.

Schumman J. TGF-b 1 of no avail as prognostic marker in Lyme disease. *Peer J.* 2014;2:e398.

Schutzer S. et al. Atypical erythema migrans in patients with PCR-positive Lyme disease. *Emerg Infect Dis. Lttr.* 2013;19(5):815-17.

Schwab J. et al. Borrelia valaisiana resist complement-mediated killing independently of the recruitment of immune regulators and inactivation of complement components. PLoS One. 2013;8(1):e53659.

Schwan TG. et al. Characterization of a novel relapsing fever spirochete in the midgut, coxal fluid, and salivary glands of the bat tick Carios kelleyi. Vector Borne Zoonotic Dis. 2009;9(6):643-7.

Schwan TG. et al. Tick-borne relapsing and Borrelia hermsii, Los Angeles County, California, USA. Emerg Infect Dis. 2009;15(7):1026-31.

Scott JD., Anderson JF. and Durden LA. Widespread dispersal of Borrelia burgdorferi- infected ticks collected from songbirds across Canada. J Parasitol. 2012 ;98(1):49-59.

Scott JD. et al. Detection of Lyme disease spirochete, Borrelia burgdorferi sensu lato, including three novel genotypes in ticks (Acari: Ixodidae) collected from songbirds (Passeriformes) across Canada. J Vector Ecol. 2010;35(1):124-39.

Scott MC. et al. High-prevalence Borrelia miyamotoi infection among [corrected] wild turkeys (Meleagris gallopavo) in Tennessee. J Med Entomol. 2010;47(60):1238-42.

Seemanapalli SV. et al. Outer surface protein C is a dissemination-facilitating factor of Borrelia burgdorferi during mammalian infection. PLoS One. 2010;5(12):e15830.

Seidel ME., Domenc AB. and Vetter H. Differential diagnoses of suspected Lyme borreliosis or post-Lyme-disease syndrome. Eur J Clin Microbiol Infect Dis. 2007;26(9):611-7.

Seling A et al. Functional characterization of Borrelia spielmanii outer surface proteins that interact with distinct members of the human factor H protein family and with plasminogen. Infect Immun. 2010;78(1):39-48.

Seppanen A. et al. Distribution of collagen XVII in the human brain. Brain Res 2007; 1158: 50-6.

Seppanen A. et al. Expression of collagen XVII and ubiquitin-binding protein p62 in motor neuron disease. Brain Res 2009; 1247: 171-7.

Seriburi V. et al High frequency of false positive LgM immunoblots for Borrelia burgdorferi in clinical practice. Clin Microbiol Infect. 2012;18(12):1236-40.

Seshu J. et al. Inactivation of the fibronection-binding adhesin gene bbk32 significantly attenuates the infectivity potential of Borrelia burgdorferi. Mol Microbiol. 2006;59(5):1591-601.

Shapiro JA. Bacteria are small but not stupid: Cognition, natural genetic engineering, and sociobacteriology. Exeter Meeting, 2006.

Shen S. et al. Treg cell numbers and function in patients with antibiotic-refractory or antibiotic-responsive Lyme arthritis. Arthritis Rheum. 2010;62(7):2127-37.

Shi C. et al. Reduced immune response to Borrelia burgdorferi in the absence of yo Tcells. Infect Immun. 2011;79(10):3940-6.

Shi Y. et al. BosR functions as a repressor of the ospAB operon in Borrelia Burgdorferi.PLOS One. 2014;9(10):e109307.

Shi Y. et al. Both decorin-binding proteins A and B are critical for the overall virulence of Borrelia burgdorferi. Infect Immun. 2008;76(3):1239-46.

Shi Y. et al. Common and unique contributions of decorin-binding proteins A and B to the overall virulence fo Borrelia burgdorferi. PLoS One. 2008;3(10):e3340.

Shin JJ., Glicksein LJ. and Steere AC. High levels of inflammatory chemokines and cytokines in joint fluid and synovial tissue throughout the course of antibiotic-refractory Lyme arthritis. Arthritis Rheum. 2007;56(4):1325-35.

Shin JJ. et al. Borrelia burgdorferi stimulation of chemokine secretion by cells of monocyte lineage in patients with Lyme arthritis. Arthritis Res Ther. 2010;12(5):R168.

Shin OS. et al. Distinct Roles for MyD88 and Toll-Like Receptors 2, 5, and 9 in Phagocytosis of Borrelia burgdorferi and Cytokine Induction. Infect Immun. 2008;76(6):2341-51.

Shin OS. et al. Downstream signals for MyD88-mediated phagocytosis of Borrelia burgdorferi can be initiated by TRIF and are dependent on PI3K. J Immunol. 2009;183(1):491-8.

Shoemaker RC. et al. Complement split products C3a and C4a are early markers of acute Lyme disease in tick bite patients in the United States. Int Arch Allergy Immunol. 2008;146(3):255-61.

Sigal LH. Musculoskeletal features of Lyme disease: understanding the pathogenesis of clinical findings helps make appropriate therapeutic choices. J Clin Rheumatol. 2011;17(5):256-65.

Signorino G. et al. Identification of OspA2 linear epitopes as serodiagnostic markers for Lyme disease. Clin Vaccine Immunol. 2014;21(5):704-11.

Sikutova S. et al. Novel spirochetes isolated from mosquitoes and black flies in the Czech Republic. J Vector Ecol. 2010;35(1):50-5.

Sikutova S. et al. Selected phenotypic features of BR01, a unique spirochaetal strain isolated from the Culex pipens mosquito. Microbiol Res. 2014;169(5-6):348-52.

Sillanpaa H., et al. Antibodies to decorin-binding protein B (DbpB) in the diagnosis of Lyme neuroborreliosis in children. Int J Infect Dis. 2014;28:160-3.

Simon JA. et al. Climate change and habitat fragmentation drive the occurrence of Borrelia burgdorferi, the agent of Lyme disease, at the Northeastern limit of its distribution. Evolut Appl ISSN 1752-4571. 2014.

Sindhava V. et al. Interleukin-10 mediated autoregulation of murine B-1 B-cells and its role in Borrelia hermsii infection. PLoS ONE. 2010;5(7):e11445.

Sirmarova J. et al. Seroprevalence of Borrelia burgdorferi sensu lato and tick-borne encephalitis viris in zoo animal species in the Czech Republic. Ticks Tick Borne Dis.2014;5(5):523-7.

Sjowall J. et al. Decreased Th-1 type inflammatory cytokine expression in the skin in associated with persisting symptoms after treatment of Erythema migrans. PLoS One. 2011;6(3):e18220.

Skogman BH. et al. Adaptive and innate immune responsiveness to Borrelia burgdorferi sensu lato in exposed asymptomatic children and children with previous clinical Lyme borreliosis. *Clin Dev Immunol.* 2012;294587.

Skotarczak B. Adaptation factors of Borrelia for host and vector. *Ann Agric Environ Med.* 2009;16(1):1-8.

Skotarczak B. Why are there several species of Borrelia burgdorferi sensu lato detected in dogs and humans? *Infect Genet Evol.* 2014;23:182-8.

Slack GA. et al. Is Tayside becoming a Scottish hotspot for Lyme borreliosis? *J R Coll Physicians Edinb.* 2011;41(1):5-8.

Slamova M. et al. Effect of tick saliva on immune interactions between Borrelia afzelii and urine dendritic cells. *Parasite Immunol.* 2011;33(12):654-60.

Smit PW. et al. Evaluation of two commercially available rapid diagnostic tests for Lyme borreliosis. *Eur J Clin Microbiol Infect Dis.* 2015;34(1):109-13.

Smith AA. and Pal U. Immunity-related genes inIxodes scapularis—perspectives from genome information. *Front Cell Infect Microbio.* 2014;4(116):1-10.

Smith BG. et al. Lyme disease and the orthopaedic implications of Lyme arthritis. *J Am Acad Orthop Surg.* 2011;19(2):91-00.

Smith GN., Gemmill I. and Moore KM. Management of tick bites and Lyme disease during pregnancy. *J Obstet Gynaecol Can.* 2012;34(11):1087-91.

Smith RP. et al. Human Babesiosis, Maine, USA. 1995-2011. *Emerg Infect Dis.* 2014;20(10):1727-30.

Sno HN. Signs and significance of a tick-bite: psychiatric disorders associated with Lyme disease. *Tijdschr Psychiatr.* 2012;54(3):235-43.

Sonderegger FL. et al. Localized production of IL-10 suppresses early inflammatory cell infiltration and subsequent development of IFN-γ-Mediated Lyme arthritis. *J Immunol.* 2012;188(3):1381-93.

Souidi Y. et al. Borrelia crocidurae in Ornithodoros ticks from Northwestern Morocco a range extension in relation to climatic change?? *J Vector Ecol.* 2014;39(2):316-20.

Sparsa L. et al. Recurrent ischemic strokes revealing Lyme menigovascularitis. *Rev Neurol (Paris).* 2009;165(3):273-7.

Sperling J. et al. Evolving perspectives on Lyme borreliosis in Canada. *Open Neurol J.* 2012;6:94-03.

Sprong H. et al. Circumstantial evidence for an increase in the total number and activity of Borrelia-infected Ixodes ricinus in the Netherlands. *Parasit Vectors.* 2012;5:294.

Sprong H. et al. Sensitivity of a point of care tick-test for the development of Lyme borreliosis. *Parasit Vectors.* 2013;6:338.

Srinivasalu H., Brescia AC. and Rose CD. Lyme chondritis presenting as painless ear erythema. *Pediatrics.* 2013;131(6):e1977-81.

Stanek G. and Reiter M. The expanding Lyme Borrelia complex—clinical significance of genomic species? *Clin Microbiol Infect.* 2011;17(4):487-93.

Stanek G. et al. Intrathecally produced IgG and IgM antibodies to recombinant VIsE, VIsE peptide, recombinant OspC and whole cell extracts in the diagnosis of Lyme neuroborreliosis. *Med Microbiol Immunol.* 2014;203(2):125-32.

Steere AC. Reply to letter by Volkman commenting on the possible onset of seronegative disease in Lyme arthritis. *Arthritis Rheum.* 2009;60(1):310.

Steere AC., Drouin EE. and Glickstein LJ. Relationship between immunity to Borrelia burgdorferi outer-surface protein A (OspA) and Lyme arthritis. *Clin Infect Dis.* 2011;52 Suppl 3:s259-65.

Steere AC. et al. Prospective study of serologic tests for Lyme disease. *Clin Infect Dis.* 2008;47(2):188-95.

Stewart PE. and Rosa PA. Transposon mutagenesis of the Lyme disease agent Borrelia burgdorferi. *Methods Mol Biol.* 2008;431:85-95.

Stinco G. et al. Borrelia infection and pityriasis rosea. *Acta Derm Venereol.* 2009;89(1):97-8.

Stinco G. et al. Clinical features of 705 Borrelia burgdorferi seropositive patients in an endemic area of Northern Italy. *Scientific World J.* 2014;2014:414505.

Stone BL. et al. The Western progression of Lyme disease: Infectious and nonclonal Borrelia burgdorferi sensu lato populations in Grand Forks County, North Dakota. *Appl Enviorn Microbiol.* 2015;81(1):48-58.

Stricker RB. Counterpoint: long-term antibiotic therapy improves persistent symptoms associated with Lyme disease. *Clinical Infectious Diseases.* 2007;45:149-57.

Stricker RB., Corson AF. and Johnson L. Reinfection versus relapse in patients with Lyme disease: Not enough evidence. *Clin Infect Dis.* 2008;46:950. Letter to the Editor.

Stricker RB. and Johnson L. Borrelia burgdorferi aggrecanase activity: more evidence for persistent infection in Lyme disease. *Front Cell Inf Microb.* 2013;3(40):1-2.

Stricker RB. and Johnson L. Chronic Lyme Disease and the "Axis of Evil." *Future Microb.* 2008;3(6):621-624.

Stricker RB. and Johnson L. Lyme disease diagnosis and treatment: lessons from the AIDS epidemic. *Minerva Med.* 2010;101(6):419-25.

Stricker RB. and Johnson L. Lyme disease: the next decade. *Infection and Drug Resistance.* 2011;4:1-9.

Stricker RB. et al. Benefit of intravenous antibiotic therapy in patients referred for treatment of neurologic Lyme disease. *IntJ Gen Med.* 2011;4:639-46.

Stricker RB. et al. Safety of intravenous antibiotic therapy in patients referred for treatment of neurologic Lyme disease. *Minerva Med.* 2010;101(1):1-7.

Stricker RB. and Johnson L. Persistent Borrelia burgorferi infection after treatment with antibiotics and anti-tumor necrosis factor. *J Infect Dis.*2008;197:1352-2.Letter to the Editor.

Stricker RB. and Johnson L. Spirochetal 'debris' versus persistent infection in chronic Lyme disease: from semantics to science. *Future Microbiol.* 2012;7(11):1243-6.

Stricker RB. and Winger E. Musical hallucinations in patients with Lyme disease. *South Medical Journal* 2003; 96(7): 711-5.

Strle F. et al. Clinical characteristics associated with Borrelia burgdorferi sensu lato skin culture results in patients with erythema migrans. *PLoS One.* 2013;8(12):e82132.

Strle F. et al. Comparison of erythema migrans caused by Borrelia burgdorferi and Borrelia garinii. *Vector Borne Zoonotic Dis.* 2011;11(9):1253-8.

Strle K. et al. Borrelia burgdorferi stimulates macrophages to secrete higher levels of cytokines and chemokines that Borrelia afzelii or Borrelia garinii. *J Infect Dis.* 2009;200(12):1936-43.

Strle K. et al. Elevated levels of IL-23 in a subset of patients with post-Lyme disease symptoms following erythema migrans. *Clin Infect Dis.* 2014;58(3):372-80.

Strle K. et al. A toll-like receptor 1 Polymorphism associated with heightened T-helper 1 inflammatory responses and antibiotic-refractory Lyme arthritis. *Arthritis Rheum.* 2012;64(5):1497-1507.

Stromdahl EY. and Hickling GJ. Beyond Lyme: aetiology of tick-borne human diseases with emphasis on the South-Eastern United States. *Zoonoses Public Health.* 2012;59 Suppl2:48-64.

Strunk T. et al. Anetoderma with positive Borrelia serology. *Hautazt* 2011;62(10):720-2.

Stubs G. et al. Acylated cholesteryl galactosides are specific antigens of Borrelia causing Lyme disease and frequently induce antibodies in late stages of disease. *J Biol Chem.* 2009;284(20):13326-34.

Stupica D. et al. Comparison of post-Lyme borreliosis symptoms in erythema migrans patients with positive and negative Borrelia burgdorferi sensu lato skin culture. *Vector Borne Zoonotic Dis.*2011;11(7):883-9.

Sullivan L. et al. Digital dermatitis treponemes associated with a severe foot disease in dairy goats. *Vet Rec* 2015; 176(11): 283.

Sullivan L. et al. The high association of bovine digital dermatitis Treponema spp. With contagious ovine digital dermatitis lesions and the presence of Fusobacterium necrophorum and Dichelobacter nodosus. *J Clin Microbiol* 2015 (March 4): epub ahead of print.

Sullivan L. at al. Presence of digital dermatitis treponemes on cattle and sheep hoof trimming equipment. *Vet Rec* 2014; 175(8): 201.

Sultan SZ. et al. Motility is crucial for the infectious life cycle of Borrelia burgdorferi. *Infect Immun.* 2013;81(6):2012-21.

Sun J. et al. Coinfection with four genera of bacteria (Borrelia, Bartonella, Anaplasma, and Ehrlichia) in Haemaphysalis longicornis and Ixodes sinensis ticks from China. *Vector Borne Zoonotic Dis.* 2008;8(6):791-5.

Sundin M. et al. Pediatric tick-borne infections of the central nervous system in an endemic region of Sweden: a prospective evaluation of clinical manifestations. *Eur J Pediatr.* 2012;171(2):347-52.

Susta L. et al. Synovial lesions in experimental canine Lyme borreliosis. *Vet Pathol.* 2012;49(3):453-61.

Svartstrom, O, et al. Genome-wide relatedness of Treponema pedis, from gingiva and necrotic skin lesions of pigs, with the human oral pathogen Treponema denticola. *PLoS One* 2013; 8(8): e71281.

Svecova D., Gavornik P. Recurrent erythema migrans as a persistent infection. *Epidemiol Mikrobiol Immunol.* 2008;57(3):97-100.

Swanson KI., Norris DE. Detection of Borrelia burgdorferi DNA in lizards from Southern Maryland. *Vector Borne Zoonotic Dis.* 2007;7(1):42-9.

Swart A. et al. Predicting tick presence by environment risk mapping. *Front Public Health.* 2014;2:238.

Swei A. et al. Effects of an invasive forest pathogen on abundance of ticks and their vertebrate hosts in a California Lyme disease focus. *Oecologia.* 2011;166(1):91-100.

Swei A. et al. Impact of the experimental removal of lizards on Lyme disease risk. *Proc Biol Sci.* 2011;278(1720):2970-8.

Swei A. et al. Impacts of an introduced forest pathogen on the risk of Lyme disease in California. *Vect Borne Zoonotic Dis.*2012;12(8):623-30.

Szulzyk T., Flisiak R. Lyme borreliosis. *Ann Parasitol.* 2012;58(6):63-9.

Takano A. et al. Characterization of reptile-associated Borrelia sp. in the vector tick, Amblyomma geomyidae, and its association with Lyme disease and relapsing fever Borrelia spp. *Environ Microbiol Rep.* 2011;3(5):632-7.

Takano A. et al. Isolation and characterization of a novel Borrelia group of tick-borne Borreliae from imported reptiles and their associated ticks. *Environ Microbiol.* 2010;12(1):134-46.

Tan Y. et al. The efficacy of antibiotics in the therapy on different types and stages of Lyme disease. *Beijing Medical Journal* 2010; 6.

Tappe J. et al. Revisited: Borrelia burgdorferi sensu lato infections in hard ticks(Ixodes ricinus) in the city of Hanover (Germany). *Parasit Vectors.* 2014;7:441.

Taragel'ova V. et al. Blackbirds and song thrushes constitute a key reservoir of Borrelia garinii, the causative agent of borreliosis in Central Europe. *Appl Environ Microbiol.* 2008;74(4):1289-93.

Tauber SC. et al. Long-term intrathecal infusion of outer surface protein C from Borrelia burgdorferi causes axonal damage. *J Neuropathol Exp Neurol.* 2011;70(9):748-57.

Tavora F. et al. Postmortem confirmation of Lyme carditis with polymerase chain reaction. *Cardiovasc Pathol.* 2008;17(2):103-7.

Tee SI. et al Acrodermatitis chronica atrophicans with pseudolymphomatous infiltrates. *Am J Dermatopathol.* 2013;35(3):338-42.

Teegler A. et al. The relapsing fever spirochete Borrelia miyamotoi resists complement-mediated killing by human serum. *Ticks Tick Borne Dis.* 2014;5(6):898-01.

Telfer, S. et al. Species interactions in a parasite community drive infection risk in a wildlife population, *Science* 2010; 330(6001): 243-6.

Thai PT. et al. Increased caspase activity primes human Lyme arthritis synovial T cells for proliferation and death. *Hum Immunol.* 2011;72(12):1168-75.

Thein M. et al. DipA, a pore-forming protein in the outer membrane of Lyme disease spirochetes exhibits specificty for the permeation of dicarboxylates. *PLoS One.* 2012;7(5):e36523.

Thein M. et al. Oms38 is the first identified pore-forming protein in the outer membrane of relapsing fever spirochetes. *J Bacteriol*. 2008;190(21):1035-42.

Tijsse-Klasen E. and Sprong H., Pandak N. Co-infection of Borrelia burgdorferi sensu lato and Rikettsia species in ticks and in an erythema migrans patient. *Parasit Vectors*. 2013; 6:347.

Tijsse-Klasen E. et al. Ability to cause erythema migrans differs between Borrelia burgdorferi sensu lato isolates. *Parasites Vectors*. 2013;6(23):1-8.

Tilly K. et al. OspC-independent infection and dissemination by host- adapted Borrelia burgdorferi. *Infect Immun*. 77(7)2672-82.

Tilly K., Bestor A. and Rosa PA. Lipoprotein succession in Borrelia burgdorferi: similar but distinct roles for OspC and VlsE at different stages of mammalian infection. *Mol Microbiol*. 2013;89(2):216-117.

Tilly K., Checroun C. and Rosa PA. Requirements for Borrelia burgdorferi plasmid maintenance. *Plasmid*. 2012;68(1):1-12.

Tilly K. et al. Biology of infection with Borrelia burgdorferi. *Infect Dis Clin North Am*. 2008;22(2):217-34.

Tjernberg I. et al. Diagnostic performance of cerebrospinal fluid chemokine CXCL13 and antibodies to the C6-peptide in Lyme neuroborreliosis. *J Infect*. 2011;62(2):149-58.

Toledo A. et al. The enolase of Borrelia burgdorferi is a plasminogen recptor released in outer membrane vesicles. *Infect Immun*. 2012;80(1):359-68.

Toledo A. et al. Phylogentic analysis of a virulent Borrelia species isolated from patients with relapsing fever. *J Clin Microbiol*. 2010;48(7):2484-9.

Toledo A. et al. Selective association of outer surface lipoproteins with the lipid rafts of Borrelia burgdorferi. *mBio*. 2014;5(2):e00899-14.

Topakian R. et al. Cerebral vasculitis and stroke in Lyme neuroborreliosis. Two case reports and review of current knowledge. *Cerebrovasc Dis*. 2008;26(5):455-61.

Tory HO., Zurakowski D. and Sundel RP. Outcomes of children treated for Lyme arthritis: Results of a large pediatric cohort. *J Rheumatol*. 2010;37(5):1049-55.

Tran PM., Waller L. Effects of landscape fragmentation and climate on Lyme disease incidence in the Northeastern United States. *Ecohealth*. 2013;10(4):394-04.

Troxell B., Xu H. and Yang XF. Borrelia burgdorferi, a pathogen that lacks iron, "gold standard" for cutaneous borreliosis? *Am J Clin Pathol*. 2007;127(2):213-22.

Troxell B. and Yang XF. Metal-dependent gene regulation in the causative agent of Lyme disease. *Front Cell Infect Microb*. 2013;3(79).

Troxell B. et al. Menganese and zinc regulate virulence determinants in Borrelia burgdorferi. *Infect Immun*. 2013;81(8):2743-52.

Troxell B. et al. Pyrovate. protects pathogenic spirochetes from H202 killing. *PLOS One*. 2014;9(1):e84625.

Troy EB. et al. Understanding barriers to Borrelia burgdorferi dissemination during infection using massively parallel sequencing. *Infect Immun*.2013;81(7):2347-57.

Tsao JI. Reviewing molecular adaptations of Lyme borreliosis spirochetes in the context of reproductive fitness in natural transmission cycles. *Vet Res*. 2009;40:36

Tschirren B. et al. Polymorphisms at the innate immune receptor TLR2 are associated with Borrelia infection in a wild rodent population. *Proc Biol Sci*. 2013;280(1759):20130364.

Ttraisk F., Lindquist L. Optic nerve involvement in Lyme disease. *Curr Opin Ophthalmol*. 2012;23(6):485-90.

Tunev SS. et al. Lymphoadenopathy during lyme borreliosis is caused by spirochete miration-induced specific B cell activation. *PL oS Pathog*. 2011; 7(5):e1002066.

Tupin E. et al. NKT cells prevent chronic joint inflammation after infectio with Borrelia burgdorferi. *PNAS*. 2008;105(50):19863-68.

Tveten AK. Exploring diversity among norwegian Borrelia strains originating from Ixodes ricinus ticks. *Int J Microbiol*.2014;2014:397143.

Tveten Y., Noraas S., Aase A. Cellular Borrelia tests. *Tidsskr Nor Laegeforen*. 2014;134(2):146-7.

Uchida, T. et al. Localizatoin of galactrocerebroside in oligodendrocytes, myelin sheath and choroid plexus. *Jpn J Exp Med* (1981); 51(1): 29-35.

Vaerma V. et al. A case of chronic progressive Lyme encephalitis as a manifestation of late Lyme neuroborreliosis. *Infect Dis Rep*. 2014;6(4):5496.

van Burgel ND. et al. Identification and functional characterization or complement regulator acquiring surface protein-1 of serum resistant Borrelia garinii OspA serotype 4. *BMC Microbiol*. 2010;10:43.

van Dam AP. Molecular diagnosis of Borrelia bacteria for the diagnosis of Lyme disease. *Expert Opin Med Diagn*. 2011;5(2):135-49.

van Dop WA. et al. Seronegative Lyme neuroborreliosis in a patient using rituximab. *BMJ Case Rep*. 2013;1013:pii bcr2012007627.

van Erp WS, Bakker NA, Aries MJ and Vroomen PC. Osoclonus and multiple cranial neuropathy as a manifestation of neuroborreliosis. *Neurology*. 2011;77(10)1013-4.

Van Laar TA. et al. Effect of levels of acetate on the mevalonate pathway of Borrelia burgdorferi. *PLOS One*. 2012;7(5):e38171.

van Maldegem F. et al. The majority of cutaneous marginal zone B-cell lymphomas expressed class-switched immunoglobulins and develops in a T-helper type 2 inflammatory environment. *Blood*2008;112(8):3355-61.

Van Snick S. et al. Acute ischaemic pontine stroke revealing Lyme neuroborreliosis in a young adult. *Acta Neurol Belg*. 2008;108(3):103-6.

Vandernesch A. et al. Incidence and hospitalisation rates of Lyme borreliosis, France, 2004-2012. *Euro Surveill*. 2014;19(34):pii20883.

Varela A. et al. First culture isolation of Borrelia lonestari, putative agent of southern tick-associated rash illness. *Journal of Clinical Microbiology* 2004; March: 1163-69.

Vasudevan B., Chatterjee M. Lyme Borreliosis and Skin. *Indian J Dermatol.* 2013;58(3):167-174.

Venclikova K. et al. Human pathogenic borreliae in Ixodes ricinus ticks in natural and urban ecosystem czech Republic. *Acta Parasitol.* 2014;59(4):717-20.

Verberkt RM., Janssen M., Wesseling J. A boy with a tight skin: Borrelia-associated early-onset morphea. *Clin Exp Rheumatol.* 2014;32(1):121-2

Vetsigian K. and Goldenfeld N. Genome rhetoric and the emergence of compositional bias. *PNAS* 2009;106(1):215-20.

Vianello M., Marchiori G. and Giometto B. Multiple cranial nerve involvement in Bannwarth's syndrome. *Neurol Sci.* 2008;29(2):109-12.

Vinodh, R, et al. Detection of Leptospira and Brucella genomes in bovine semen using polymerase chain reaction. *Trop Anim Health Prod* 2008; 40(5): 323-9.

Vojdani A. et al. Novel diagnosis of Lyme disease: potential for CAM intervention. *eCAM.* 2009;6(3):283-295.

vol Baehr V. et al. The lymphocyte transformation test for Borrelia detects active Lyme borreliosis and verifies effective antibiotic treatment. *Open Neurol J.* 2012;6:104-12.

Volkman DJ. Seronegative disease after inadequate therapy in Lyme arthritis: comment on the article by Kanian et al. Letter to the Editor:2212-13.

Voordouw MJ. Co-feeding transmission in Lyme disease pathogens. *Parasitology.* 2014:1-13.

Vrethem M. et al. Clinical, diagnostic and immunological characteristics of patients with possible neuroborreliosis without intrathecal Ig-synthesis against Borrelia antigen in the cerebrospinal fluid. *Neurol. Int.* 2011;3(1):e2.

Vrinkerhoff RJ. et al. Genotypic diversity of Borrelia burgdorferi strains detected in Ixodes scapularis larvae collected from North American songbirds. *Appl Environ Microbiol.* 201;76(24):8265-8.

Wagemakers A. et al. The relapsing fever spirochete Borrelia miyamotoi is cultivable in modified Kelly-Pettenkofer medium, and is resistant to human complement. *Parasit Vectors.* 2014;7:418.

Wagh, D, et al, Borreliacidal activity of Borrelia metal transporter A (BmtA) binding small molecules by manganese transport inhibition, *Drug Design, Development and Therapy* 2015; 9: 805-16.

Wagner V. et al. Acute atrioventricular block in chronic Lyme disease. *Orv Hetil.* 2010; 151 (39):1585-90.

Walia R., Chaconas G. Suggested role for G4 DNA in recombinational switching at the antigenic variation locus of the Lyme disease spirochete. *PLoS One.* 2013;8(2):e57792.

Walid MS., Ajjan M. and Ulm AJ. Subacute transverse myelitis with Lyme profile dissociation. *Ger Med Sci.* 2008;6:Doc04.

Wallet F. et al. Molecular diagnosis of a bilateral panuveitis due to Borrelia burgdorferi sensu lato by cerebral spinal fluid analysis. *Jpn J Infect Dis.* 2008;61(3):214-5.

Wang G. et al. Pattern of pro-inflammatory cytokine induction in RAW264.7 mouse macrophages

is identical for virulent and attenuated Borreia burgdorferi. *J Immunol.* 2008;180(12):8306-15.

Wang J. et al. Lipid binding orientation within CD1d affects recognition of Borrelia burgdorferi antigens by NKT cells. *Proc Natl Acad Sci U S A.* 2010;107(4):1535-40.

Wang P. et al. Emergence of Ixodes scapularis and Borrelia burgdorferi the Lyme disease vector and agent, in Ohio. *Front Cell Infect Microbiol.* 2014;4:70.

Wang P. et al. A novel iron-and copper-binding protein in the Lyme disease spirochaete. *Mol Microbiol.* 2012;86(6):1441-51.

Wang X. et al. T cell infiltration is associated with increased Lyme arthritis in TLR2-/- mice. *FEMS Immunol Med Microbiol.* 2008;52(1):124-33.

Watanabe S. et al. Glycosphingolipid synthesis in cerebellar Purkinje neurons: roles in myelin formation and axonal homeostasis. *Glia* 2010; 58(10): 1197-207.

Weinstein A. Laboratory testing for Lyme disease: Time for a change? *Clinical Infectious Diseases.* 2008;47:196-7.

Wendling D. et al. Parsonage-Turner syndrome revealing Lyme borreliosis. *Joint Bone Spine.* 2009;76(2):202-4.

Wenger N. et al. Atrial fibrillation, complete atrioventricular block and escape rhythm with bundle-branch block morphologies: an exceptional presentation of Lyme carditis. *Int J Cardiol.* 2012;160(1):e12-4.

Widhe M. et al. Up-regulation of Borrelia-specific IL-4- and IFN-gamma-secreting cells in cerebrospinal fluid from children with Lyme neuroborreliosis. *Int Immunol.* 2005;17(10):1283-91.

Wilhelmsson P. et al. Prevalence, diversity, and load of Borrelia species in ticks that have fed on human in regions of Sweden and Aland Islands, Finland with different Lyme Borreliosis incidences. *PLoS One.* 2013;8(11):e81433.

Wilking H. et al. Antibodies against Borrelia burgdorferi sensu lato among adults, Germany, 2008-2011. *Emerg Infect Dis.* 2015;21(1):107-10.

Wilson JM. Concerns regarding the Infectious Diseases Society of America Lyme Disease clinical practice guidelines. *Clin Infect Dis. (LTE).* 2007;44(4):1135-7.

Wilson-Welder, J, et al. Biochemical and molecular characterization of Treponema phagedenis-like spirochetes isolated from a bovine digital dermatitis lesion. *BMC Microbiology* 2013; 13: 280.

Winter EM., Rothbarth PH., Delfos NM. Misleading presentation of acute Lyme neuroborreliosis. *BMJ Case Rep.* 2012;2012:pii bcr2012006840.

Wojcik-Fatla A. et al. Leptospirosis as a tick-borne disease? Detection of Leptospira spp. in Ixodes ricinus ticks in Eastern Poland. *Ann Agric Environ Med.* 2012;19(4):656-9.

Wolanska-Klimkiewicz E. et al. Orofacial symptoms related to borreliosis—case report. *Ann Agric Environ Med.* 2010;17(2):319-21.

Wood E. et al. BB0172, a Borrelia burgdorferi outer membrane protein that binds integrin a3b1. *J Bacteriol.* 2013;195(15):3320-30.

Woodman ME. et al. Borrelia burgdorferi binding of host complement regulator factor H is not required for efficient mammalian infection. *Infect Immun.* 2007;75(6):3131-9.

Woodman ME. et al. Roles for phagocytic cells and complement in controlling relapsing fever infection. *J Leukoc Biol.* 2009;86(3):727-36.

Wormser GP., Halperin JJ. Toward a better understanding of European Lyme neuroborreliosis. *Clin Infect Dis.* 2013;57(4):510-2.

Wormser GP. and Schwartz I. Antibiotic treatment of animals infected with Borrelia burgdorferi. *Clin Microbiol Rev.* 2009;22(3):387-95.

Wormser GP. and Shapiro ED. Implications of gender in chronic Lyme disease. *J Womens Health (Larchmt).* 2009;18(6):831-4.

Wormser GP. et al. Anti-Tumor necrosis factor-alpha activation of Borrelia burgdorferi Spirochetes in antibiotic-treated murine Lyme borreliosis: An unproven conclusion. *J Infect Dis.* 2007;196:1865-6.

Wormser GP. et al. Impact of clinical variable on Borrelia burgdorferi-specific antibody seropositivity in acute-phase sera from patients in North America with culture-confirmed early Lyme disease. *Clin Vaccine Immunol.* 2008;15(10):1519-22.

Wright WF. et al. Diagnosis and management of Lyme disease. *AAFP.* 2012;0601:1086-93.

Wu J. et al. Invasion of eukaryotic cells by Borrelia burgdorferi requires b(1) integrins and Src kinase activity. *Infect Immun.* 2011;79(3):1338-48.

Wutte N. et al. CXCL13 chemokine in pediatric and adult neuroborreliosis. *Acta Neurol Scand.* 2011;124(5):321-8.

Wutte N. et al. Laboratory diagnosis of Lyme neuroborreliosis is influenced by the test used: Comparison of two ELISAs, immunoblot and CXCL13 testing. *J Neurol Sci.* 2014;347(1-2):96-103.

Wutte N. et al. Serum cxcl13 chemokine is not a marker for activity Lyme borreliosis. *Acta Derm Venereol.* 2011;91.

Wy L. et al. Invariant natural killer T cells act an extravascular cytotoxic barrier for joint-invading Lyme Borrelia. *Proc Natl Acad Sci U S A.* 2014;111(38):139376-41.

Wywial E. et al. Fast, adaptive evolution at a bacterial host-resistance locus: the PFam54 gene array in Borrelia burgdorferi. *Gene.* 2009;445(1-2):26-37.

Xu Q., McShan K. and Liang FT. Essential protective role attributed to the surface lipoproteins of Borrelia burgdorferi against innate defenses. *Mol Microbiol.* 2008;69(1):15-29.

Xu Q., McShan K. and Liang FT. Modification of Borrelia burgdorferi to overproduce OspA or VlsE alters its infectious behaviour. *Microbiology.* 2008;154(Pt11):3420-9.

Xu Q. et al. Increasing the interaction of Borrelia burgdorferi with decorin significantly reduces the 50 percent infectious dose and severely impairs dissemination. *Infect Immun.* 2007;75(9):4272-81.

Xu Q. et al. Increasing the recruitment of neutrophils to the site of infection dramatically attenuates Borrelia burgdorferi infectivity. *J Immunol.* 2007;178(8):5109-15.

Yakimchuk K. et al. Borrelia burgdorferi infection regulates CD1 expression in human cells and tissues via IL-1b. *Eur J Immunol.* 2011;41(3):694-05.

Yang X. et al. Borrelia burgdorferi lipoprotein BmpA activates pro-inflammatory responses in human synovial cells through a protein moiety. *Microbes Infect.* 2008;10(12-13):1300-08.

Yang X. et al. A chromosomally encoded virulence factor protects the Lyme disease pathogen against host-adaptive immunity. *PLoS Pathog.* 2009;5(3):e1000326.

Yegutkin GG. et al. Disordered lymphoid purine metabolism contributes to the pathogenesis of persistent Borrelia garinii infection in mice. *J Immunol.* 2010;184(9):5112-20.

Yimer M. et al. Prevalence and risk factors of louse-bourne relapsing fever in high risk populations in Bahir Dar city Northwest, Ethiopia. *BMC Res Notes.* 2014;7:615.

Yossepowitch O. et al. Aseptic meningitis and adult respiratory distress syndrome caused by Borrelia persica. *Infection.* 2012;40(6):695-7.

Yrjanainen H. et al. Anti-Tumor necrosis factor-alpha treatment activates Borrelia burgdorferi spirochetes 4 weeks after ceftriaxone treatment in C3H/He mice. *J Infect Dis.* 2007;195(10):1489-96.

Yrjanainen H. et al. Persistence of borrelial DNA in the joints of Borrelia burgdorferi-infected mice after ceftriaxone treatment. *APMIS.* 2010;118(9):665-73.

Yrjanainen H. et al. Persistent joint swelling and Borrelia-specific antibodies in Borrelia garinii-infected mice after eradication of vegetative spirochetes with antibiotic treatment. *Micobes Infect.* 2006;8(8):2044-51.

Yrjanainen H. et al. Reply to Wormser et al. and to McSweegan. *J Infect Dis.* 2007;196:1866-7. Letter to the Editor.

Zachaus M. Mesangioproliferative IgA-nephritis in a patient with Lyme borreliosis. *MMW Fortschr Med.* 2008;150(13):38-40.

Zajkowska J. et al. Clinical forms of neuroborreliosis—the analysis of patients diagnosed in department of infectious diseases and neuroinfection medical academy in Bialystok between 2000-2005. *Przegl Epidemiol.* 2007;61(1):59-65.

Zajkowska J. et al. Lyme Borreliosis: From pathogenesis to diagnosis and treatment. *Clin Develp Immunol.* 2012;231657:1-2.

Zajkowska J. et al. New aspects of pathogenesis of Lyme borreliosis. *Przegl Epidemiol.* 2006;60Suppl1:167-70.

Zajkowska JM. et al. Peripheral neuropathies in Lyme borreliosis. *Pol Merkur Lekarski.* 2010;29(170):115-8.

Zakovska A., et al. Isolation of Borrelia afzelii from overwintering Culex pipiens biotype molestus mosquitoes. *Ann Agric Environ Med.* 2006;13(2):345-8.

Zamani Z. et al. Culture of Borrelia persica and its flagella antigen in vitro. *Pak J Biol Sci.* 2014;17(2):190-7.

Zanchi AC. et al. Necrotizing granulomatous hepatitis as an unusual manifestation of Lyme disease. *Dig Dis Sci.* 2007;52(10):2629-32.

Zeidner N. et al. A borreliacidal factor in Amblyomma americanum saliva is associated with phospholipase A2 activity. *Exp Parasitol.* 2009;121(4):370-5.

Zeidner NS. et al. Suppression of Th2 cytokines reduces tick-transmitted Borrelia burgdorferi load in mice. *J Parasitol.* 2008;94(3):767-9.

Zelger B. et al. Detection of spirochetal micro-organisms by focus-floating microscopy in necrobiotic xanthogranuloma. *J Am Acad Dermatol.* 2007;57(6):1026-30.

Zhang XC. et al. The composition and transmission of microbiome in hard tick, Ixodes persulcatus, during blood meal. *Ticks Tick Borne Dis.* 2014;5(6):864-70.

Zhao Z. et al. Borrelia burgdorferi-induced monocyte chemoattractant protien-1 production in vivo and in vitro. *Biochem Biophs Res Commun.* 2007;358(2):528-33.

Zhao Z. et al. CD14 mediates cross talk between mononuclear cells and fibroblasts for upregulation of matrix metalloproteinase 9 by Borrelia burgdorferi. *Infect Immun.* 2007;75(6):3062-69.

Zhi H. et al. The BBA33 lipoprotein binds collagen and impacts Borrelia burgdorferi pathogenesis. *Mol Microbiol.* 2015;6.

Zhou W., Brisson D. Potentially conflicting selective forces that shape the vls antigenic variation system in Borrelia burgdorferi. *Infect Genet Evol.* 2014;27:559-65.

Ziemer M. et al. Granuloma annulare—a manifestation of infection with Borrelia? *J Cutan Pathol.* 2008;35(11):1050-7.

Zotter S. et al. Neuropsychological profile of children after an episode of neuroborreliosis. *Neuropediatrics.* 2013;44(6):346-53.

Zuckert WR. A call to order at the spirochetal host-pathogen interface. *Mol Microbiol.* 2013;8992):2017-11.

Zuckert WR. Secretion of bacterial lipoproteins: through the cytoplasmic membrane, the periplasm and beyond. *Biochim Biophys Acta.* 2014;1843(8):1509-16.

Chlamydia

Abdelsamed H., Peters J. and Byrne GI. Genetic variation in Chlamydia trachomatis and their hosts: impact on disease severity and tissue tropism. *Future Microbiol.* 2013;8(9):1129-46.

Aigelsreiter A. et al. Chlamydia psittaci infection in nongastrointestinal extranodal MALT lymphomas and their precursor lesions. *Am J Clin Pathol.* 2011;135(1):70-5.

Aiyar A. et al. Influence of the tryptophan-indole-IFNg axis on human genital Chlamydia trachomatis infection: role of vaginal co-infections. *Front Cell Inf Microbiol,* 2014;4(72):1-9.

ATP/ADP Translocases: A common feature of obligate intracellular amoebal symbionts related to Chlamydiae and Rickettsiae. *J Bacteriol.* 2004;186(3):683-91.

Baud D., Greub G. Intracellular bacteria and adverse pregnancy outcomes. *Clin Microbiol Infect.* 2011; 17(9):1312-22.

Bonner CA., Byrne GI., Jensen RA. Chlamydia exploit the mammalian tryptophan-depletion defense strategy as a counter-defensive cue to trigger a survival state of persistence. *Front Cell Inf Microb.* 2014;4(17):1-17.

Cai T. et al. Semen quality in patients with Chlamydia trachomatis genital infection treated concurrently with prulifloxacin and a phytotherapeutic agent. *J Androl.* 2012l33(4):615-23.

Caldwell HD., Belden EL. Studies of the role of Dermacentor occidentalis in the transmission of Bovine Chlamydial abortion. *Infect Immun.* 1973;7(2):147-51.

Campbell LA., Rosenfeld ME. Persistent C. pneumoniae infection in atherosclerotic lesions: rethinking the clinical trails. *Front Cell Infect Microb.* 2014;4(34):1-4.

Capmany A., Damiani MT. Chlamydia trachomatis intercepts Golgi-derived sphingolipids through a Rab 14-mediated transport required for bacterial development and replication. *PLoS One.* 2010;5(11):e14084.

Chen J. et al. Chlamydia pneumoniae infection and cerebrovascular disease: a systematic review and meta-analysis. *BMC Neurology.* 2013;13(183):1-13.

Choroszy-Krol I. et al. Characteristics of the Chlamydia trachomatis species – Immunopathology and infections. *Adv Clin Exp Med.* 2012;21(6):799-808.

Circella E. et al. Chlamydia psittaci infection in canaries heavily infested by Dermanyssus gallinae. *Exp Appl Acarol.* 2011;55(4):329-38.

Cocchiaro JL., Valdivia RH. New insights into Chlamydia intracellular survival mechanisms. *Cell Microbiol.* 2009;11(11):1571-78.

Collina F. et al. Chlamydia psittaci in ocular adnexa MALT lymphoma: a possible role in lymphomagenesis and a different geographical distribution. *Infect Agent Cancer.* 2012;7:8.

Corsaro D., et al. Novel Chlamydiales strains isolated from a water treatment plant. *Environ Microbiol.* 2009;11(1):188-200.

Croxatto A. et al. Presence of Chlamydiales DNA in ticks and fleas suggests that ticks are carriers of Chlamydiae. *Ticks Tick Borne Dis.* 2014;292:1-7.

Darville T., Hiltke TJ. Pathogenesis of genital tract disease due to Chlamydia trachomatis. *J Infect Dis.* 2010;201(Suppl 2):S114-S125.

Dean D. Chlamydia trachomatis today: treatment, detection, immunogentics and the need for a greater global understanding of chlamydial disease pathogenesis. *Drugs Today (Barc).* 2009;45(Suppl B):25-31.

Dielissen PW., Teunissen DA., Largro-Janssen AL. Chlamydia prevalence in the general population: is there a sex difference? A systematic review. *BMC Infect Dis.* 2013;13:534.

Eddie B. Isolation of a PL agent (Chlamydi, Bedsonia) from ticks (Argas (P.) arboreus) parasitic on the white-necked cormorant (Phalacrocorax carbo) in Ethiopia. *J Med Entomol.* 1970;7(6):745-46.

Eddie B. et al. Psittacosis-lymphogranuloma venereum (PL) agents (Bedsonia, Chlamydia) in ticks, fleas, and native mammals in California. *Am J Epidemiol.* 1969;90(5):449-60.

Elwell CA. and Engel JN. Lipid acquisition by intracellular Chlamydiae. *Cell Microbiol.* 2012;14(7):1010-18.

Elwell CA. et al. Chlamydia trachomatis co-opts GBF1 and CERT to acquire host sphingomyelin for distinct roles during intracellular development. *PLoS Path.* 2011;7(9):e1002198.

Fabris M. et al. High prevalence of Chlamydophila psittaci subclinical infection in Italian patients with Sjogren's syndrome and parotid gland marginal zone B-cell lymphoma of MALT-type. *Clin Exp Rheumatol.* 2014;32(1):61-5.

Facco F. et al. Chlamydial and rickettsial transmission through tick bite in children. *Lancet.* 1992;339(8799):992-3.

Forsey T., Darougar S. Transmission of Chlamydiae by the housefly. *Br J Ophthalmol.* 1981;65(2):147-50.

Frohlich KM. et al. Membrane vesicle production by Chlamydia trachomatis as an adaptive response. *Front Cell Infect Microbiol.* 2014;4(73):1-9.

Geng Y. et al. Chlamydia pneumoniae inhibits apoptosis in human peripheral blood mononuclear cells through induction of -10. *J Immunol.* 2000;164:5522-29.

Hackstadt T. and Scidmore MA., Rockey DD. Lipid metabolism in Chlamydia trachomatis-infected cells: Directed trafficking of Golgi-derived sphingolipids to the Chlamydial inclusion. *Proc Natl Acad Sci. USA.* 1995;92:4877-81.

Hackstadt T. et al. Chlamydia trachomatis interrupts an exocytic pathway to acquire endogenously synthesized sphingomyelin in transit from the Golgi apparatus to the plasma membrane. *EMBO J.* 1996;15(5):1996.

Han JJ. et al. Long-term outcomes of first-line treatment with doxycycline in patients with previously untreated ocular adnexal marginal zone B cell lymphoma. *Ann Hemamtol.* 2014;24:1-2.

Han X. et al. Chlamydia infection induces ICOS ligand-expressing and IL-10-producing dendritic cells that can inhibit airway inflammation and mucus overproduction elicited by allergen challenge in BALB/c Mice. *J Immunol.* 2006;176:5232-39.

Hao X-F. et al. Advance in the chemical and immunological controls of ticks. *Prog Veterin Med.* 2008;12:1-2.

He X. et al. Inflammation and fibrosis during Chlamydia pneumoniae infection is regulated by IL-1 and the NLRP3/ASC inflammasome. *J Immunol.* 2010;184(10):5743-54.

Hu VH., Holland MJ., Burton MJ. Trachoma: Protective and pathogenic ocular immune responses to Chlamydia trachomatis. *PLOS Neglec Trop Dis.* 2013;7(2):e2020.

Huang B. et al. Anaplasma phagocytophilum APH-1387 is expressed throughout bacterial intracellular development and localized to the pathogen-occupied vascular membrane. *Infect Immun.* 2010;78(5):1864-73.

Huston WM. et al. Evolution to a chronic disease niche correlates with increased sensitivity to tryptophan availability for the obligate intracellular bacterium Chlamydia pneumoniae. *J Bacteriol.* 2014;196(11):1915-24.

Jendro MC. et al. Cytokine profile in serum and synovial fluid of arthritis patients with Chlamydia trachomatis infection. *Rheumatol Int.* 2005;(1):37-41.

Jongejan F. et al. The tick-borne rickettsia Cowdria ruminantium has a Chlamydia-like developmental cycle. *Onderstepoort J Vet Res.* 1991;58(4):227-37.

Judson FN. Assessing the number of genital Chlamydial infections in the United States. *J Reprod Med.* 1985;30(Suppl):269-72.

Kalmar ID. et al. Zoonotic infection with Chlamydia psittaci at an avian refuge centre. *Vet J.* 2014;199(2):300-2.

Khader SA., Gopal R. IL-17 in protective immunity to intracellular pathogens. *Virulence.* 2010;1(5):423-27.

Korman Tm., Turnidge JD., Grayson ML. Neurological complications of chlamydial infections: case report and review. *Clin Infect Dis.* 1997;25(4):847-51.

Kotake S., Nanke Y. Chlamydia-associated arthritis and enteropathic arthritis--two important spondyloarthritides. *Nihon Rinsho Menki Gakkai Kaishi.* 2011;34(3):121-30.

Kuipers JG. et al. Reactive and undifferentiated arthritis in North Africa: use of PCR for detection of Chlamydia trachomatis. *Clin Rheumatol.* 2009;28(1):11-6.

Lagae S. et al. Emerging Chlamydia psittaci infections in chickens and examination of transmission to human. *J Med Microbiol.* 2014;63(Pt 3):399-407.

Leite-Browning ML. Causes of infectious abortions in goats. *ACES Pub.* 2006;UNP-0079.

Ling Y. et al. Epidemiology of Chlamydia psittaci infection in racing pigeons and pigeon fanciers in Beijing, China. *Zoonoses Public Health.* 2014;22.

Lo CC. et al. The alternative translational profile that underlies the immune-evasive state of persistence in Chlamydiaceae exploits differential tryptophan contents of the protein repertoire. *Microbiol Mol Biol Rev.* 2012;76(2):405-43.

Malhotra M. et al. Genital Chlamydia trachomatis: An update. *Indian J Med Res.* 2013;138(3):303-16.

Mantovani E. et al. Description of Lyme disease-like syndrome in Brazil. Is it a new tick borne disease or Lyme disease variation? *Braz J Med Biol Res.* 2007;40(4):443-56.

Marks E., Tam MA., Lycke NY. The female lower genital tract is a privileged compartment with IL-10 producing dendritic cells and poor Th1 immunity following Chlamydia trachomatis infection. *PLoS Path.* 2010;6(11):e1001179.

Marrazzo J., Suchland R. Recent advanced in understanding and managing Chlamydia trachomatis infections. *F1000 Prime Rep.* 2014;6(120):1-7.

McCoy AJ. et al. L,L-diaminopimelate aminotransferase, a trans-kingdom enzyme shared by Chlamydia and plants for synthesis for Diaminopimelate/Lysine. *Proc Natl Acad Sci USA.* 2006;103(47):17909.

McKercher DG. Assay of experimental transmission with an argaside (Ornithodoros coriaceus), of a Chlamydia, associated with Bovine Abortion. *Bull L-Acad Veterin France.* 2981.

McKercher DG. et al. Preliminary studies on transmission of Chlamydia to cattle by ticks (Ornithodoros coriaceus). *Am J Vet Res.* 1980;41(6):922-4.

Mediannikov O., Fenollar F. Looking in ticks for human bacterial pathogens. *Microbial Path.* 2014;77:142-48.

Mehlitz A., Rudel T. Modulation of host signaling and cellular responses by Chlamydia. *Cell Communic Signal.* 2013;11(90):1-11.

Moustafa A., Reyes-Prieto A., Bhattacharya D. Chlamydiae has contributed at least 55 gene to plantae with predominantly plastid functions. *PLoS One.* 2008;3(5):e2205.

Mueller KE., Plano GV. and Fields KA. New frontiers in Type III secretion biology: The Chlamydia perspective . *Infect Immun.* 2014;82(1):2-6.

Myer GS. et al. Evidence that human Chlamydia pneumoniae was zoonotically acquired. *J Bacteriol.* 2009;191(23):7225-33.

Nakao R. et al. A novel approach, based on BLSOMs (Batch Learning Self-Organizing Maps), to the microbiome analysis of ticks. *ISME J.* 2013;7:1003-15.

Osman KM. et al. Antimicrobial susceptibility and molecular typing of multiple Chlamydiaceae species isolated from genital infection of women in Egypt. *Microb Drug Resist.* 2012;18(4):440-5.

Pazniak AL. et al. Acute Chlamydial lesions of the nervous system: etiology, diagnosis, clinical aspects. *Klin Med (Mosk).* 2002;80(9):31-4.

Penate Medina TA. et al. Identification of sphingomyelinase on the surface of Chlamydia pneumoniae: Possible role in the entry into its host cells. *Interdiscripl. Perspect. Inf Dis.* 2014;412827:1-12.

Pierzchalski JL., Bretl DA., Matson SC. Phthirus pubis as a predictor for Chlamydia infections in adolescents. *Sex Transm Dis.* 2002;29(6):331-4.

Pietro MD. et al. Chlamydia pneumoniae infection in atherosclerotic lesion development through oxidative stress: A brief overview. *Int J Mol Sci.* 2013;14:15105-20.

Pokrovskaya ID. et al. Chlamydia trachomatis hijacks intra-Golgi COG complex-dependent vesicle trafficking pathway. *Cell Microbiol.* 2012;14(5):656-68.

Puolakkainen M. Laboratory diagnosis of persistent human chlamydial infection. *Front Cell Inf Microbiol.* 2013;3(99).

Qiu Y. et al. Microbiome population analysis of the salivary glands of Ticks; A possible strategy for the surveillance of Bacterial pathogens. *PLOS One.* 2014;9(8):e103961.

Rank RG., Yeruva L. Hidden in plain sight: Chlamydial gastrointestinal infection and its relevance to persistence in human genital infection. *Infect Immun.* 2014;82(4):1362-71.

Rasmussen SJ. et al. Secretion of proinflammatory cytokines by epithelial cells in response to Chlamydia infection suggests a central role for epithelial cells in response to Chlamydial pathogensis. *J Clin Invest.* 1997;99(1):77-87.

Redgrove KA., McLaughlin EA. The role of the immune response in Chlamydia trachomatis infection of the male genital tract: A double-edged sword. *Front Immunol.* 2014;5(534):1-13.

Rockey DD. Unraveling the basic biology and clinical significance of the chlamydial plasmid. *J Exp Med.* 2011;208(11):2159-62.

Sabtil A., Coolingro A., Horn M. Tracing the primordial Chlamydiae: Extinct parasites of plants? *Trends Plant Sci.* 2014;19(1):36-43.

Saka HA., Valdivia RH. Acquisition of nutrients by Chlamydiae: Unique challenges of living in an intracellular compartment. *Curr Opin Microbiol.* 2010;13(1):4-10.

Sandoz KM., Rockey DD. Antibiotic resistance in Chlamydiae. *Future Microbiol.* 2010; 5(9):1427-42.

Schnarr S. et al. Chlamydia and Borrelia DNA in synovial fluid of patients with early undifferentiated oligoarthritis: results of a prospective study. *Arthritis Rheum.* 2001 44(11):2679-85.

Schoborg RV. Chlamydia persistence – a tool to dissect Chlamydia-Host interactions. *Microbes Infect.* 2011;13(7):649-62.

Scidmore MA. Recent advances in Chlamydia subversion of host cytoskeletal and membrane trafficking pathways. *Microbes Infect.* 2011;13(6):527-35.

Scidmore MA., Fischer ER. and Hackstadt T. Sphingolipids and glycoproteins are differentially trafficked to the Chlamydia trachomatis inclusion. *J Cell Biol.* 1996;134(2):363-74.

Sessa R. et al. Infectious burden and atherosclerosis: A clinical issue. *World J Clin Cases.* 2014;2(7):240-9.

Shao R. et al. Nitric oxide synthases and tubal ectopic pregnancies induced by Chlamydia infection: Basic and clinical insights. *Mol Human Reprod.* 2010;16(12):907-15.

Shima K. et al. Impact of a low-oxygen environment of the efficacy of antimicrobials against intracellular Chlamydia trachomatis. *Antimicrob Agents Chemother.* 2011;55(5):2319-24.

Shimada K., Crother TR. and Arditi M. Innate immune responses to Chlamydia pneumoniae infection: Role of TLRs, NLRs, and the inflammasome. *Microbes Infect.* 2012;14(4):1301-07.

Shimada K. et al. Caspase-1 dependent IL-1b secretion is critical for host defense in a mouse model of Chlamydia pneumoniae lung infection. *PLoS One.* 2011;6(6):e21477.

Somboonna N. et al. Discovering and differentiating new and emerging clonal populations of Chlamydia trachomatis with a novel shotgun cell culture harvest assay. *Emerg Infect Dis.* 2008;14(3):445-453.

Steel I N , Balsara ZR., Starnback MN. Hematopoietic cells are required to initiate a Chlamydia trachomatis-specific CD8-T cell response. *J Immunol.* 2004;173:6327-37.

Stephens AJ., Aubuchon M., Schust DJ. Antichlamdial antibodies, human fertility, and pregnancy wastage. *Infect Dis Obstet Gynecol.* 2011;2011:525182.

Stratton CW., Wheldon DB. Multiple sclerosis: an infectious syndrome involving Chlamydophila pneumoniae. *Trends Microbiol.* 2006;14(11):474-9.

Sullivan JL., Weinberg ED. Iron and the Role of Chlamydia pneumoniae in Heart disease. *Emerging Inf Dis.(LTTE)* 1999:5(5):724-26.

Tiwari V. et al. Role of heparan sulfate in sexually transmitted infections. *Glycobiology.* 2012;22(11):1402-12.

Trentmann O. et al. Enlightening energy parasitism by analysis of an ATP/ADP transporter from Chlamydiae. *PLoS Bio.*2007;5(9):e231.

Vainshenker LuL. Chlamydial infection of the central nervous system. Laboratory diagnosis and clinic and morphological features. *Arkh Patol.* 2014;76(1):57-62.

Wang C. Multivariate analysis of Chlamydia pneumoniae lung infection in two inbred mouse strains. *Auburn Univ Dissertation.* 2005;12(16).

Wang SA. et al. Evaluation of antimicrobial resistance and treatment failures for Chlamydia trachomatis: A meeting report. *J Inf Dis.* 2005;191:917-23.

Weyer F. Zur Frage der Rolle von Arthropoden als Reservoir des Psittakoseerregers. *Zeits Tropenmed Parasito.* 1970;T448:146-53.

Wheelhouse N. et al. Chlamydia trachomatis and Chlamydophila abortus induce the expression of secretory leukocyte protease inhibitor in cells of the human female reproductive tract. *Microbiol Immunol.* 2008;52(9):465-8.

Wixel B. et al. Role of CD8+ T cells in the host response to Chlamydia. *Microbes Infect.* 2008;10(14-15-):1420-30.

Wolf K., Hackstadt T. Sphingomyelin trafficking in Chlamydia pneumoniae-infected cells. *Cellular Microbiol.* 2001;3(3):145-52.

Xuiqin H. et al. Clinical observation on prenatal Chlamydia trachomatis infection. *Chinese J Obstetric Gynecol.* 1995;08:1-2.

Yang X. et al. IL-10 Gene knockout mick show enhanced Th1-like protective immunity and absent granuloma formation following Chlamydia trachomatis lung infection. *J Immunol.*1999;162:1010-17.

Ying S. et al. Premature apoptosis of Chlamydia-infected cells disrupts chlamydial development. *J Infect Dis.* 2008;198(10):1536-44.

Yoshinari NH. et al. Brazilian Lyme-like disease or Boggio-Yoshinari syndrome: exotic and emerging Brazilian tick-borne zoonosis. *Rev Assoc Med Bras.*2010;56(3):363-9.

Yucesan C., Sriram S. Chlamydia pneumoniae infection of the central nervous system. *Curr Opin Neurol.* 2001;14(3):355-9.

Zhong G. et al. Killing me softly: Chlamydial use of proteolysis for evading host defenses. *Trends Microbiol.* 2009;17(10):467-74.

Rickettsia

Abdad MY., Stenos J., Graves S. Rickettsia felis, and emerging flea-transmitted human pathogen. *Emerg Health Threats J.* 2011;4:1-6.

Andersson SGE. et al. The genome sequence of Rickettsia prowazekii and the origin of mitochondria. *Nature.* 1998;396(12):133-40.

Arguello AP. et al. A fatal urban case of Rocky Mountain spotted fever presenting an eschar in San Jose, Costa Rica. *Am J Trop Med Hyg.* 2012;87(2):345-8.

Astrup E. et al. A Complex Interaction between Rickettsia conorii and Dickkopf-1 – Potential role in immune evasion mechanisms in endothelial cells. *PLoS One.* 2012;7(9):e43638.

Azad AF., Beard CB. Rickettsial pathogens and their arthropod vectors. *Emerg Infect Dis.*1998;4(2):178-86.

Bacci MR., Namura JJ. Association between sepsis and Rocky Mountain spotted fever. *BMJ Case Rep.* 2012;6:pii:bcr2012007024.

Baganz MD., Dross PE., Reinhardt. Rocky Mountain spotted fever encephalitis: MR findings. *Amer Soc Neurorad.* 1993;16:919-22.

Bal AK., Kairys SW. Kawasaki disease following Rocky Mountain spotted fever a case report. *J Med Case Rep.* 2009;6(3):7320.

Baltadzhiev I., Balchev S. Changes of bel-2, bax and caspase-3 expression in the dermal microvascular endothelial cells and the epidermal layers of the eschar (tache noire) in patients with Mediterranean spotted fever. *Polish Soc Histochem Cytochem.* 2013;51(2):121-26.

Bechelli JR. et al. Rickettsia rickettsii infection protects human microvascular endothelial cells against staurosporine-induced apoptosis by a cIAP(2)-independent mechanism. *J Infect Dis.* 2009;199(9):1389-98.

Beselga D. et al. A rare case of retinal artery occlusion in the context of Mediterranean spotted fever. *Case Rep Ophthalmol.* 2014;5(1):22-7.

Bhavnani SK. et al. How cytokines co-occur across Rickettsioses patients: from bipartite visual analytics to mechanistic inferences of a cytokine storm. *AMIA Jt Summits Transi Sci Proc.* 2013;Mar:15-9.

Blair PJ. et al. Characterization of spotted fever group Rickettsiae in flea and tick specimens from Northern Peru. *J Clin Microbiol.* 2004;42(11):4961-7.

Bonawitz C., Castillo., Mukherji SK. Comparison of CT and MR features with clinical outcome in patients with Rocky Mountain spotted fever. *Amer J Neurorad.* 1997;18:459-464.

Bonoldi VL. et al. First report of mild Brazilian spotted fever associated to arthritis. *Rev Bras Reumatol.* 2014;54(3):237-40.

Boppana VD. et al. Blood feeding by the Rocky Mountain spotted fever vector, Dermacentor andrsoni, induces interleukin-4 expression by cognate antigen responding CD4+T cells. *Parasit Vectors.* 2009;2(1):47.

Breitschwerdt EB. et al. Rickettsia rickettsii transmission by a lone star tick, North. *Emerg Infect Dis.* 2011;17(5):873-5.

Centers for Disease Control and Prevention (CDC). Fatal cases of Rocky Mountain spotted fever in family clusters – three states, 2003. *MMWR Morb Mortal Wkly Rep.* 2004;53(19):407-10.

Clark I.A. et al. Pathogenesis of malaria and clinically similar conditions. *Clinical Microbiology Reviews* 2004; 17(3): 509-39.

Clifton DR. et al. NF-kappaB activation during Rickettsia rickettsii infection of endothelial cells involves the activation of catalytic ikappaB kinases IkBalpha and IkBbeta and phosphorylation-proteolysis of the inhibitor protein IkappaBalpha. *Infect Immun.* 2005;73(1):155-65.

Clifton DR. et al. NF-kB-dependent inhibition of apoptosis is essential for host cell survival during Rickettsia rickettsii infection. *Proc Natl Acad Sci.* 1998;95:4646-51.

Colomba C. et al. First case of Mediterranean spotted fever-associated rhabdomyoysis leading to fatal acute renal failure and encephalitis. *Int J Infect Dis.* 2014;26:12-3

Colonne PM. Interferon-B-mediated innate host defense in Rickettsia conorii-infected human endothelium. *Depart Pathol Lab Med School Med Dent.* 2012:1-137.

Dahlgren FS. et al. Fatal Rocky Mountain spotted fever in the United States, 1999-2007. *Am J Trop Med Hyg.* 2012;86(4):713-19.

Demma LJ. et al. Rocky Mountain spotted fever from an unexpected tick vector in Arizona. *N Engl J Med.* 2005;353(6):587-94.

Devamanoharan PS. et al. Infection of human endothelial cells by Rockettsia rickettsii causes a significant reduction in the levels of key enzymes involved in protection against oxidative injury. *Infect Immun.* 1994;62(6):2619-21.

DiNubile M. Reliving a Nightmare: A hard (and tragic) lesson in humility. *Clin Infect Dis.*1996;23:160-4.

Drancourt M. et al. Secretion of tissue type plasminogen activator and plasminogen activator by Rickettsia conorii- and Rickettsia rickettsii-infected cultured endothelial cells. *Infect Immun.* 1990;58(8):2459-63.

Dubourg G. et al. Scalp eschar and neck lyphadenopathy after tick bite: an emerging syndrome with multiple causes. *Eur J Clin Microbiol Infect Dis.* 2014;33(8):1449-56.

Eloubeidi MA., Burton CS., Sexton DJ. The great imitator: Rocky Mountain spotted fever occurring after hospitalization for unrelated illnesses. *South Med J.* 1997;90(9):943-5.

Eremeeva ME., Dasch GA., Silverman DJ. Quantitative analyses of variations in the injury of endothelial cells elicited by 11 isolates of Rickettsia rickettsii. *Clin Diagn Lab Immun.* 2001;8(4):788-96.

Eremeeza ME., Silverman DJ. Rickettsia rickettsii infection of the EA.hy 926 endothelial cell line: morphological response to infection and evidence for oxidative injury. *Microbio.* 1998;144(Pt 8):2037-48.

Faccini-Martinez AA. et al. Probable case of flea borne spotted fever (Rickettsia felis). *Biomedica.* 2013;33(Suppl 1):9-13.

Feng H., Popov VI., Walker DH. Depletion of gamma interferon and tumor necrosis factor alpha in mice with Rickettsia conorii-infected endothelium: impairment of rickettsicidal nitric oxide production resulting in fatal, overwhelming rickettsial disease. *Infect Immun.* 1994;62(5):1952-60.

Feng HM., Walker DH. Mechanisms of intracellular killing of Rickettsia conorii in infected human endothelial cells, hepatocytes, and macrophages. *Infect Immun.* 2000;68(12):6729-36.

Folkema AM. et al. Trends in clinical diagnoses of Rocky Mountain spotted fever among American Indians, 2001-2008. *Am J Trop Med Hyg.* 2012;86(1):152-8.

Fornadel CM. et al. High rates of Rickettsia parkeri infection in Gulf Coast tricks (Amblyomma maculatum) and identification of "Candidatus Rickettsia andeanae" from Fairfax County, Virginia. *Vector Borne Zoonotic Dis.* 2011;11(12):1535-39.

Fourier PE. et al. Evidence of Rickettsia helvetica infection in humans, Eastern France. *Emerg Inf Dis.* 2000;6(4):389-92.

Gar-Yun Chan Y., Riley SP., Martinez JJ. Adherence to and invasion of host cells by spotted fever group Rickettsia species. *Front Micrbio.* 2010;1(139):1-10.

Germanakis A. et al. Rickettsia aeschlimannii infection in a man, Greece. *Emerg Infect Dis.* 2013;19(7):1176-7.

Gillespie JJ. et al. Plasmids and rickettsial evolution: Insight from Rickettsia. *PLoS One.* 2007;2(3):e266.

Gillespie JJ. et al Rickettsia phylogenomics: Unwinding the intricacies of obligate intracellular life. *PLoS One.* 2008;3(4):1-2.

Giudice E. et al. A molecular survey of Rickettsia felis in fleas from cats and dogs in Sicily (Southern Italy). *PLoS One.* 2014;9(9):106820.

Gong B. et al. Compartmentalized, functional role of angiogenin during spotted fever group Rickettsia-induced endothelial barrier dysfunction: Evidence of possible mediation by host tRNA-derived small noncoding RNAs. *BMC Infect Dis.* 2013;13(285):1-16.

Gong B. et al. Rickettsiae induce microvascular hyperpermeability via phosphorylation of VE-cadherins: Evidence from atomic force microscopy and biochemical studies. *PLoS One.* 2012;6(6):e1699.

Grasperge BJ. et al Feeding by Amblyomma maculatum (Acari: Ixodidae) enhances Rickettsia parkeri (Rickettsiales: Rickettsiaceae) infection in the skin. *J Med Entomol.* 2014;51(4):855-63.

Gupta R., Singh V. Indian tick typhus – an uncommon cause of hepatitis: A case report. *J Clin Diagn Res.*2014;8(5):MD02-1.

Holman RC. et al. Analysis of risk factors for fatal Rocky Mountain spotted fever: evidence for superiority of tetracyclines for therapy. *J Infect Dis.* 2001;184(11):1437-44.

Jia N. et al. Human infection with Candidatus Rickettsia tarasevichiae. *N Engl J Med.* 2013;369:1178-80.

Joshi SG. et al. Nuclear factor kB protects against host cells Apoptosis during Rickettsia rickettsii infection by inhibiting activation of apical and effector caspases and maintaining mitochondrial integrity. *Infect Immun.* 2003;71(7):4127-36.

Kularatne SA. et al. A case series of spotted fever rickettsiosis with neurological manifestations in Sri Lanka. *Int J Infect Dis.* 2012;16(7):e14-7.

Kummerfeldt CE., Huggins JT., Sahn SA. Unusual bacterial infections and the pleura. *Open Respir Med J.* 2012;6:75-81.

Kundavaram A. et al. Acute infectious purpura fulminans due to probable spotted fever. *J Postgrad Med.* 2014;60(2):198-9.

Kushawaha A. et al. Hitch-hiker taken for a ride: an unusual cause of myocarditis, septic shock and adult respiratory distress syndrome. *BMJ Case Rep.* 2013;pii:bcr2012007155.

Levin ML. et al. Clinical presentation, convalescence, and relapse of Rocky Mountain spotted fever in dogs experimentally infected via tick bite. *PLoS One.* 2014;9(12):1-19.

Luciani F. et al. Spotted fever from Rickettsia typhi in an older woman: A case report from a geographic area where it would not be expected. *Int J Infect Dis.* 2014;27:10-12.

Mays RM. et al. Rocky Mountain spotted fever in a patient treated with anti-TNF-alpha inhibitors. *Dermatol Online J.*2013;19(3):7.

Mendese G., Grande D. Asymptomatic petechial eruption on the lower legs. *J Clin Aesthet Dermatol.* 2013;6(9):48-9.

Moncaya AC. et al. Absence of Rickettsia rickettsii and occurrence of other spotted fever group rickttsiae in ticks from Tennessee. *Am J Trop Med Hyg.* 2010;83(3):653-7.

Mosites E. et al. Knowledge, attitudes, and practices regarding Rocky Mountain spotted fever among healthcare providers, Tennessee, 2009. *Am J Trop Med Hyg.* 2013;88(1):162-6.

Myers T. et al. Detecting Rickettsia parkeri infection from eschar swab specimens. *Emerg Infect Dis.* 2013;19(5):778-80.

Nakata R. et al. A case of Japanese spotted fever complicated with central nervous system involvement and multiple organ failure. *Intern Med.* 2012;51(7):783-6.

Nesbit RM. Myocarditis, pericarditis, and cardiac tamponade associated with Rocky Mountain spotted fever. *J Americ Coll Card.* 2011;57(24):1.

Nilsson K., Lindquist O., Pahlson C. Association of Rickettsia helvetica with chronic perimyocarditis in sudden cardiac death. *Lancet.* 1999;354(9185):1169-73.

Nilsson K. et al. Bell's palsy and sudden deafness associated with Rickettsia spp. infection in Sweden. A retrospective and prospective serological survey including PCR findings. *Eur J Neurol.* 2014;21(2):206-14.

Nilsson K. et al. Demonstration of intracellular microorganisms (Rickettsia spp., Chlamydia pneumoniae, Bartonella spp.) in pathological human aortic valves by PCR. *J Infect* 2005;50(1):46-52.

Nwariaku FE. et al. The role of p38 map kinase in tumor necrosis factor-induced redistribution of vascular endothelial cadherin and increased endothelial permeability. *Shock.* 2002;18(1):82-5.

Openshaw JJ. et al. Rocky Mountain spotted fever in the United States, 2000-2007: Interpreting contemporary increases in incidence. *Am J Trop Med Hyg.* 2010;83(1):174-82.

Paddock CD. et al. Assessing the magnitude of fatal Rocky Mountain spotted fever in the United States comparison of two national data sources. *Am J Trop Med Hyg.* 2002;67(4):349-54.

Paddock CD. et al. Isolation of Rickettsia akari from eschars of patients with rickettsialpox. *Am J Trop Hyg.* 2006;75(4):732-8.

Paddock CD. et al. Isolation of Rickettsia parkeri and identification of a novel spotted fever group Rickettsia sp. from Gulf Coast ticks (Amblyomma maculatum) in the United States. *Appl Environ Microbiol.* 2010;76(9):2689-96.

Paddock CD. et al. Rickettsia parkeri: A newly recognized cause of spotted fever rickettsiosis in the United States. *Clin Infect Dis.* 2004;38(6)805-11.

Paddock CD. et al. Rickettsia parkeri rickettsiosis and its clinical distinction from Rocky Mountain spotted fever. *Clin Infect Dis.* 2008;47:1188-96.

Parola P. et al. Update on tick-borne Rickettsioses around the world: a geographic approach. *Clin Microbiol Review.* 2013;26(4):657-702.

Perlman SJ., Hunter MS., Zchori-Fein E. The emerging diversity of Rickettsia. *Proc R Soc B.* 2006;273:2097-2106.

Perotti MA. et al Rickettsia as obligate and mycetomic bacteria. *FASEB J.* 2006;20:E1646-E1655.

Pornwiroon W. et al. Comparative microbiota of Rickettsia felis-infected and colonized cat fleas, Ctenocephalides felis. *ISME J.* 2007;1:394-02.

Premaraina R. et al. A patient with spotted fever group rickettsiosis mimicking connective tissue disease. *Ceylon Med J.* 2012;57(3):127-8.

Radulovic S. et al. Rickettsia-macrophage interactions: Host cells responses to Rickettsia akari and Rickettsia typhi. *Infect Immun.*2002;70(5):2576-82.

Raoult D., Paddock CD. Rickettsia parkeri infection and other spotted fevers in the United States. *New Engl J Med.* 2005;353(6):626-27.

Reed S C.O., Serio AW., Welch MD. Suppressor of cytokine signaling protein SOCS1 and UBP43 regulate the expression of type I interferon-stimulated genes in human microvascular endothelial cells infected with Rickettsia conorii. *Cell Microbiol.* 2012;14(4):529-45.

Ren V., Hsu S. Why sulfonamides are contraindicated in Rocky Mountain spotted fever. *Derma. Online J.* 2014;20(2):1-3.

Richards AL. et al. Human infection with Rickettsia felis, Kenya. *Emerg Infect Dis.* 2010;16(7):1081

Romer Y. et al. Rickettsia parkeri rickettsiosis, Argentina. *Emerg Infect Dis.* 2011;17(7):1169-73.

Rydkina E. et al. Infection of human endothelial cells with spotted fever group Rickettsiae stimulates cyclooxygenase 2 expression and release of vasoactive prostaglandins. *Infect Immun.* 2006;74(9):5067-74.

Rydkina E. et al. Rickettsia rickettsii infection of cultured human endothelial cells induces heme oxygenase 1 expression. *Infect Immun.* 2002;70(8):4045-52.

Sahni SK. and Rydkina E. Host-cell interactions with pathogenic Rickettsia species. *Future Microbiol.* 2005;April 4:323-39.

Sahni SK. et al. Involvement of protein kinase C in Rickettsia rickttsii-induced transcriptional activation of the host endothelial cell. *Infect Immun.*1999;67(12):6418-23.

Sahni SK. et al. Proteasome-independent activation of nuclear factor kappaB in cytoplasmic extracts from human endothelial cells by Rickettsia rickettsii. *Infect Immun.* 1998;66(5):1827-33.

Sahni SK. et al. Recent molecular insights into rickettsial pathogenesis and immunity. *Future Microbiol.* 2013;8(10):1265-88.

Santucci LA., Gutierrez PL., Silverman DJ. Rickettsia rickettsii induces superoxide radical superoxide dismutase in human endothelial cells. *Infect Immun.* 1992;60(12):5113-8.

Saraiva DG. et al. Feeding period required by Amblyomma aureolatum ticks for transmission of Rickettsia rickettsii to vertebrate hosts. *Emerg Infect Dis.*2014;20(9):1504-10.

Sexton DJ., Kirkland KB. Rickettsial infections and the central nervous system. *Clin Inf Dis.* 1998;26:247.

Shaked Y. et al. Relapse of rickettsial Mediterranean spotted fever and murine typhus after treatment with chloramphenicol. *J Infect.* 1989;18(1):35-7.

Shapiro MR. et al. Rickettsia 364D: A newly recognized cause of eschar-associated illness in California. *Clin Infect Dis.* 2010;50:541-8.

Shi RJ. et al. Transcrptional regulation of endothelial cell tissue factor expression during Rickettsia rickettsii infection: involvement of the transcription factor NF-kappaB. *Infect Immun.* 1998;66(3):1070-5.

Speed RR., Winkler HH. Acquisition of polyamines by the obligate intracytoplasmic bacterium Rickettsia prowazekii. *J Bacteriology.* 1990;174(10):5690-96.

Sporn LA. E-selectin-dependent neutrophil adhesion to Rickettsia rickettsii-infected endothelial cells. *Blood* 1993;81(9):2406-12.

Sporn LA. and Marder VJ. Interleukin-1 alpha production during Rickettsia rickettsii infection of cultured endothelial cells: Potential role in autocrine cell stimulation. *Infect Immun.* 1996;64(5):1609-13.

Sporn LA. et al. Rickettsia rickettsii infection of cultured human endothelial cells induces NF-kappaB activation. *Infect Immun.* 1997;65(7):2786-91.

Sporn LA. et al. Rickettsia rickettsii infection of cultured human endothelial cells induces tissue factor expression. *Blood.* 1994;83(6):1527-34.

Sporn LA. et. al. Rickettsia rickettsii infection of cultured endothelial cells induces release of large von Willebrand factor multimers from Weibel-Palade bodies. *Blood* 1991;78(10):2595-602.

Stothard DR., Clark JB., Fuerst PA. Ancestral divergence of Rickettsia bellii from the spotted fever and typhus groups of Rickettsia and antiquity of the genus Rickettsia. *Intern J System Bacterio.* 1994;44(4):798-04.

Switaj K. et al. Spotted fever rickettsiosis caused by Ricketsia raoultii – case report. *Przegl Epidemiol.* 2012;66(2):347-50.

Szabo MR., Pinter A., Lebruna MB. Ecology, biology and distribution of spotted-fever tick vectors in Brazil. *Front. Cell Inf Microb.* 2013;3(27)1-9.

Tai K. et al. Significantly higher cytokine and chemokine levels in patients with Japanese spotted fever than in those with Tsutsugamushi disease. *J Clin Microbiol.* 2014;52(6):1938-46.

Thorner AR., Walker DH., Petri WA Jr. Rocky Mountain spotted fever. *Clin Infect Dis.* 1998;27:1353-60.

Tribaldos M. et al. Rocky Mountain spotted fever in Panama: a cluster description. *J Infet Dev Ctries.* 2011;5(10):737-41.

Turco J., Winkler HH. Role of the nitric oxide synthase pathway in inhibition of growth of interferon-sensitive and interferon-resistant Rickettsia prowazekii strains in L929 cells treated with tumor necrosis factor alpha and gamma interferon. *Infect Immun.* 1993;61(10):4317-25.

Turner RC., Chaplinski TJ., Adams HG. Rocky Mountain spotted fever presenting as thrombotic thrombocytopenic purpura. *Am J Med.* 1986;81(1):153-7.

Uchiyama T. Tropism and pathogenicity of rickettsiae. *Frontier Microbio.* 2012;3(23):1-7.

Valbuena G., Bradford W., Walker DH. Expression analysis of the T-cell-targeting chemokines CXCL9 and CXCL10 in mice and humans with endothelial infections caused by Rickettsiae of the spotted fever group. *Amer J Pathol.* 2003;163(4):1357-69.

Valbuena G., Walker DH. Effect of blocking the CXCL9/10-CXCR3 chemokine system in the outcome of endothelial-target Rickettsial infections. *Am J Trop Med.* 2004;71(4):393-99.

Vitorino L. et al. Rickettsiae phylogeny: A multigenic approach. *Microbio.*2007;153:160-68.

Walker DH. The realities of biodefense vaccines against Rickettsia. *Vaccine.* 2009;27(Suppl 4):D52-D55.

Walker DH. Rickettsia Rickettsii: As virulent as ever. *Am J Trop Med Hyg.* 2002;66(5):448-9. Editorial.

Walker DH. Rickettsiae. *Med Microbio.-NCBI.*1996.

Walker DH. Rickettsiae and rickettsial infections: The current state of knowledge. *Clin Infect Dis.* 2007;45:539-44.

Walker DH. et al. Cytokine-induced, nitric oxide-dependent, intracellular antirickettsial activity of mouse endothelial cells. *Lab Invest.* 1997;76(1):129-38.

Wallmenius K. et al. Spotted fever Rickettsia species in Hyalomma and Ixodes ticks infesting migratory birds in the European Mediterranean area. *Parasit Vectors.* 2014;7:318.

Weinert LA. et al Evolution and diversity of Rickettsia bacteria. *BMC Biology.* 2009;7(6):1-15

Woods ME. Host defenses to Rickettsia rickttsii infection contribute to increased microvascular permeability in human cerebral endothelial cells. *J Clin Immunol.* 2008;28(2):174-85.

Woods ME., Wen G., Olano JP. Nitric oxide as a mediator of increased microvascular permeability during acute rickettsioses.*Ann N Y Acad Sci.* 2005;1063:239-45.

Woodward T. Remember Rocky Mountain spotted fever – A lesson in ethical principles. *Clin Infect Dis.*1996;23:165-6. Editorial.

Polygonum cuspidatum

Agarwal B. et al. Resveratrol for primary prevention of atherosclerosis: clinical trial evidence for improved gene expression in vascular endothelium. *Int J Cardiol.* 2013;166(1):246-48.

Azachi M. et al. A novel red grape cells complex: health effects and bioavailability of natural resveratrol. *Int J Food Sci Nutr.* 2014;65(7):848-55.

Bailey J. The Japanese knotweed invasion viewed as a vast unintentional hybridisation experiment. *Heredity (Edinb).*2013;110(2):105-10.

Ban SH. et al. Effects of a bio-assay guided fraction from Polygonum cuspidatum root on the viability, acid production and glucosyltranferase of mutans streptococci. *Fitoterapia.* 2010;81(1):30-4.

Benova B. et al. Analysis of selected stilbenes in Polygonum cuspidatum by HPLC coupled with CoulArray detection. *J Sep Sci.* 2008;31(31):2404-9.

Bhatt JK., Thomas S., Nanjan MJ. Resveratrol supplementation improves glycemic crol in type 2 diabetes mellitus. *Nutr Res.* 2012;32(7):537-41.

Bo S. et al. Anti-inflammatory and antioxidant effects of resveratrol in healthy smokers a randomized, double-blind, placebo-controlled, cross-over trial. *Curr Med Chem.*2013;20(10):1323-31.

Bralley EE. et al. Topical anti-inflammatory activity of Polygonum cuspidatum extract in the TPA model of mouse ear inflammation. *J Inflamm.* 2008;5:1.

Brasnyo P. et al. Resveratrol improves insulin sensitivity, reduces oxidative stress and activates the Akt pathway in type 2 diabetic patients. *Br J Nutr.* 2011;106(3):383-9.

Breen, DM, et al, Resveratrol inhibits neointimal formation after arterial injury through an endothelial nitric oxide synthase-dependent mechanism. *Atherosclerosis* 2012; 222(2): 375-81.

Buluc, M and Demirel-Yilmaz, E. Resveratrol decreases calcium sensitivity of vascular smooth muscle and enhances cytosoliccalcium increase in endothelium. *Vascular Pharmacology* 2006; 44(4): 231-7.

Campos-Toimil, M, et al, Trans- and cis-resveratrol increase cytoplasmic calcium levels in A7r5 vascular smooth muscle cells. *Molecular Nutrition and Food Research* 2005; 49(5): 396-404.

Chang JS. et al. Ethanol extract of Polygonum cuspidatum inhibits hepatitis B virus in a stable HBV-producing cell line. *Antiviral Res.* 2005;66(1):29-34.

Chanim H. et al. A resveratrol and polyphenol preparation suppresses oxidative and inflammatory stress response to a high-fat, high-carbohydrate meal. *J Clin Endocrinol Metab.* 2011;96(5):1409-14.

Chen KT. et al. Active neuraminidase constituents of Polygonum cuspidatum against influenza A(H1N1) influenza virus. *Zhongguo Zhong Yao Za Zhi.* 2012;37(20):3068-73.

Chen Y. et al. Anti-oxidant polydatin (piceid) protects against substantia nigral motor degeneration in multiple rodent models of Parkinson's disease. *Mol Neurodegener.* 2015;10(1):4.

Chen YB., Sun BX., Chen JX. Study on the stability of resveratrol in rhizoma polygoni cuspidati. *Zhong Yao Cai.* 2007;30(7):805-7.

Cheng Y. et al. Involvement of cell adhesion molecules in polydatin protection of brain tissues from ischemia-reperfusion injury. *Brain Res.* 2006;1110(1):193-200.

Chi YC., Lin SP., Hou YC. A new herb-drug interaction of Polygonum cuspidatum, a resveratrol-rich nutraceutical, with carbamazepine in rats. *Toxicol Appl Pharmacol.* 2012;263(3):315-22.

Chueh FS. Crude extract of Polygonum cuspidatum stimulates immune responses in normal mice by increasing the percentage of Mac-3-positive cells and enhancing macrophage phagocytic activity and natural killer cell cytotoxicity. *Mol Med Rep.* 2015;11(1):127-32.

Clark, D, et al, Protection against recurrent stroke with resveratrol: Endothelial protection. *PloS One* 2012; 7(10): e47792.

Coenye T. et al Eradication of Propionibacterium acnes biofilms by plant extracts and putative identification of icariin, resveratrol and salidroside as active compounds. *Phytomedicine.* 2012;19(5):409-12.

Crandall JP. et al. Pilot study of resveratrol in older adults with impaired glucose tolerance. *J Gerontol A Biol Sci Med Sci.* 2012;67(12):1307-12.

Cudic M. et al. Analysis of flavonoid-based pharmacophores that inhibit aggrecanases (ADAMTS-4 and ADAMTS-5) and matrix metalloproteinases through the use of topologically constrained peptide substrates. *Chem Biol Drug Des.* 2009;74(5):473-82.

Deng YH. et al. Inhibition of TNF-a-mediated endothelial cell-monocyte cell adhesion and adhesion molecules expression by the resveratrol derivative, trans-2,5,4'-trimethoxystilbene. *Phytother Res.* 2011;25(3):451-7.

Dommanget F. et al. Differential allelopathic effects of Japanese knotweed on willow and cottonwood cuttings used in riverbank restoration techniques. *J Environ Manage.* 2014;132:71-8.

Dong J. et al. Identification and determination of major constituents in Polygonum cuspidatum Sieb. et Zucc. by high performance liquid chromatography/electrospray ionization-ion trap-time-of-flight mass spectrometry. *Se Pu.* 2009;27(4):425-30.

Dong, M, et al, Effects of emodin on expression of Smad3 in rats with hepatic fibrosis induced by carbon tetrachloride. *Chinese Journal of Traditional Chinese Medicine and Pharmacy;* 2013-02.

Dorbrydneva Y., Williams RL., Blackmore PF. Trans-resveratrol inhibits calcium influx in thrombin-stimulated human platelets. *Br J Pharmacol.* 1999;128(1):149-57.

Du J. et al. Lipid-lowering effects of polydatin from Polygonum cuspidatum in hyperlipidemic hamsters. *Phytomedicine.* 2009;16(6-7):652-8.

Estrov Z. et al, Resveratrol blocks interleukin-1B-induced activation of the nuclear transcription factor Nf-kB, inhibits proliferation, causes S-phase arrest and induces apoptosis of acute myeloid leukemia cells. *Blood* 2003; 102(3): 987-95.

Fan P., Zhang T., Hostettmann K. Anti-inflammatory activity of the invasive neophyte Polygonum cuspidatum Sieb. and Zucc. (Polygonaceae) and the chemical comparison of the invasive and native varieties with regard to resveratrol. *J Tradit Complement Med.* 2013;3(3):182-187.

Fan P. et al. Rapid separation of three glucosylated resveratrol analogues from the invasive plant Polygonum cuspidatum by high-speed countercurrent chromatography. *J Sep Sci.* 2009;32(17):2979-84.

Fujitaka K. et al. Modified resveratrol Longevinex improves endothelial function in adults with metabolic syndrome receiving standard treatment. *Nutr Res.* 2011;31(11):842-7.

Gao JP et al. Effects of polydatin on attenuating ventricular remodeling in isoproterenol-induced mouse and pressure-overload rat models. *Fitoterapia.* 2010;81(7):953-60.

Ghanim H. et al. An anti-inflammatory and reactive oxygen species suppressive effects of an extract of Polygonum cuspidatum containing resveratrol. *J Clin Endocrinol Metab.* 2010;95(9):E1-8.

Gocmen AY., Burgucu D., Gumuslu S. Effect of resveratrol on platelet activation in hypercholesterolemic rats: CD40-CD40L system as a potential target. *Appl Physiol Nutr Metab.* 2011;36(3):323-30.

Goh KP. et al. Effects of resveratrol in patients with type 2 diabetes mellitus on skeletal muscle SIRT1 expression and energy expenditure. *Int J Sport Nutr Exerc Metab.* 2014;24(1):2-13.

Han JH. et al. Analgesic and anti-inflammatory effects of ethyl acetate fraction of Polygonum cuspidatum in experimental animals. *Immunopharmacol Immunotoxicol.* 2012;34(2):191-5.

Han SY. et al. Resveratrol inhibits lgE-mediated basophilic mast cell degranulation and passive cutaneous anaphylaxis in mice. *J Nutr.* 2013;143(5):632-9.

Hsu CY., Chan YP., Chang J. Antioxidant activity of extract from Polygonum cuspidatum. *Biol Res.* 2007;40(1):13-21.

Hu B. et al. Polygonum cuspidatum extract induces anoikis in hepatocarcinoma cells associated with generation of reactive oxygen species and downregulation of focal adhesion kinase. *Evid Based Complement Alternat Med.* 2012;2012:607675.

Huang T. et al. Resveratrol inhibits oxygen-glucose deprivation-induced MMP-3 expression and cell apoptosis in primary cortical cells via the NF-kB pathway. *Molecular Medicine Reports* 2014; 10(2): 1065-71.

Huang W. et al. Piperine potentiates the antidepressant-like effect of trans-resveratrol: involvement of monoaminergic system. *Metab Brain Dis.* 2013;28(4):585-95.

Huang WY. et al. Comparative analysis of bioactivities of four Polygonum species. *Planta Med.* 2008;74(1):43-9.

Ji Q. et al. Resveratrol inhibits invasion and metastasis of colorectal cancer cells via MALAT1 mediated Wnt/B-catenin signal pathway. *PLoS One.* 8(11):e78700.

Jiang QL. et al. Variances of leptin mRNA in the adipose tissue of NAFLD rats intervened with the extracts of Polygonum cuspidatum compound. *Zhong Yao Cai.* 2007;30(8):974-7.

Kennedy DO. et al. Effects of resveratrol on cerebral blood flow variables and cognitive performance in humans: A double-blind, placebo-controlled, cross-over investigation. *Am J Clin Nutr.* 2010;91(6):1590-7.

Kim J. et al. Key compound groups for the neuroprotective effects of roots of Polygonum cuspidatum on transient middle cerebral artery occlusion in Sprague-Daley Rats. *Nat Prod Res.* 2010;24(13):1214-26.

Kim JR. et al. Protective effect of polygoni ciuspidati radix and emodin on Vibrio bulnificus cytotoxicity and infection. *J Microbiol.* 2008;46(6):737-43.

Kim KW. et al. Polygonum cuspidatum, compared with baicalin and berberine, inhibits inducible nitric oxide synthase and cyclooxygenase-2 gene expressions in RAW 264.7 macrophages. *Vascul Pharmacol.* 2007;47(2-3):99-107.

Kim YS. et al. Polygonum cuspidatum inhibits pancreatic lipase activity and adipogenesis via attenuation of lipid accumulation. *BMC Complement Altern Med.* 2013;13:282.

Kirino A. et al. Analysis and functionality of major Polyphenolic components of Polygonum cuspidatum (Itadori). *J Nutr Sci Vitaminol.* 2012;58:278-86.

Kumar, A, et al, Emodin (3-methyl-1, 6, 8-trihydroxyanthraquinone) inhibits TNF-induced NF-kappaB activation, IkappaB degradation, and expression of cell surface adhesion proteins in human vascular endothelial cells. *Oncogene* 1998; 17: 913-8.

Kuo YC. et al. Regulation of cell proliferation, inflammatory cytokine production and calcium mobilization in primary human T lymphocytes by emodin from Polgonum hypoleucum Ohwi. *Inflamm Res.* 2001;50(2):73-82.

Kurita S. et al. Content of resveratrol and glycoside and its contribution to the antioxidative capacity of Polygonum cuspidatum (Itadori) harvested in Kochi. *Biosci Biotechnol Biochem.* 2014;78(3):499-502.

Lee CC. et al. Polygonum cuspidatum extracts as bioactive antioxidation, anti-tyrosinase, immune stimulation and anticancer agents. *J Biosci Bioeng.* 2014;pii:S1389-1723(14)00343-0.

Lee MH. et al. Comparison of the antioxidant and transmembrane permeative activities of the different Polygonum cuspidatum extracts in phospholipid-based microemulsions. *J Agric Food Chem.* 2011;59(17):9135-41.

Leu YL. et al. Anthroquinones from Polygonum cuspidatum as tyrosinase inhibitors for dermal use. *Phytother Res.* 2008;22(4):552-6.

Li F. et al. Polyflavanostilbene A, a new flavanol-fused stilbene glycoside from Polygonum cuspidatum. *Org Lett.* 2013;15(3):674-7.

Li RP. et al. Polydatin protects learning and memory impairments in a rat model of vascular dementia. *Phytomedicine.* 2012;19(8-9):677-81.

Li W. et al, Intra-articular resveratrol injection prevents osteoarthritis progression in a mouse model by activating SIRT1 and thereby silencing HIF-2a. *Journal of Orthopedic Research* 2015; 33(7): 1061-70.

Li X. et al. The action of resveratrol, a phytoestrogen found in grapes, on the intervertebral disc. *Spine (Phila Pa 1976).* 2008;33(24):2586-95.

Li Y. et al. Inhibitory effect of polydatin on expression of toll-like receptor 4 in ischemia-reperfusion injured NRK-52E cells. *Zhongguo Zhong Yao Za Zhi.* 2014;39(16):3157-61.

Li YB. et al. Protective, antioxidative and antiapoptotic effects of 2-methoxy-6-acetyl-7-methyljuglone from Polygonum cuspidatum in PC12 cells. *Planta Med.* 2011;77(4):354-61.

Lim BO. et al. Polygoni cuspidati radix inhibits the activation of Syk kinase in mast cells for antiallergic activity. *Exp Biol Med (Maywood).* 2007;232(11):1425-31.

Lin CJ. et al. Polygonum cuspidatum and its active components inhibit replication of the influenza virus through toll-like receptor 9-induced interferon beta expression. *PLoS One.* 2015;10(2):e0117602.

Lin HW. et al. Anti-HIV activities of the compounds isolated from Polygonum cuspidatum and Polygonum multiflorum. *Planta Med.* 2010;76(9):889-92.

Lin QQ. et al. SIRT1 regulates TNF-a-induced expression of CD40 in 3T3-L1 adipocytes via NF-kB pathway. *Cytokine* 2012; 60(2): 447-55.

Lin SP. et al. Pharmacokinetics and tissue distribution of resveratrol, emodin and their metabolites after intake of Polygonum cuspidatum in rats. *J Ethnopharmacol.* 2012;144(3):671-6.

Lin YL. et al. Resveratrol protects against oxidized LDL-indicated breakage of the blood-brain barrier by lessening disruption of tight junctions and apoptotic insults to mouse cerebrovascular endothelial cells. *J Nutr.* 2010;140:2187-92.

Lin YW. et al. Free radical scavenging activity and antiproliferative potential of Polygonum cuspidatum root extracts. *J Nat Med.* 2010;64(2):146-52.

Liu D. et al. Resveratrol prevents impaired cognition induced by chronic unpredictable mild stress in rats. *Prog Neuropsychopharmacol Biol Psychiatry.* 2014;49:21-9.

Liu F. et al. Neuroprotective naphthalene and flavan derivatives from Polygonum cuspidatum. *Phytochemistry.* 2015110:150-9.

Liu GS. et al. Resveratrol attenuates oxidative damage and ameliorates cognitive impairment in the brain of senescence-accelerated mice. *Life Sci.* 2012;91(17-18):872-7.

Liu J. et al. Small-molecule STAT3 signaling pathway modulators from Polygonum cuspidatum. *Planta Med.* 2012;78(14):1568-70.

Liu K. et al. Effect of resveratrol on glucose control and insulin sensitivity: A meta-analysis of 11 randomized controlled trials. *Am J Clin Nutr.* 2014;99(6):1510-9.

Liu LT. et al. Clinical study on treatment of carotid atherosclerosis with extraction of polygoni cuspidati rhizoma et radix and crataegi fructus: A randomized controlled trail. *Zhonogguo Zhong Yao Za Zhi.* 2014;39(6):1115-9.

Liu T. et al. Neuroprotective effects of emodin in rat cortical neurons against beta-amyloid-induced neurotoxicity. *Brain Res.* 2010;1347:149-60.

Liu Z. et al. In vitro and in vivo studies of the inhibitory effects of emodin isolated from Polygonum cuspidatum on Coxsakievirus B4. *Molecules.* 2013;18(10):11842-58.

Liu Z. et al, Resveratrol reduces intracellular free calcium concentration in rat ventricular myocytes. *Shen li xue bao [Acta Physiologia Sinica]* 2005; 57(5): 599-604.

Liu ZO. et al. Effects of tans-resveratrol from Polygonum cuspidatum on bone loss using the ovariectomized rat model. *J Med Food.* 2005;8(1):14-9.

Long J. et al. Grape extract protects mitochondria from oxidative damage and improves locomotor dysfunction and extends lifespan in a Drosophila Parkinson's disease model. *Rejuvenation Res.* 2009;12(5):321-31.

Ma C. et al. Anti-inflammatory effect of resveratrol through the suppression of NF-kB and JAK/STAT signaling pathways. *Acta Biochim Biophys Sin (Shanghai).* 2015;pii:gmu135.

Mabrouk ME. et al. Curcumin, nordihydroguiaretic acid, quercetin and resveratrol inhibit interleukin-1-induced ADAMTS-4 (Aggrecanase-1) gene expression in articular chondrocytes: Natural products as potential anti-arthritic agents. *Parmacologyonline 3.* 2006:601-610.

Macedo RC. et al. Effects of chronic resveratrol supplementation in military firefighters undergo a physical fitness test – placebo-controlled, double blind study. *Chem Biol Interact.* 2015;227:89-95.

Magyar K. et al. Cardioprotection by resveratrol: A human clinical trial in patients with stable coronary artery disease. *Clin Hemorheol Microcirc.* 2012;50(3):179-87.

Miao Q. et al. Cardioprotective effect of polydatin against ischemia/reperfusion injury: roles of protein kinase C and mito K(ATP) activation. *Phytomedicine.* 2011;19(1):8-12.

Militaru C. et al. Oral resveratrol and calcium fructoborate supplementation in subjects with stable angina pectoris: effects on lipid profiles, inflammation markers, and quality of life. *Nutrition.* 2013;29(1):178-83.

Mobasheri A. et al. Scientific evidence and rationale from the development of cucumin and resveratrol as nutraceutricals for joint health. *Int J Mol Sci.* 2012;13:4202-32.

Pandit S. et al. Enhancement of fluoride activity against Streptococcus mutans biofilms by a substance separated from Polygonum cuspidatum. *Biofouling.* 2012;28(3):279-87.

Park CE. et al. Resveratrol stimulates glucose transport in C2C12 myotubes by activating AMP-activated protein kinase. *Exp Mol Med.* 2007;39(2):222-9.

Patel KR. et al. Clinical pharmacology of resveratrol and its metabolites in colorectal cancer patients. *Cancer Res.* 2010;70(19):7392-9.

Peng W. et al. Botany, phytochemistry, pharmacology, and potential application of Polygonum cuspidatum Sieb.et Zucc.: A review. *J Ethnopharmacol.* 2013;148(3):729-45.

Pitozzi V. et al. Chronic resveratrol treatment ameliorates cell adhesion and mitigates the inflammatory phenotype in senescent human fibroblasts. *J Germatol Biol Med Sci.* 2013;68(4):371-81.

Potter KA. et al. The effect of resveratrol on neurodegeneration and blood brain barrier stability surrounding intracortical microelectrodes. *Biomaterials.* 2013;34:7001-15.

Poulsen MM. et al. High-dose resveratrol supplementation in obese men: An investigator-initiated, randomized, placebo-controlled clinical trial of substrate metabolism, insulin sensitivity, and body composition. *Diabetes.* 2013;62(4):1186-95.

Qian Y. et al. A geochemical study of toxic metal translocation in an urban brownfield wetland. *Environ Pullut.* 2012;166:23-30.

Quin G. et al. Optimization and validation of a chromatographic method for the simultaneous quantification of six bioactive compounds in Rhizoma et Radix Polygoni cuspidati. *J Pharm Pharmacol.* 2008;60(1):107-13.

Richards CL., Schrey AW., Pigliucci M. Invasion of diverse habitats by few Japanese knotweed genotypes is correlated with epigenetic differentiation. *Ecol Lett.* 2012;15(9):1016-25.

Richer S. et al. Observation of human retinal remodeling in octogenarians with a resveratrol based nutritional supplement. *Nutrients.* 2013;5(6):1989-05.

Rouifed S. et al. Invasive knotweeds are highly tolerant to salt stress. *Environ Manage.* 2012;50(6):1027-34.

Saha A. et al. The blood-brain barrier is disrupted in a mouse model of infantile neuronal ceroid lipofuscinosis: Amelioration by resveratrol. *Human Molecular Gen.* 2012;10.1093:1-12.

Sareen D., et al. Mitochondria, calcium, and calpain are key mediators of resveratrol-induced apoptosis in breast cancer. *Mol Parmacol.* 2007;72(6):1466-75.

Shen B. et al. An in vitro study of neuroprotective properties of traditional Chinese herbal medicines thought to promote healthy ageing and longevity. *BMC Complement Altern Med.* 2013;13:373.

Shen MY. et al. Combined phytochemistry and chemotaxis assays for identification and

mechanistic analysis of anti-inflammatory phytochemicals in Fallopia japonica. *PLoS One.* 2011;6(11):e27480.

Shin JA. et al. Apoptotic effect of Polyonum cuspidatum in oral cancer cells through the regulation of specificity protein 1. *Oral Dis.* 2011;17(2):162-70.

Shiyu S. et al. Polydatin up-regulates Clara cell secretory protein to suppress phospholipase A2 of lung induced by LPS in vivo and in vitro. *BMC Cell Biol.* 2011;12:31.

Song JH. In vitro effects of a fraction separated from Polygonum cuspidatum root on the viability, in suspension and biofilms, and biolflim formation of mutans streptococci. *J Ethnopharmacol.* 2007;112(3):419-25.

Song JH. et al. In vitro inhibitory effects of Polygonum cuspidatum on bacterial viability and virulence factors of Streptococcus mutans and Streptococcus sobrinus. *Arch Oral Biol.* 2006;51(2):1131-40.

Storniolo CE. et al. Piceid presents antiproliferative effects in intestinal epithelial Caco-2 cells, effects unrelated to resveratrol release. *Food Funct.* 2014;5(9):2137-44.

Su JL. et al. Resveratrol induces FasL-related apoptosis through Cdc42 activation of ASK1-JNK-dependent signaling pathway in human leukemia HL-60 cells. *Carcinogenesis.* 2005;26(1):1-10.

Sun J. et al. Protective effect of polydatin on learning and memory impairments in neonatal rats with hypoxic-ischemic brain injury by up-regulating brain-derived neurotrophic factor. *Mol Med Rep.* 2014;10(6):3047-51.

Svajger, U, et al, Dendritic cells treated with resveratrol during differentiation from monocytes gain substantial tolerogenic properties upon activation. *Immunology* 2010; 129(4): 525-35.

Tian C. et al. Resveratrol ameliorates high-glucose-induced hyperpermeability mediated by caveolae via VEGF/KDR pathway. *Genes Nutr.* 2013;8(2):231-9.

Tian J. et al. Resveratrol inhibits TNF-a-induced IL-1B, MMP-3 production in human rheumatoid arthritis fibroblast-like synoviocytes via modulation of PI3kinase/Akt pathway. *Rheumatol Int.* 2013;33(7):1829-35.

Tome-Carneiro J. et al. One-year consumption of a grape nutraceutical containing resveratrol improves the inflammatory and fibrinolytic status of patients in primary prevention of cardiovascular disease. *Am J Cardiol.* 2012;110(3):356-63.

Tome-Carneiro J. et al. One-year supplementation with a grape extract containing resveratrol modulates inflammatory-related microRNAs and cytokines expression in peripheral blood monocuclear cells of type 2 diabetes and hypertensive patients with coronary artery disease. *Pharmacol Res.* 2013;72:69-82.

Varinska L. et al. Antiangongenic effect of selected phytochemicals. *Pharmazie.* 2010;65:57-63.

Wang C. et al. Neuroprotective effects of emodin-8-O-beta-D-glucoside in vivo and in vitro. *Eur J Pharmacol.* 2007;577(1-3):58-63.

Wang D., Xu Y., Liu W. Tissue distribution and excretion of resveratrol in rat after oral administration of Polygonum cuspidatum extract (PCE). *Phtomedicine*. 2008;15(10):859-66.

Wang L. et al. Effects of resveratrol on calcium regulation in rats with severe acute pancreatitis. *Eur J Pharmacol*. 2008;580(1-2):271-6.

Wang W. et al. The protective effect of fenofibrate against TNF-a-induced CD40 expression through SIRT1-mediated deacetylation of NF-kB in endothelial cells. *Inflammation* 2014; 37(1): 177-85.

Wang Y. et al. Protective effect of resveratrol derived from Polygonum cuspidatum and its liposomal form on nigral cells in parkinsonian rats. *J Neurol Sci*. 2011;304(1-2):29-34.

Wightman EL. et al. Effects of resveratrol alone or in combination with piperine of cerebral blood flow parameters and cognitive performance in human subjects: A randomized, double blind, placebo-controlled, cross-over investigation. *Br J Nutr*. 2014; 112(2):203-13.

Witte AV. et al. Effects of resveratrol on memory performance, hippocampal functional connectivity, and glucose metabolism in healthy other adults. *J Neurosci*. 34(23):7862-70.

Wu XB. et al. The effect of Polygonum cuspidatum extract on wound healing in rats. *J Ethnopharmacol*. 2012;141(3):934-7.

Wuertz, K, et al. The red wine polyphenol resveratrol shows promising potential for the treatment of nucleus pulposus-mediated pain in vitro and in vivo. *Spine* 2011; 36(21): e1373-84.

Xia L. et al. Resveratrol reduces endothelial progenitor cells senescence through augmentation of telemerase activity by Akt-dependent mechanisms. *Brit J Pharmacol*. 2008;155:387-94.

Xiao K. et al. Constituents from Polygonum cuspidatum. *Chem Pharm Bull*. 2002;50(5):605-08.

Xie Q. et al. Resveratrol-4-O-D-(2'galloyl)-glucopyranoside isolated from Polygonum cuspidatum exhibits anti-hepatocellular carcinoma viability by inducing apoptosis via the JNK and ERK pathway. *Molecules*. 2014;19(2):1592-602.

Xio HT. et al. Membrane permeability-guided identification of neuroprotecive components from Polygonum cuspidatun. *Pharm Biol*. 2014;52(3):356-61.

Xu Y. et al. Antidepressant-like effect of trans-resveratrol: Involvement of serotonin and noradrenaline system. *Eur Neuropsychopharmacol*. 2010;20(6):405-13.

Xue Y., Liang J. Screening of bioactive compounds in Rhizoma Polygoni Cuspidati with hepatocyte membranes by HPLC and LC-MS. *J Sep Sci*.2014;37(3):250-6.

Yang L. et al. Sirt1 regulates CD40 expression induced by TNF-a via NF-kB pathway in endothelial cells. *Cellular Physiology and Biochemistry* 2012; 30(5): 1287-98.

Yang YM. et al. Resveratrol attenuates adenosine diphosphate-induced platelet activation by reducing protein kinase C activity. *Am J Chin med*. 2008;36(3):603-13.

Yiu CY. et al. Inhibition of Epstein-Barr lytic cycle by an ethyl acetate subfraction separated from Polygonum cuspidatum root and its major component, emodin. *Molecules*. 2014;19(1):1258-72.

Yu SH. et al. Contents comparison of resveratrol and polydatin in the wild Polygonum cuspidatum plant and its tissue cultures. *Zhongguo Zhong Yao Za Zhi*. 2006;31(8):637-41.

Yu Y. et al. Antidepressant-like effect of trans-resveratrol in chronic stress model: behavioral and neurochemical evidences. *J Psychiatr Res*. 2013;47(3):315-22.

Zahedi HS. et al. Effects of Polygonum cuspidatum containing resveratrol on inflammation in male professional basketball players. *Int J Prev Med*. 2013;4(Suppl 1):S1-4.

Zhang H. et al. A review of the Pharmacological effects of the dried root of Polygonum cuspidatum (Hu Zhang) and its constituents. *Evidence Based Complement Altern Med*. 2013;208349:1-13.

Zhang J. et al. Polydatin alleviates non-alcoholic fatty liver disease in rats by inhibiting the expression of TNF-a and SREBP-1c. *Mol Med Rep*. 2012;6(4):815-20.

Zhang L. et al. Resveratrol inhibits enterovirus 71 replication and pro-inflammatory cytokine secretion in Rhabdosarcoma cells. *PLoS One*. 2015;10(2):e0116879.

Zhang Q. et al. Polydatin supplementation ameliorates diet-induced development of insulin resistance and hepatic steatosis in rats. *Mol Med Rep*. 2015;11(1):603-10.

Zhang Y. et al. Polydatin inhibits growth of lung cancer cells by inducing apoptosis and causing cell cycle arrest. *Oncol Lett*. 2014;7(1):295-301.

Zuo K. et al. FTIR specta-pricial component analysis of roots of Polygonum cuspidatum from different areas. *Guang Pu Xue Yu Guang Pu Fen Xi*. 2007;27(10):1989-92.

Uncaria

Ahn SM. et al. Neuroprotective effect of 1-methoxyoctadecan-1-ol from Uncaria sinensis on glutamate-induced hippocampal neuronal cell death. *J Ethnopharmacol*. 2014;155(1):293-9.

Bednarek D. et al. Analysis of phenotype and functions of peripheral blood leukocytes in cellular immunity of calves treated with Uncaria tomentosa. *Bull Vet Inst Pulawy*. 2004;48:289-96.

Chik SC. et al. Pharmacological effects of active compounds on neurodegenerative disease with gastrodia and Uncaria decoction, a commonly used poststroke decoction. *ScientificWorldJournal*. 2013;896873:1-2.

Cowden WL. et al. Pilot study of pentacyclic alkaloid-chemotype of Uncaria tomentosa for the treatment of Lyme disease. *Presented Internat Sympos Nat Treatment Intracell Micro Organisms*. 2003;March(29).1-7.

Datar A. et al. In vitro effectiveness of Samento and Banderol herbal extracts on the different Morphological forms of Borrelia Burgdoferi. *Townsend Lett. Exam Altern Med*. 2010;07:1-9.

de Caires S., Seenkamp V. Use of Yokukansan (TJ-54) in the treatment of neurological disorders: A review. *Phytother Res.* 2010;24(9):1265-70.

Fernandes Vattimo NMF., Oliveira da Silva N. et al. Uncaria tomentosa and acute ischemic kidney injury in rats. *Rev Esc Enferm USP.* 2011;45(1):189-93.

Fuiwara H. et al. Uncaria rhynchophylla, a Chinese medicinal herb, has potent antiaggregation effects on Alzheimer''s B-Amyloid protein. *J Neurosci Res.* 2006;84:427-33.

Gan R. et al. Protective effects of isorhynchophylline on cardiac arrhythmia in rats and guinea pigs. *Planta Med.* 2011;77(13):1477-81.

Ge Z. et al.. Pharmacokinetic comparative study of gastrodin and rhynchophylline after oral administration of different prescriptions of Yizhi tablets in rats by an HPLC-ESI/MS method. *Evid Base Complement Altern Med.* 2014;167253:1-1-10.

He Y. et al. Effects of rhynchophylline on GluN1 and GluN2B expressions in primary cultured hippocampal neurons. *Fitoterapia.* 2014;98:166-73.

Heitzman ME. et al. Ethnobotany, phytochemistry and pharmacology of Uncaria (Rubiaceae). *Phytochem.* 2004;66:5-29.

Ho TY. et al. Uncaria rhynchophylla and rhynchophylline improved kainic acid-induced epileptic seizures via IL-1B and brain-derived neurotrophic factor. *Phytomedicine.* 2014;21(6):893-900.

Hsieh CL. et al. Uncaria rhynchophylla and rhynchophylline inhibit c-Jun N-terminal kinase phosphorylation and nuclear factor-kappaB activity in kainic acid-treated rats. *Am J Chin Med.* 2009;37(2):351-60.

Hsieh SL. et al. Anticonvulsant effect of Uncaria rhynchophylla (Miq) Jack. in rats with kainic acid-induced epileptic seizure. *Am J Chin Med.* 1999;27(2):257-64.

Huang H. et al. Neuroprotective effects of rhynchophylline against ischemic brain injury via regulation of the Akt/mTOR and TLRs signaling pathways. *Molecules.* 2014;19:11196-11210.

Huang ZQ. et al. A study on the chemical change in the decoction of Uncaria hook. *J NW Univ.(Nat Sci Edition.* 2008;05:1.

Jang JY. et al. Hexane extract from Uncaria sinensis exhibits anti-apoptotic properties against glutamate-induced neurotoxicity in primary cultured cortical neurons. *Int J Mol med.* 2012;30(6):1465-72.

Jung HY. et al. Hirsutine, an indole alkaloid of Uncaria rhynchophylla, inhibits inflammation-mediated neurotoxicity and microglial activation. *Mol Med Rep.* 2013;7(1):154-8.

Kanno I I. et al. Glycyrrhiza and Uncaria Hook contribute to protective effect of traditional Japanese medicine yokukansan against amyloid B oligomer-induced neuronal death. *J Ethnopharmacol.* 2013;149(1):360-70.

Keplinger K. et al. Uncaria tomentosa (Willd.) DC.– Ethnomedicinal use and new pharmacological, toxicological and botanical results. *J Ethnopharmacol.* 1999;64:23-34.

Kim DY. et al. Oral administration of Uncaria rhynchophylla inhibits the development of DNFB-induced atopic dermatitis-like skin lesions via IFN-gamma down-regulation in NC/Nga mice. *J Ethnopharmacol.* 2009;122(3):567-72.

Kim JH. et al. Uncaria rhynchophylla inhibits the production of nitric oxide and interleukin-1B through blocking nuclear factor kB, Akt, and mitogen-activated protein kinase activation in macrophages. *J Med Food.* 2010;13(5):1133-40.

Kushida H. et al. Simultaneous quantitative analyses of indole and oxindole alkaloids of Uncaria Hook in rat plasma and brain after oral administration of the traditional Japanese medicine Yokukansan using high-performance liquid chromatography with tandem mass spectrometry. *Biomed Chromatogr.* 2013;27(12):1647-56.

Lee CJ. et al. Determination of protein-unbound rhynchophylline brain distribution by microdialysis and ultra-performance liquid chromatography with tandem mass spectrometry. *Biomed Chromatogr.* 2014;28(6):901-6.

Lee J. et al. Alkaloid fraction of Uncaria rhynchophylla protects against N-methyl-D-aspartate-induced apoptosis in rat hippocampal slices. *Neurosci Lett.* 2003;348(1):51-5.

Lee J. et al. Protective effect of methanol extract of Uncaria rhynchophylla against excitotoxicity induced by N-Methyl-D-Aspartate in rat hippocampus. *J Pharmacol Sci.* 2003;92:70-73.

Li SG. et al. Non-alkaloid components from Uncaria sinensis (Oliv.) Havil. and their chemotaxonomic significance. *J Med Plant Res.* 2011;5(19):4962-67.

Lin YW., Hsieh CL. Oral Uncaria rhynchophylla (UR) reduces kainic acid-induced epileptic seizures and neuronal death accompanied by attenuating glial cell proliferation and S100B proteins in rats. *J Ethnopharmacol.* 2011;135(2):313-20.

Liu W. et al. Protective effect of Uncaria rhynchophylla total alkaloids pretreatment on hippocampal neurons after acute hypoxia. *Zhongguo Zhong Yao Za Zhi.* 2006;31(9):763-5.

Lu WY. et al. Uncaria rhynchophylla upregulates the expression of MIF and cyclophilin A in kainic acid-induced epilepsy rats: A proteomic analysis. *Am J Chin Med.* 2010;38(4):745-59.

Lu JH. et al. Isorhynchophylline, a natural alkaloid, promotes the degradation of alpha-synuclein in neuronal cells via inducing autophagy. *Autophagy.* 2012;8(1):98-108.

Mai QX. et al. Study on effects of Uncaria tomentosa on CNS. *Strait Pharma J.* 2009;02:1.

Masumiya H. et al. Effects of hirsutine and dihydrocorynantheine on the action potentials of sino-atrial node, atrium and ventricle. *Life Sci.* 1999;65(22):2333-41.

Matsumoto K. et al. Kampo Formulations, Chotosan, and Yokukansan, for dementia therapy: Existing clinical and preclinical evidence. *J Pharmacol Sci.* 2013;122:257-69.

Mizoguchi K. et al. Specific binding and characteristics of geissoschizine methyl ether, an indole alkaloid of Uncaria Hook, in the rat brain. *J Ethnopharmacol.* 2014;158 Pt.A:264-70.

Morita S. et al. Geissoschizine methyl ether, an alkaloid from the Uncaria hook, improves remyelination after cuprizone-induced demyelination in medial prefrontal cortex of adult mice. *Neurochem Res.* 2014;39(1):59-67.

Nishi A. et al. Geissoschizine methyl ether, an alkaloid in Uncaria hook, is a potent serotonin 1A receptor agonist and candidate for amelioration of aggressiveness and sociability by yokukansan. *Neuroscience.* 2012;207:124-36.

Pilarski R. et al. Antiproliferative activity of various Uncaria tomentosa preparations on HL-60 promyelocytic leukemia cells. *Parmacol Rep.* 2007;59:565-72.

Qin F. The clinical effects comparision of Tianmagoutengyin and Tianmagouteng particle on treating hypertension. *Chin Mod Med.* 2010;10:1-2.

Qu J. et al. Comparative study of fourteen alkaloids from Uncaria rhynchophylla hooks and leaves using HPLC-Diode array detection-atmospheric pressure chemical ionization/MS method. *Chem Pharm Bull.* 2012;60(1):23-30.

Reinhard KH. Uncaria tomentosa (Willd.) D.C.: Cat's Claw, Una de Gato, or Saventaro. *J Altern Comp Med.* 1999;5(2):143-51.

Sheng Y. et al. Induction of apoptosis and inhibition of proliferation in human tumor cells treated with extracts of Uncaria tomentosa. *Anticanacer Res.* 1998;18(5A):3363-8.

Shi JS. et al. Pharmacological actions of Uncaria alkaloids, rhynchophylline and isorhynchophylline. *Acta Pharmacol Sin.* 2003;24(2):97-101.

Shim JS. et al. Effects of the hook of Uncaria rhynchophylla on neurotoxicity in the 6-hydroxydopamine model of Parkinson's disease. *J Ethnopharmacol.* 2009;126(2):361-5.

Shin SC., Lee DU. Ameliorating effect of new constituents from the hooks of Uncaria rhynchophylla on scopolamine-induced memory impaiment. *Chin J Nat Med.* 2013;11(4):391-5.

Song Y. et al. Rhynchophylline attenuates LPS-induced pro-inflammatory responses through down-regulation of MAPK/NF-kB signaling pathways in primary microglia. *Phytother Res.* 2012;26(10):1528-33.

Suk K. et al. Neuroprotection by methanol extract of Uncaria rhynchophylla against global cerebral ischemia in rats. *Life Sci.* 2002;70(21):2467-80.

Tanaka Y., Sakiyama T. Potential usefulness of the kampo medicine Yukukansan, containing Uncaria hook, for paediatric emotional and behavioural disorders: A case series. *Evid Base Complem Altern Med.* 2013;502726:1-4.

Tang NY. et al. Uncaria rhynchophylla (miq) Jack plays a role in neuronal protection in kainic acid-treated rats. *Am J Chin Med.* 2010;38(2):251-63.

Tao ZY. et al. Studies on the chemical constituents of Uncaria yunanensis Hsia. C.C. *Yao Xue Xue Bao.* 2001;36(2):120-2.

Wang HB. et al. Qualitative and quantitative analyses of alkaloids in Uncaria species by UPLC-ESI-Q-TOF/MS. *Chem Pharm Bull.* 2014;62(11):1100-09.

White G., Bourbonnais-Spear N., Garner F. Antibacterial constituents from Uncaria tomentosa. *Phytopharmacology.* 2011;1(2):16-19.

Winkler C. et al. In vitro effects of two extracts and two pure alkaloid preparations of Uncaria tomentosa on peripheral blood mononuclear cells. *Planta Med.* 2004;70:205-10.

Wu JY., Li GC., Wang DY. Chemical constituents of the non-alkaloid fraction of Uncaria macrophylla. *Nan Fang Yi Ke Da Xue Xue Bao.* 2007;27(2):226-7.

Wu LX. et al. Protective effects of novel single compound, hirsutine on hypoxic neonatal rat cardiomyocytes. *Eur J Pharmacol.* 2011;650(1):290-7.

Wu YT., Lin LC., Tsai TH. Determination of rhynchophylline and hirsutine in rat plasma by UPLC-MS/MS after oral administration of Uncarcia rhynchophylla extract. *Biomed Chromatogr.* 2014;28(3):439-45.

Wurm M. et al. Pentacyclic oxindole alkaloids from Uncaria tomentosa induce human endothelial cells to release a lymphocyte-proliferation-regulating factor. *Planta Med.* 1998;64(8):701-4.

Xian YF. et al. Bioassay-guided isolation of neuroprotective compounds from Uncaria rhynchophylla against beta-amyloid-induced neurotoxicity. *Evid Bas Complement Altern Med.* 2012;802625:1-8.

Xian YF. et al. Isorhynchophylline improves learning and memory impairments induced by D-galactose in mice. *Neurochem Int.* 2014;76:42-9.

Xian YF. et al. Protective effect of isorhynchophylline against B-amyloid-induced neurotoxicity in PC 12 cells. *Cell Mol Neurobiol.* 2012;32(3):353-60.

Xian YF. et al. Uncaria rhynchophylla ameliorates cognitive deficits induced by D-galactose in mice. *Planta Med.* 2011;77(18):1977-83.

Xu DD. et al. Rhynchophylline protects cultured rat neurons against methamphetamine cytotoxicity. *Evid Base Complement Altern Med.* 2012;636091:1-7.

Yang J., Song CQ., Hu ZB. Studies on constituents in Uncaria macrophylla Wall. *Zhongguo Zhong Yao Za Zhi.* 2000;25(8):484-5.

Ye ST. et al. Efficacy of compound Uncaria hypotensive tablet on hypertensive disease with left ventricular hypertrophy of complex syndrome of yin deficiency yang excess and blood stasis: a clinical research of 31 cases. *Guid J Trad Chin Med Pharm.* 2013;05:1-3.

Yimam M. et al. UP3005, a botanical composition containing two standardized extracts of Uncaria gambir and Morus alba, improves pain sensitivity and cartilage degradation in monosodium iodoacetate-induced rat OA disease model. *Evid Base Complement Altern Med.* 2015;785638:1-10.

Yu Z. et al. Survey on traditional medicinal resources of Uncaria distributed in China. *Zhongguo Zhong Yao Za Zhi.* 1999;24(4):198-202,254.

Yuan D. et al. Alkaloids from the leaves of Uncaria rhynchophylla and the inhibitory activity on NO production in lipoplysaccharide-activated microglia. *J Nat Prod.* 2008;71(7):1271-4.

Yuan D. et al. Anti-inflammatory effects of rhynchophylline and isorhynchophylline in mouse N9 microglial cells and the molecular mechanism. *Int Immunopharmacol.* 2009;9(13-14):1549-54.

Zhang C. Effects of gastrodia and Uncaria decoction on blood pressure and nitric oxide in patients with hypertension of liver yang hyperactivity. *J Integrat Trad Chin West Med.* 2011;28:1-2.

Andrographis paniculata

Akbar S. Andrographis paniculata: a review of pharmacological activities and clinical effects. *Altern Med Rev.* 2011;16(1):66-75.

Akbarsha MA. et al. Antifertility effect of Andrographis paniculata (Nees) in male albino rat. *Indian J Exp Biol.* 1990;28(5):421-6.

Arifullah M. et al. Evaluation of anti-bacterial and anti-oxidant potential of andrographolide and echiodinin isolated from callus culture of Andrographis paniculata Nees. *Asian Pac J Trop Biomed.* 2013;3(8):604-10.

Bera R. et al. Pharmacokinetic analysis and tissue distribution of andrographolide in rat by a validated LC-MS/MS method. *Pharm Biol.* 2014;52(3):321-9.

Bhatter P. et al. Antimycobacterial Efficacy of Andrographis paniculata leaf extracts under intracellular and hypoxic conditions. *J Evid Based Complementary Altern Med.* 2015;20(1):3-8.

Chao WW., Lin BF. Isolation and identification of bioactive compounds in Andrographis paniculata. *Chinese Med.* 2010;5:1-17.

Chen HW. et al. Inhibition of TNF-a-induced inflammation by andrographolide via down-regulation of the P12K/Akt signaling pathway. *J Nat Prod.* 2011;74(11):2408-13.

Chen YY. et al. Andrographolide inhibits nuclear factor-kB activation through JNK-Akt-p65 signaling cascade in tumor necrosis factor-a-stimulated vascular smooth muscle cells. *ScientificWorldJournal.*

Chien CF. et al. Herb-drug interaction of Andrographis paniculata extract and andrographolide on the pharmacokinetics of theophylline in rats. *Chem Biol Interact.* 2010;184(3):458-65.

Chu W. et al. Effect of traditional Chinese herbal medicine with antiquorum sensing activity on pseudomonas aeruginosa. *Evid based Complement Alternat Med.*

Coon JT., Ernst E. Andrographis paniculata in the treatment of upper respiratory tract infections: a systematic review of safety and efficacy. *Planta Med.* 2004;70:293-98.

Dua VK. et al. Andrographis paniculata. *J Ethnopharmacol.* 2004;95(2-3):247-51.

Hossain S. et al. Andrographis paniculata (Burm.f.) Wall. ex Nees: a review of ethnobotany, phytochemistry and pharmacology. *Sci World J.* 2014;274905:1-28.

Jarukamjorn K., Nemoto N. Pharmacological aspects of Andrographis paniculata on health and its major diterpenoid constituent Andrographolide. *J Health Sci.* 2008;54(4):370-81.

Jayakumar T. et al. Experimental and clinical pharmacology of Andrographis paniculata and its major bioactive phytoconstituent andrographolide. *Evident Base Complem Altern Med.* 2013;846740:1-16.

Jua Z. et al. Andrographolide inhibits intracellular Chlamydia trachomatis multiplication and reduces secretion of proinflammatory mediators produced by human epithelial cells. *Pathog Dis.* 2015;73(1):1-11.

Kale RS. et al. Anti-scorpion venom activity of Andrographis paniculata: a combined and comparative study with anti-scorpion serum in mice. *Anc Sci Life.* 2013;32(3):156-60.

Lee W. et al. Andrographolide inhibits HMGB1-induced inflammatory responses in human umbilical vein endothelial cells and in urine polymicrobial sepsis. *Acta Physiol (Oxf).* 2014;211(1):176-87.

Lee WR. et al. Suppression of matrix metalloproteinase-9 expression by andrographolide in human monocytic THP-1 cells via inhibition of NF-kB activation. *Phytomedicine.* 2012;19(3-4):270-7.

Low M. et al. An in vitro study of anti-inflammatory activity of standardized Andrographis paniculata extracts and pure andrographolide. *BMC Complement Altern Med.* 2015;15:18.

Lu CY. et al. Andrographolide inhibits TNFa-induced ICAM-1 expression via suppression of NADPH oxidase activation and induction of HO-1 and GCLM expression through the P13K/Akt/Nrf2 and P13K/Akt/AP-1 pathways in human endothelial cells. *iochem Pharmacol.* 2014;91(1):40-50.

Luo LK. Andrographolide enhances proliferation and prevents dedifferentiation of rabbit articular chondrocytes: an in vitro study. *Evid Based Complement Alternat Med.* 2015;2015:984850.

Malahubban M. et al. Phytochemical analysis of Andrographis paniculata and Orthosiphon stamineus leaf extracts for their antibacterial and antioxidant potential. *Trop Biomed.* 2013;30(3):467-80.

Mishra K. et al. Anti-malarial activities of Andrographis paniculata and Hedyotis corymbosa extracts and their combination with curcumin. *Malaria J.* 2009;8(26):1-9.

Mishra SK. et al. Andrographolide and analogues in cancer prevention. *Front Biosci (Elite Ed).* 2015;7:255-66.

Mishra US. et al. Antibacterial activity of ethanol extract of Andrographis paniculata. *Indian J Pharm Sci.* 2009;71(4):436-38.

Misra P. et al. Antimalarial activity of Andrographis paniculata (kalmegh) against Plasmodium berghei NK 65 in Mastomys natalensis. *Pharmaceutical Bio.* 1992;30(4):263-74.

Ojha SK. et al. Protective effect of hydroalcoholic extract of Andrographis paniculata on ischaemia-reperfusion induced myocardial injury in rats. *Indian J Med Res.* 2012;135:414-21.

Panossian A. et al. Pharmacokinetic and oral bioavailability of andrographolide from Andrographis paniculata fixed combined Kan Jang in rats and human. *Phytomed.* 2000;7(5):351-64.

Premendran SJ. et al. Anti-cobra venom activity of plant Andrographis paniculata and its comparison with polyvalent anti-snake venom. *J Nat Sci Biol Med.* 2011;2(2):198-204.

Radhika P., Annapurna A., Rao SN. Immunostimulant, cerebroprotective & nootropic activities of Andrographis paniculata leaves extract in normal & type 2 diabetic rats. *Indian J Med Res.* 2012;135(5):636-41.

Rao YK. et al. Flavonoids and andrographolides from Andrographis paniculata. *Phytochem.* 2004;65:2317-2321.

Serrano FG. et al. Andrographolide reduces cognitive impairment in young and mature AbetaPPswe/PS-1 mice. *Mol Neurodegener.* 2014;9(1):61.

Suwankesawong W. et al. Characterization of hypersensitivity reactions reported among Andrographis paniculata users in Thailand using health product vigilance center (HPVC) database. *BMC Complement Alt Med.* 2014;14(515):7-7.

Tang LI. et al. Screening of anti-dengue activity in methanolic extracts of medicinal plants. *BMC Complement Altern Med.* 2012;12:1-3.

Thakur AK. et al. Protective effects of Andrographis paniculata extract and pure andrographolide against chronic stress-triggered pathologies in rats. *Cell Mol Neurobiol.* 2014;34(8):1111-21.

Wong SY. et al. Andrographolide attenuates interleukin-1B-stimulated upregulation of chemokine CCL5 and glial fibrillary acidic protein in astrocytes. *Neuroreport.* 2014;25(12):881-6.

Yu Z. et al. Andrographolide ameliorates diabetic retinopathy by inhibiting retinal angiogenesis and inflammation. *Biochem Biophys Acta.* 2015;1850(4):824-31.

Zein U., Fitri LE., Saragih A. Comparative study of antimalarial effect of sambiloto (Andrographis paniculata) extract, chloroquine and artemisinin and their combination against plasmodium falciparum in-vitro. *Acta Med Indones.* 2013;45(1):38-43.

Zhang WX. et al. Andrographolide induced acute kidney injury: analysis of cases reported in Chinese literature. *Nephrology (Carlton).* 2014;19(1):21-6.

Zhu T. et al. Andrographolide protects against LPS-induced acute lung injury by inactivation of NF-kB. *PLoS One.* 2013;8(2):e56407.

Herbs, General

Abdelmonem AM., Rasheed SM., Mohamed ASh. Bee-honey and yogurt: a novel mixture for treating patients with vulvovaginal candidiases during pregnancy. *Arch Gynecol Obstet.* 2012;286(1):109-14.

Achaieb K. et al. Antibacterial activity of thymoquinone, and active principle of Nigella sativa and its potency to prevent bacterial biofilm formation. *BMC Complement Altern Med.* 2011;11:29.

Adonizio A. et al. Inhibition of Quorum sensing-controlled virulence factor production in Pseudomonas aeruginosa by South Florida plant extracts. *Antimicrob Agents Chemotherapy.* 2008;52(1):198-203.

Adonizio AL. et al. Anti-quorum sensing activity of medicinal plants in southern Florida. *J Ethno Pharmacol.* 2006;105:427-35.

Akagi M. et al. Anti-allergic effect of tea-leaf saponin (TLS) from tea leaves (Camellia sinensis var. sinensis). *Biol Pharm Bull.* 1997;20(5):565-7.

Al-Sahaibani S., Murugan K. Anti-biofilm activity of Salvadora persica on cariogenic isolates of Streptococcus persica on cariogenic isolates of Streptococcus mutans: In vitro and molecular docking studies. *Biofouling.* 2012;28(1):19-38.

Alternative Medicine Review. Berberine Monograph. *Alt Med Rev.* 2000;5(2):175-177.

Amin K. et al. Binding of Galanthus nivalis lectin to Chlamydia trachomatis and inhibition of in vitro infection. *APMIS.* 1995;103(10):714-20.

Andreotti R. et al. Protection action of Targets minuta (Asteraceae) essential oil in the control of Rhipicephalus microplus (Canestrini, 1887) (Acari: Ixodide) in a cattle pen trial. *Vet Parasitol.* 2013;197(1-2):341-5.

Arakawa M., Ito Y. N-acetylcysteine and neurodegenerative diseases: basic and clinical pharmacology. *Cerebellum.* 2007;6(4):308-14.

Arena A. et al. Antiviral and immunomodulatory effect of a lyophilized extract of Capparis spinosa L. buds. *Phytother Res.* 2008;22(3):313-7.

Arfan M. et al. Analgesic and anti-inflammatory activities of 11-0-galoylbergenin. *J Ethnopharmacol.* 2010;131(2):502-4.

Azam MM. et al. Pharmacological potentials of Melia azedarach L. – a review. *Amer J BioSci.* 2013;1(2):44-49.

Bae MJ. et al. Inhibitory effect of unicellular green algae (Chlorella vulgaris) water extract on allergic immune response. *J Sci Food Agric.* 2013;93(12):3133-6.

Baek EB. et al. Inhibition of arterial myogenic responses by a mixed aqueous extract of Salvia miltiorrhiza and Panax notoginseng (PASEL) showing hypertensive effects. *Korean J Physiol Pharmacol.* 2009;13:287-93.

Balogh EP. et al. Anti-chlamydial effect of plant peptides. *Acta Microbiol Immunolog Hungarica.* 2014;61(2):231-41.

Banaclocha MM. Therapeutic potential of N-acetylcysteine in age-related mitochondrial neurodegenerative diseases. *Med Hypotheses.* 2001;56(4):472-7.

Bhengraj AR. et al. Assessment of antichlamydial effects of a novel polyherbal tablet Basant. *Sex Transm Infect.* 2009;85(7):561.

Birdsall TC., Kelly GS. Berberine: Therapeutic potential of an alkaloid found in several medicinal plants. *Altern. Med Rev.* 1997;2(2):97-103.

Bubik MF. et al. A novel approach to prevent endothelial hyperpermeability: The Crataegus extract WS 1442 targets the cAMP/Rap1 pathway. *J Mol Cell Cardiol.* 2012;52(1):196-205.

Cao Y. et al. In vitro activity of baicalein against Candida albicans biofilms. *Int J Antimicrob Agents.* 2008;32(1)73-7.

Chai OH. et al. Inhibitory effects of Morus alba on compound 48/80-induced anaphylactic reactions and anti-chicken gamma globulin IgE-mediated mast cell activation. *Biol Pharm Bull.* 2005;28(10):1852-8.

Chang C-Z., Wu S-C., Kwan A-L. Magnesium lithospermate B, and active extract of Salvia miltiorrhiza, mediates sGC/cGMP/PKG translocation in experimental vasospasm. *BioMed Res Internat.* 2014;272101:1-9.

Chen MK. et al. Effects of Salvia miltiorrhiza on Chlamydia trachomatis mice of salpingitis. *Zhongguo Zhong Yao Za Zhi.* 2007;32(6):523-5.

Chen PN. et al. Silibinin inhibits invasion of oral cancer cells by suppressing the MAPK pathway. *J Dent Res.* 2006;85(3):220-5.

Chen PN. et al. Silibinin inhibits cell invasion through inactivation of both P13K-Akt and MAPK signaling pathways. *Chem Biol Interact.* 2005;156(2-3):141-50.

Cheng HJ. et al. Effects of compound Baifuqing on biofilm formation and the recurrence rate in the rat model with bacterial vaginosis. *Chinese Archiv Trad Chinese Med.* 2007;02:1-3.

Cheng HJ. et al. The in vitro effects of heartleaf houttuynia herb decoction against Pseudomonas aeruginosa biofilms and its synergism with azithromycin on planktonic Pseudomonas aeruginosa. *Lishizhen Med Materia Medica Res.* 2012;07:1-3.

Cheng Q. et al. Comparison of the effects of Gingko biloba extract and minocycline hydrochloride on periodontitis. *Zhonghua Kou Qiang Yi Xue Za Zhi.* 2014;49(6):347-51.

Cheng Q. et al. Effects of Gingko biloba extract on periodontal pathogens and its clinical efficacy as adjuvant treatment. *Chin J Integr Med.* 2014;20(10):729-36.

Chiu JH. et al. Cordyceps sinensis increases the expression of major histocompatibility complex class II antigens on human hepatoma cell line HA22T/VGH cells. *Am J Chin Med.* 1998;26(2):159-70.

Choi IY. et al. Observations of Forsythia koreana methanol extract on mast cell-mediated allergic reactions in experimental models. *In Vitro Cell Dev Biol Anim.* 2007;43(7):215-21.

Choi JH. et al. Effects of SKI 306X, a new herbal agent, on proteoglycan degradation in cartilage explant culture and collagenase-induced rabbit osteoarthritis. *Osteoarthritis Cartilage.* 2002;10:471-78.

Choi YH. and Yan GH. Pycnogenol inhibits immunoglobulin E-mediated allergic response in mast cells. *Rhytother Res.* 2009;23(12):1691-5.

Choi YH. and Yan GH. Silibinin attenuates mast cell-mediated anaphylaxis-like reactions. *Biol Pharm Bull.* 2009;32(5):868-75.

Choi YH. et al. Inhibitory effects of Agaricus blazei on mast cell-mediated anaphylaxis-like reactions. *Biol Pharm Bull.* 2006;29(7):1366-71.

Dai Y. et al. Effects of oleanolic acid on immune system and type I allergic reaction. *Zhongguo Yao Li Xue Bao.* 1989;10(4):381-4.

Dai Y. et al. Inhibition of immediate allergic reactions by ethanol extract from Plumbago zeylanica stems. *Biol Pharm Bull.* 2004;27(3):429-32.

Dean O., Giorlando F., Berk M. N-acetylcysteine in psychiatry: Current therapeutic evidence and potential mechanisms of action. *J Psychiatry Neurosci.* 2011;36(2):78-86.

Dietrich G. et al. Repellent activity of fractioned compounds from Chamaecyparis nootkatensis essential oil against nymphal Ixodes scapularis (Acari: Ixodidae). *J med Entomol.* 2008;43(5):957-61.

Ding X. et al. Screening for novel quorum-sensing inhibitors to interfere with the formation of Pseudomonas aeruginosa biofilm. *J Med Microbiol.* 2011;60:1827-34.

Dolan MC. et al. Ability of two natural products, nootkatone and carvacrol, to suppress Ixodes scapularis and Amblomma americanum (Acari:Ixodidae) in a Lyme disease endemic area of New Jersey. *J Econ Entomol.* 2009;102(6):2316-24.

Dulak J. Nutraceuticals as anti-angiogenic agents: Hopes and reality. *J Physiol Pharmac* 2005;56 (Suppl 1):51-69.

Dumlao DS. et al. Dietary fish oil substitution alters the eicosanoid profile in ankle joints of mice during Lyme infection. *J Nutr.* 2012;142(8):1582-9.

Dwivedi D., Singh V. Effects of the natural compounds embelin and piperine on the biofilm-producing property of Streptococcus mutans. *J Trad Complement Med.* 2015:1-15.

Elisabetsky, E. Phytotherapy and the new paradigm of drugs mode of action, *Scientia et Technica* 2007; 12(33): 459-64.

El-Nakeeb MA. et al. Membrane permeability alteration of some bacterial clinical isolates by selected anthihistaminics. *Brazil J Microbio.* 2011;42:992-1000.

Fan C. ct al. Exploration of inhibitors for diaminopimelate aminotransferase. *Bioorg Med Chem.* 2010;18(6):2141-51.

Fan TP. et al. Angiogenesis: From plants to blood vessels. *TRENDS Pharmacolog Sci.* 27(60):301.

Figueieredo NL. et al. The inhibitory effect of Plectranthus barbatus and Plectranthus ecklonii leaves on the viability, glucosyltransferase activity and biofilm formation of Streptococcus sobrinus and Streptococcus mutans. *Food Chem.* 2010;119(2):664-68.

Frekiaer H. et al. Astragalus root and elderberry fruit extracts enhance the IFN-B stimulatory effects of Lactobacillus acidophilus in murine-derived dendritic cells. *PLoS One.* 2012;7(10):e47878.

Fukui H. et al. Novel functions of herbal medicines in dendritic cells: role of Amomi semen in tumor immunity. *Microbiol. Immunol.* 2007;51(11):1121-33.

Furumoto T. et al. Mallotus philippinensis bark extracts promote preferential migration of mesenchymal stem cells and improve wound healing in mice. *Phytomedcine.* 2014;21(3):247-53.

Gangwar M., Goel R.K., Nath G. Mallotus philippinensis Muell. Arg (Euphorbiaceae): Ethnopharmacology and phytochemistry review. *BioMed. Resear Intern.* 2014;213973.1-13.

Gangwar M. et al. Antioxidant capacity and radical scavenging effect of polyphenol rich Mallotus philippenensis fruit extract on human erythrocytes: an in vitro study. *Scientific World J.* 2014;279451.

Gangwar M. et al. In-vitro scolicidal activity of Mallotus philippinensis (Lam.) Muell arg. fruit glandular hair extract against hydatid cyst echinococcus granulosus. *Asian Pac J Trop Med.* 2013; 6(8):595-601.

Gardulf A., Wohlfart I., Gustafson R. A prospective cross-over field trial shows protection of lemon eucalyptus extract against tick bites. *J Med Entomol.* 2004;41(6):1064-7.

Girish, KS and Kemparaju, K. Inhibition of Naja naja venom hyaluronidase by plant-derived bioactive components and polysaccharides, *Biochemistry* 2005; 70(8): 948-52.

Haide UK., Wake R., Patil N. Genus Sida: The plants with ethnomedicinal & therapeutic potential. *Golden Research THoughts.* 2011;1(V):1-4.

Hallahan TW. et al. Importance of asparagine-61 and asparagine-109 to the angiogenic activity of human angiogenin. *Biochemistry.* 1992;31(34):8022-9.

Han EH. et al. Houttuynia cordata water extract suppresses anaphylactic reaction and IgE-mediated allergic response by inhibiting multiple steps of FcepsilonRI signaling in mast cells. *Food Chem Toxicol.* 2009;47(7):1659-66.

Hao H. et al. Baicalin suppresses expression of Chlamydia protease-like activity factor in Hep-2 cells infected by Chlamydia trachomatis. *Fitoterapia.* 2009;80(7):448-52.

Hao H. et al. Baicalin suppresses expression of TLR2/4 and NF-kB in Chlamydia trachomatis-infected mice. *Immunopharmacol Immunotoxicol.* 2012;34(1):89-94.

Hao H. et al. Effects of baicalin on Chlamydia trachomatis infecion in vitro. *Planta med.* 2010;76(1):76-8.

Hasan S. et al. Efficacy of E. officinalis on the cariogenic properties of Streptococcus mutans: A novel and alternative approach to suppress quorum-sensing mechanism. *PLoS One.* 2012;7(7):e40319.

Hei Z-q. et al. Emodin inhibits dietary induced atherosclerosis by antioxidation and regulation of the sphingomyelin pathway in rabbits. *Chin Med J.* 2006:119(10):868-870.

Henrotin Y., Sanchez C., Reginster JY. The inhibition of metalloproteinases to treat osteoarthritis: Reality and new perspectives. *Expert Opin Therapeu Patents.* 2002;12(1):29-43.

Homer KA. et al. Inhibition of peptidase and glycosidase activities of Porphyromonas gingivalis, Bacteroides intermedius and Treponema denticola by plant extracts. *J Clin Periodontol.* 1992;19(5):305-10.

Hong Q. et al. Anti-tuberculosis compounds from Mallotus phiippinensis. *Nat Prod Commun.* 2010;5(2):211-7.

Hu W. et al. Puerarin inhibits adhesion molecule expression in TNF-alpha-stimulated human endothelial cells via modulation of the nuclear factor kappaB pathway. *Pharmacol.* 2010;85(1):27-35.

Huang H. et al. Clinical study of TCM combined with Western medicine treatment on Lyme disease. *Practic Preven Med.* 2005;02:1.

Huang Q. et al. Emodin inhibits tumor cell adhesion through disruption of the membrane lipid raft-associated integrin signaling pathway. *Cancer Res.* 2006;66(11):5807-15.

Huh JE. et al. Combined prescription (OAH19T) of Aralia cordata Thunb and Cimicifuga heracleifolia Komar and its major compounds inhibit matrix proteinases and vascular endothelial growth factor through the regulation of mitogen-activated protein kinase pathway. *J Ethnopharmacol.* 2011;135(2):414-21.

Hui-Chun Ho J., Hong C-Y. Salvianolic acids: Small compounds with multiple mechanisms for cardiovascular protection. *J BioMed Sci.* 2011;18(30):1-5.

Hutschenreuther A., et al. Growth inhibiting activity of volatile oil from Cistus creticus L. against Borrelia burgdorferi s.s. in vitro. *Pharmazie.* 2010;65(994):290-5.

Imada K. et al. Anti-arthritic action mechanisms of natural chondroitin sulfate in human articular chondrocytes and synovial fibroblasts. *Biol Pharm Bull.* 2010;33(3):410-4.

Imada K. et al. Nobiletin, a citrus polymethoxy flavonoid, suppresses gene expression and production of aggrecanases-1 and -2 in collagen-induced arthritic mice. *Biochem Biophys Res Commun.* 2008;373(2):181-5.

Ippoushi K. et al. Evaluation of inhibitory effects of vegetables and herbs on hyaluronidase and identification of rosmarinic acid as a hyaluronidase inhibitor in Lemon Balm (Melissa Officinalis L.) *Food Sci Tech Res.* 2000;6(1):74-77.

Issac Abraham SV. et al. Antiquorum sensing and antibiofilm potential of Capparis spinosa. *Arch Med Res.* 2011;42(8):658-68.

Jadhav S. et al. Inhibitory activity of yarrow essential oil on listeria planktonic cells and biofilms. *Food Control.* 2013(29):125-30.

Jang SI. et al. Tanshinone IIA inhibits LPS-induced NF-kB activation in RAW 264.7 cells: Possible involvement of the NIK-IKK, ERK1/2,p38 and JNK pathways. *Europ J Pharmacology.* 2006;542:1-7.

Jaenson TG., Palsson K., Borg-Karlson AK. Evaluation of extracts and oils of tick-repellent plants from Sweden. *Med Vet Entomol.* 2005;19(4):345-52.

Jafari S. et al. Cytotoxic evaluation of Melia azedarach in comparison with Azadirachta indica and its phytochemical investigation. *DARU J Pharmaceutical Sci.* 2013;21(37):1-7.

Jeong HJ. et al. Inhibitory effects of mast cell-mediated allergic reactions by cell cultured Siberian Ginseng. *Immunopharmacol Immunotoxicol.* 2001;23(1):107-17.

Jian LY. et al. In vitro activity and related mechanisms of action of baicalin in combination with levofloxacin on Pseudomonas aeruginose biofilms. *Chinese J Hospit Pharm.* 2012;14:1-3.

Jiang S-J. et al. Retinoic acid prevents Chlamydia pneumoniae induced foam cell development in a mouse model of atheroscelosis. *Microbes Infect.* 2008;10(12-13):1393-97.

Jordan RA. et al. Suppression of host-seeking Ixodes scapularis and Amblyomma americanum (Acari:Ixodidae) nymphs after dual applications of plant-derived acaricides in New Jersey. *J Econ Entomol.* 2011;104(2):659-64.

Kakegawa H., Matsumoto H., Satoh T. Inhibitory effects of some natural products on the activation of hyaluronidase and their anti-allergic actions. *Chem Pharm Bull (Tokyo)*. 1992.40(6):1439-42.

Kang B. et al. Abolition of anaphylactic shock by Solanum iyratum Thunb. *Int J Immunopharmacol*. 1997;19(11-12):729-34.

Kang TH. et al. Ailanthus altissima swingle has anti-anaphylactic effect and inhibits inflammatory cytokine expression via suppression of nuclear factor-kappaB activation. *In Vitro Cell Dev Biol Anim*. 2010;46(1):72-81.

Karthikeya A. et al. Antibiofilm activity of Dendrophthoe falcata against different bacterial pathogens. *Planta Med*. 2012;78(18):1918-26.

Kaul-Ghanekar R., Raina P. Potential of Nutraceuticals and medicinal plants in the management of osteoarthritis. *Acta Biologica Indica*. 2012;1(1):27-46.

Kemppainen T. et al. No observed local immunological response at cell level after five years of oats in adult coeliac disease. *Scand J Gastroenterol*. 2007;42(1):54-9.

Khan AV. et al. In vitro antibacterial potential of Melia azedarach crude leaf extracts against some human pathogenic bacteria strains. *Ethnobotanical leaflets*. 2008;12:439-45.

Khizer M., Reshma K. "Pomegranate" One more herbal agent against dental plaque/biofilm. *J Pearldent*. 2014;5(3):18-22.

Kim H. et al. Effect of Rehmannia glutinosa on immediate type allergic reaction. *Int J Immunopharmacol*. 1998;20(4-5):231-40.

Kim H. et al. Effect of Sophora flavescens Aiton extract on degranulation of mast cells and contact dermatitis induced by dinitrofluorobenzene in mice. *J Ethnopharmacol*. 2012;142(1):253-8.

Kim HM. et al. Antianaphylactic properties of eugenol. *Pharmacol Res*. 1997;36(6):475-80.

Kim HM. et al. Effect of Syzygium aromaticum extract on immediate hypersensitivity in rats. *J Ethnopharmacol*. 1998;60(2):125-31.

Kim HM. et al. The evaluation of the antianaphylactic effect of Oryza sativa L. subsp. Hsien Ting in rats. *Pharmacol Res*. 1999;40(1):31 6.

Kim HM. et al. Inhibitory effect of mast cell-mediated immediate-type allergic reactions by Cichoium intybus. *Pharmacol Res*. 1999;40(1):61-5.

Kim HM. et al. Inhibitory effect of mast cell-mediated immediate-type allergic reactions in rats by spirulina. *Biochem Pharmacol*. 1998;55(7):1071-6.

Kim HM. et al. Salviae radix root extract inhibits immunoglobulin E-mediated allergic reaction. *Gen Pharmacol*. 1999;32(5):603-8.

Kim HM. et al. The stem of Sinomenium acutum inhibits mast cell-mediated anaphylactic reactions and tumor necrosis factor-alpha production from rat peritoneal mast cells. *J Ethnopharmacol*. 2000;70(2):135-41.

Kim HM., Cho SH. Lavender oil inhibits immediate-type allergic reaction in mice rats. *J Pharm Pharmacol*. 1999;51(2):221-6.

Kim HM., Hong DR., Lee EH. Inhibition of mast cell-dependent anaphylactic reactions by the pigment of Polygonum tinctorium (Chung-Dae) in rats. *Gen Pharmacol*. 1998;31(3):361-5.

Kim HM., Yi JM., Lim KS. Magnoliae flos inhibits mast cell-dependent immediate-type allergic reactions. *Pharmacol Res*. 1999;39(2):107-11.

Kim KM. et al. HMCO5, herbal extract, inhibits NF-kB expression in lipopolysaccharide treated macrophages and atherosclerotic lesions in cholesterol fed mice. *J Ethno Pharmacology*. 2007;114(2007):316-24.

Kim SH. et al. Paeonol inhibits anaphylactic reaction by regulating histamine and TNF-a. *Interna Immunopharmacol*. 2004;4:279-87.

Kim SY. et al. Isodon japonicus inhibits mast cell-mediated immediate-type allergic reactions. *Immunoparmacol Immunotoxicol*. 2004;26(2):273-84.

Kitazato, K et al, Viral infectious disease and natural products with antiviral activity, *Drug Discov Ther* 2007; 1(1):14-22.

Koo H. et al. Apigenin and tt-farnesol with fluoride effects on S. mutans biofilms and dental caries. *J Dent Res*. 2005;84(11):1016-20.

Koo H. et al. Effects of apigenin and tt-farnesol on glucosyltransferase activity, biofilm viability and caries development in rats. *Oral Microbiol Immunol*. 2002;17(6):337-43.

Koo H. et al. Inhibition of Streptococcus mutans biofilm accumulation and polysaccharide production by apigenin and tt-farnesol. *J Antimicrob Chemother*. 2003;52(5):782-9.

Kuang Z. et al. Effect of baicalin on expression of adhesion molecules on human endothelial cells induced by Chlamydia pneumoniae. *J Guangzhou Univ Tradit Chinese Med*. 2004;06:1-4.

Lakhdar L. et al. Antibacterial activity of essential oils against periodontal pathogens: a qualitative systematic review. *O.S.T.-T.D.J*. 2012;35(N°140):38-46.

Lau D., Plotkin BJ. Antimicrobial ad biofilm effects of herbs used in traditional Chinese medicine. *Nat Prod Commun*. 2013;8(11):1617-20.

Lee EJ., Kim WJ., Moon SK. Cordycepin suppresses TNF-alpha-induced invasion, migration and matrix metalloproteinase-9 expression in human bladder cancer cells. *Phytother Res*. 2010;24(12):1755-61.

Lei L., Li Z., Zhong G. Rottlerin-mediated inhibition of Chlamydia trachomatis growth and uptake of sphingolipids is independent of p28-regulated/activated protein kinase (PRAK). *PLOS One*. 2012;7(9):e44733.

Li GZ. et al. Inhibitory effects of Houttuynia cordata water extracts on anaphylactic reaction and mast cell activation. *Biol Pharm Bull*. 2005;28(10):1864-8.

Li GZ., Chai OH., Song CH. Inhibitory effects of epigallocatechin gallate on compound 48/80-induced mast cell activation and passive cutaneous anaphylaxis. *Exp Mol Med*. 2005;37(4):290-6.

Li JJ. et al. Inhibitory activity of Dianthus superbus L. and 11 kinds of diuretic Traditional Chinese medicines for urogential Chlamydia trachomatis in vitro. *Zhongguo Zhong Yao Za Zhi*. 2000;25(10):628-30.

Li-Weber M. New therapeutic aspects of flavones: t\The anticancer properties of Scutellaria and its main active constituents wogonin, baicalein and baicalin. *Cancer Treat Rev.* 2009;35(!):57-68.

Lin CJ. et al. Bai-Hu-Tang, ancient Chinese medicine formula, may provide a new complementary treatment option for sepsis. *Eviden Bas Complemen Altern Med.* 2013;193084:1-8.

Liu Y. et al. Aqueous extract of rhubarb stabilizes vulnerable atherosclerotic plaques due to depression of inflammation and lipid accumulation. *Phythother Res.* 2008;22(7):935-42.

Machiah DK., Girish KS., Gowda V. A glycoprotein from a folk medicinal plant, Withania somnifera, inhibits hyaluronidase activity of snake venoms. *Comparat Biochem Physiol Pt.C: Toxicol Pharmacol.* 2006;143(2):158-61.

Maioli E. et al. Rollerin inhibits Ros formation and prevents NfkappaB activation in MCF-7 and HT-29 cells. *J Biomed Biotechnol.* 2009;2009:742936.

Malcomb, Jacob. Can an invasive herb affect Lyme disease risk? Examining the interactions between garlic mustard, entomopathogenic fungi, and blacklegged ticks, Bard College, online paper, 2010.

Marino A. et al. In vitro effect of branch extracts of Juniperus species from Turkey on Staphylococcus aureus biofilm. *FEMS Immunol Med Microbiol.* 2010;59(3):470-6.

Mehlhorn H., Schmahl G., Schmidt J. Extract of the seeds of the plant Vitex agnus castus proven to be highly efficacious as a repellent against ticks, fleas, mosquitoes and biting flies. *Parasitol Res.* 2005;95(5):363-5.

Meng F. et al. Research progress of the herbs of Senecio scandens. *J Northeast Agr Univ.* 2010;09:1.

Miyataka H. et al. Evaluation of propolis (II): e\ Effects of Brazilian and Chinese propolis on histamine release from rat peritoneal mast cells induced by compound 48/80 and concanavalin A. *Biol Pharm Bull.* 1998;21(7):723-9.

Mladenov IV. et al. Characterization of 20-kDa lectin-spermagglutinin from Arum maculatum that prevents Chlamydia pneumoniae infection of L-929 fibroblast cells. *FEMS Immunol Med Microbiol.* 2001;32(3):249-54.

Moncada-Pazos A. et al. The nutraceutical flavonoid luteolin inhibits ADAS4 and ADAMTS-5 aggrecanase activities. *J Mol Med.* 2011;155-163.

Murata T. et al. Hyaluronidase inhibitors from Takuran, Lycopus lucidus. *Chem Pharma Bull.* 2010;58(3):394-97.

Murugan K. et al. Antibiofilm and quorum sensing inhibitory activity of Achyranthes aspera on cariogenic Streptococcus mutans: an in vitro and in silico study. *Pharm Biol.* 51(6):728-36.

Murugan K. et al. In vitro and in silico screening for Andrographis paniculata quorum sensing mimics: New therapeutic leads for cystic fibrosis Pseudomonas aeruginosa biofilms. *Plant Omics.* 2013;20133364888:1-4.

Neelakantan P. et al. Effectiveness of curcumin against Enterococcus faecalis biofilm. *Acta Odontologica Scandinavica.* 2013:1-5.

Nelson J. et al. Cytomorphological changes and inhibition of inclusion body formation in Leptospira interrogans on treatment with fifteen extracts of Adhatoda vasica. *Adv Tech Biol Med.* 2013;1(1):1000101.

Nicolson GL., Settineri R., Ellithorpe RR. Neurodegenerative and fatiguing illnesses infections and mitochondrial dysfunction: use of natural supplements to improve mitochondrial function. *Funct Foods Health Dis.* 2014;4(1):23-65.

Nogami M. et al. Studies on Ganoderma lucidum. IV. Anti-allergic effect. (1). *Yakugaku Zasshi.* 1986;106(7):594-9.

Oh JY. et al. The ethyl acetate extract of Cordyceps militaris inhibits IgE-mediated allergic responses in mast cells and passive cutaneous anaphylaxis reaction in mice. *J Ethnopharmacol.* 2011;135(2):422-9.

Orlando KA., Pittman RN. Rho kinase regulates phagocytosis, surface expression of GlcNAc, and Golgi fragmentation of apoptotic PC12 cells. *Exp Cell Res.* 2006;312(17):3298-311.

Panella NA. et al. Susceptibility of immature Ixodes scapularis (Acari:Ixodidae) to plant-derived acaricides. *J Med Entomol.* 1997;34(3):340-5.

Park HJ. et al. Quercetin regulates Th1/Th2 balance in a murine model of asthma. *Int Immunopharmacol.* 2009;9(3):261-7.

Parzonko A., Naruszewicz M. Silymarin inhibits endothelial progenitor cells senescence and protects against the antiproliferative activity of rapamycin: Preliminary study. *Cardiovasc Pharmacol.* 2010;56(6):610-18.

Patidar A. et al. A review on advantages of natural analgesics over conventional synthetic analgesics. *CODEN(USA):IJPLCP.* 2014;5(5):3534-3539.

Piesman J. et al. Efficacy of an experimental azithromycin cream for prophylaxis of tick-transmitted Lyme disease spirochete infection in a murine model. *Antimicrob Agents Chemother.* 2014;58(1):348-51.

Politi FA. Acaricidal activity of ethanolic extract from aerial parts of Tagetes patula L. (Asteraceae) against larvae and engorged adult females of Rhipicephalus sanguineus (Latreille, 1806). *Parasit Vector.* 2012;5:295.

Politi FA. et al. Chemical characterization and acaricide potential of essential oil from aerial parts of Tagetes patula L. (Asteraceae) against engorged adult females of Rhipicephalus sanguineus (Latreille, 1806). *Parasitol Res.* 2013;112(6):2261-8.

Poovendran P., Ramanathan N., Prabhu N. Evaluation of the antibacterial activity of Aegle marmelos and Cassia siamea extracts against biofilm and extended spectrum B-lactamase producing uropathogenic Escherichia coli. *Internat J Microbiolog Res.* 2014;5(3):217-221.

Poovendran P., Vidhya N., Murugan S. Antimicrobial activity of Coccinia grandis against biofilm and ESBL producing uropathogenic E. coli. *Glob J Pharmacol.* 2011;5(1):23-26.

Prabhu N. et al. In vitro evaluation of Eclipta alba against serogroups of Leptosira interrogans. *Indian J Pharm Sci.* 2008;70(6):788-91.

Puolakkainen M. et al. Retinoic acid inhibits the infectivity and growth of Chlamydia pneumoniae in epithelial and endothelial cells through different receptors. *Microb Pathog.* 2008;44(5):410-16.

Quingchang H. Study of activities of five kinds of antimicrobial Chinese traditional medicine against Chlamydia trachomatis in Vitro. *Chine J Fam Planning.* 1998:05:1-2.

Ren XP. et al. Effects of Glycyrrhiza physic liquor and Glabrous crazyweed herb liquor on biofilm formation by Staphylococcus epidermidis. *Chinese J Veterin Sci.* 2013;01;1-4.

Saising J., Ongsakul M., Voravuthikunchai SP. Rhodomyrtus tomentosa (Aiton) Hassk ethanol extract and rhodomyrtone: A potential strategy for the treatment of biofilm-forming staphylococci. *J Med Microbiol.* 2011;60(PT12):1793-800.

Salin O. et al. Corn Mint (Mentha arvensis) extract diminishes acute Chlamydia pneumoniae infection in vitro and in vivo. *J Agric Food Chem.* 2011;59(24):12836-42.

Samprasit W. et al. Antibacterial activity of Garcinia mangostana extracts on oral pathogens. *Minerva Stomatol.* 2014;63(7-8):249-57.

Sandasi M. et al. Peppermint (Mentha piperita) inhibits microbial biofilms in vitro. *S African J Bot.* 2011;77(1):80-85.

Sandasi M., Leonard CM., Viljoen AM. The in vitro antibiofilm activity of selected culinary herbs and medicinal plants against Listeria monocytogenes. *Letters Appl Microbiol.* 2010;50(1):30-35.

Sandasi M., Viljoen A., Leonard C. The in vitro antimicrobial and antibiofilm activity of herbal extracts. *African J Trad Complemt Altern Med(AJTCAM).* 2008;nov(capetown):1-2.

Saravanan R., Saradhi P., Rani E. Effect of Phyllanthus amarus extract on SphH gene of Leptospira autumnalis studied by an in-house PCR. *Indian J Appl Microbiol.* 2012;15(2):40-45.

Sarkar R. et al. Anti-biofilm activity of Marula – a study with the standardized bark extract. *J Ethnopharmacol.* 2014;154(1):170-5.

Seesom W. et al. Antileptospiral activity of xanthones from Garcinia mangostana and synergy of gamma-mangostin with penicillin G. *BMC Complement Altern Med.* 2013;13:182.

Sessa R. et al. Effects of Mentha suaveolens essential oil on Chlamydia trachomatis. *BioMed Res Intern.* 2014;508071.

Shahripour RB., Harrigan MR., Alexandrov AV. N-acetylcysteine (NAC) in neurological disorders: mechanisms of action and therapeutic opportunities. *Brain Behavior.* 2014;4(2):108-22.

Shi TY., Kim HM. Inhibition of immediate-type allergic reactions by the aqueous extract of Salvia plebeia. *Immunopharmacol Immunotoxicol.* 2002;24(2):303-14.

Shin TY. Inhibition of immunologic and nonimmunologic stimulation-mediated anaphylactic reaction by the aqueous extract of Mentha arvensis. *Immunopharmacol Immunotoxicol.* 2003;25(2):273-83.

Shin TY., Kim YK., and Kim HM. Inhibition of immediate-type allergic reactions by Prunella vularis in a murine model. *Immunopharmacol Immunotoxicol.* 2001;23(3):423-35.

Shin TY. et al. Anti-allergic effects of Lycopus lucidus on mast cell-mediated allergy model. *Toxicol Appl Pharmacol.* 2005;209(3):255-62.

Shin TY. et al. Antiallergic action of Magnolia officinalis on immediate hypersensitivity reaction. *Arch Pharm Res.* 2001;24(3):249-55.

Shin TY. et al. Effect of Schizonepeta tenuifolia extract on mast cell-mediated immediate-type hypersensitivity in rats. *Immunopharmacol Immunotoxicol.* 1999;21(4):705-15.

Shin TY. et al. Inhibitory effect of mast cell-mediated immediate-type allergic reactions in rats by Perilla frutescens. *Immunopharmacol Immunotoxicol.* 2000;22(3):489-500.

Shin Y. et al. Inhibitory effect of anaphylactic shock by caffeine in rats. *Int J Immunopharmacol.* 2000;22(6):411-8.

Shin YW. et al. In vitro and in vivo antiallergic effects of Glycyrrhiza glabra and its components. *Planta Med.* 2007;73(3):257-61.

Shivshankar P. et al. Rottlerin inhibits chlamydial intracellular growth and blocks chlamydial acquisition of sphingolipids from host cells. *Appl Enviorn Microbiol.* 2008 74(4):1243-9.

Sinclair M. Environmental costs of pain management: Pharmaceuticals vs. physical therapies. *Integrat Med.* 2012;11(5):38-45.

Sohn Y. et al. Angelicae Gigantis Radix regulates mast cell-mediated allergic inflammation in vivo and in vitro. *Food Chem Toxicol.* 2012;50(9):2987-95.

Song Q. et al. Effect of Ginseng and Angelica sinensis decoction (GASD) on learning and memory of dementia rat with hippocampal lesions induced by quinolinic acid. *Chin Trad Herb Drugs.* 1994;09:1.

Spelman, et al, Modulation of cytokine expression by traditional medicines: A review of immunomodulators, *Alternative Medicine Review* 2006; 11(2): 128-50.

Sudati JH. et al. In vitro antioxidant activity of Valeriana officinalis against different neurotoxic agents. *Neurochem Res.* 2009;34(8):1372-9.

Sumantran, VN, et al. Hyaluronidase and collagenase inhibitory activities of the herbal formulatin Triphala guggulu. *Journal of Biosciences* 2007; 32(4): 755-61.

Takada K. et al. Ursolic acid and oleanolic acid, members of pentacyclic triterpenoid acids, suppress TNF-a-induced E-selectin expression by cultured umbilical vein endothelial cells. *Phytomedicine.* 2010;17(14):1114-9.

Talwar GP. et al. Praneem polymherbal cream and pessaries with dual properties of contraception and alleviation of genital infections. *Current Sci.* 1995;68(4):437-40.

Tang FY., Nguyen N., Meydani M. Green tea catechins inhibit VEGF-induced angiogenesis in vitro through suppression of VE-cadherin phosphorylation and inactivation of Akt molecule. *Int J Cancer.* 2003;106(6):871-8.

Taweechaisupapong S. et al. Antimicrobial effects of Boesenbergia pandurata and Riper sarmentosum leaf extracts on planktonic cells and biofilm of oral pathogens. *Pak J Pharm Sci.* 2010;23(2):224-31.

Tsai HR. et al. Andrographolide acts through inhibition of ERK1/2 and Akt phosphorylation to suppress chemotactic migration. *Eur J Pharmacol.* 2004;498(1-3):45-52.

Tsang CM. et al. Berberine inhibits Rho GTPases and cell migration at low doses but induces G2 arrest and apoptosis at high doses in human cancer cells. *Int J Mol Med.* 2009;24(1):131-8.

Tsuruga T. et al. Biologically active constituents of Magnolia salicifolia: Inhibitors of induced histamine release from rat mast cells. *Chem Pharm Bull(Tokyo).* 1991;39(12):3265-71.

Venier M. et al. Action of crude extracts of Melia azedarach L on the multiplication of Chlamydia in distinct cellular systems. *Rev Argent Microbiol.* 1999;31(Suppl 1):24-6.

Wang CZ. et al. In vitro activity of andrographolide against Candida albicans biofilms. *Chinese J Mycolog.* 2009;03:1-3.

Wang Q-Q. et al. In vitro inhibitive effects of 28 Chinese herbs on Chlamydia trachomatis and herpes simplex virus. *J China AIDS/STD.* 2004;04:1-3.

Wang Y., Hu Z., Lu W. Danhong injection: A modulator for Golgi structural stability after cerebral ischemia-reperfusion injury. *Neural Regen Res.* 2013;8(25):2343-49.

Wang X. et al. Berberine inhibits Staphylococcus epidermidis adhesion and biofilm formation on the surface of titanium alloy. *J Orthop Res.* 2009;27(11):1487-92.

Wang X. et al. Effect of berberine on Staphylococcus epidermidis biofilm formation. *Int J Antimicrob Agents.* 2009; 34(1):60-6.

Wang Y. et al. Anti-biofilm activity of TanReQing, a traditional Chinese medicine used for the treatment of acute pneumonia. *J Ethnopharmacol.* 2011;134(1)165-70.

Wang Z., Luo D. Chinese herbs and anti-infection immunity. *Internation J Biosci.* 2012;2(11):18-29.

Wang Z. et al. Melatonin alleviates secondary brain damage and neurobehavioral dysfunction after experimental subarachnoid hemorrhage: possible involvement of TLR4-mediated inflammatory pathway. *J Pineal Res.* 2013;55(4):399-408.

Wei H. et al. Traditional Chinese medicine Astragalus reverses predominance of Th2 cytokines and their up-stream transcript factors in lung cancer patients. *Oncol Rep.* 2003;10(5):1507-12.

Weniger B. et al. Antiprotozoal activities of Colombian plants. *J Ethnopharmacol.* 2001;78(2-3):193-200.

Wojnicz D. et al. Medicinal plants extracts affect virulence factors expression and biofilm formation by the uropathogenic Escherichia coli. *Urol Res.* 2012;40:683-97.

Xie GY. et al. The effects of compound baifuqing against mixed biofilms of vulvovaginal candidiasis. *Lishizhen Med Meteria Medica Res.* 2012;09:1-3.

Xing HC. et al. Effects of Salvia miltiorrhiza on intestinal microflora in rats with ischemia/reperfusion liver injury. *Hepatob Pancreat Dis Int.* 2005;4(2):274-80.

Xu Y. et al. The effect of herbal Sapanwood on the biofilm of Entercocus faecalis in starvation phase. *Chinese J Microecol.* 2013;07:1-2.

Xu Y. et al. Treatment with SiMiaoFang, an anti-arthritis Chinese herbal formula, inhibits cartilage matrix degradation in osteoarthritis rat model. *Rejuvenation Res.* 2013;16(5):364-76.

Yan F. et al. Berberine promotes recovery of colitis and inhibits inflammatory responses in colonic macrophages and epithelial cells in DSS-treated mice. *Am J Physiol Gastrointest Liv Physiol.* 2012;302:G504-G514.

Yang HN., Lee EH., Kim HM. Spirulina platensis inhibits anaphylactic reaction. *Life Sci.* 1997;61(13):1237-44.

Yang JH. et al. Anti-allergic activity of an ethanol extract from Salvia miltiorrhiza. *arch Pharm Res.* 2008;31(12):1597-603.

Yang L. et al. The effect of breviscapine on the pulmonary arterial pressure and the expression of Rho-kinase in pulmonary arterioles of hypoxic rats. *Zhonghua Jie He He Hu Xi Za Zhi.* 2008;31(11):826-30.

Yi JM. et al. Acanthopanax senticosus root inhibits mast cell-dependent anaphylaxis. *Clin Chim Acta.* 2001;312(1-2):163-8.

Yi JM. et al. Effect of Acanthopanax senticosus stem on mast cell-dependent anaphylaxis. *J Ethnopharmacol.* 2002;79(3):347-52.

Yoon TJ. et al. Inhibitory effect of chaga mushroom extract on compound 48/80-induced anaphylactic shock and IgE production in mice. *Int Immunopharmacol.* 2013;15(4):666-70.

Yoshikawa M. et al. Bioactive constituents of Chinese natural medicines. IV. Rhodiolae radix. (2): On the histamine release inhibitors from the underground part of Rhodiola sacra (Prain ex Hamet) S.H. Fu (Crassulaceae): Chemical structures of rhodiocyanoside D and sacranosides A and B. *Chem Pharm Bull (Tokyo).* 1997;45(9):1498-503.

Yuan XL. Effect of anti-Pseudomonas aeruginosa biofilm by combining Chinese and western medicine. *J Schaanxi Univ Sci Tech.* 2010;01:1-3.

Yuk HJ. et al. Profiling of neuraminidase inhibitory polyphenols from the seeds of Paeonia lactiflora. *Food Chem Toxicol.* 2013;55:144-9.

Zaidi SFH. et al. Potent bactericidal constituents from Mallotus philippinensis against clarithromycin and metronidazole resistant strains of Japanese and Pakistani Helicobacter pyloi. *Biol. Pharm Bull.* 2009;32(4):631-36.

Zhang H. et al. Anti-anaphylactic pharmacological action of water-soluble constituents of Ginkgo biloba L. episperm. *Zhongguo Zhong Yao Za Zhi.* 1990;15(8):496-7,513.

Zhang LJ. et al. Berberine inhibits Hep-2 cell invasion induced by Chlamydophila pneumoniae infection. *J Microbiol.* 2011; 49(5):834-40.

Zhang LR., Ma TX. Antagonistic effect of oleanolic acid on anaphylactic shock. *Zhongguo Yao Li Xue Bao.* 1995;16(6):527-30.

Zhang W., Dai SM. Mechanisms involved in the therapeutic effects of Paeonia Iactiflora Pallas in rheumatoid arthritis. *Int Immunopharmacol.* 2012;14(1):27-31.

Zhang XD. et al. Study on the immunocompetence of polysaccharide extracted from root of Salvia miltiorrhiza. *Zhong Yao Cai.* 2012;35(6):949-52.

Zhang Z-Q. et al. Inhibitory impacts of Niaoluquing on urogenital Chlamydia trachomatis in vitro. *Nation J Androlog.* 2005;11:1-3.

Zhao S. et al. Pretreatment with Scutellaria baicalensis stem-leaf total flavonoid prevents cerebral ischemia-reperfusion injury. *Neural Regen Res.* 2013;8(34):3183-92.

INDEX

Page numbers in italics refer to charts, tables, or sidebars.